Unlocking the Brain

Unlocking the Brain

VOLUME I: CODING

GEORG NORTHOFF

OXFORD
UNIVERSITY PRESS

OXFORD
UNIVERSITY PRESS

Oxford University Press is a department of the University of Oxford.
It furthers the University's objective of excellence in research, scholarship,
and education by publishing worldwide.

Oxford New York
Auckland Cape Town Dar es Salaam Hong Kong Karachi
Kuala Lumpur Madrid Melbourne Mexico City Nairobi
New Delhi Shanghai Taipei Toronto

With offices in
Argentina Austria Brazil Chile Czech Republic France Greece
Guatemala Hungary Italy Japan Poland Portugal Singapore
South Korea Switzerland Thailand Turkey Ukraine Vietnam

Published in the United States of America by
Oxford University Press
198 Madison Avenue, New York, NY 10016

Library of Congress Cataloging-in-Publication Data

Northoff, Georg. Unlocking the brain / Georg Northoff.
p. ; cm.
Includes bibliographical references and indexes.
ISBN 978-0-19-982698-8 (alk. paper)—ISBN 978-0-19-982699-5 (alk. paper)
I. Title. [DNLM: 1. Brain—physiology. 2. Brain Mapping—psychology.
3. Cognition—physiology. 4. Neural Pathways—physiology. 5. Neuropsychiatry. WL 335]

612.8—dc23
2012029357

9 8 7 6 5 4 3 2 1
Printed in the United States of America
on acid-free paper

CONTENTS

PREFACE

What is the brain? Though many answers have been suggested, we simply do not know at this point in time. Let's compare the situation with other organs. We know what the heart is; the heart is an organ that pumps blood. We know what the stomach is; it is a digestive organ that extracts the relevant nutrients from food. And one could expand that list to other organs.

Let's compare the current situation in neuroscience to the following imaginary scenario about the heart. Imagine that we do not know yet that the heart is a pumping organ. All we know is that the heart is a muscle, that it uses much energy to run that muscle, and that plenty of blood is accumulated periodically in the heart. But—and this is essential—we cannot yet ascribe any purpose to all of this; we know plenty of the details, but we cannot make sense of them. We do not know, for instance, why the heart is designed as muscle and why it accumulates blood periodically.

Even more important, this lack of insight into the heart's purpose may prevent us from having not only a better understanding of the heart's overall purpose and role in the organism, but also a more detailed insight into its physiological processes. For instance, we do not investigate the rhythmic nature of the heart's contractions and its underlying electrophysiological activity; that makes sense only if we know that the heart is continuously contracting in order to maintain its pumping function. Accordingly, the lack of an answer to the "what" question may be not only philosophically but also empirically relevant, and thus physiologically relevant, in order to get a better grip on the heart's "how."

I now argue that current neuroscience is in exactly the same state with regard to the brain as just stated in the thought experiment about the heart. We currently know a lot about the brain's regions, its networks and their metabolic, hormonal, and immunological processes, and their genetic regulation. In contrast, we do not know why these neuronal processes and various mechanisms take place in the way they do and thus what overall purpose they serve.

Accordingly, we currently have plenty of knowledge about the "how" of the brain but still lack an answer to the "what" of the brain. We thus remain blind to its main and overarching purpose. Once we get a tighter grip of the brain's main and overarching purpose, the "what," we may also be able to more specifically tailor our experimental designs to better investigate its various functions—the "how."

My starting point in this book is the brain itself: what the brain is, and, even more important, what the brain does. I postulate that, in order to understand what the brain does, we need to investigate the features that define the brain *as* brain. These intrinsic features include the brain's neural code and its intrinsic activity, as I suggest. This volume is about the brain's intrinsic features and more specifically how the brain's neural code and its intrinsic activity operate and impact the subsequent neural processing of extrinsic stimuli from body and environment. Why do I put such emphasis on the intrinsic features of the brain, its resting-state activity and neural code, here in Volume I? Only by revealing the brain's intrinsic features will we be able to understand what the brain is and why and how the brain does what it does.

What is analogous to the heart's pumping of blood in the case of the brain? I suppose that the heart's pumping of blood may find its analogue on the brain's side in its ability to associate its own neural activity with consciousness. That will be the focus in Volume II. To understand that, though, we first need to understand the brain itself and how it encodes its neural activity. This is the focus in this volume. Accordingly, Volume II complements the neuronal groundwork laid in Volume I by showing how the brain and its intrinsic features predispose the generation of consciousness.

I want to thank several people. First and foremost, I want to thank Catharine Carlin from Oxford University Press, who supported me very much in the early stages by giving excellent advice. Her editorial role was taken over later by Joan Bossert, who was extremely supportive of this rather complex project. Many thanks to Joan and her excellent help and advice! Her assistants, Jennifer Milton and Miles Osgaard, provided excellent support and encouragement in the later stages. A big thank-you to all of you for making possible such a complex project with two volumes.

Several anonymous reviewers also need to be thanked for providing very thoughtful comments, with one of them even suggesting I split my ideas into two volumes. My institution, the Institute of Mental Health Research in Ottawa, Canada, and its generous director, Zul Merali, shall also be thanked for the freedom and mental space they provide me to tackle such a complex organ as the brain in such extensive ways. I also want to explicitly thank Xuchu Weng and his Center for Cognition and Brain Disorders at Hangzhou Normal University/China for the generous support and the many inspirations. A great thank you also goes to Dr Xuehai Wei in Shanghai who introduced me to the clinical phenomenology of vegetative state patients which served as basis for several ongoing collaborative studies on the loss of consciousness. The same generosity was also made possible in Bologna and Dr Marina Farinelli where we conduct EEG studies on vegetative state patients.

My friend and dear colleague Jaak Panksepp should also be thanked. I cherish my discussions with him, his out-of-the-box thinking and his excellent ideas and understanding. Thank-you, Jaak. The members of my research group also deserve a big thank-you for their wonderful discussion of my ideas in their often wild and immature *gestalt*; hence, my special thanks go to Pengmin Qin, David Hayes, Niall Duncan, Takashi Nakao, Christine Wiebking, Zirui Huang, and Chao-Yi. Others who must be thanked are Timothy Lane, Alexander Heinzel, Simone Grimm, Alexander Sartorius, Jianfeng Zang, Shihui Han, and Fan Yan.

For excellent support in some editorial work, my thanks goes to Giles Holland, my research coordinator, who took pains to go through the proofs with me and to make suggestions for further improvement. For financial support, I have to thank the Canada Institute of Health Research (CIHR) and the Michael Smith Foundation, who granted me two endowed chairs. Further, I have to thank the Hope of Depression Research Foundation (HDRF) for financial support. Finally, I need to give a big thank-you to my partner, John Sarkissian. He has to endure my rather frequent mental (and physical) absence when my own brain's intrinsic activity "prefers" to drift away from the outer world and let me muse about the inner world of the brain by associating its own purely neuronal states with a phenomenal state; that is, consciousness.

LIST OF FIGURES

INTRODUCTION

Prelude I: Why Do We Need to Know the Brain's Neural Code?

We know much about the brain these days. Neuroscience has explored its various molecular, cellular, and biochemical mechanisms. Much progress has also been made in understanding the regional and network levels of neural activity. Functional imaging allows us to investigate how the neural activity of specific regions and networks is related to particular sensory, motor, affective, cognitive, or social functions. This has even brought consciousness and other mental features, whose neural correlates we search for intensely, into the realm of neuroscience.

One feature of the brain remains elusive, however. We do not know the brain's neural code: the currency the brain uses to generate and process its neural activity. This may hinder progress and block our insight into the brain's various functions.

We recall from biology Francis Crick and James Watson's discovery of the DNA molecule, as the genetic code has opened new pathways in our understanding of life and has put biology on a new platform. Analogously, unraveling the brain's neural code may enable us to understand why the brain works in the way it does and how it can generate the various sensory, motor, affective, cognitive, and social functions. To put it in a nutshell, the detection of the brain's neural code may provide a novel, much-needed ground for neuroscience.

Prelude II: Code as Common Metric or Measure of Different Kinds of Neural Activity

What does the term "code" stand for? The term "code" is often used to mean a metric or measure that captures and reflects purposeful and biologically or teleologically meaningful activity in a system (DeCharms and Zador 2000; Friston and Dolan 2000). As such, the term "code" describes a specific processing algorithm or instruction set according to which information is processed in a system.

Such processing algorithm as metric or measure remains purely formal by itself; this means that it is as yet devoid and prior to the constitution of any contents such as, for instance, sensory, motor, cognitive, affective, or social contents as related to the respective functions of the brain. The term "code" is used from here on in a purely formal way (see also Freeman 2007, 2011). Taken in this sense, a code allows the transformation of information from one particular form into another form in order to make possible the subsequent processing of that information.

For instance, the computer codes any kind of incoming stimuli according to 0 and 1, a format that allows the computer to further process the stimuli and their information. While we do know very well the basic code and its format in the case of the computer, we are currently at a loss when it comes to the basic code of the brain, the "neural code," and the kind of format it entails. To put it in a nutshell, we currently lack the knowledge of the neural code—that is, the metric or measure—the brain applies to the encoding and processing of its own neural activity.

I propose that such a basic metric or measure applies to any neural activity in the brain, whether it is stimulus-induced activity or the brain's resting-state activity (see later sections in this introduction for more details on that distinction). The basic metric or measure provides a common code or, more metaphorically put, a common currency or language for all kinds of neural activities in the brain. This makes possible, for instance, the direct interaction between the different associated functions (sensory, motor, affective, cognitive, social, etc.) and their respective neural networks as it is often observed these days in functional brain imaging in affective, cognitive, and social neuroscience.

Prelude III: Different Suggestions for the Neural Code of the Brain

Matters are far from simple, however. Searching for the term "neural code" in the current Internet databases will reveal an abundant and almost inflationary use of this term. The term "code" is used on different levels, ranging from the molecular to the cellular, and population levels to the regional and network levels of the brain's neural activity.

Most often the term "neural code" is intended to describe activity changes at the cellular level as observed in single- or multi-unit electrophysiological recordings. This is, for instance, the case in the concept of *rate coding* that describes the carrying (and representing) of information in the neurons' firing rates as the rate of the latter varies with the changes in the former (see Singer 1999, 2009; Friston 2009; and see Parts I and IV of this volume for a more detailed discussion).

The term "neural code" is also often used to describe the temporal constellation of neural activity especially on the population level of neural activity. This is, for instance, the case when one speaks of "temporal" or "synchrony coding": *temporal coding* describes the neuronal synchronization of different neuron populations and regions across time as observed in recording studies in both primates and humans (Singer 1999, 2009; Engel and Singer 2001; Rodriguez et al. 1999; Lutz et al. 2002; and see Part IV of this volume for details).

The situation is even more complex, however. While often being associated with the cellular and population levels of neural activity, the term "code" can also be used on the level of regions and neural networks: the regional and network level. One recent example is the concept of *predictive coding* that is often used in the context of functional imaging of different regions during reward and mirror neurons, for example (see Friston 1995, 1997, 2000, 2010; Montague et al. 2006; see Chapters 7–9 in this volume for details and references).

The concept of predictive coding postulates that neural activity in particular regions like the ventral striatum (as for instance during reward) stems from the comparison between predicted and actual inputs. The measure or metric determining neural activity on a regional level thus pertains to a difference: predictive coding implies that the neural activity in particular regions is based on the encoding of a difference, the difference between predicted and actual input.

Prelude IV: Neural Code as "Common Currency" Between the Different Levels of Neural Activity

How do these different forms of neural coding stand in relation to each other? Rate coding, temporal coding, and predictive coding are suggestions for a neural code on specific levels of neural activity—cellular, population, and regional.

What remains unclear, though, is how these different levels of neural activity can communicate and interact with each other. For that, they must share the same code so that, for instance, the single cell's number of spikes translates into population activity and ultimately into the activation of a specific region or even network. Hence, the interaction between different levels of neural activity requires what may be described as a "common currency."

What does this "common currency" consist of? Such a common currency needs to link the different levels of the brain's neural activity—cellular, population, and regional (and network)—in order to make possible their direct interaction. Only if (metaphorically put) the different levels of the brain's neural activity "speak the same language" and "use the same currency" can they interact with each other. What is the "common currency" or "language" of the brain that links and glues its different levels of neural activity together? We currently do not know.

Prelude V: Encoding Versus Decoding

We have so far determined the concept of the neural code as a purely formal measure/metric and as "common currency" between the different levels of neural activity. There is yet another feature that needs to be mentioned. The concept of the neural code can be understood in terms of either "encoding" or "decoding" (Naselaris et al. 2009, 2011; Kay et al. 2008; Friston 2010; Haynes 2009, 2011).

The concept of "encoding" concerns how stimuli and their features are transformed and translated into neural activity. The focus is here on how information from the outside of the brain, as from the world, generates neural activity: How must the neural activity in the inside of the brain be generated in order to contain some information about the stimuli and their features from the outside world? Accordingly, encoding describes the strategy the brain itself applies to generate its own neural activity during the encounter with stimuli from the outside of the brain.

This is different in "decoding." Unlike in "encoding," the focus here is not so much on the generation of neural activity by stimuli from the outside of the brain. Instead, decoding focuses on the information that is contained in the brain's neural activity itself (see Haynes 2009, 2011; Friston 2009). The guiding question here is: What information about the outside world and their stimuli and features is contained in the brain's neural activity?

Decoding refers to the information about the outside world as it is contained in the brain's neural activity. This distinguishes it from *encoding.* Rather than focusing on the information itself as it is contained in neural activity, encoding searches for how the neural activity itself is generated. The brain must generate and thus encode its neural activity in a particular way in order to contain some information about the outside world. Encoding thus precedes decoding in very much the same way the older twin precedes the younger one.

The difference between encoding and decoding goes along with different methodological strategies in, for instance, the analysis of brain imaging data like that obtained from functional magnetic resonance imaging (fMRI). This is well expressed in the following quote by Naselaris et al. (2011, p. 401):

Most current understanding has been achieved by analysing fMRI data from the mirror perspectives of encoding and decoding. When analysing the data from the encoding perspective, one attempts to understand how activity varies when there is concurrent variation in the world. When analysing data from the decoding perspective, one attempts to determine how much can be learned about the world (which includes sensory stimuli, cognitive state, and movement) by observing activity.

For instance, Kay and colleagues (2008) observed that the three-dimensional space of the stimuli from natural scenes, the "input space," is mirrored in the space of the stimulus-induced different activity (the voxels as measured in fMRI) in visual cortex, the "activity space." How is the transformation of the "input space" and thus the natural scenes into the "activity space" of the brain's neural activity possible? Kay et al. (2008) assume what they describe as "feature space" that, on the basis of the feature of the stimuli and their encoding by the neurons, provides the transformation between stimuli and neural activity (see Chapter 1–3 for details as well as Naselaris et al. 2009).

Prelude VI: Narrow Versus Wide Version of Encoding

One may distinguish between "narrow" and "wide" versions of the concept of encoding. Most generally, encoding describes a formal measure or metric for how neural activity is generated in relation to stimuli and their features. Usually, these stimuli and their features are understood to originate in the environment, thus concerning exteroceptive stimuli (see Kay et al. 2008; Naselaris et al., 2009, 2011). This is the narrow version of encoding that concerns the encoding of exteroceptive stimuli into neural activity.

In addition to exteroceptive stimuli from the environment, the interoceptive stimuli from one's own body also generate neural activity and thus need to be encoded, too. Furthermore, as it will become clear later, the intrinsic activity in the brain itself, its spontaneous or resting-state activity (see Chapters 4–6), is undergoing continuous changes that also need to be encoded into neural activity. Accordingly, besides exteroceptive stimuli from the environment, interoceptive stimuli from the body and the intrinsic activity changes within the brain itself require some kind of encoding.

This means that the encoding of neural activity cannot be restricted to exteroceptive stimuli alone. Instead, we need to understand the concept of encoding in a wider way that includes all extrinsic stimuli, intero- and exteroceptive, from both the body and the environment. In addition, we also need to consider the encoding of activity changes that are induced by the brain itself and its intrinsic activity. We therefore need to opt for a wide version of encoding that pertains to any kind of neural activity generated in the brain, independently of its origin in either environment, body, or brain.

The overarching aim in this volume is to investigate how the brain generates and thus encodes neural activity. Rather than focusing on decoding information from neural activity, my focus is on the encoding and thus generation of neural activity. This pertains to neural activity in general, irrespective of its origin in either brain, body, or environment. I thus presuppose the wide version of the concept of encoding throughout this volume.

Therefore, I will investigate how different forms of neural activity are generated. Part I concerns the encoding of exteroceptive stimuli; Part II focuses on the encoding of the brain's intrinsic activity changes; Part III touches upon the encoding of the body's interoceptive stimuli; and Part IV discusses the encoding of extrinsic activity: namely, stimulus-induced activity.

Fugue I: Encoding of Differences into Neural Activity on the *Cellular* Level

In music, every prelude is followed by a fugue. The famous composer Johann Sebastian Bach told us that the fugue is supposed to spell out and develop the material introduced in the prelude. I consequently have to determine the nature of the neural code and to spell out the exact mechanisms by means of which the brain generates neural activity.

The purpose of the next few sections will be to introduce a particular hypothesis about the brain's neural code. I propose that the brain's neural activity is based on the encoding of spatial and temporal differences between different (or the same) stimuli into neural activity, rather than on encoding the single stimuli themselves in an isolated and independent way. Such encoding of differences between stimuli rather than the stimuli themselves is supposed to hold true on different levels of neural activity: on cellular, population, and regional levels. Therefore, I will now go into some empirical detail by discussing paradigmatic examples from the single-cell level, the population level, and the regional level of neural activity.

Let us start with the cellular level of neural activity. Fiorillo and colleagues (2008) consider the single neuron and characterize it by the neural coding of differences. Based on the neuron's biophysical properties, like its K^+ and Cl^- channels, Fiorillo and colleagues (2008, pp. 3–4) argue that the single neuron in general will "integrate current information about its stimulus from one pool of ion channels and synapses, and prior information from another pool. Its membrane potential signals prediction error." The single cell's actual membrane potential—that is, its activity—is determined by the difference between current and prior states; this is signaled by the differences in activity levels between different ion channels and synapses (see also Rolls and Treves 2011).

Fiorillo and colleagues (2008) thus apply and extend the concept of predictive coding (see earlier discussion and Chapters 7–9) beyond the regional level to the level of the single neuron. Analogous to the regional level of neural activity, the single neuron's goal is to minimize prediction error and thus to keep the difference between anticipated and actual activity levels (i.e., between predicted and actual input) as low as possible (see Chapter 8 for details). Even the selection of both prior and current information sources is very much oriented to keeping this difference low. Only the actual inputs from the various stimuli that can contribute to minimizing the difference between anticipated and actual activity levels are selected. This implies that the neuron produces output signals (as changes in its activity level) only when there is a difference between anticipated and actual activity level: if the actual activity level is higher, exceeding its prediction or anticipation, the output signal is positive, while in the reverse case the output signal may be negative. The single cell's activity, its membrane potential, is thus based on the encoding of a difference, the difference between previous/predicted and actual inputs.

Fugue II: Encoding of Differences into Neural Activity on the *Population* Level

Let's move on from the cellular level to the population level, and more specifically to the neurons in the motor cortex. Georgopoulus and colleagues (1986) demonstrated that the activity of a given motor cortical neuron is changed depending on the function of other motor neurons. While each single neuron from the primary motor cortex encodes a given, or preferred, direction of a movement, it encodes this in relation to the other neurons' preferred directions. This means that the single neuron also contains at least some of the information from the respective others via encoding its own activity relative to them.

This is further supported by Grammont and Riehle (2003). They demonstrated that each motor cortical neuron within a neuronal assembly depends on its relationship to its respective neighboring neuron. Whether, for instance, the single neuron might synchronize its activity with the other neurons' activity depends on the single neuron's relationship to its respective neighboring neurons, while the latter's degree of synchronizing activity depends, in turn, on the activity of the former, and so on. Accordingly, the single neuron's activity cannot be considered by itself, independent of and in isolation from the other neurons. Instead, the single neuron's activity can be understood only when considering its relationship to, that is, difference from, the other neurons.

Another example for the encoding of differences into neural activity is a study by Selezneva and colleagues (2006) that concerns the sensory rather than the motor cortex. They undertook single-cell recordings in monkey's auditory cortex during a decision task where only certain stimuli were associated with reward. The data were analyzed in two different ways. The single-cell recordings were first analyzed and grouped across trials, categorized according to the different stimuli. Since this did not yield any correlation between the recorded neuronal activities and the behavioral effects (i.e., the decisions about rewarding trials), they analyzed their data in a different way. They no longer grouped the neuronal activities according to the different categories of stimuli presented across trials. Instead, they calculated the ratios between the actual and the respectively preceding trials in a serial way.

Interestingly, the ratios—that is, the differences in the firing rates between actual and preceding trials—correlated with the behavioral, or rewarding, effects. This means that what is behaviorally relevant is not so much the neural activity associated with a particular stimulus by itself, but the difference in neural activity between actual and preceding stimuli. In short, behavioral relevance is here encoded in terms of differences rather than in terms of the stimuli themselves independent and isolated from each other (see Chapter 3 for more detailed discussion of this study and how it relates to difference-based coding).

Fugue III: Encoding of Differences into Neural Activity on the *Regional* Level

Let us move on from the cellular/population level to the regional level of neural activity. Kayser and colleagues (2005) investigated cross-modal interaction in monkeys using functional magnetic resonance imaging. They tested for the effects of tactile stimuli on neural activity in auditory cortex while concurrently presenting auditory stimuli. Signifying cross-modal interaction, neural activity, especially in the auditory cortex, was significantly enhanced by the concurrent presentation of tactile stimuli.

Most importantly, the resulting neural activity in auditory cortex was higher than could be accounted for by the mere addition or superposition of the ones associated with each—that is, tactile and auditory—stimulus alone. They concluded that there must be some non-linear interaction in the auditory cortex during the concurrent presentation of tactile and auditory stimuli.

How is such non-linear interaction possible? "Non-linear" interaction implies that the resulting neural activity during the interaction between two (or more) different stimuli is either stronger or weaker than the activity associated with each stimulus alone. This implies that the resulting neural activity cannot be based on the encoding of the single stimulus alone and the mere addition of the different stimuli's activities during their interaction. Such non-linear interaction implies that there must be some extra ingredient that allows, enhances, or weakens the resulting stimulus-induced activity beyond the mere addition or summation of the different stimuli's activities. Where does this extra ingredient come from? It cannot come from the stimuli themselves. Instead, it must come from the interaction itself: how the two stimuli interact with each other and how their interaction is encoded into neural activity.

The only way for their interaction to yield non-linear stimulus-induced activity is by encoding the spatial and temporal differences between the different stimuli, the tactile and auditory stimuli, into the neural activity of the auditory cortex. The encoding of the spatial and temporal differences between the auditory and tactile stimuli may thus make possible the observation of non-linear changes in the subsequent stimulus-induced activity.

In contrast, this would remain impossible if both stimuli, auditory and tactile, were encoded into neural activity by themselves in an independent and isolated and way. Accordingly, non-linear interaction during cross-modal interaction presupposes the encoding of differences between stimuli into neural activity on a regional level rather than the encoding of the stimuli themselves (see Chapters 10–12 for extensive discussion of non-linearity and difference-based coding).

Fugue IV: Encoding of Spatial and Temporal *Differences* between Different Stimuli into Neural Activity

What do these different examples share? They all concern the encoding of differences into neural activity by linking and binding different stimuli. In the case of the cell, different ions were integrated and computed against each other. On the population level, the spatially separated and/or temporally preceding inputs or stimuli from the other neurons were integrated into the neural activity of the single neuron. Finally, auditory and tactile stimuli were integrated and encoded against each other in the auditory cortex on the regional level of neural activity.

What is common among the various examples is the encoding of differences between different inputs or stimuli into neural activity. Rather than encoding the stimuli themselves independently and isolated from each other, the differences between different stimuli are encoded into neural activity. By encoding their differences into neural activity, the different stimuli are linked and integrated like, as in our examples, the stimuli from the preceding trial, the stimuli from other motor neurons, or the stimuli from another sensory modality.

How are such linkage and integration between different stimuli possible? The stimuli occur at different points in physical space and time. This means that their underlying different points in physical time and space must be linked and integrated in order to encode the difference between different stimuli into neural activity.

Rather than the discrete points in physical time and space themselves, the spatial and temporal differences between the different stimuli and their discrete points in physical time and space are then encoded into neural activity. Accordingly, the differences encoded into neural activity can be further specified as temporal and spatial differences between the different stimuli's discrete points in physical time and space.

Before going on, we have to make a brief remark about the notion of "physical time and space" as understood here. When I speak about "different stimuli's discrete points in physical time and space," I presuppose a very simple determination of the concept of "physical time and space." Physical time and space are here meant to denote the way we observe the stimuli in time and space from the outside in a third-person perspective in an objective way. This means that the concept of "physical time and space" is closely tied to objective third-person observation.

That is to be distinguished from the way physics investigates and considers the various processes of how time and space themselves are generated as such. Throughout this and the second volume, the concept of "physical time and space" is supposed to signify an observer-based notion, while it does not pertain to the generation of time and space as investigated in physics.

Fugue V: Low-Frequency Fluctuations and Functional Connectivity Encode Spatial and Temporal *Differences* on the *Regional* Level of Neural Activity

How can the brain encode temporal and spatial differences between different stimuli into its neural activity on a regional level? I postulate that this is possible by neuronal measures like functional connectivity and low-frequency fluctuations that operate in the spatial and temporal dimensions on the regional level of neural activity.

I suggest that low-frequency fluctuations are one neuronal measure that encodes temporal differences between different stimuli into neural activity. The phrase "low-frequency fluctuations" describes spontaneous changes or fluctuations in the neural activity in a frequency range from around 0.001 to 1Hz. By showing such a low-frequency range, low-frequency fluctuations can be characterized by relative long phase durations, which may be ideally suited to integrate and thus encode temporal differences between different stimuli into neural activity. We will see later that such temporal integration is indeed central in constituting the brain's intrinsic activity (see Chapter 5) as well as consciousness, especially "inner time consciousness" (see Chapters 14 and 15).

In addition to temporal integration, there is also spatial integration, for which functional connectivity may be central. Functionally, *connectivity* describes the correlation between two or more different, spatially distant regions' neural activities across time. Such correlation, or functional connectivity, can, as I suggest, be considered the result of prior encoding of spatial differences between different stimuli into neural activity (as it will be detailed in Chapters 4 and 11; see also Chapter 16 in Volume II with regard to consciousness).

Fugue VI: Difference-Based Coding as *"Common Currency"* of the Brain's Neural Activity on Different Levels

One may now wonder why I described these different examples. Despite describing different levels—cellular, population, and regional—they all share the characteristic that the resulting neural activity is based on the encoding of differences between different stimuli rather than being based on the stimuli themselves. Differences may thus be the shared and common metric or measure between the different levels of neural activity. Therefore, one may speak of "difference-based coding" (see Fig. I1-1a).

What do I mean by "differences" as common metric or measure? The notion of difference applies to different kinds of differences: the difference between different stimuli, as in cross-modal interaction; the difference between previous and actual states of the single cell; or the difference between different cells. Though describing different levels of neural activity, the formal metric or measure determining and constituting the respectively resulting neural activity is the same in all instances. Accordingly, spatial and temporal differences are the formal metric or measure that applies throughout the different levels of neural activity.

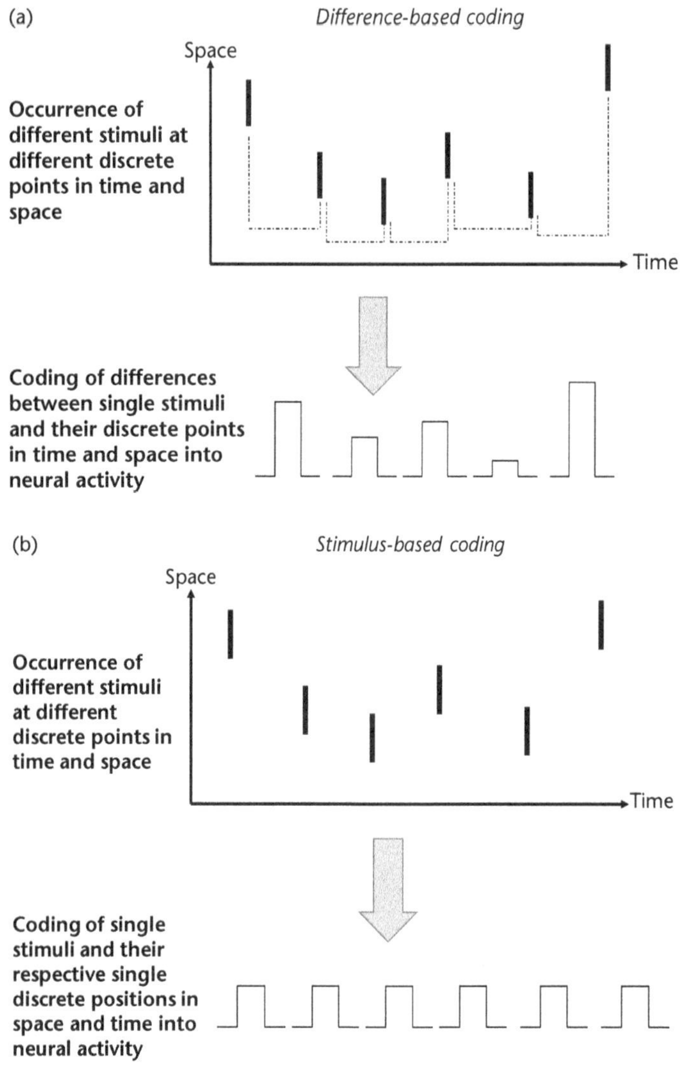

Figure I1-1 Different Models of Neural Coding. The figure depicts two different models of neural coding: difference-based coding (*a*) and stimulus-based coding (*b*). The upper part in each figure illustrates the occurrence of stimuli across their different discrete points in physical time and space, indicated by the vertical lines. The lower part in each figure (with the bars) stands for the action potentials/firing rates/regional activity levels as elicited by the stimuli, with the blue arrow describing the link between stimuli and neural activity. (*a*) In the case of difference-based coding, the stimuli and their discrete points in physical time and space are compared, matched, and integrated with each other. In other terms, the spatial and temporal differences between the different stimuli are computed as indicated by the dotted lines. The degree of spatial and temporal difference between the different stimuli's spatial and temporal positions does in turn determine the degree of the resulting neural activity. The different stimuli are thus dependent on each other during their encoding into neural activity. Hence, there is no longer a one-to-one correspondence but rather a many-to-one relationship between stimulus and neural activity. (*b*) This is different in the case of stimulus-based coding. Here each stimulus, including its respective discrete point in physical space and time, is encoded into the brain's neural activity. Most importantly, unlike in difference-based coding, each stimulus is encoded by itself, isolated and independent of the respective other stimuli. This results in one-to-one matching between stimuli and neural activity.

Based on these considerations, I suggest the following hypothesis. I postulate that spatial and temporal differences between different stimuli rather than the stimuli themselves are the common measure or metric in the brain's encoding of neural activity. This amounts to what I describe as *difference-based coding* as the brain's general encoding strategy. Difference-based coding can thus be considered the "common code," "common currency," or "common language" between the different levels of neural activity.

Let me explicate what exactly I mean by "common code" or "common currency." It does not matter whether the encoding concerns the difference between two regions' neural activities, the difference between preceding and actual states, the differences between different cells, the differences between rest and stimuli, and so forth. What instead is important here is the purely formal measure or metric that the brain applies to all kinds of stimuli, levels, and functions in order to encode them into neural activity.

I suppose difference-based coding to be such a formal measure or metric. Therefore, I postulate that difference-based coding applies to the different levels, the different functions, and all kinds of stimuli during their generation of neural activity. In short, I suggest that any neural activity in the brain is generated on the basis of difference-based coding.

How can we illustrate the central role I attribute to difference-based coding as the brain's neural code? Let us consider an analogous example from biology. The DNA molecule is considered *the* genetic code, the code that transmits the information of our genes and, to be more precise, how any kind of information is encoded into our genes. In short, DNA is the "currency" of our genes. As we all know, this opened the door for us to understand the nature of life.

Analogously, I regard difference-based coding to be *the* neural code, the code that transmits and transfers and therefore encodes any kind of information into the neural activity of the brain. Such encoding of spatial and temporal differences into neural activity needs to be distinguished from the encoding of the stimuli themselves, which would amount to stimulus-based coding (see Chapter 1 and 2 in this volume).

To put this in a nutshell, differences rather than stimuli are the "currency" of our brain's neural activity. This will open the door for us to understand, not only the nature of our brain, but also how it generates consciousness, as I will claim in Volume II.

Objection Ia: Difference-Based Coding Versus Stimulus-Based Coding

How, now, can we distinguish difference-based coding from other forms of neural coding? Differences as formal measures or metrics are characterized by linking and connecting different discrete points in physical time and space; the encoded neural activity is thus based on spatial and temporal differences. Such encoding of temporal and spatial differences into neural activity is the hallmark feature of what I described as difference-based coding.

However, neural activity could also be encoded in ways other than in terms of spatial and temporal differences. Instead of being based on the spatial and temporal differences between different discrete points in physical time and space, neural activity may rather be traced back to the discrete and single points themselves as they are related to the occurrence of the stimuli. The encoded neural activity would then be based on the single stimuli themselves rather than on their spatial and temporal differences. This entails stimulus-based coding rather than difference-based coding.

What is "stimulus-based coding"? The concept of stimulus-based coding posits that the formal metric or measure that encodes neural activity is the stimulus itself. Very much like the concept of difference (see earlier), the term "stimulus" applies here to different levels, functions, and stimuli of different origins. The notion of "stimulus" is thus understood here in a purely formal way, in the sense of an input.

Unlike difference-based coding that refers to temporal and spatial differences between different stimuli, stimulus-based coding is based on the encoding of the single stimuli: This means that the single stimulus' discrete temporal and spatial point in physical time and space is encoded by itself, independently of other stimuli and their respective spatial and temporal positions (see Fig. I1-1b).

Is such stimulus-based coding empirically plausible? Given the examples discussed earlier, one is inclined to opt in favor of difference-based coding rather than stimulus-based coding. This will be further supported by the various examples I will cite and describe throughout this volume that all serve the purpose of lending empirical plausibility to the hypothesis that difference-based coding is the neural code of the brain.

Objection Ib: Balance Between Difference-Based Coding and Stimulus-Based Coding

However, as we all know only too well, nothing is easy when it comes to the brain. Difference-based coding can occur in different degrees and thus in a "more-or-less" and continuous way, rather than in an all-or-nothing way. This means that there may neither be 100% difference-based coding and 0% stimulus-based coding, nor 0% and 100% stimulus-based coding. We will see later that difference-based coding may indeed occur in different degrees and is thereby reciprocally related to the degree of stimulus-based coding. Their balance is supposedly modulated by the resting-state activity level that provides a threshold for the possible degree of difference-based coding (see Chapter 11).

Higher degrees of difference-based coding entail lower degrees of stimulus-based coding, and vice versa. While this may be not important in the healthy subjects, it may, however, be highly relevant in neurological and psychiatric disorders. For instance, psychiatric disorders like schizophrenia and depression may be characterized by an abnormal balance between difference-based coding and stimulus-based coding (see Chapters 22 and 27 in Volume II). I will hypothesize that the balance between difference- and stimulus-based coding may be central in generating the kind of rather bizarre behavior and symptoms that schizophrenic patients, especially, show (see Chapter 22).

Besides such behavioral relevance, the balance between difference- and stimulus-based coding may also be phenomenally relevant; that is, relevant for consciousness. A neurological disorder like the vegetative state (VS), where patients lose consciousness, may be characterized by an abnormally high degree of stimulus-based coding. The degree of difference-based coding and its balance with stimulus-based coding may thus be highly relevant for consciousness; that is, phenomenally relevant. Why that is so and how this is neuronally mediated will be discussed in full detail in Chapters 28 and 29 in Volume II.

Objection IIa: Dualism Between Difference- and Stimulus-Based Coding

One may now be rather puzzled that I suppose the brain's neural activity to be based on differences across various, discrete points in physical time and space rather than on the stimuli themselves and their single discrete points in physical time and space. Why is that puzzling? It sounds rather counterintuitive that the brain encodes its neural activity in terms of differences between stimuli rather than encoding the stimuli themselves.

Why counterintuitive? One would intuitively suggest that the stimuli are first encoded by themselves, for example, in a stimulus-based way, on the lower level of the sensory cortex before any differences between stimuli, such as difference-based coding, can be generated as, for instance, on a higher level of neural activity in prefrontal cortex. Stimulus-based coding must precede difference-based coding. In other words, difference-based coding may well be possible, but only in higher-order regions on the basis of prior stimulus-based coding in lower-order regions. One would thus propose dualism between difference- and stimulus-based coding rather than difference-based coding as the sole neural code of the brain.

Does stimulus-based coding indeed precede difference-based coding? No!. I will argue that there is difference-based coding right from the very beginning of the brain's neural processing. This implies that any neural activity is encoded (to a higher or lower degree) in terms of spatial and temporal differences. To recruit empirical support for that rather radical hypothesis, I will discuss various lines of evidence on both the cellular and the regional levels of neural activity in this volume. This will lend support to the hypothesis that difference-based coding already holds in sensory cortex during the encoding of sensory stimuli (see Chapters 1–3 and 10–12).

Objection IIb: Difference-Based Coding is a Statistically Based Encoding Strategy

What is encoded into neural activity in sensory cortex is not the single stimulus itself and its distinct features in an isolated and independent way. Instead, what is encoded into sensory cortical activity (and any kind of neural activity by default, as I suggest) are the spatial and temporal differences between the same or different sensory stimuli (and their features).

The encoding of spatial and temporal differences mirrors the statistical frequency distribution of the stimuli and thus their "natural statistics" (Barlow 2001; and see Chapter 1 in this volume for details). I will show in detail in Chapters 1 and 2 how such encoding of the stimuli's natural statistics is possible only on the basis of the encoding of spatial and temporal differences—that is, difference-based coding—into neural activity on the cellular level.

I postulate that the encoding of neural activity in terms of difference-based coding is closely aligned with the encoding of the stimuli's statistical frequency distribution, their natural statistics. Therefore difference-based coding must be considered a statistically based encoding strategy.

This is to be distinguished from stimulus-based coding. Rather than encoding the stimuli's natural statistics, the stimuli themselves and their physical features are here encoded into neural activity. Stimulus-based coding can thus be characterized as a physically based encoding strategy as distinguished from a statistically based encoding strategy.

Objection IIIa: Differences Cannot Encode the Brain's Neural Activity

One may want to bring forth another argument against difference-based coding by reverting to physics. Since the brain is a physical organ and determined by physical processes, it must conform to the laws of physics. Usually, one would assume that physical processes and activities are based on the encoding of single physical variables and their respective physical measures in an isolated and independent way. For instance, one would expect that single discrete points in time and space are encoded separately and independently of each other. The respective physical variables are this encoded as isolated and non-relational entities.

What does this imply for the neural code within the context of the brain? Since the brain's neural activity is physical, the neural code must abide to the laws of physics and encode the stimuli as isolated and non-relational entities into neural activity. That, however, is possible only when presupposing stimulus-based coding rather than difference-based coding as a relationally determined encoding strategy. Accordingly, physics itself seems to make the assumption of stimulus-based coding necessary.

This, however, is to neglect the fact that physics is not as simple as we often think. Physical processes and activities can well be based on relations between different physical variables and thus be relationally determined. This is well described in the following quote by Wolfgang Koehler (1887–1967), the founder of Gestalt psychology, who was born in Germany and moved later to the United States:

> "I will therefore add that relationally determined processes are extremely common in physics. For instance, if temperatures differ in two parts of a system, a current of heat energy is established which tends to equalize the temperatures. The direction of the flow depends upon the direction of the difference, and in the absence of any difference, there is no flow. Similarly, if a solution which contains certain molecules is surrounded by a second solution which contains these molecules in a different concentration, a current of diffusion will be observed, unless the solutions are separated by an impermeable barrier. The current flows as long as the concentration differ[s]. Thus it is again a relation of inequality between the two parts of the system which maintains the process." (W. Koehler 1967, pp. 209–210)

Objection IIIb: Difference-Based Coding is a Relationally Determined Encoding Strategy

What does the quote from Koehler tell us? He is saying that physical processes and their respective activities can well be constituted by and based on differences and thus be relationally determined. Most important, we can apply that lesson to the brain. In the same way as physical activity can be relationally determined, the brain can encode its neural activity in a relationally determined way.

Such relationally determined encoding strategy is suggested by difference-based coding when it postulates the encoding of spatial and temporal differences that signify the relations between different stimuli into neural activity. In sum, physics does not exclude difference-based coding as a relationally determined encoding strategy but rather supports it, by showing the existence of relationally determined processes and activities in the physical world.

How about the counterintuitive nature of the relationally determined nature of the brain's neural activity? The encoding of neural activity in terms of spatial and temporal differences between different stimuli may seem rather repugnant to common sense. Why is this? Before differences between stimuli can be yielded in neural activity, the single stimuli themselves must be encoded into neural activity.

Stimulus-based coding should thus precede difference-based coding. That, however, is neither empirically implausible as indicated earlier, nor is it really counterintuitive, given that both quantum mechanics and general relativity theory in physics are supposed to be highly counterintuitive to common sense (see the philosopher P. M. Churchland 2012, p. 274, who makes this argument).

Objection IVa: "Theory of Brain Activity" Versus "Theory of Brain Function"

My focus in this volume is on how the brain's neural activity is generated by using a particular encoding strategy: difference-based coding as distinguished from stimulus-based coding. As detailed earlier, I suppose that any kind of neural activity is generated by encoding spatial and temporal differences between different stimuli rather than the stimuli themselves and their different discrete points in physical time and space. Since it concerns the generation of the brain's neural activity as such, my hypothesis of difference-based coding amounts to a "theory of brain activity."

What do I mean by "theory of brain activity"? The concept of "theory of brain activity" describes how the brain generates and encodes neural activity. The theory of brain activity is thus about neural activity as such. A theory of brain activity in this sense must be distinguished from a "theory of brain function." Rather than concerning the generation and encoding of neural activity, a theory of brain function focuses on how the brain's neural activity generates and constitutes different functions like sensory, motor, cognitive, and affective functions, as well as consciousness.

Recent theories of brain function include, for instance, re-entrant processing (Edelman 2003, Seth et al. 2006); information integration (Tononi 2004; Tononi and Koch 2008); global workspace and global neuronal workspace (Baars 2005; Dehaene and Changeux 2011); the concept of free energy (Friston 2010); prediction generation (Llinas 1998, 2002; Friston 2010); and neuronal synchronization (Crick and Koch 2003; Singer 1999, 2009; Llinas 1998), to name just a few. Since most of these theories of brain function have been developed in close relationship to consciousness, I will discuss them and how they stand compared to difference-based coding in Volume II of *Unlocking the Brain*.

Objection IVb: "Theory of Brain Activity" Precedes "Theory of Brain Function"

How does a "theory of brain function" stand in relation to a "theory of brain activity"? Any theory of brain function presupposes a certain kind of neural activity, since, without the brain's neural activity, no function including consciousness could be performed at all. By focusing on how the brain yields the various functions like sensory, motor, cognitive, or affective functions, their neural activity is simply taken for granted and thus, as given.

The mechanisms and encoding strategy that allow the generating of the observed neural activity during these functions are thus neglected and not investigated by themselves in a theory of brain function. This is different in a "theory of brain activity." Here, the brain's neural activity and how it is generated and encoded come under scrutiny by themselves. For that purpose, different encoding strategies like difference- and stimulus-based coding are discussed and investigated with regard to their empirical plausibility; that is, their neuronal plausibility.

Moreover, we will investigate whether the observed behavior and the various sensory, motor, affective, and cognitive functions of the brain and their respective stimulus-induced or task-related activities presuppose a particular encoding strategy. The different functions of the brain can thus serve to illustrate the brain's encoding strategy. This distinguishes a "theory of brain activity" from a "theory of brain function" where the brain's various functions are by themselves the primary target and thus the departure point.

Objection V: Criteria for a Future Theory of Brain Activity

How could a future theory of brain activity look like? I want to briefly discuss the hallmark features and criteria for a future theory of brain activity. Following David Marr (1982), a "general computational theory of the nervous system" should meet three criteria:

(1) The theory needs to determine a single computational mechanism; that is, a specific neural code, that is broad and general enough to apply to the nervous system across different domains and levels (see also Logothetis 2008, 2010; Logothetis et al. 2009).
(2) The theory should be specific enough to define such a computational mechanism in terms of both format and algorithm so as to account for how any kind of neural activity is realized and implemented.
(3) The theory should sufficiently specify the cellular, biochemical, molecular, and physical processes underlying the observed neural activity with respect to the postulated computational mechanism (that is, the proposed coding mechanism).

The hypothesis of difference-based coding aims to tentatively meet the following three criteria:

(1) It is broad and general enough to apply to the different levels of neural activity—cellular, population, and regional—of the brain. This is possible because it does not describe specific contents (see Chapters 18 and 19 in Volume II for a more exact determination of the notion of "content") but rather a formal metric or measure (i.e., spatial and temporal differences) as the computational mechanism that constitutes and generates and thus encodes any kind of neural activity in the brain.
(2) At the same time, difference-based coding is specific enough to describe the neuronal and computational mechanisms that are at work in the different functions of the brain: sensory, motor, cognitive, affective, and social. While this will not be described here in a systematic way, it at least will be illustrated by various examples from different functions throughout this (and the second) volume of *Unlocking the Brain.*
(3) Finally, I postulate that difference-based coding in this sense is constituted by the excitation-inhibition balance (EIB), which biochemically is closely related to the biochemical substances GABA and glutamate (see Chapters 2, 6, and 12 of this work). I postulate that GABA and glutamate are central in constituting spatial and temporal differences, so I will here focus on these two transmitters. In contrast, I will neglect the many others transmitter (serotonin, dopamine, acetylcholine, etc.) that may modulate the degree of differences rather than constitute the encoding of spatial and temporal differences by themselves (as GABA and glutamate) into neural activity.

Objection VI: No Need for "Theory" in the "Theory of Brain Activity"

One may now want to complain that difference-based coding as the brain's neural code is way too abstract and theoretical and thus too removed from the empirical data. However, reading through the different parts of this book will put the hypothesis of difference-based coding as the brain's neural code into a more empirical context. I will provide more empirical detail in the four parts in this volume whereas its relevance for consciousness will be discussed in Volume II.

But why start with all the theory instead of just describing the empirical data? Any theory is, after all, only as good as the empirical data that support it. However, it is often forgotten that the reverse holds true, too; namely, that the empirical data are only as good as the theory.

Despite the enormous increases in empirical data in neuroscience these days, we still lack a coherent theory, a theory of brain activity. Such theoretical deficit has been observed by some of the most prominent neuroscientists of our time, like N. Logothetis (2010), G. Buzsáki (2006, pp. xii–xiii), E. R. John (2006), W. J. Freeman (2007, 2011), and R. G. Shulman (van Eijsden et al. 2009). As Nikos Logothetis puts it: "But, as I said in the beginning, in the end what we need are not necessarily more data but a theory and a plausible theoretical context within which data can be better (and more intelligently) interpreted" (2010, p. 175).

Therefore, sometimes it may be better to think about the theoretical background assumptions than to conduct the next experiment. Why? This is not just to resolve a deficit in theory and to interpret the same data in different ways. Even more importantly, it is to reveal some hidden presuppositions that may lead to novel and different kinds of experimental designs. That is the prime and major aim of this book: to let novel hypotheses and different experimental ideas evolve from theoretical reflection about the brain's encoding of neural activity.

We recall from physics at the beginning of the twentieth century. At that time, ground-breaking empirical discoveries were closely linked with novel theoretical assumptions, as, for instance, in the relativity theory and quantum physics. Another example of the tight linkage between theoretical reflection and empirical discoveries is the science of the other organs of the body. Once we had an established theory of the heart as a pumping organ, or a theory of the kidney's function as blood-washing organ, we could much better understand why the heart and the kidney do what they do, which in turn led to novel experimental designs and research.

I now propose the same to hold in the case of the brain. Here, too, empirical discovery and theoretical reflection have to go hand-in-hand. This is the aim and purpose of this volume. That in turn provides the groundwork for a novel approach, both experimentally and theoretically, to consciousness as one of the main puzzles and mysteries in current neuroscience. This will be the focus in Volume II.

Approach to the Brain Ia: Extrinsic Versus Intrinsic *Features* of the Brain

I characterize the brain by the application of a particular encoding strategy, difference-based coding as distinguished from stimulus-based coding. Such an encoding strategy must be traced back to the brain itself: it is the input that the brain itself provides to the generation and processing of its own neural activity. Since it can be traced back to the brain itself, its encoding strategy—namely, difference-based coding—must be considered an intrinsic feature of the brain.

The brain's intrinsic input to its neural activity must be distinguished from the intero- and exteroceptive stimuli and their origin in the body and the environment. Since they originate outside the brain, their input can be characterized as extrinsic rather than intrinsic. The stimulus-induced activity as related to the various stimuli and functions must therefore be considered an extrinsic rather than intrinsic feature of the brain. While the extrinsic features of the brain, and thus its stimulus-induced or task-related activity, are extensively investigated these days, my focus is more on the brain's intrinsic features and how they impact the extrinsic features.

What are the intrinsic features of the brain? The intrinsic features are the characteristics or aspects of the brain's neural processing (like its encoding strategy) whose origin must be traced back to the brain itself and its insides. This is to be distinguished from extrinsic features whose origin is "located" outside of the brain, as in body or environment (see also the Introduction in Volume II of this book for more details on the distinction between intrinsic and extrinsic features of the brain).

There is yet another intrinsic feature of the brain besides its encoding strategy. The brain shows spontaneous activity that remains independent of any extrinsic stimulus input. Such spontaneous activity has also been called "intrinsic activity" or "resting-state activity" (see Chapter 4 for conceptual and empirical details). The brain's resting-state activity has recently become particularly relevant, especially in the context of neuroimaging and its detection of the default-mode network (DMN) (see Raichle et al. 2001; Raichle 2009, 2010; Northoff et al. 2010; Northoff and Bermpohl 2004) (and see Chapter 4 for details).

Since it originates in the inside of the brain and remains independent of extrinsic stimuli, the brain's intrinsic activity may be considered an intrinsic feature of the brain. The exact role and function of the brain's intrinsic activity and how it is related to its extrinsic activity, the stimulus-induced or task-related activity, remain unclear these days, however. Interestingly, the debate about their relation can be traced back to different views of the brain in neuroscience at the turn of the nineteenth–twentieth century.

Approach to the Brain Ib: Extrinsic Versus Intrinsic *Views* of the Brain

One view of the brain, favored by the British neurologist Sir Charles Sherrington (1857–1952), proposed the brain and the spinal cord to be primarily *reflexive*. "Reflexive" means that the brain reacts in predefined and automatic ways to stimuli: the stimuli from the outside of the brain, originating extrinsically in either body or environment, are assumed to determine completely and exclusively the subsequent neural activity. The resulting stimulus-induced activity, and more generally, any neural activity, in the brain is then traced back to the extrinsic stimuli. One may therefore speak of what I describe as the "extrinsic view" of the brain (see Fig. I12-a).

An alternative view, however, was already suggested by one of Sherrington's students, Thomas Graham Brown. In contrast to his teacher, he suggested that the brain's neural activity—that is, in spinal cord and brain stem—is not primarily driven and sustained by extrinsic stimuli from the outside of the brain; that is, the body and environment. Instead, he held that the spinal cord and brain stem do show spontaneous activity that originates within the brain and thus intrinsically.

Other neuroscientists, like Karl Lashley, Kurt Goldstein, and Wolfgang Koehler, followed Brown's line of thought and proposed that the brain shows intrinsic activity. This leads me to speak of an "intrinsic view" of the brain. The distinction between extrinsic and intrinsic views of the brain is nicely illustrated in the following quote by the early German neurologist Kurt Goldstein in his book *The Organism*, which appeared originally in 1934 (Goldstein 2000):

> The system is never at rest, but in a continual state of excitation. The nervous system has often been considered as an organ at rest, in which excitation arises only as a response to stimuli. This was due to the fact that only those phenomena that became particularly pronounced on stimulation were considered as expression of the processes in the nervous system. The fact that the nervous system is continuously under the influence of stimuli and is continually excited was overlooked. It was not recognized that events that follow a definite stimulus are only an expression of a change of excitation in the nervous system, that they represent only a special pattern of the excitation process. This assumption of a system at rest was especially favoured by the fact that only the external stimuli were considered. Too little attention was given to the fact that the organism is continuously exposed, even in the apparent absence of outward stimuli, to the influence of internal stimuli—influences that may be of highest importance for its activity, for example, the effect

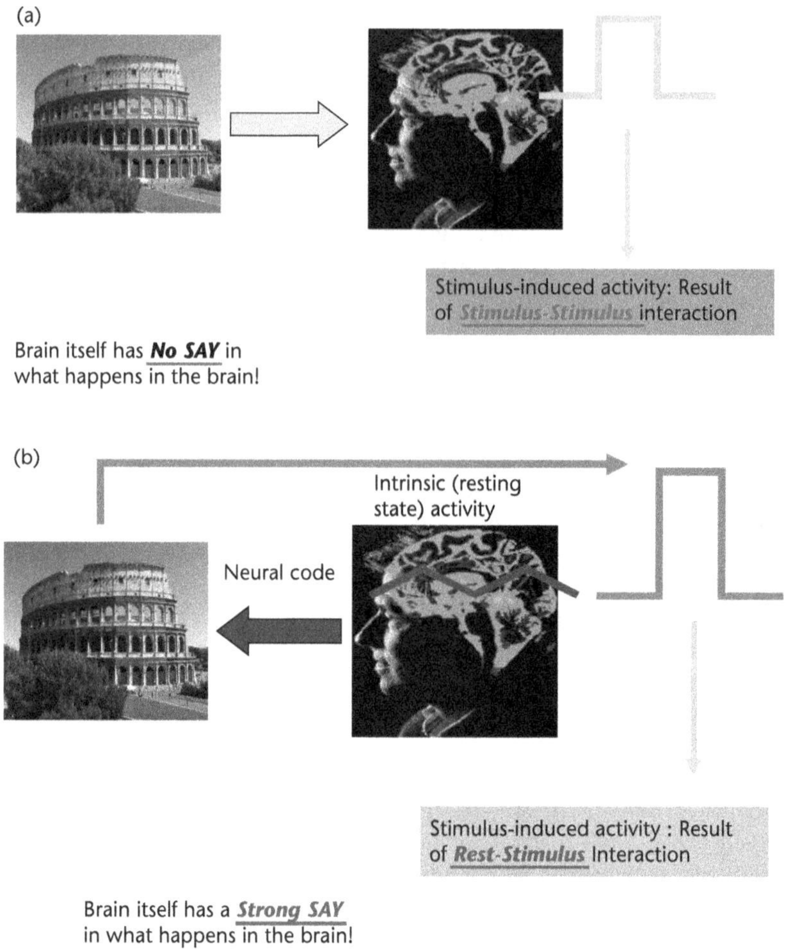

Figure I1-2 Extrinsic Versus Intrinsic View of the Brain. The figure illustrates two views of the brain, the brain's neural activity as purely determined by the extrinsic stimuli (*a*), and by both the brain's intrinsic activity and the extrinsic stimuli from the environment (*b*). The painting on the left in both figures shall illustrate the stimuli from the environment, while the brain in the middle stands for the brain. The grey line within the brain itself in (*b*) shall symbolize the brain's intrinsic activity, its resting-state activity, which as such remains independent of extrinsic stimuli from the environment. The bar diagram on the far right on both figures stands for the neural activity we observe once the person and its brain encounter the stimuli from the environment. (*a*) In the case of a purely extrinsic view of the brain, the observed stimulus-induced activity is exclusively and completely determined by the stimulus itself; the brain is passive and functions more or less like an automatic and reflex-like machine. Any neural activity in the brain can be traced back to stimuli and their interactions with each other; i.e., stimulus–stimulus interaction. The brain itself has thus no say in what happens in the brain. (*b*) This is different once one assumes intrinsic activity in the brain itself; i.e., in the resting state. In this case, the observed stimulus-induced activity results from the interaction between brain and stimuli amounting to rest–stimulus interaction. The brain itself has thus a strong say in what actually happens in the brain during its encounter with extrinsic stimuli from the environment (and the body).

of stimuli issuing from the blood, the importance of which was particularly pointed out by Thomas Graham Brown. Our view has received support by the investigation of the action currents of the brain, for as has been shown that even while the organism is not exposed to any external stimuli regular excitation processes occur in the brain. Stimulation appears in the curves rather as a disturbance of the regularity of the currents. (Goldstein 2000, pp. 95–96).

Why is the distinction between intrinsic and extrinsic views of the brain relevant? The assumption of intrinsic activity generated inside the brain itself has major implications for how we conceive of, view, and approach the brain's neural activity. What we as outside observers describe as "stimulus-induced" activity and usually associate with the extrinsic stimulus itself must, from the inside of the brain itself, be regarded as the hybrid result of a specific interaction between the brain's intrinsic activity and the extrinsic stimulus. In other words, stimulus-induced activity must be traced back to what we recently described as "rest–stimulus interaction" (see Northoff et al. 2010; see also Chapters 11 and 12 in this Volume for details) (see Fig. I12-b).

Which view of the brain do I follow here? Rather than subscribing to either the intrinsic or extrinsic view, my aim is to understand the brain's intrinsic features and thus how the brain encodes neural activity in general and how that affects both intrinsic and extrinsic activity. I postulate that we can understand the brain's extrinsic features, its stimulus-induced or task-related activity, only when we sufficiently investigate its intrinsic features; that is, its encoding strategy and intrinsic activity. This, I claim, will not only shed a novel light on the brain's neural activity but also on consciousness and how it is yielded by the brain, as will be discussed in Volume II.

Approach to the Brain IIa: Energy and Intrinsic Activity

This has been a rather abbreviated history of neuroscience. How about the present? The dichotomy between intrinsic and extrinsic views of the brain is still as controversial and has most recently resurfaced, especially in functional brain imaging (see, for instance, Raichle 2009, 2010). Let's start with the extrinsic view.

Many domains of neuroscience, ranging from cellular, to regional, to behavioral levels of the brain, rely on the experimental application of specific stimuli and tasks to probe neural activity. By comparing different stimuli and tasks, the resulting differences in neural activity are associated with the respective stimuli or tasks. This means that the experimental requirements may predispose and pull us toward an extrinsic view. The extrinsic view has been most predominant in behaviorism, which, according to authors like Jaak Panksepp (see Panksepp 1998, 2011a and 2011b; Cromwell and Panksepp 2011), finds its continuation in the cognitive and social neuroscience of our days.

However, the extrinsic view of the brain has most recently been challenged on metabolic-energetic and neuronal (and behavioral) grounds. Even in the resting state—that is, in the absence of any specific extrinsic stimuli from either body or environment—the brain shows a rather high degree of metabolic-energetic consumption, with about 20% of the body's overall energy budget (and oxygen fraction) (see Shulman et al. 2003, 2009b; Hyder et al. 2006; van Eijsden et al. 2009; Raichle et al. 2001; Raichle 2009, 2010).

This is even more remarkable given that the brain accounts for only 2% of the total body weight. Most important, the major part of that 20%—namely, 80% of the total brain's energy budget—is invested in the resting-state activity, while the stimulus-induced activity only requires an incremental increase of up to 20%. If the brain's invests so much energy to do its own intrinsic activity, there must be something special about it.

Approach to the Brain IIb: Intrinsic Activity and Spatial (and Temporal) Structure

The assumption of the special nature of the brain's intrinsic activity has been further propelled by the detection of a particular set of regions, the *default-mode network* (DMN), which includes various anterior and posterior cortical midline structures as well as the bilateral posterior parietal cortex (see Raichle et al. 2001; Raichle and Gusnard 2005; Gusnard and Raichle 2001; Buckner et al. 2008). The DMN shows high metabolism in the resting state that is defined by the absence of any specific extrinsic stimuli; such high metabolism is accompanied by a particular configuration of functional connectivity that distinguishes it from other neural networks (salience network, executive network, sensorimotor networks, etc.; see Menon 2011; see Chapters 4–6 in this volume for details).

However, spontaneous and thus intrinsic activity in the brain is not limited to the DMN. Other regions outside the DMN also show spontaneous neural activity that is independent of any extrinsic stimuli. This has been, for instance, demonstrated in the auditory and visual cortex, the thalamus, the hippocampus, the olfactory cortex, the cortical midline regions, the prefrontal cortex, the motor cortex, and other subcortical regions like the brain stem and the midbrain (Hunter et al. 2006; Wang et al. 2008; Freeman 2007, 2011; Buzsaki 2004, 2006, 2007; Buzsaki and Draguhn 2004; Llinas 1998, 2002; Panksepp 1998, 2011a and 2011b; Arieli et al. 1996; Singer 1999, 2009; Fries et al. 2007; Fries 2005, 2009; Raichle et al. 2001; Greicius and Menon 2004; Fox and Raichle 2007; Fox et al. 2005, 2006).

What can we take away from this quick glance (see Chapters 4–6 herein for more details) over the most recent results about the brain's intrinsic activity? There is plenty of empirical evidence for intrinsic activity throughout the whole brain. The intrinsic activity seems to show though a certain spatial structure as it is evidenced by different neural networks like the default-mode network, the sensorimotor network, the salience networks, and the central executive network (see for instance Menon 2011 as well as Chapter 4 in this volume). Furthermore there seems to be a temporal structure where low and high frequency fluctuations of neural activity are linked and integrated with each other (see Lakatos et al. 2008 as well as Chapter 5 for details).

The intrinsic activity's spatial and temporal structure remains to be determined, as it will be the focus in Chapters 4 through 6. Most importantly, I will postulate in Volume II that the spatial and temporal structure of the brain's intrinsic activity proves crucial in understanding how the brain can associate consciousness and its phenomenal features with the otherwise purely neuronal stimulus-induced activity.

Approach to the Brain III: "Intrinsic-Extrinsic View" of the Brain

Which view holds—the intrinsic or the extrinsic one? Rather than cashing out one view at the expense of the other, the brain itself may force us to go beyond and reconcile both views. Any given neural activity in the brain may be suggested to result from the interaction between the brain's intrinsic activity and the extrinsic stimuli from either the body—that is, interoceptive stimuli; or the environment—that is, exteroceptive stimuli. What I previously described as "rest–stimulus interaction" (Northoff et al. 2010), the neuronal mechanisms underlying the encounter between resting state and stimulus may thus be central in understanding the brain's neural activity in general.

Why is such rest–stimulus interaction so important? This question can be answered from both sides, the side of the resting-state activity and the side of the stimulus (and its stimulus-induced activity). Let us start with the resting-state activity itself.

Even in an apparent resting state, such as during sleep, the seemingly intrinsic activity of the brain is nevertheless still exposed to continuous extrinsic input from the body, or interoceptive stimuli, and the environment, or unspecific sensory stimuli (from all sensory modalities except the visual sense). For instance, the continuous action of our heart sends interoceptive stimuli to the brain during sleep, as do the continuous tactile, auditory, olfactory, and gustatory inputs from the environment.

The brain's resting-state activity may thus not be as purely intrinsic in its origin as is suggested by the term "intrinsic activity" (see Chapter 4 for the discussion of the concepts of "intrinsic activity" and "resting state"). Instead, the brain's resting activity may be hybrid rather than purely intrinsic, in that it results from a particular constellation between different stimuli from different origins: brain, body, and environment. The hybrid nature of the brain's resting-state activity will be pivotal in understanding why and how it constitutes some kind of spatial (and temporal) structure, as indicated earlier (see Chapters 4 and 5 for details).

Conversely, any extrinsic stimulus first encounters the brain's intrinsic activity before it can be processed at all and associated with sensorimotor, affective, cognitive, and social functions. The resulting stimulus-induced activity can therefore not be associated exclusively with the particular stimulus or task alone. Instead, the stimulus-induced activity must be considered a hybrid that results from the relationship of the stimulus in question to the other stimuli that are processed in the brain's resting-state activity at that particular point in time. Analogous to the brain's resting-state activity, the stimulus-induced activity is therefore hybrid rather than being purely extrinsic (see Chapter 12 for details on the hybrid nature of stimulus-induced activity).

What does the hybrid characterization of both resting-state and stimulus-induced activity imply for the view of the brain? Rather than opposing intrinsic and extrinsic views, we may need to investigate how the brain's resting-state activity and the extrinsic stimuli from body and environment interact with each other during both resting-state and stimulus-induced activity. What we described as rest–stimulus interaction in the empirical context may thus find its conceptual analogue in what I refer to as an "intrinsic-extrinsic view" of the brain.

Approach to the Brain IVa: Need for a "Common Currency" Between Intrinsic Activity and Extrinsic Stimuli

The "intrinsic-extrinsic view" postulates direct interaction between the brain's intrinsic activity and the extrinsic stimuli from body and environment. Both intrinsic activity and extrinsic stimuli are very different, however. Despite their differences, both intrinsic activity and extrinsic stimuli can nevertheless directly interact with each other.

How is such direct interaction possible? For that, both intrinsic resting-state activity and extrinsic stimuli must be encoded into neural activity in the same format, utilizing the same metric or measure. Only if both intrinsic resting-state activity and extrinsic stimuli are processed in the same format, i.e., metric or measure, are they compatible and therefore able to directly interact with each other.

If, in contrast, they are not computed in the same format, like two different computer software programs, they remain incompatible, which makes their direct interaction impossible. More metaphorically put, there must be a "common code" working as a "common currency" or "common language" between the brain's intrinsic activity and the extrinsic stimuli from body and environment.

How can we further illustrate the need for such a "common currency"? For that, I turn to the example of a market and two merchants. One merchant coming from the city may use money as currency for exchanging the bread he wants to trade, with one loaf costing, for instance, $5. Another merchant coming from the mountains uses chickens as currency for trading the meat, with 1 kilo of meat for 5 chickens.

How, now, is it possible for the two to do business? The mountain merchant needs bread, while the one from the city wants the meat. How can they exchange their goods? They are lacking a common currency unless they are able to negotiate the value of both bread and chicken relative to a common standard or measure.

Approach to the Brain IVb: Difference-Based Coding as "Common Currency" Between Intrinsic Activity and Extrinsic Stimuli

How does the example with our two merchants relate to the brain? The distinction between the two trading merchants corresponds to the distinction between intrinsic activity and extrinsic stimuli. In the same way the two merchants want to interact and trade their goods, the extrinsic stimuli from body and environment "want to interact and trade" with the brain's intrinsic activity.

The analogy goes even further. The two merchants meet on a common ground, the market place, to trade their goods. What is the common ground, the "market place," in the case of the encounter between intrinsic activity and extrinsic stimuli? Very simply, it is the brain itself where the encounter between intrinsic activity and extrinsic stimuli takes place.

This, however, is the point where the commonalities end and the differences start. Unlike in the case of our two merchants with their incompatible currencies, intrinsic activity and extrinsic stimuli are well able to directly interact with each other: "they can trade their information to the respective other and converge and merge with each other." This is possible, though, only because intrinsic activity and extrinsic stimuli share a "common currency," something our poor merchants are lacking.

What does this "common currency" consist of? In the case of today's merchants, it is easy. Money is the "common currency" in our markets. What now is the "common currency" that allows us to "trade and cash in" intrinsic activity and extrinsic stimuli with each other in the marketplace called "brain"? We currently do not know.

I suppose that the "common currency" between intrinsic activity and extrinsic stimuli can be found in what I earlier described as difference-based coding. The brain encodes the differences between different discrete points in physical time and space; that is, spatial and temporal differences into neural activity. I now postulate that such difference-based coding applies to the encoding of both the brain's intrinsic activity (see Chapters 4–6) and the extrinsic stimuli from body and environment (see Chapters 1–3).

Both intrinsic activity and extrinsic stimuli are encoded into neural activity in the same way: namely, in terms of spatial and temporal differences. Such spatial and temporal differences may then be constituted not only within, but also across intrinsic activity and extrinsic stimuli. What is then encoded during rest–stimulus interaction are the spatial and temporal differences between the intrinsic activity and the extrinsic stimuli (see Chapters 10–12 for details).

Differences as encoded into neural activity via difference-based coding are consequently the "common currency" between intrinsic activity and extrinsic stimuli. This means that differences as "common currency" provide the very basis for the here advocated "intrinsic-extrinsic view" of the brain.

Approach to the Brain V: "Code- Versus Content-Based View" of the Brain

My hypothesis is a rather strong one, since it claims that *any* neural activity in the brain, whether resting-state or stimulus-induced activity, is encoded in terms of difference-based coding rather than stimulus-induced activity. This means that I consider difference-based coding the neural code of the brain, the code that signifies and characterizes the brain as distinguished from, for instance, other organs like heart, kidney, etc., as well as from the computer (see my Epilogue in this volume for the comparison of the brain to other organs). In short, I consider difference-based coding to characterize and define the brain and its specific way of generating and processing neural activity.

I therefore base the characterization of the brain and its neural activity on a particular code, difference-based coding. One may thus want to speak of a "code-based view of the brain." A code-based view of the brain characterizes the brain by a particular code rather than some other features such as, for instance, behavioral, phenomenal, or mental contents (see the next paragraphs). We must thus distinguish the here-suggested "code-based view of the brain" from a "content-based view of the brain" (see Fig. I1-3).

What do I mean by "content-based view of the brain"? In that case, the brain and its neural activity are no longer characterized by a particular code but by the kinds of contents and their associated functions and neural networks. The brain's neural activity triggers various kinds of behavior—affective, sensorimotor, cognitive, or social—that are associated with the

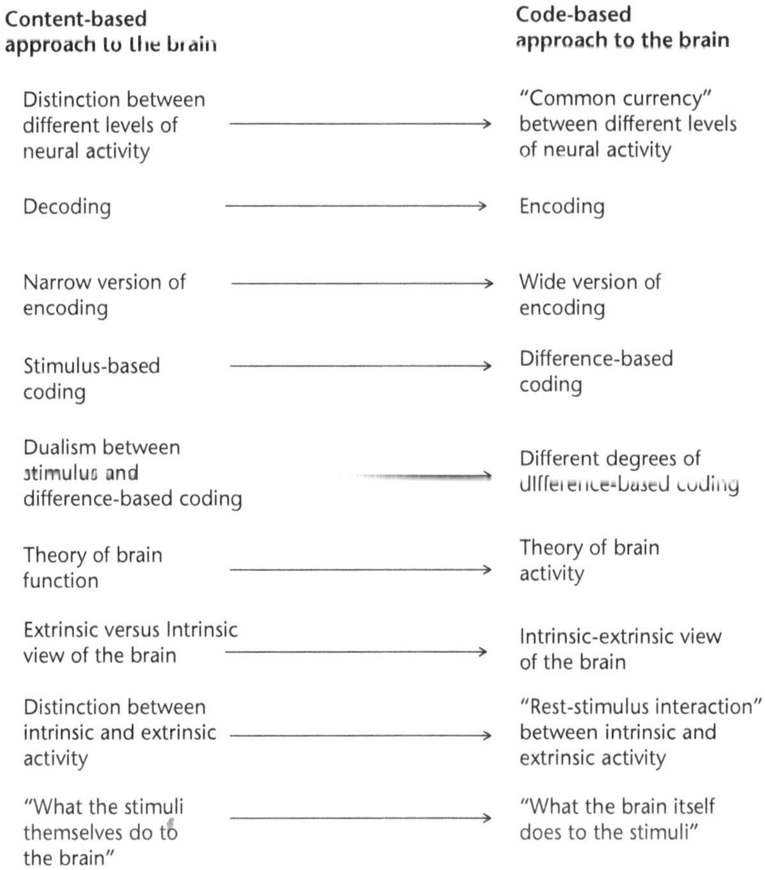

Figure I1-3 Content- Versus Code-Based Approach to the Brain. The figure illustrates the comparison between a content- and code-based approach to the brain. The figure presents a summary of the main features discussed and outlined in this introduction. This general theoretical overview will be supported by specific empirical data in the different parts of this volume.

corresponding functions and their underlying neural networks (and modules) in the brain. The different functions and their respective neural networks thus constitute behavioral contents.

However, the constitution of such behavioral contents by the various sensorimotor, affective, cognitive, and social functions and their respective neural networks is very much dependent on the brain's resting-state activity and how it interacts with the various stimuli and tasks (see especially Chapter 11 for details on that). This means that the constitution of behavioral contents is based on and presupposes a particular kind of encoding strategy; namely, difference-based coding, as I will argue. Before pursuing a "content-based view of the brain," we therefore need to address the "code-based view of the brain."

In addition to behavioral contents, one may also want to consider phenomenal and mental contents in order to signify a "content-based view of the brain." Though not yet fully understood, consciousness and both its phenomenal contents (like subjective experience) and mental contents (like our thoughts) are these days often taken as hallmark features of the brain and its neural activity.

As in the case of behavioral contents, I argue that phenomenal and mental contents do very much presuppose a particular encoding strategy in the generation of the brain's neural activity in order for them to be possible. More technically put, I propose difference-based coding as necessary condition of possible consciousness and its phenomenal and mental contents. This leads me to develop what I describe as the "coding hypothesis of consciousness," which will be elaborated in full detail in Volume II.

Approach to the Brain VI: "What the Brain Itself Does to the Stimuli" Versus "What the Stimuli Themselves Do to the Brain"

The focus in this volume is on developing a "code-based view of the brain" on a purely neuronal basis, independent of its behavioral, phenomenal, and mental functions. I therefore discuss how both stimuli from body and environment (see Chapters 1–3) and the brain's resting-state activity (see Chapters 4–6) are encoded into neural activity. This is complemented by showing how their interaction, rest–stimulus interaction, is encoded into neural activity (see Chapters 10–12) and, most importantly, predisposed by the resting-state activity itself (see Chapters 7–9).

Rather than focusing on particular functions and their respective neural networks, I discuss the neuronal mechanisms underlying the encoding of spatial and temporal differences into neural activity; that is, difference-based coding. For that purpose, I will discuss several different functions and neural regions and networks, taking them as paradigmatic examples of how neural activity is encoded in terms of difference-based coding.

My approach to the brain taken in this volume differs from the one usually taken these days. The commonly accepted approach starts with particular stimuli or tasks from body and environment and investigates how they affect the brain's various functions and networks. The movement is thus from stimuli and tasks to the brain. This is different in my approach. Rather than starting with the extrinsic stimuli (and tasks), I start with the brain itself and its intrinsic features. To put it slightly differently, I start with the code rather than the contents of the brain, thus pursuing a code- rather than content-based approach to the brain.

Neuronally, such a code-based approach to the brain entails a shift from stimulus-induced activity to resting-state activity in order to investigate how the latter affects the encoding of the former. Therefore, I start with the investigation of the brain's resting-state activity itself and its particular way of encoding (see Chapters 4–6 and 7–9) before turning to stimulus-induced activity (see Chapters 10–12) that then, as I claim, can be understood as a "natural outflow" of the former.

Such a characterization of stimulus-induced as the "natural outflow" of the ongoing resting-state activity and its particular spatial and temporal structure has already been espoused by one of the earlier major neuroscientists, Karl Lashley (1949):

A second point of major importance is that the nervous system is not a neutral medium on which learning imposes any form of organization whatsoever. On the contrary, it has definite predilections for certain forms of organization and imposes these upon the sensory impulses which reach it.... In its functional organisation the nervous system seems to consist of schemata or basic patterns within which new stimuli are fitted. (Lashley 1949, p. 35)

Following Lashley's footsteps, and putting it metaphorically, I am more interested in "what the brain itself does to the stimuli" than in "what the stimuli themselves do to the brain." This will open a novel door to our understanding of the brain: namely, why and how it works the way it does rather than in some other way. Most important, this will also open the door to reveal the neuronal mechanisms that make possible the association of consciousness and its phenomenal features to the otherwise purely neuronal stimulus-induced activity.

Outline of the Book I: Parts I and II

The main and overarching aim of this book is to discuss the hypothesis of difference-based coding as *the* neural code of the brain. As outlined in this introduction, this makes necessary a shift in our view on the brain from a content- to a code-based approach. In order to investigate the brain's neural code and, more specifically, its encoding of neural activity, I will discuss the brain's neural activity in different stages, ranging from its encounter with extrinsic stimuli (Part I), to its intrinsic activity (Part II), to its own preparation to extrinsic stimuli (Part III), and to its modulation by extrinsic stimuli (Part IV) (see Fig. I1-4).

In Part I, I discuss how the brain encodes its neural activity when encountering stimuli. Single recordings in especially sensory cortical regions observed that stimuli are not represented one-to-one in neural activity. Instead, the neural activity of, for instance, one neuron may be involved in the representation of more than one stimulus, implying a many-to-one relationship between stimuli and neurons. This is possibly only when the neural activity is temporally and spatially made sparser compared to the number of stimuli, which has led to the hypothesis of *sparse coding* (Olshausen and Fields 1996).

Sparse coding implies a many-to-one relationship with regard to the number of neurons recruited per stimulus; this implies that a lower number of neurons is actually recruited compared to the number of those that could possibly be recruited. This means that the resulting neural activity is spatially and temporally "sparsened," reflecting what is described as "lifetime sparseners" and "population sparseness" (Part I).

Sparse coding has been predominantly investigated on the cellular level. I will here extend its central claim to the regional level, taking results from perceptual decision-making as the paradigmatic example. As on the cellular level, the findings suggest that neural activity on the regional level can only result when encoding the difference between different stimuli rather than the stimuli themselves. Hence, I will

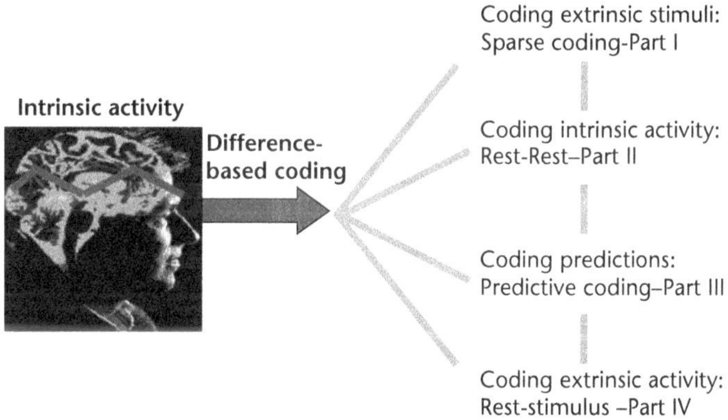

Figure I1-4 **Overview of the Brain The figure illustrates the main parts of the book and how they are based on each other. On the far left, the main assumption is described by assuming intrinsic activity in the brain; i.e., resting-state activity. This in turn is supposed to entail a particular way of neural coding: difference-based coding as distinguished from stimulus-based coding. That means that any change in neural activity must be encoded relative to the brain's actual resting-state activity level. Hence, what is encoded is the virtual difference between the actual resting-state activity level and the possible neural activity elicited by the stimulus independently of any resting-state activity. I propose that difference-based coding is the basic code of the brain, *the* neural code. If so, difference-based coding should be manifested in the various neural operations of the brain and thus in its different forms of neural activity. This is indicated on the far right. First, I show that difference-based coding must underlie the encoding of stimuli from the environment into the brain's neural activity; this will be discussed in Part I. Second, I propose difference-based coding to be central in encoding spontaneous changes in the resting-state activity itself; this will be discussed in Part II. Third, I suggest difference-based coding to make possible the encoding of predictions or anticipations of possible stimuli from the environment in the brain's neural activity; this is currently subsumed under the theory of predictive coding, which will be discussed in Part III. Finally, I demonstrate that difference-based coding allows for the direct interaction of the brain's intrinsic activity with the extrinsic stimuli from body and environment amounting to rest–stimulus interaction; this will be discussed in Part IV.**

propose that sparse coding on both cellular and regional levels is possible only when presupposing difference-based coding (rather than stimulus-based coding).

The second part shifts the focus from the encoding of stimuli by the brain to the brain itself and its intrinsic activity. I will here focus exclusively on the brain's intrinsic activity, which recently has been much debated, especially in the functional imaging literature. The description of the brain's resting state and its high metabolic-energetic and neural activity has led to much research into the spatial and temporal features of the resting-state activity as manifested in functional connectivity and low-frequency fluctuations.

My focus is especially on the neuronal mechanisms of how such functional connectivity and low-frequency fluctuations are generated. What kind of neuronal processes and coding strategies must be presupposed in order to make possible the kind of functional connectivity and low-frequency fluctuations we observe in the brain's resting state? This leads me to describe the spatiotemporal dynamics of the resting state.

I postulate that the resting state is a highly dynamic, that is, non-static state wherein plenty of interactions across different discrete points in physical time and space are going on. There are, for example, interactions across the different regions in the resting state itself, as reflected in functional connectivity. And there is continuous interaction between different frequency ranges (like low-frequency fluctuations and gamma oscillations; see Chapter 5 in this volume for details). In short, there is plenty of continuous interaction across different discrete points in physical time and space in the intrinsic activity and thus in the resting state itself.

Following my main hypothesis, I hypothesize that the resting state and its encoding of neural activity can be characterized by difference-based coding. I will show that the brain's intrinsic activity is encoded in terms of spatial and temporal differences between different discrete points in physical time and space. This presupposes difference-based coding rather than stimulus-based coding in the encoding of the brain's resting-state activity.

Outline of the Book II: Parts III and IV

After having discussed the encoding of extrinsic stimuli (Part I) and the more intrinsic activity (Part II) into neural activity, we next shift our focus to how both of them, and especially the brain's intrinsic activity, impact subsequent stimulus-induced activity. This will be investigated in two different steps: first, how the brain's intrinsic activity "prepares itself" for its potential encounter with extrinsic stimuli; this is discussed in the current literature under the concept of *predictive coding* (see Part III). Such predictive coding sets the stage for the actual interaction of the extrinsic stimuli with the brain's intrinsic activity, which is supposed to be based on difference-based coding (see Part IV).

Part III focuses on predictive coding and how it stands in relation to difference-based coding. Predictive coding claims that neural activity results from the matching and comparison between a predicted input and the actual input, with this difference being the prediction error. The amount of prediction error may then determine the degree of the subsequent stimulus-induced activity. This makes it clear that the prediction error is based on the encoding of spatial and temporal differences, the difference between predicted and actual input. Hence, predictive coding is not only well compatible with difference-based coding but presupposes it.

How, though, is the predicted input generated? The theory of predictive coding implies a hierarchical model of organization wherein each layer functions as either predicted or actual input for the respectively next-higher and -lower layers (see Part III for details). This neglects, however, the central role of the brain's intrinsic activity.

I will here target those neuronal mechanisms that are central in generating the predicted input on the basis of the brain's intrinsic activity and the encoding of its own neural activity in terms of spatial and temporal differences; that is, difference-based coding. Since reward is one of the main functions where predictive coding has been demonstrated, I devote two chapters (see Chapters 8 and 9) to it, in which I will discuss how difference-based coding and predictive coding complement each other.

How about the actual stimulus-induced activity by itself? This is the focus in Part IV. Volume I ends with the discussion of the neuronal mechanisms underlying stimulus-induced activity and more specifically rest–stimulus interaction as the interaction between extrinsic stimuli and intrinsic activity. The insights from the interaction between different stimuli—that is, stimulus–stimulus interaction (see Chapter 10)—serve as a template to gain insight into the neuronal mechanisms underlying rest–stimulus interaction (see Chapter 11). I suppose that such rest–stimulus interaction, including its behavioral (and phenomenal) effects, is possible only by encoding the extrinsic stimulus into neural activity relative to the actual level of the brain's intrinsic activity, thus presupposing difference-based coding rather than stimulus-based coding.

I propose that the excitation-inhibition balance (EIB) is central in making possible the encoding of spatial and temporal differences into stimulus-induced activity during rest–stimulus interaction. Since the EIB is based on GABA and glutamate, I discuss the most recent results on how resting-state levels of both GABA and glutamate predict the degree of stimulus-induced activity and its associated behavioral effects (see Chapter 12).

I postulate that the EIB is central in constituting spatial and temporal differences and their subsequent encoding into any kind of neural activity. Without the interplay and balance between GABA and glutamate and thus between neural inhibition and excitation, the brain would remain unable to constitute spatial and temporal differences at all and thus to use difference-based coding as its basic coding strategy. I therefore focus on the role of GABA and glutamate in different neuronal contexts during stimulus-induced activity (Chapter 2), resting-state activity (Chapter 6), and rest–stimulus interaction (Chapter 12).

Outline of the Book III: Epilogue and Appendix

The book concludes with an epilogue. Comparing the brain to other organs of the body like the stomach, the heart, and the kidney, I summarize the main points and hypotheses postulated here. For that I use some basic questions regarding the what, how, where, and why of the brain as a template, which helps me in sketching a first tentative outline of a future "theory of brain activity."

In addition to the four parts, the book also contains four appendices. Each appendix discusses a particular theoretical issue relevant for a more thorough understanding of difference-based coding. Appendix 1 extends Chapters 10–12 when discussing the presumed relationship between resting-state activity and stimulus-induced activity, thereby assuming what I describe as "continuity hypothesis."

Appendix 2 picks up the question of localizationism versus holism as an important theoretical debate that has long lingered and still is highly prevalent in neuroscience in general and functional imaging in particular. Finally, Appendix 3 raises some epistemological questions concerning the relationship between brain and observer, including some principal experimental and epistemological limits in our possible investigation and knowledge of the brain.

Reading Instructions I: Individual Preferences

This Volume I contains four parts. Each part of the book can be read on its own, however. If readers are mainly interested in sparse coding, for instance, they may want to focus on the first part. In the case of a strong interest in the resting state, the brain's intrinsic activity, readers may want to read Part II and, if their interest extends further, Part IV, which focuses on rest–stimulus interaction. Readers focusing on predictive coding may find Part III of interest. Finally, those who are more interested in stimulus-induced activity may find the most useful material in Part IV.

More theoretically inclined readers from, for instance, neurophilosophy or philosophy may want to focus more on the sections where I discuss conceptual issues. While being rather infrequent and scattered within the main text, these issues are discussed in more detail in the four appendices. The empirically minded reader may be sometimes puzzled about why I discuss and raise these more conceptual and theoretical issues in either the main text or the appendices.

As I said before, I am convinced that neuroscience needs to tackle these theoretical and conceptual issues if it ever wants to find out how the brain works and encodes stimuli and its own resting state into neural activity. Neuroscience may here want to learn its lesson from, for example, physics and biology, where experimental discoveries and theoretical-conceptual reflections went hand in hand.

To give the reader some signposts in each chapter, I indicate by the title what each section is about. I therefore distinguish different sections: "Neuronal Findings," "Neuronal Hypothesis," "Neuroempirical Background." This and the respective section titles serve to orient the reader to what each section is about. Moreover, each chapter starts with a summary and the key concepts and topics, while it ends with a section that addresses open questions.

If the reader wants to get a general overview, I recommend reading the Introduction and the Epilogue. The Introduction will provide a general overview of the kind of future theory of brain activity I envision here. Rather than summarizing the main empirical findings in the Epilogue, I there discuss more theoretical issues like the what, how, and why of the brain and its characterization as distinguished from other organs like the heart, stomach, and kidney.

Reading Instructions II: General Limitations

While I raise many issues, the number of questions and findings I leave out is much greater. First, I do not discuss higher-order cognition such as attention, executive functions, memory, and so forth, in detail. Since my focus is more on neuronal mechanisms and coding strategies, I intend to reveal what must happen in the brain underpinning all of these cognitive functions. However, future investigations may show how the neuronal mechanisms and coding strategies discussed here may apply and predispose to cognitive and other functions. This, however, is beyond the scope of this book.

Second, I do not go into detail about cellular and molecular processes, since this would simply transcend the context of this book. Moreover, my biochemical account is rather limited, focusing only on GABA and glutamate while neglecting the many other transmitters like dopamine, serotonin, and so on. I am well aware that these aspects require attention in the future.

More specifically, I would hypothesize that cellular, molecular, and biochemical processes function according to the same principles outlined here, meaning that they are also subject to difference-based coding. This will be a task for the future, and I am sure that the regional level as the main target here will surely benefit from such investigation of the cellular-molecular-biochemical and microscopic levels.

Third, coding specialists may miss mathematical models and formulae that are essential to account for a particular coding strategy. I here focus on describing difference-based coding in various contexts, while leaving out completely the mathematization of difference-based coding (see, for instance, Friston and Dolan 2010). This must be left for future specialists, who are versatile in mathematical and subsequent neural network modeling.

Fourth, it should be mentioned that due to the wide range of topics covered here, I will not be able to cover the whole literature on each topic. Instead of giving a full-blown overview (which is the purpose of review papers), I will often point out certain examples that I consider to be paradigmatic. That being said, as I often do not provide examples without competing data, one may therefore accuse me of "cherry picking" by focusing on certain viewpoints only, while neglecting competing ones. However, a discussion of all viewpoints would simply exceed the context of this book.

Hence, the focus here is on developing my own ideas about how the brain could possibly function. For that, I rely on several studies, which I often discuss in a paradigmatic way. Explication of my main hypothesis of difference-based coding is accompanied by the hope that it will stir plenty of controversial discussions in the future and, even more importantly, experimental testing of the many hypotheses I suggest. In the meantime, I have to beg the forgiveness of all authors whose data and positions I neglect and do not give sufficient credit.

Reading Instructions III: Coding and Consciousness

Finally, one may wonder how this Volume I, about the brain's neural code, is related to Volume II, about consciousness. In short, Volumes I and II share the work. Volume I focuses only on neuronal processes and how the brain must process and encode its neural activity in order to yield the kind of neuronal (and behavioral) results we observe. With this in mind, functions like perception, reward, and perceptual decision-making serve only to illustrate the neuronal mechanisms in question.

The focus changes in Volume II from such purely neuronal account of the brain to the phenomenal features of consciousness. I focus no longer on the purely neuronal mechanisms but on how these yield the kind of phenomenal (and ultimately mental) features that characterize consciousness; that is, phenomenal consciousness and its various features (see Introduction in Volume II for a more detailed description).

Thereby I propose that difference-based coding, as hypothesized in Volume I, predisposes the association of the brain's purely neuronal states during either the resting state or stimulus-induced activity with consciousness and its phenomenal features. Accordingly, Volume I lays the groundwork, the purely neuronal floor, without which the phenomenal furniture called consciousness could not possibly be set in Volume II.

To understand the full implications of the here-suggested neural code, difference-based coding, the reader should not limit herself or himself to Volume I but take at least a look into Volume II—for instance, its Introduction and Epilogue. From there on, you may decide. Either you immerse yourself in the purely neuronal floor of the brain itself and its neural code in Volume I; or, you prefer to explore right away the phenomenal (taken both literally and figuratively) furniture of consciousness in Volume II and how it stands on the neuronal floor of the brain and its neural code.

PART I
Encoding Extrinsic Stimuli

General background:

The brain is exposed to continuous stimulation from the environment. What does the brain do with all of these stimuli? The brain reacts to stimuli by modulating its intrinsic neural activity. Such changes in neural activity yield what we as observers call "stimulus-induced activity." Now the question is how the brain translates and transforms the stimuli from the environment into neural activity.

What are the rules and principles that guide the translation and transformation of mere stimuli into neural activity? How does the brain itself determine and modulate its own neural activity? Which features of the stimuli are central to the brain's determination of its own neural activity?

These questions touch upon a common theme, the kind of neural algorithm or neural code the brain itself applies in order to encode and determine its own neural activity when being exposed to the stimuli from the environment. The question of the neural code is a central theme in current neuroscience, especially on the cellular level of single and multiple neurons, as it will be discussed in this and subsequent chapters.

However, the importance of the question of the brain's neural code extends far beyond that, into almost philosophical relevance. By deciphering the kind of neural code the brain itself applies to encode stimuli from the environment (and the body), we learn much about the brain and how it can—and, even more important, cannot—process stimuli from the environment. This will tell us not only about the brain's neural functions but also much about the kind of relationship the brain can (and cannot) establish in relation to its environment (and the body of which the brain is a part).

Such an understanding of the brain's neural (or "neuro-ecological," if one wants to say so) code is important in order to understand the various functions that are usually associated with the brain, like sensory, motor, affective, cognitive, and even social functions (see Part IV in this volume for some discussion in this regard). Most important, deciphering the neural code of the brain will, as we will see in Volume II, also prove vital to understanding how the brain can associate its purely neuronal stimulus-induced activity with consciousness and its phenomenal features.

Let us, though, return to the brain's neural code independent of any particular function. The question of the neural code is often raised in the context of the investigation of single neurons and a population of neurons using single- and multi-cell recordings. Recent investigations show that what is encoded into the single neuron's (and a population of neurons') stimulus-induced activity is not the single stimulus by itself, isolated and independent of other stimuli. This means that the single discrete point in physical time and space as associated with a particular stimulus does not seem to surface as such—in a one-to-one way—in the encoded neural activity.

Instead, the stimulus-induced activity seems to encode the single stimulus' frequency of occurrence across different, discrete points in physical space and time in relation to other stimuli. This means that the statistical frequency distribution of the stimulus, its so-called natural statistics, rather than the stimulus' physical features themselves, that is its discrete points in physical time and space, is encoded in stimulus-induced activity. Therefore, the relationship between the number of the stimuli's discrete points in physical time and space on one hand, and the number of the encoding neurons on the other is no longer one-to-one but rather many-to-one, with many stimuli being encoded in the activity of one neuron. There is thus a rather sparse representation of the stimulus in the activity pattern of the neurons, amounting to what is called "sparse encoding."

How is such sparse encoding of the stimuli's statistical frequency distribution into the neurons' activity possible? For that, as I will argue, the neurons must encode the spatial and temporal differences between the different discrete points in physical time and space as associated with the different stimuli. Such encoding of spatial and temporal differences rather than the single stimulus' discrete points in physical time and space themselves; i.e., stimulus-based coding, signifies what I described as "difference-based coding" (see Introduction for a definition). In short, I postulate that sparse coding presupposes difference-based coding rather than stimulus-based coding.

General overview:

The goal of Part I of this volume is to discuss the empirical findings supporting sparse coding, including its more precise neuronal mechanisms. This serves as a starting point to develop the first major hypothesis: that sparse coding is possible only on the basis of difference-based coding, as described in the Introduction.

Chapter 1 focuses on the neuronal mechanisms underlying sparse coding in single cells and a population of neurons and how that presupposes difference-based coding.

Chapter 2 extends sparse coding to the biochemical dimension, focusing especially on GABA and glutamate as the main constituents of the "excitation-inhibition balance" (EIB); especially GABAergic-mediated neural inhibition is shown to have a central role in sparsening neural activity in response to stimuli. While the first two chapters remain almost completely on the level of single cells and a population of neurons, the third chapter aims to apply the principles underlying sparse coding to the regional level.

Chapter 3 therefore focuses on empirical evidence from recent imaging studies on perceptual decision making (taken as paradigmatic example). The reported regional activation pattern observed in these studies is shown to be possible only on the basis of difference-based and sparse coding on a regional level, while they are not compatible with stimulus-based coding and a non-sparse form of neural coding (like local or dense coding).

CHAPTER 1
Sparse Coding and Natural Statistics

Summary

The brain is exposed to continuous sensory input from the environment (and the body). How does the brain encode such continuous sensory input and translate it into neural activity; for example, stimulus-induced activity? Results from cellular recordings show that single neurons and a population of neurons represent the stimulus in a rather sparse way so that many stimuli are represented in one neuron's (or one population of neurons') activity. This amounts to a many-to-one relationship between stimuli and neurons entailing sparse coding. As such, sparse coding must be distinguished from other coding strategies like dense and local coding that imply a one-to-many and one-to-one relationship between stimuli and neurons. How is such sparse coding possible? The neurons' (and population of neurons') activity seems to encode the statistical frequency distribution of stimuli across their different discrete points in physical time and space; that is, their natural statistics. However, this is possible only when presupposing that differences between the stimuli's different discrete points in physical space and time are encoded into neural activity. In other words, spatial and temporal differences (between the different discrete points in physical time and space) must be encoded into neural activity in order for sparse coding as a many-to-one relationship between stimuli and neurons to be possible. This is empirically supported by empirical findings of single neuron and by population recordings that show "stretching" and "adaptive rescaling" of neuronal activity in response to the stimuli's temporal (velocity) and spatial (classical and non-classical receptive fields) features. Such stretching and adaptive rescaling can occur only within the maximal and minimal possible biophysical and computational limits, signifying what I call the "biophysical-computational spectrum" of the neurons (and the population of neurons), which may vary between different species. I therefore postulate the degree of sparse coding to be dependent on and related to the biophysical-computational spectrum of the particular organism, i.e., species. Taken together, I demonstrate empirical evidence for the close linkage of sparse coding to difference-based coding in both spatial and temporal terms on a single-neuron and population level of neural activity.

Key Concepts and Topics Covered

Coding strategies of sensory input, sparse coding, local coding, dense coding, single neuron and population level, non-linearity, biophysical-computational features of neurons, schizophrenia, different species

Neuroempirical background IA: Encoding of stimuli in terms of sparse coding

We are bombarded with a multitude of inputs from the environment: for instance, sensory stimuli, such as various forms of light intensity and changes in sound pressure; gustatory and olfactory stimuli; and so on. How does the brain process all of these stimuli? Different possibilities exist.

The brain could, for instance, process each stimulus by itself, independently of any others. In this case, the multitude of stimuli would correspond to the number of active neurons, implying a one-to-one relationship between stimuli and neurons. Such a coding strategy is described as "local coding." Roughly, the concept of local coding describes that each stimulus and, more specifically, its physical features like color, motion, and so on, are encoded separately in different neurons. Local coding thus implies a one-to-one relationship between the number of stimuli and the number of active neurons.

However, as I will demonstrate later in detail, such a one-to-one relationship between stimuli and neurons cannot be observed in nature. Instead, the various sensory stimuli are represented by a relatively small number of simultaneously active neurons when compared to the large number of neurons present in the brain. Thus, there is a many-to-one relationship between sensory stimuli and active neurons, amounting to what is called "sparseness" in the neuronal representation of sensory input. The sensory inputs are processed and coded in a sparse way; that is, by a number of active neurons lower than the number of stimuli, entailing what is called "sparse coding" (for reviews, see Simoncelli and Olshausen 2001; Rolls and Treves 2011; Olshausen and Fields 2004; Jacob et al. 2012; Molotchnikoff and Rouat 2012).

Let us now describe sparse coding in further detail (see later discussions for more empirical details) and, in particular, let us explore why such sparse encoding of sensory stimuli may be beneficial. When encountering our environment, our brain is confronted with a multitude of stimuli. Not every stimulus is relevant to the organism, however.

If, for instance, we hear a bird singing the same tone over and over, it is relevant the first time (if at all) but becomes increasingly irrelevant with each repetition. There are thus plenty of irrelevant stimuli; that is, redundancies. Coding each of these redundant stimuli on a one-to-one basis, as described in local coding, would be highly inefficient. One could hear the brain saying (if it could speak by itself): "Why should I waste my precious neural and energetic resources on stimuli that are irrelevant for my owner?"

Neuroempirical background Ib: Redundancy of sensory inputs and different possible encoding strategies

How does our brain deal with redundancies in sensory input? British neuroscientist Horace Barlow, born in 1921 and a great-grandson of Charles Darwin, focused on this question. Barlow (1972, 2001) suggests that such redundancies in sensory inputs are central and provide important knowledge about our environment that is processed and coded in the activity changes of the brain and more specifically in the sensory cortex.

This model, however, makes it even more difficult for the brain. The brain is confronted with a "difficult choice," as one may want to say in a figurative way: There is plenty of redundancy in the sensory inputs that needs to be reduced, but at the same time, such redundancy may contain some useful information. The brain is thus torn between discarding redundant information and retaining information that could be relevant.

How can the brain "deal" with the contradictory requirement of discarding and retaining information at the same time? We already discarded local coding as one possible option, since it requires too much effort to encode seemingly redundant information.

Another possible coding strategy could be to select or compress the multitudes of sensory inputs, amounting to what Barlow calls "selective coding" or "compressive coding" (see Barlow 2001, p. 243). Such selective coding retains certain inputs while discarding others. This entails that the latter ones, the discarded inputs, are lost irreversibly; this is problematic, however, because these inputs may potentially be relevant in the future. Hence, "selective or compressive coding" may be an insufficient coding strategy to deal with the problem of redundancy.

Neuroempirical background Ic: Encoding of the stimuli's "natural statistics" in sparse coding

Barlow suggests an alternative strategy to both "local and selective coding." Rather than coding each stimulus by itself, as in local coding, or selecting stimuli, as in selective coding, he suggests that the brain codes and represents chunks of stimuli and their details together; for example, as "gathered details" (Barlow 2001, p. 248). Let us explain what exactly is meant by "gathered details." These gathered details may, for instance, concern the sensory inputs' frequency of occurrence across the different discrete points in physical time and space. In our earlier example of the singing bird, this raises the question of whether the stimulus occurs with a certain temporal regularity (i.e., the same tone over and over again) and whether the bird's tone occurs in conjunction with other stimuli, such as the moving of leaves (due to the bird's efforts while singing).

How can we specify such an encoding strategy? Let us start with what is *not* encoded into neural activity, since that will make it easier for us to better understand the brain's actual encoding strategy. Barlow proposes that the sensory cortex does not encode each tone by itself, including its respective discrete point in physical time and space; that is, its respective temporal and spatial position. The single tone and its respective spatial and temporal features are not encoded by themselves and thus separately and in isolation from the other tones, as described in local coding.

After having shown how the brain does not encode, we now we can turn our focus to the brain's actual encoding strategy. Instead of encoding single stimuli by themselves, the brain seems to encode the distribution of the stimulus, the tone during the bird's singing, across its different discrete points in physical time and thus the frequency distribution of the tone. And the brain may also encode the spatial position of the bird's tone relative to, for instance, the tree's moving leaf.

What is encoded into neural activity is thus the statistical frequency distribution of stimuli—the tone—across different discrete points in physical time and space. This is what Barlow describes as the encoding of the stimuli's "natural statistics," the statistical frequency distribution of a stimulus across different discrete positions in time and space.

Neuroempirical background Id: inefficiency of dense and local coding

Encoding of the stimuli's natural statistics implies that several stimuli are encoded by the neural activity of one neuron, entailing a many-to-one relationship and thus sparse coding. Accordingly, sparse coding can tentatively (at this point) be defined as the neural coding of the stimuli's natural statistics across different discrete points in physical time and space. Before going into empirical detail, I will briefly contrast sparse coding with other possible coding strategies with regard to how they stand in relation to the earlier mentioned problem of redundancy (see Fig. 1-1).

Instead of only a few neurons' being recruited during multiple sensory inputs, a higher number of neurons may respond to most stimuli. For instance, one stimulus may then induce the activity of several neurons. This implies a one-to-many relationship between stimuli and neurons and amounts to what is called "dense coding" (see Vinje and Gallant 2000).

However, such dense coding is highly redundant in that it codes the same sensory input in the activities of many neurons while each neuron contains only a little information. The high redundancy and the little information encoded in the neurons' activity make such dense coding rather inefficient (see Vinje and Gallant 2000). One may thus want to speak of the "informational inefficiency" of "dense coding."

Alternatively, each sensory input may be coded separately by one specific neuron in a one-to-one way, amounting to what is described as "local coding" (see Vinje and Gallant 2000). The neurons would then be tuned to give highly selective responses to extremely specific sensory inputs. Given the almost unlimited number of possible sensory inputs, this would require an implausibly large number of neurons.

In addition, each neuron would also need to show extremely specific computational properties as being tuned to only one particular sensory input, if not to only one specific physical feature. However, this is not only empirically implausible but also highly inefficient with regard to

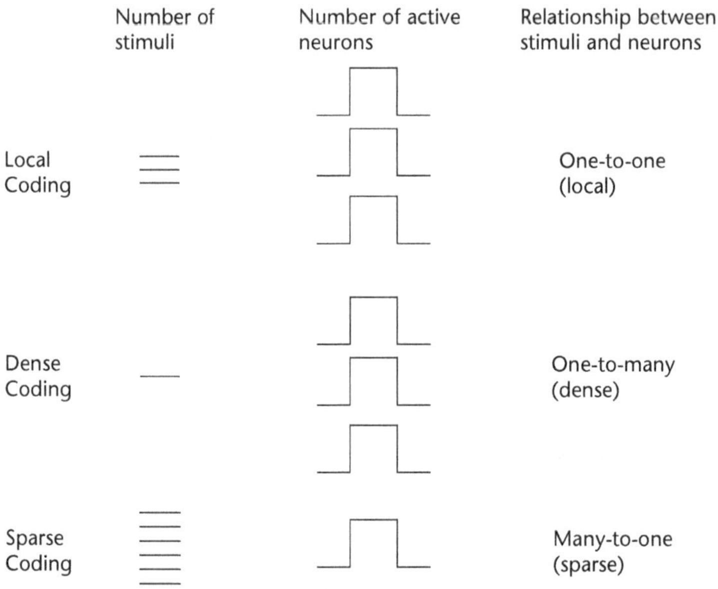

Figure 1-1 Different coding strategies of sensory input. This figure shows different possible strategies of encoding stimuli into the neurons' activity. Thereby, the relationship between the number of stimuli and the number of active neurons is central. If their relationship is one to one, one speaks of "local coding." If the number of active neurons exceeds the number of stimuli in a. one-to-many way, one speaks of "dense coding." If the reverse is the case, the number of stimuli exceeding the number of active neurons in a many-to-one way, sparse coding must be proposed. Finally, all three forms of coding occur more or less on a continuum, as discussed in Figure 1-5.

the number of required computations and the amount of energy needed for each of the different computations. "Informational inefficiency" may thus be closely linked to "computationally and energetically inefficiency."

Neuroempirical background Ie: Sparse coding as efficient encoding strategy

The inefficiency of both dense and local coding must be distinguished from the apparent efficiency of sparse coding. Sparse coding allows for maximum information to be encoded when generating neural activity on the basis of the natural statistics and thus the spatiotemporal structure across sensory inputs, rather than encoding single sensory inputs. Such sparse coding requires the recruitment of only a few neurons that encode the sensory inputs' statistical structure.

Unlike dense and local coding, sparse coding may therefore be considered a rather efficient way of neural coding by allowing for a good if not maximally high ratio between the amount of coded information and the number of neurons that need to be recruited. Since it allows for maximal information transfer and minimal involvement of active neurons, sparse coding is also described as "efficient coding" (see, for instance, Olshausen and Field 1996; Simoncelli and Olshausen 2001; Lewicki 2002; Olshausen and O'Connor 2002).

Such "informational efficiency" of sparse coding may be closely linked to both "computational and energetic efficiency." The number of computations required for the processing of stimuli is lower than the number required in both local and dense coding, so sparse coding may be more computationally efficient. That in turn implies lower energy demands and thus "energetic efficiency."

Accordingly, sparse coding may be described as "efficient coding strategy" in informational, computational, and energetic demands. After this more general overview, we now need to into empirical detail to better understand how exactly sparse coding works on a cellular and population level of neural activity.

Neuronal findings Ia: Encoding of the stimuli's standard deviation into neural activity in visual cortex

How can we lend empirical support to sparse coding? Most work on sparse coding has been done in the visual domain and hence in the visual cortex (see Olshausen and Field 1996; Simoncelli and Olshausen 2001; Lewicki 2002; David et al., 2004; Olshausen and O'Connor 2002; Zylberberg et al. 2011; Lőrincz et al. 2012; Willmore et al. 2011; Rozell et al. 2008). To better understand the neuronal mechanisms underlying sparse coding, I focus on the visual cortex in this chapter and discuss other sensory and non-sensory regions in the second and third chapters. Let me here proceed with a study by Brenner et al. (2000) as an example of sparse coding on the cellular and population level (while not going into detail on the other studies cited earlier; see also Friedlander and Brenner 2009).

Brenner et al. (2000) recorded activity in the H1 neurons in the visual system of the blowfly. H1 neurons are sensitive to horizontal motion across the visual field. These neurons generate action potentials during motion in the preferred direction, whereas motion in the opposite direction inhibits the neurons. The spike trains of H1 thus carry information about the horizontal velocity across time. Experimentally, Brenner et al. (2000) stimulated the H1 neurons with bar patterns whose velocity and acceleration were varied in order to test how the action potentials of H1 react to such changes.

In a first step, Brenner et al. (2000) manipulated the velocity (and later the acceleration) of the stimulus to which the fly and its H1 neuron were exposed. The stimulus—for example, the bar pattern—was presented with different velocities, either rapidly or slowly varying while all other stimulus parameters remained the same. Hence, only velocity variance differed among the stimulus ensembles presented. This allowed Brenner to investigate how the H1 neurons' activity reacted to the changes in the stimulus ensembles' velocity variance.

What are their results? The absolute firing rate followed the velocity of the stimulus presentation, with slower velocity inducing fewer spikes, and higher velocity being accompanied by a higher number of spikes. The firing rate was then plotted as a function of the stimulus velocity; more precisely, the firing rate at each time bin was plotted as a function of the stimulus velocity 30 ms earlier. This showed an almost non-linear exponential dependence of the firing rate on the velocity (and also the acceleration) changes of the stimulus. How about the timing relation between velocity changes and the neurons' activity? The neurons' activity integrated velocity changes in the stimulus within the time range of 20–300 ms. The authors then tested whether the neurons' activity would also adapt to velocity changes in the stimulus within a longer time frame, using the same stimulus ensemble with a different standard deviation in its velocity changes.

This yielded the same neuronal response; for example, the same spike to time curve, i.e., a non-linear exponential dependence of the firing rate on the velocity as in the first experiment: the single neurons' activity was again dependent upon the standard deviation of the velocity changes. These results indicate that the neurons' activity really encodes the standard deviation of the stimulus' velocity changes across different time frames rather than the velocity itself, as isolated variable, within a particular time frame.

Neuronal findings Ib: Encoding of the stimuli's "natural statistics" into neural activity in visual cortex

What does the standard deviation of the stimulus' velocity changes stand for? The standard deviation of the stimulus' velocity changes reflects the statistical range of the stimulus' velocity in the environment and thus, more generally, the statistical frequency distribution—that is, natural statistics—of that stimulus across different discrete points in time. This, more generally taken, allows the neuron to encode stimulus' fluctuations within the stimulus ensemble standard deviations and thus to rescale its neural response according to the natural statistics of the stimulus. What determines the neurons' activity is not so much the stimulus' physical features themselves in an absolute way; that is, velocity or acceleration in a particular time frame. Instead, the neurons' activity encodes the statistical variance of the velocity and acceleration across different time frames and thus the standard deviation of the stimulus across different discrete points in physical space and time in a relative way.

The dependence of the neurons' activity upon the standard deviation of the stimulus means that the former can adapt to the variations of the latter. This is made possible by a non-linear response function of the neuron, which allows for what Brenner et al. (2000) call "the stretch factor" (see also Friedlander and Brenner 2009).

The stretch factor allows for rescaling of the neurons' activity in orientation on the stimulus' variance; for example, the standard deviation. However, the stretch factor breaks down for very large variances where the stimulus' velocities are either too fast or too slow for the neuron to follow because the detection of such extremely slow or fast velocities is beyond the neurons' physical detection threshold (see Fig. 1-2).

Taken together, Brenner et al. (2000) (see also Friedlander and Brenner 2009) demonstrate that the neurons' activity adapts to the natural statistics of the stimuli within the environment rather than encoding the stimuli themselves and their physical features (like its associated velocity). There is consequently no fixed or ideal response

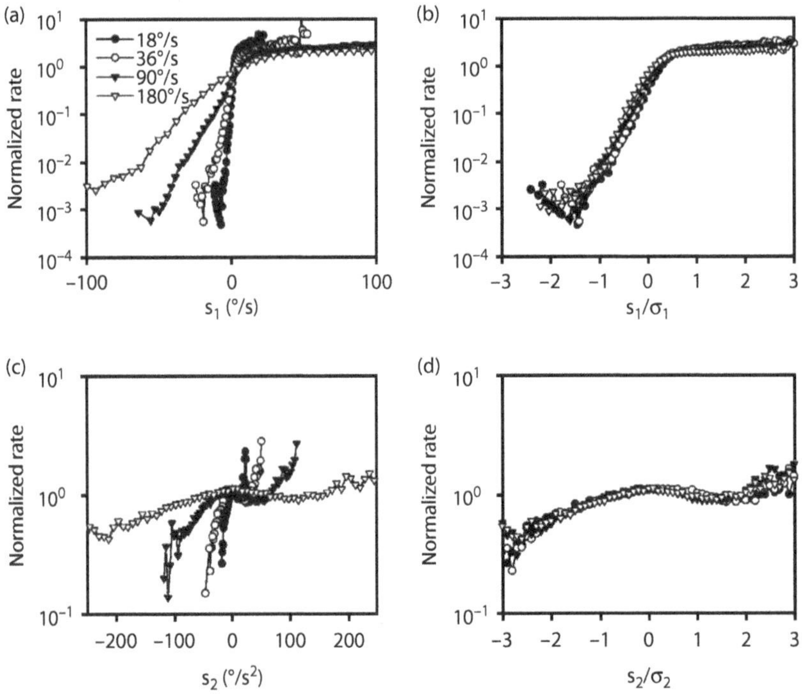

Figure 1-2a **Sparse coding: rescaling of responses to dynamic inputs. Adaptive rescaling of the input/output relations along the two leading dimensions. (*a* and *c*): Response as a function of stimulus velocity as seen through the first (*a*) and second (*c*) filter. (*b* and *d*): Response as a function of stimulus projections, each normalized by its standard deviation. (Reprinted with permission from Brenner N, Bialek W, de Ruyter van Steveninck R. (2000) Adaptive rescaling maximizes information transmission. *Neuron*. 2000 Jun;26(3):695–702.)**

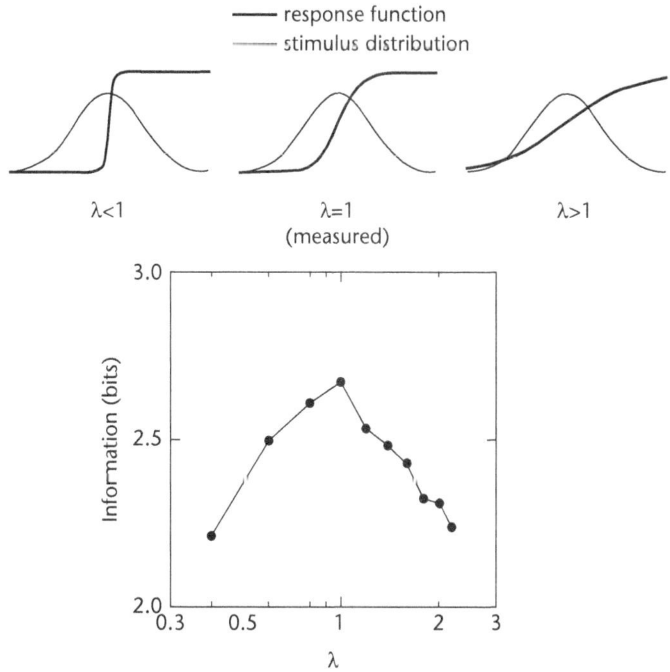

Figure 1-2b Optimizing information transmission: information as a function of the stretch factor λ. The input/output relation measured in the experiment was artificially stretched or contracted by a factor λ, simulating the rescaling that occurs during adaptation. This is illustrated schematically in the three top panels. For each value of l, the stretched input/output relation and the distribution of stimuli used in the experiment determine a distribution of rates, which in turn determines the information with Equation 2. The point λ = 1 corresponds to the stretch factor measured in the experiment. The maximum at this point indicates that the process of adaptation selects a stretch factor that maximizes the information transmission. (Reprinted with permission from Brenner N, Bialek W, de Ruyter van Steveninck R. (2000) Adaptive rescaling maximizes information transmission. *Neuron*. 2000 Jun;26(3):695–702.)

or tuning curve of the neurons' activity as fitted to specific physical features of the stimulus (like velocity).

Instead, the neurons' response or tuning curves change—for example, stretch or compress—and are thus tuned according to the statistical variance in the occurrence, i.e., frequency distribution, of the stimuli and their physical features (such as, for instance, velocity or acceleration). In other terms, the sensory stimuli's physical features are rescaled and normalized by the neurons according to the inputs' standard deviation, reflecting their statistical frequency distribution across different discrete points in physical time and space; that is, their natural statistics.

Neuronal hypothesis IA: statistically versus physically based encoding strategies

Sparse coding implies that the neurons' activity adapts to the statistical frequency distribution of the stimulus within the environment rather than to the stimulus itself and its physical features (like velocity and acceleration at their discrete points in physical time and space). How is such adaptive rescaling possible? The time scales of adaptive rescaling and normalization may vary from milliseconds over seconds, to hours and years if not thousands of years, with the stimuli's natural statistics being the common denominator in tuning the neurons' responses (and response curves).

Brenner et al. (2000) propose that such adaptive rescaling across different time scales may itself be an adaptation to the frequency in the occurrence of signals and inputs within the natural world (see also Barlow 2001). This adaptation is possible only by encoding the stimuli's statistical features, the statistical frequency distribution, i.e., variance, of their physical features (like velocity and acceleration), rather than the physical features themselves.

How is it possible for the neuron to encode the variance of the stimulus' physical features, the standard deviation, rather than the physical features themselves? For the neurons' activity to be dependent upon the stimulus' variance, or standard deviation, they must encode an integral or difference of the stimulus' physical features across their occurrence at different discrete points in physical time and space.

The encoding of the stimuli and their physical features is thus based on the statistics of the stimuli, for which reason one may want to speak of "statistically based encoding" strategy. As mentioned, such statistically based encoding implies the encoding of the integrals or differences between different discrete points in physical time and space as associated with the stimuli and their physical features.

Such statistically based encoding of stimuli must be distinguished from a more physically based encoding strategy, where the stimuli's physical features themselves, including their different discrete points in physical time and space, are encoded into neural activity by themselves, separately and in isolation from each other (rather than their statistical differences across different discrete points in physical time and space) (see Fig. 1-3a, b).

Neuronal hypothesis Ib: Encoding of temporal and spatial differences into neural activity during sparse coding

Let us be more detailed about the statistically based encoding strategy. The encoding of the stimuli's physical features across their different points in physical time and space means that temporal and spatial differences or integrals must be encoded into neural activity. For instance, the neurons must encode the temporal difference value of the physical features between the occurrence of the stimulus *a* at time point *x* and its repetition at a later time point, *y*.

This temporal difference value between the time points x and y reflects the stimulus' frequency of occurrence across time: its statistically based temporal structure. Since the neurons encode this temporal difference value, i.e., x–y, their activity corresponds to and thus mirrors the stimulus' statistically based temporal structure (see later for more details about the term "temporal [and also spatial] structure").

Due to the encoding of statistically based temporal differences, each single neuron is able to encode more than one stimulus into its activity.

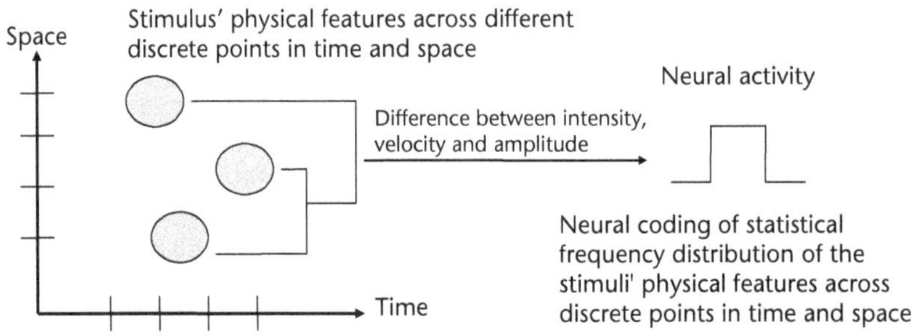

Figure 1-3a Difference-based coding as statistically based coding strategy. The figure shows the physical features of the stimuli (gray spots) in time and space (x- and y-coordinates). What is now encoded from the stimuli in the brain are not the physical features themselves at their respective single discrete points in physical time and space, but rather the statistically based differences in their frequency distribution across different discrete points in physical time and space as indicated by the brackets. Neural activity is illustrated on the *right*, indicating one active neuron whose action potential is related to the spatial and temporal difference in the statistical frequency distribution of the stimuli's physical features.

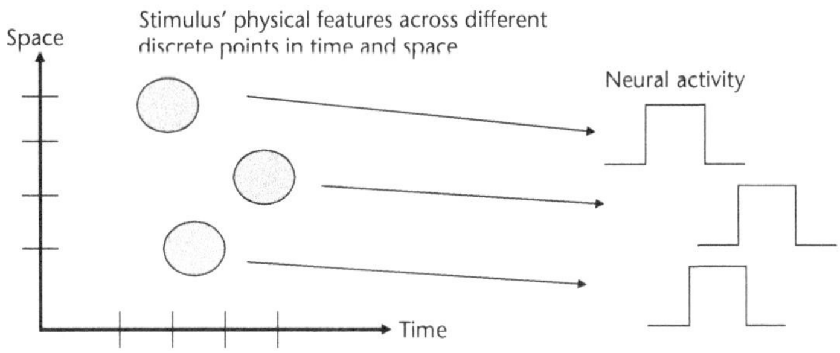

Figure 1-3b Stimulus-based coding as physically based coding strategy. This figure illustrates stimulus-based coding, or more correctly, the encoding of the stimuli's physical features at their different discrete positions in physical time and space into the activity of the neurons. Unlike in difference-based coding, one physical feature and its respective single discrete position in physical time and space are encoded into the activity of one neuron; the encoding of three physical features thus entails the activity of three different neurons, as indicated on the *right*.

This means that the number of neurons activated is lower than the number of stimuli, entailing a many-to-one relationship between stimuli and neurons. There is thus sparseness in the number of the recruited neurons when compared to the number of stimuli. This entails sparse coding rather than local or dense coding.

The sparseness in the encoding of the stimulus' occurrence across different discrete points in physical time corresponds on the neural side—that is, at the level of the single neuron—to what is described as "lifetime sparseness." "Lifetime sparseness" describes that one and the same neuron is only sparsely recruited during its lifetime when compared to the number of occurrences of a particular stimulus across time that could recruit this neuron at different discrete points in physical time (Fig. 1-3c; Weliky et al. 2003).

In addition to the temporal difference, the neurons must also encode the spatial difference in the occurrence of the physical features of a stimulus *a* at the point v and the ones of stimulus *b* occurring at point w. This spatial difference value, v–w, reflects the stimulus' spatial configuration, its statistically based structure (see later for definition of the term "spatial structure").

What is encoded into the neurons' activity is no longer the single discrete points in physical space that are associated with stimulus *a* and *b* respectively, i.e., v and w. Instead, the difference value between the two different discrete points in physical space as associated with the stimuli *a* and *b* and their respective physical features, v–w, is encoded into the neurons' activity. Accordingly, as in the temporal dimension, there is also sparse coding in the spatial dimension, as manifested in the encoding of spatial integral or difference values between two different discrete positions in physical space.

The sparse coding of the stimulus' statistical frequency distribution across different discrete points in physical space corresponds on the neural side, that is, on the level of the single neuron, to what is described as "population sparseness." Population sparseness describes the fact that only a sparse number of neurons are recruited from the total pool of possible neurons during the encoding of different stimuli and their distinct discrete positions in space (Fig. 1-3d; see also Olshausen and Field 2004).

NEURONAL HYPOTHESIS IC: SPARSE CODING PRESUPPOSES DIFFERENCE-BASED CODING

Taken together, the encoding of the stimulus' statistical properties is possible only when encoding relative values of physical parameters (like velocity or acceleration) rather than their absolute values. This is well reflected in the

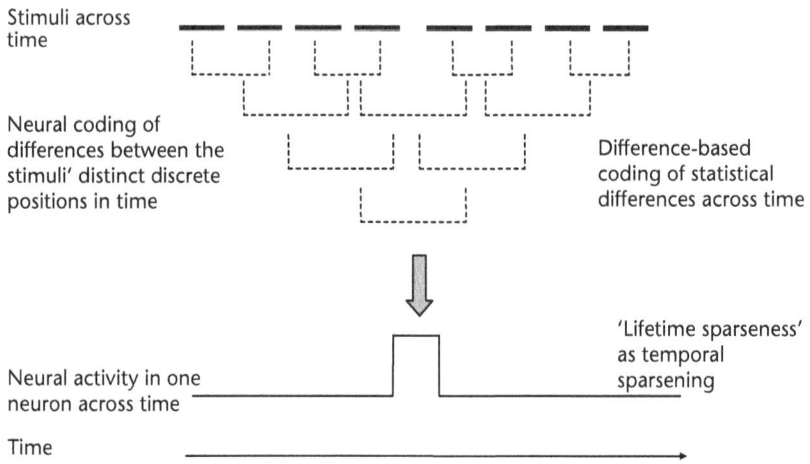

Figure 1-3c **Temporal difference-based coding and "lifetime sparseness." The figure shows how difference-based coding operates in the temporal domain. Different stimuli occur across time as indicated in the *upper* part. What is now encoded in the neurons' activity is not each single stimulus at its specific single discrete point in physical time. Instead, the brain encodes the statistical frequency distribution of the stimulus (and its physical features) across different single discrete points in physical time as indicated by the differences and brackets in the *middle* part of the figure. That, in turn, implies that one neuron's activity may integrate the stimuli's temporal differences across time, resulting only in one activity at one particular discrete point in physical time (in the life of the neuron) (*lower* part). Hence, difference-based coding in the temporal domain goes along with sparseness of the neuron's neural activity across time—this is called "lifetime sparseness."**

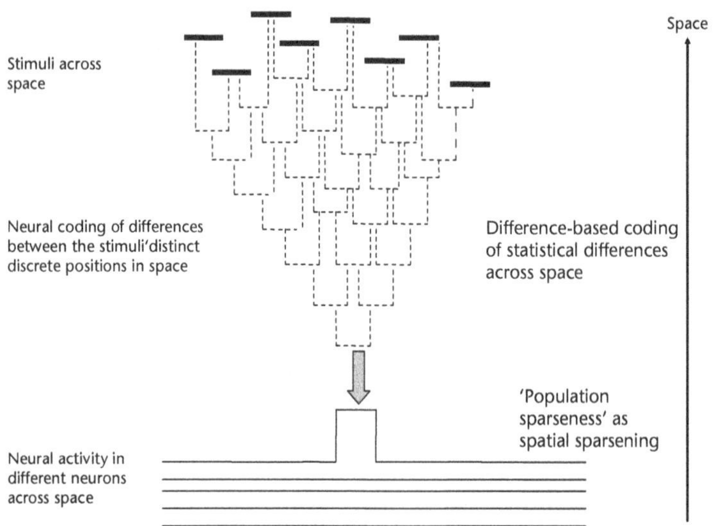

Figure 1-3d **Spatial difference-based coding and "population sparseness." The figure shows how difference-based coding operates in the spatial domain. The *upper* part indicates how different stimuli occur in different single discrete positions in space. The statistical frequency distribution is signified by the spatial differences between the different single discrete spatial positions are indicated in the *middle* of the figure by the brackets. Among the many neurons (as indicated in the *lower* part), only one becomes active, as indicated in the *lower* part of the figure; this sparseness of activity is called "population sparseness."**

encoding of the physical parameter's variance as shown in the study by Brenner et al. (2000).

Most important, these relative values reflect spatial and temporal difference values that signify the occurrence of the stimulus's physical features across different discrete points in physical time and space, rather than the stimulus's physical features themselves at their single different discrete points in physical time and space. In other words, the neurons' activity must encode differences, or spatial and temporal difference values, in order to account for the stimuli's statistical frequency distribution across different discrete points in physical time and space, or their spatiotemporal structure. This leads to sparse coding as distinguished from local and dense coding.

On the whole, sparse coding presupposes and is therefore possible only on the basis of difference-based coding. I consequently hypothesize that sparse coding presupposes difference-based coding: sparse coding is supposed to be based on the encoding of spatial and temporal difference values as extracted from the stimuli's statistical frequency distribution across different discrete points in physical time and space. In short, I postulate that sparse coding presupposes difference-based coding.

Neuronal hypothesis Id: dependence of the degree of sparseness on the degree of difference-based coding

I hypothesize that sparse coding is based on encoding spatial and temporal difference values. There is sparseness of the single neuron across time and space, amounting to "lifetime sparseness" and "population sparseness."

How now is such sparse coding in both spatial and temporal dimensions manifested in the various functions associated with the brain, like sensory function and perception? Empirical evidence shows that lifetime and population sparseness can predict the local contrast structure in natural scenes in our perception; this shall be further illustrated by the following empirical example.

Bruno Olshausen is a computational neuroscientist who, located in Berkeley in California, is one of the main driving forces behind the development of sparse coding. Together with a colleague (Olshausen and Field 1996, 1997), he trained a network on approximately half a million image patches (all of the same size), which were extracted from whole images of natural scenes. The network's receptive fields that emerged from training were spatially localized, oriented, and band-pass (i.e., selective to spatial structure) in very much the same way as it has been described for neurons in primary visual cortex, or "V1."

While the neural network receives many visual inputs, the output is much sparser in both regards: spatially, for example, number of recruited neurons; and temporally, activity of a neuron in time. The few or sparse outputs represent the difference between the various sensory inputs within the natural scenes rather than each sensory input by itself (see also Rozell et al. 2008; Zhao 2004; Zylberberg et al. 2011; Lörincz et al. 2012; Willmore et al. 2011). This is possible only, as I suppose, if there is difference-based coding rather than stimulus-based coding. Hence, for sparse coding to be possible, there must be difference-based coding.

Future studies are needed, however, to lend further empirical support to the suggested dependence of sparse coding on difference-based coding. One may, for instance, vary (in real or modeling contexts) the amount of spatial or temporal differences between stimuli. The degree of temporal and spatial sparsening in neural activity may vary depending on the degree of spatial or temporal differences.

That may lead one to propose that larger spatial and temporal differences (within a biophysically and computationally realistic limit) in the stimuli's statistical frequency distribution may induce larger degrees of sparse coding in the resulting neural activity. This suggests that sparse coding is indeed dependent upon difference-based coding: "Difference-based coding" may refer to the process of encoding, while "sparse coding" may rather signify the outcome or results of such encoding.

However, we should be aware that sparse coding is then not to be understood in an absolute, all-or-nothing way, but rather in a relative, more-or-less way. Sparse coding in neural activity may then occur in different degrees on a continuum, depending on the degree of spatiotemporal differences encoded between the different stimuli (see later discussion for further details).

Neuronal hypothesis Ie: Sparse coding and schizophrenia

The prediction of local contrast scenes by sparse coding raises the question of how such an encoding strategy impacts our perception. While perception will be discussed in more detail in Part IV of this volume and also in Volume II, I nevertheless want to present a brief outline here. For that, let's conduct a thought experiment and imagine the consequences of the opposite coding strategy holding sway in your brain.

Your neurons would not encode spatial and temporal differences between stimuli. Instead, your neurons would encode the exact spatial and temporal position of each stimulus separately from each other. You would be flooded with a multitude of unrelated spatial and temporal positions of the various stimuli. But, since they are coded separately from each other, you would not be able to link and relate them to each other.

What does that imply for your perception of, for instance, a bird on a tree? The bird's spatial position on top of the tree would be completely unrelated to the tree you perceive. Because tree and bird always occur together, you would wonder why they are always together. You would recruit your cognitive apparatus to dwell on and think about this and would develop some ideas and theories. And all this would occur because your brain does not encode the spatial (and temporal) differences between the bird and the tree. Hence, what is usually given as evident and tacit knowledge in our perception becomes suddenly questionable and bizarre once one presupposes an encoding strategy other than sparse coding.

One may now argue that this is a purely logical thought experiment with no correspondence in empirical reality. This, however, may not be true, as I will discuss in further detail in Chapter 22 in Volume II. Let me briefly explain here. Patients with schizophrenia suffer from perceptual abnormalities with fragmentation and lack of linkage between different stimuli and their respective contents; this may come close to the aforementioned scenario (see especially Volume II, Chapter 22, for details on schizophrenia).

These patients seem to encode the spatial and temporal features of different stimuli in isolation from each other, rather than as spatial and temporal integral or difference values. Hence, their encoding of the stimuli's statistical frequency distribution across time and space may be disrupted. This means that their degrees of both difference-based coding and sparse coding may be abnormally reduced, which is indeed plausible given the recent empirical findings. However, this is, at this point, a speculative hypothesis, which will be discussed in full detail in Volume II (see Chapters 22 and 27), since it spills over into the phenomenal domain of consciousness.

Neuronal findings IIa: Stimulation of classical receptive fields and sparse coding

Up to this point, I have discussed how stimuli are encoded by the brain's sensory cortex and have argued for difference-based coding that results in sparse coding. This shows that, instead of single stimuli by themselves, the brain's sensory cortex encodes the stimuli's statistical frequency distribution across different discrete points in physical time and space; that is, their natural statistics.

The encoding of the stimulus's natural statistics implies that a particular stimulus is encoded in relation to other stimuli that occur either at the same or different discrete time points at a different or the same discrete position in space. This means that what is encoded in sensory cortical activity is not the single stimulus itself (in an absolute way), but rather its difference or relationship (i.e., relative) to other stimuli. This is possible only if the brain encodes the relationship and thus the interaction between the different stimuli across different discrete points in time and space; I call this stimulus–stimulus interaction. How does the brain encode such stimulus–stimulus interaction? Stimuli or specific physical features of the stimuli may correspond on the neural side to the receptive fields of the neuron. However, stimuli from the environment do not occur in isolation, but rather in a specific context entailing other stimuli that may go beyond the receptive field of the respective neuron. If there is sparse coding, one would expect the context and its respective stimuli to impact the processing of the stimulus in question.

This means that stimulation outside the neuron's receptive field may impact the neuronal activity related to the inside of the receptive field by sparsening it. The classical receptive field (CRF) may then be modulated in a non-linear way by the surrounding non-classical receptive field (nCRF), thereby promoting sparseness. This was tested and experimentally addressed by Vinje and Gallant (2000, 2002), which shall be described next (see also David et al. 2004; Kay et al. 2008; Willmore et al. 2011; Naselaris et al. 2011, for other studies from the group around Gallinat). Their results have been replicated and extended by others, such as, for instance, Haider et al. (2010) in cat's visual cortex (see Chapter 2 for a detailed discussion of the study by Haider et al. 2010).

Neuronal findings IIb: Stimulation of non-classical receptive fields and the sparsening of neural activity

Vinje and Gallant (2000, 2002) recorded 61 neurons in V1 in two awake macaques, and stimulated the monkeys with natural images in a movie. The size of the image patches was manipulated, varying the diameter of the CRF from one to four so that the effect of stimulation outside the CRF on neuronal activity could be observed. The action potentials across the 61 recording sites were plotted in a peri-stimulus-time histogram and compared between stimulation inside and outside the CRF.

Let us describe the main results. Stimulation inside the CRF led to a rather dense distribution of action potentials in many neurons, with a sparseness of 16%. This changed once the movie was presented, with stimuli four times the CRF diameter; here the distribution of action potentials became rather sparse, with a sparseness of 53%. How about the single neuron? This will be the focus of the next section.

The distribution of action potentials also becomes sparse for the single neuron. Sparseness is described by the variable *S*; *S* is 0% when a neuron responds equally to all frames or image patches of the movie, while *S* is 100% in the case of the neuron responding only to a single specific frame.

An increase in *S* consequently indicates an increase in the sparseness of the single neuron's response to stimuli. Do the different sizes of the image patches—one, two, three, or four times the diameter of the CRF—go along with different values of *S*? Sparseness values, that is, *S*, increased from 41% over 52% and 61% to 62% for stimuli one, two, three, and four times the CRF diameter.

The shift in sparseness between the different stimulus's sizes was also calculated by the ratio of the observed shift in *S* to the maximum possible shift as a function of the stimulation outside the receptive field, the non-classical receptive field (nCRF). This yielded values for the shift in sparseness from 18% over 32% to 36% for stimuli two, three, and four times the CRF diameter, respectively. Hence, many neurons display a shift toward sparser responses when increasing stimulation outside their respective CRF. Which purpose does the sparseness of action potentials and single neuron's activity serve? By sparsening their responses, neurons may decorrelate their various neuronal responses and thus the different stimuli from each other. This may be especially necessary if there are increasing contextual demands, such as during stimulation outside the classical receptive field. If so, one would propose that increased stimulation outside the classical receptive field goes along with an increase in decorrelation.

Neuronal findings IIc: Statistical structure of natural scenes and the sparsening of neural activity

To test this assumption, Vinje and Gallant (2000) calculated what they call the "separation angle," which is inversely proportional to the similarity of responses between randomly selected V1 neurons as recorded in separate sessions. The higher the separation angle, the more different and thus decorrelated the neurons' activities during stimulation. Stimulation with stimuli four times the diameter of the CRF led to a separation angle of 67 degrees, while the one for stimuli inside the CRF, for example, generated a lower separation angle of only 51 degrees.

Hence, stimulation outside the CRF—for example, the stimuli four times the diameter of the CRF—led to increased differences, i.e., increased separation angles, and thus decorrelation in the neuron's activities. This means that with the increasing size of the stimuli and their increasing stimulation outside the neurons' classical receptive field, neuronal activities across the different neurons became increasingly decorrelated and independent from each other.

Only single neurons and their action potentials were considered so far. How does the sparseness of single neurons affect the population of neurons? For that, Vinje and Gallant (2000, 2002) calculated the response distribution, the histogram of action potentials pooled over all cells and all stimuli for each stimulus type: for example, one, two, three, and four times the diameter of the CRF. With increasing stimulus size, response distribution became sparser; the number of moderate responses decreased across neurons, while smaller and larger responses increased. The sparseness of responses, as measured by Kurtosis, increased from 4.1 over 5.2 and 8.7 to 10.2 with stimuli one, two, three, and four times the CRF diameter (see Fig. 1-4).

Taken together, these findings clearly demonstrate that the sparseness of neural activity—for example, sparse coding of both single neurons'

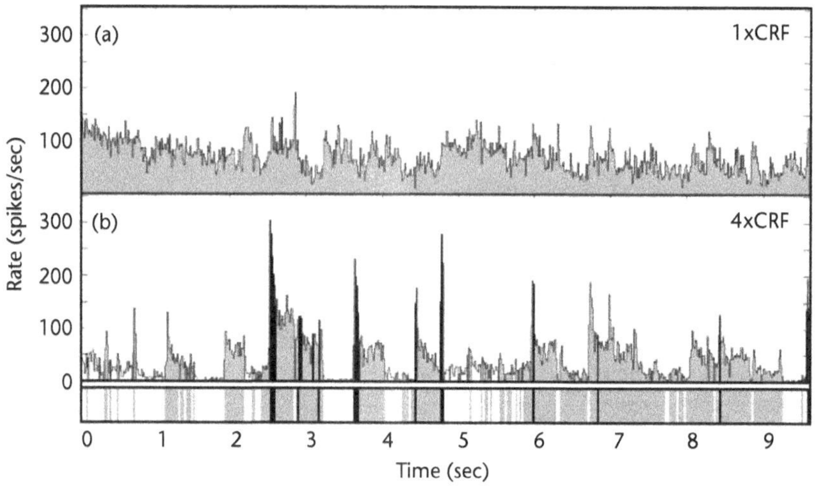

Figure 1-4 Sparse coding of stimulus–stimulus interaction. The non-classical receptive field (nCRF) modulates responses during natural vision. (*a*) Post-stimulus time histogram obtained from one V1 neuron in response to a natural-vision movie confined to the classical receptive field (CRF). Responses are weakly modulated by the simulated fixations (information per second, 13.1 bits/s; information per spike, 0.18 bits/spike; efficiency, 10%; selectivity index, 13%). (*b*) Responses of the same cell to a natural-vision movie composed of the CRF stimulation used in (*a*) plus a circular surrounding region. The overall stimulus size was 4x CRF diameter. Stimulation of the nCRF dramatically increases variation of responses across fixations (information per second, 28.4 bits/s; information per spike, 0.67 bits/spike; efficiency, 26%; selectivity index, 51%). Responses to some stimuli are significantly enhanced (*black* bins; $p \leq .01$). For this neuron, enhancement is concentrated in the onset transients occurring at the beginning of simulated fixations. Other responses are strongly suppressed (*white* bins; $p \leq .01$). The underbar highlights those time bins where significant enhancement and suppression occur. (Reprinted with permission of *Science* from Vinje WE, Gallant JL. Sparse coding and decorrelation in primary visual cortex during natural vision. *Science*. 2000 Feb 18;287(5456):1273–6.)

activity and population activity—is a function of the stimulus size in relation to the neurons' classical receptive fields. The more the stimulus size stimulates outside the neurons' classical receptive fields, the more the neurons' activities and responses are sparsened.

This means that the neurons' responses, such as the degree of sparseness of their neuronal activity, are matched to the statistical structure of natural scenes. The degree of sparseness is thus directly dependent on and thus is a function of the statistical structure of the stimuli in the natural scenes. Such encoding of natural scenes allows us to link and integrate classical and non-classical receptive fields into a single computational unit for which non-linear interaction seems to be central (see Chapter 2 for details on non-linear interaction, as well as Olshausen and Field 1996).

Neuronal hypothesis IIa: Difference-based coding and non-linearity

The results by Vinje and Gallant (2000, 2002) (and more recent ones by others like Haider et al. 2010, and Park et al. 2012a and 2012b) highlight the crucial role of stimulus–stimulus interaction in constituting sparseness of neuronal responses. The more complex, that is, spatially and temporally extended, the stimulus–stimulus interaction, the higher the degree of sparseness of the neurons' activities; this means that the degree of sparse coding on the neuronal side may be directly dependent upon the degree of spatiotemporal complexity on the side of the stimuli. The term "spatiotemporal complexity" describes here the degree and number of spatial and temporal differences between the different stimuli and their physical features at their respective different discrete points in physical time and space.

What is encoded into the sensory cortical neurons' activity is the degree of spatiotemporal complexity of stimulus–stimulus interaction. This, in turn, determines the degree of non-linearity during stimulus–stimulus interaction and ultimately the degree of sparseness as encoded into the resulting neural activity. In short, the degree of sparse coding may be dependent upon the degree of spatiotemporal complexity during stimulus–stimulus interaction.

Recall that I proposed that sparse coding, the temporal and spatial sparsening of neural activity, is dependent on difference-based coding of the spatiotemporal features of stimuli. The results by Vinje and Gallant confirm this hypothesis, especially in the spatial regard, due to their focus on the interaction between classical and non-classical receptive fields.

Stimulation in the non-classical receptive field significantly increases the degree of sparseness in a non-linear way when compared to stimulation inside the classical receptive field. Since sparse coding presupposes difference-based coding, both are closely and intrinsically linked to non-linear interaction. How does such non-linear interaction work? Nonlinear interaction seems to be central in constituting differences between, for instance, the spatial positions of two stimuli (as in classical and non-classical receptive fields). Hence, the demonstration of non-linear interaction by Vinje and Gallant in the context of sparse coding may shed more light on the mechanisms by means of which spatiotemporal differences between stimuli are constituted (see also Part IV).

Neuronal hypothesis IIb: Encoding of differences and the "stretch factor"

I will now elaborate on the mechanisms of how differences are constituted. How is it possible for the neurons to sparsen their activity temporally and spatially with regard to the stimuli and other neurons' activity? I discussed the neurons' encoding strategy and suggested difference-based coding to enable and predispose such temporal and spatial sparsening of their activity. But I left open the exact physiological mechanism. For that, we may want to go back briefly to the results by Brenner, as described earlier.

Based on their results, Brenner et al. (2000, p. 697) propose what they call the "stretch factor." By exerting a non-linear rather than linear response function, the neurons are able to stretch or compress their neuronal activity maximally across the whole range within their respective biophysical-computational spectrum. And such stretching or compressing of the neurons' own biophysical-computational features allows the neuron to adapt and thus encode the statistical frequency distribution of the stimulus.

Using Brenner's (et al. 2000) terms, the neurons' activity can be characterized by "adaptive rescaling" (see also Park et al. 2012a and 2012b; Díaz-Quesada and Maravall 2008). Such adaptive rescaling via the stretch factor makes it possible for the neurons' activity to encode the stimulus's statistical frequency distributions rather than their (i.e., the neurons') own biophysical-computational features (as induced by stimuli with the same physical features as the respective neurons).

Adaptive rescaling in orientation on the stimulus's statistical frequency distribution is possible, however, only within the biophysical-computational range of the neurons. At the borders close to the neurons' maximal and minimal biophysical-computational range, as well as outside that range, however, the mechanisms of adaptive rescaling may be postulated to decrease considerably and ultimately to break down.

This may, for instance, be the case when there are very large variances of the stimuli and thus high standard deviations, indicating extremely high difference values in the stimulus's physical features across different discrete points in physical time and space (see also Brenner et al. 2000, p. 697). Such large difference values may then exceed the degree of spatial and temporal differences than can possibly be encoded by the neuron on the basis of its biophysical-computational spectrum.

NEURONAL HYPOTHESIS IIC: "STRETCH FACTOR" AND NON-LINEARITY

In other words, the large (or also possibly minimal) difference values of the stimuli force the neurons to operate at the maximal (or minimal) limits of their biophysical-computational spectrum. That in turn decreases the possible extension of their "stretch factor" and consecutively the possible degree of their "adaptive rescaling" including the possible degree of non-linearity (that then is transformed into mere linearity). Finally, if the to-be-encoded spatial and temporal differences are too large, ranging beyond the neurons' biophysical-computational spectrum, no activity is elicited anymore in the neuron.

For instance, the velocities or accelerations of the stimuli tested in the Brenner study may be extremely rapid with very small temporal difference values; they may therefore touch upon the limits of temporal resolution and thus the minimal range of the neurons' biophysical-computational spectrum. Velocity may simply be too high and the associated temporal difference values may be too low and "located" too much toward the minimal extreme of the neurons' biophysical-computational spectrum to allow the neurons' "stretch factor" to operate. Any non-linearity and consequently adaptive rescaling may then become impossible.

The neurons may still respond but may no longer be able to adaptively rescale their activity in a non-linear way, showing instead a merely linearly determined neural activity. The responses of the neurons may consecutively no longer be able to encode the stimuli's statistical frequency distribution; for example, the standard deviation of their velocity and acceleration as signified by spatial and temporal differences between different discrete points in physical time and space (see Fig. 1-5a). Instead, the neurons may show some activity oriented on the stimuli's physical features; for example, on the absolute values of their velocity and accelerations including the respectively associated different discrete points in physical time and space.

This is the case if the stimulus' velocity and acceleration still fall within the neurons' biophysical-computational spectrum but in the maximal or minimal border regions of the respective range. This is what happens when the stimuli themselves show abnormally large or small temporal and spatial difference values. However, the same, and thus a merely linear rather than non-linear, response can also happen when the neurons themselves are changed and receive, for instance, less energy, which may artificially shrink and limit their biophysical-computational spectrum.

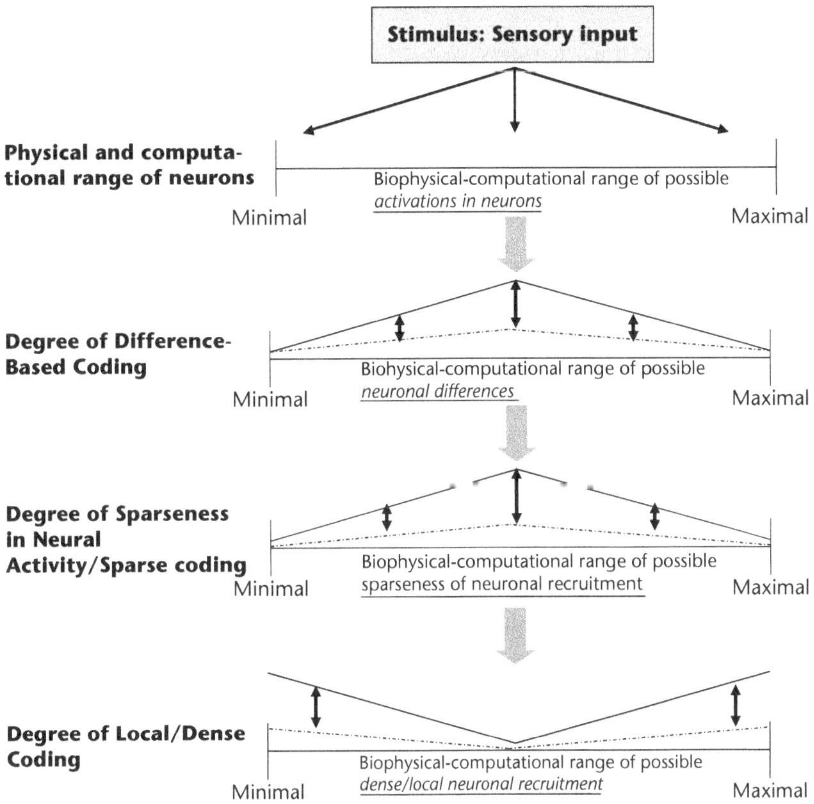

Figure 1-5a Biophysical-computational constraints and sparse coding. The figure shows the relationship between the neurons' biophysical-computational demands and the degree of sparse coding in humans (a and b) and nonhuman species (*c*). (*a*) Physical and computational constraints and the degree of sparse coding. (*First step*): The figure shows the different steps, four steps as intermediated by the big arrows, in the encoding of a stimulus in the neural activity of the brain's neurons, given the latter's biophysical and computational demands. The brain's intrinsic biophysical equipment shows a continuum between the minimally and maximally possible ranges within the neurons' biophysical-computational spectrum within which it can process stimuli and their spatial and temporal differences; this is indicated by the horizontal line. The physical features of the stimuli and especially their spatial and temporal differences may now match with either the optimal range (in the *middle*) or the less optimal range of the neurons' biophysical-computational spectrum as indicated by the different arrows. (*Second step*): If the stimuli and their spatial and temporal differences match with the optimal (and thus medium) range of the brain's biophysical-computational spectrum, the degree of difference-based coding is the highest, as indicated by the main line. The more closely, in contrast, the stimuli and their spatial and temporal differences match with the less optimal ranges, that is, the minimal and maximal ends of the neurons' biophysical-computational spectrum, the lower the degree of difference-based coding. The dotted line represents stimulus-based coding as distinguished from difference-based coding, with both curves showing different directions. (*Third step*): Difference-based coding goes along with sparse coding. The higher the degree of difference-based coding, the more sparsely the stimulus is encoded in neural activity. That, in turn, implies that the curve of sparse coding is similar to the one of difference-based coding and deviates in the same way from the dotted line that signifies stimulus-based coding. (*Fourth step*): Difference-based coding stands in a reverse relationship to local or dense coding (see Fig. 1-3). The higher the degree of difference-based coding, the lower the degree of local and dense coding in neural activity. That, in turn, implies that the curve of local/dense coding is opposite to the one of difference-based coding and deviates as much, though in an opposite way, from the dotted line that signifies stimulus-based coding.

That is the case, for instance, in what clinically is called "disorders of consciousness" like persistent vegetative state (VS). Patients with VS lost their consciousness and seem to suffer from a vastly decreased energy supply to their brain. The extreme energy reduction seems to make it much more difficult, if not impossible, for the neurons to impose the "stretch factor" and thus non-linearity and "adaptive rescaling" to their own processing of stimuli.

This may lead to loss of non-linearity during the purely neuronal stimulus-induced activity that therefore can apparently no longer be associated with consciousness. While this example demonstrates the potential clinical relevance of the "stretch factor," non-linearity, and adaptive rescaling, it exceeds far beyond the purely neuronal scope of the current chapter into the phenomenal domain of consciousness. Therefore, I will discuss the example of VS (and other states) in full detail, including all the recent findings, in Part VIII in Volume II.

Neuronal hypothesis IIIa: "Adaptive rescaling" and the neuron's biophysical-computational spectrum

How can we put together all these different findings and observations into a coherent neuronal hypothesis? I hypothesize that there are mainly two different types of possible neuronal responses (and a third type of response that is rather a non-response; see below).

The first type of neuronal response concerns the case when the stimulus's physical features correspond well to the middle range of the neurons' biophysical-computational spectrum. In this case, the stretch factor may be able to operate in a maximally possible way and thus allow for the highest degree of non-linearity and the best possible adaptive rescaling with maximum information transmission. Hence, there is both adaptive rescaling and adaptive response.

The second type of neuronal response is proposed to describe those cases where the stimulus's physical features correspond to those in the neurons that lie at either extreme, such as either the maximum or minimum, of their biophysical-computational spectrum. The stretch factor may then no longer be able to operate in a maximal possible way with the degree of both non-linearity and adaptive rescaling decreasing; however, this means that what is encoded in the neurons' activity corresponds less to the stimulus's statistical frequency distribution across different discrete points in physical time and space than to the different stimuli themselves and their various discrete points in physical time and space.

This leads me to the following hypothesis. I hypothesize that the more the stimulus's physical features and their respective temporal and spatial difference values fall within the maximal or minimal ranges of the neurons' biophysical-computational spectrum, the less the stimuli's statistical frequency distribution and the more their physical features themselves including their single discrete points in time and space are encoded by the neurons. Hence, there would be neural response but no adaptive rescaling.

Neuronal hypothesis IIIb: The neuron's biophysical-computational spectrum and consciousness

Why is that relevant at all? At the minimal and maximal ranges of their biophysical-computational spectrum, neurons may be less able to encode spatial and temporal difference values into their neural activity. The degrees of both difference-based and sparse coding may consequently decrease, whereas there may be an abnormally high degree of stimulus-based coding (see later for more details).

As indicated earlier, such a response pattern possibly holds in the case of patients in the vegetative state: Neuronal responses are still obtained, but they seem to show a low degree of difference-based coding and an abnormally high degree of stimulus-based coding. Since these patients suffer from loss of consciousness, the type of neuronal response and its "location" on the biophysical-computational spectrum seem to matter quite a lot when it comes to the phenomenal domain that is consciousness. This topic, however, will be discussed in Volume II.

Finally, one may propose a third type of possible neuronal response that is rather a non-response. If the stimulus's physical features, including the respective spatial and temporal difference values, do fall outside the neurons' possible biophysical-computational range, no neuronal response and thus activity can be elicited at all in the neurons.

There is thus no neuronal response, nor are the stretch factor, non-linearity, and adaptive rescaling at work. Nothing is possible anymore in such brain. The stimuli no longer induce any response at all, whether linear or non-linear. Neither the stimulus itself nor differences between stimuli are encoded into neural activity anymore. Nothing is encoded at all. Clinically this means that one is not even in vegetative state anymore, but already in coma if not brain-dead (see Part VIII in Volume II).

NEURONAL HYPOTHESIS IIIC: SPARSE CODING AND THE NEURONS' BIOPHYSICAL-COMPUTATIONAL SPECTRUM

How is this hypothesis of the three types of neuronal responses related to sparse coding and difference-based coding? Based on the results reported by Brenner et al. (2000), I hypothesize the following: The better the stretch factor operates and thus the higher the degrees of non-linearity and adaptive rescaling, the more likely the stimuli's spatial and temporal difference values can fall within an intermediate range (i.e., medium standard deviations) of the neurons' biophysical-computational spectrum.

This makes possible higher degrees of non-linear interaction, which in turn results in consecutively higher degrees of sparseness in the encoding of the stimuli's statistical frequency distribution into the neurons' activity. I thus postulate higher degrees of both difference-based coding and sparse coding within the middle ranges of the neurons' biophysical-computational spectrum.

The possibility of adaptive rescaling implies that sparse coding can occur in different degrees. Rather than being an absolute all-or-nothing coding strategy, sparse coding may then need to be considered in a relative, more-or-less way, presupposing a continuum of different degrees. The higher the degree of adaptive rescaling and thus the more the stretch factor operates, the higher the degrees of both difference-based coding and sparse coding.

NEURONAL HYPOTHESIS IIID: BALANCE BETWEEN SPARSE CODING AND LOCAL/DENSE CODING WITHIN THE NEURONS' BIOPHYSICAL-COMPUTATIONAL SPECTRUM

We may, however, need to consider not only different degrees of sparse coding, but also its balance with other coding strategies like dense and local coding (see earlier discussion). Higher degrees of sparse coding may then go along with lower degrees of local and dense coding, and conversely. Hence, we may need to search for the balance between sparse coding and local/dense coding.

I hypothesize that this balance may very much be dependent upon the degree of spatial and temporal differences between different stimuli that are to be encoded into neural activity: encoding of larger spatial and temporal differences may tilt the balance toward sparse coding at the expense of local and dense coding. In contrast, encoding of smaller spatial and temporal differences may shift the balance from sparse coding toward higher degrees of local and dense coding (see Fig. 1-5a).

If, in contrast, the stretch factor cannot operate maximally, resulting in lower degrees of non-linearity and adaptive rescaling, I hypothesize the following: the more the amount of the stimuli's spatial and temporal difference values to be encoded by the neurons falls within the extreme, for example, maximal and minimal, ranges (i.e., high or low standard deviations) of the neurons' biophysical-computational spectrum, the lower the degree of non-linear interaction and the lower the degree of sparseness and sparse coding in subsequent neural activity. Accordingly, sparse coding and local (and dense) coding are reciprocally related to each other. The degree of sparse coding with its many-to-one relationship between stimulus and neurons decreases, while the degree of local coding with a one-to-one relationship increases (see Fig. 1-5a, b).

Why is all that relevant? We already indicated that the degree of difference-based coding and sparse coding may be significantly decreased in

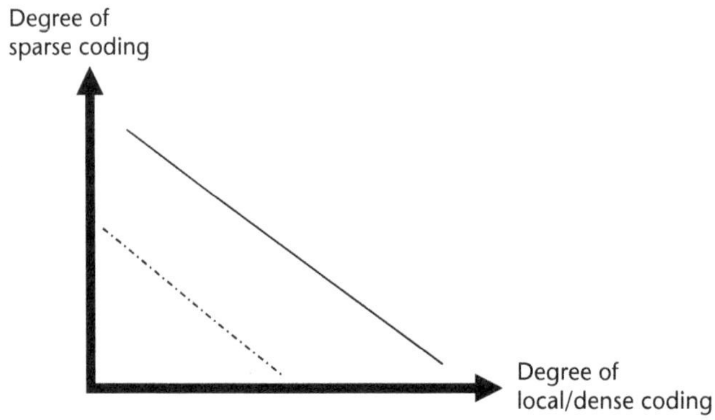

Figure 1-5b Reciprocal relationship between sparse coding and local/dense coding. Like difference-based coding, sparse coding also stands in a reverse or reciprocal relationship to local/dense coding, which is now illustrated in a graph (which I could have also done for difference-based coding and local/dense coding). The x-axis describes the degree of local/dense coding, while the y-axis stands for the degree of sparse coding. The higher the degree of sparse coding, the lower the degree of local/dense coding.

disorders like VS and schizophrenia. While I will provide the details in Volume II, this makes it clear that the encoding strategy, and especially the neural balance between difference- and stimulus-based coding, is highly relevant for consciousness and its various phenomenal features. Before venturing into the phenomenal domain of consciousness, though, we need to better understand the neuronal mechanisms the brain itself applies to its own neural processing, as it is the focus in this volume.

Neuronal hypothesis IIIe: sparse coding and the neurons' biophysical-computational spectrum in different species

Finally, one may also want to note that sparse coding is not limited to humans but also operates in the brains of non-human species. This is well documented in the results described earlier that were mostly obtained in non-human species. I postulate that the brain in non-human species also operates the same coding and encoding strategy; namely, difference-based coding and sparse coding.

The difference between human and non-human species and thus between the different species in general may then not be found so much in the presence or absence of a particular encoding strategy, which may rather be shared across species and their respective brains (such as all relying on a statistically based rather than physically based encoding; see earlier). Instead, the difference may then be found in the range of the biophysical-computational spectrum, which may be species-specific, as based on the different biophysical features of the brains in the different species. These biophysical-computational differences may enable the different species to encode species-specific temporal and spatial difference values into their neurons' activity in a difference-based and sparse way (see Fig. 1-5c).

For instance, monkeys show different physical and computational features of their neurons when compared to humans. Where there is non-response and no adaptive rescaling in humans, in monkeys there may be some response with possibly even the stretch factor, non-linearity, and adaptive rescaling at work in biophysical-computational ranges that remain impossible in humans.

This means that we need to consider the neurons' response properties and, for instance, the degree to which the stretch factor, non-linearity, and adaptive rescaling (can possibly) operate in relation to the respective species and their neurons' biophysical-computational spectrum. To extend the scope further, one may even consider the different species and their neurons'

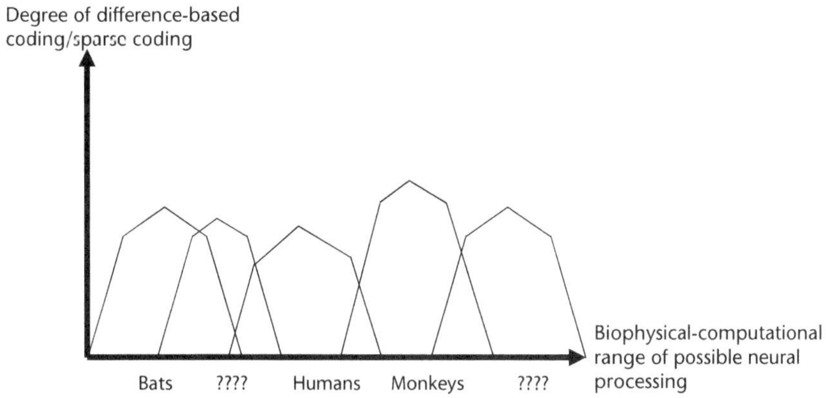

Figure 1-5c **Species-dependence of the neuron's physical-computational ranges and difference-based coding. The figure describes the relationship between different biophysical-computational spectra in different species and their respective degrees of difference-based coding. Thereby, different species may show different biophysical-computational ranges, depending on the physical (and biophysical) features of their brains. That, in turn, may go along with different degrees of difference-based coding, as indicated by the heights of their respective spectrum. Moreover, the shape of the distribution of the degree of difference-based coding along the respective species' specific biophysical-computational spectrum may vary between different species.**

biophysical-computational spectrum in their respective ecological and hence ultimately evolutionary context. This, however, is far beyond the scope of this book, which I therefore leave to others to pursue in the future.

Open Questions

One of the main questions concerning sparse coding is how the neurons can encode spatial and temporal differences between different stimuli and their physical features; that is, their statistical frequency distribution across different discrete points in physical time and space. Neurons do not encode the stimuli's physical features at their particular discrete points in physical time and space, but rather their statistical frequency distribution across different discrete points in physical time and space.

The question is now why and how the neurons' activity is tuned to encode the statistical frequency distribution of the stimuli's physical features rather than encoding the physical features themselves. This question remains open for future studies, for which the evolutionary roots and context may need to be considered.

Specifically, sparse coding yields the question why and how the neurons' activity is more tuned to spatial and temporal difference values between different stimuli rather than to one stimulus alone. Current neuroscience does not seem to provide an answer to that, as I see it. But we have to be careful. As suggested by the empirical data, the encoding strategy of sparse encoding is not as absolute as all or nothing. Rather, it seems to be continuous and thus reciprocally balanced with the degrees of dense and local coding.

The results described earlier focused only on the degree of sparse coding, while its reciprocal balance with local and dense coding was more or less neglected. Future studies may thus want to develop measures—that is, variables or indexes—of the neural balance between the different encoding strategies. I hypothesize that the neural balance between the degrees of sparse and local/dense coding, rather than either index by itself, may best predict subsequent behavioral as well as cognitive performances.

Furthermore, how the neural balance between sparse and local/dense coding is determined and modulated remains completely unclear at this point. One could, for instance, imagine that the neurons' baseline activity, their resting state or intrinsic activity, may be central in modulating the threshold for the possible degree of difference-based and sparse coding during subsequent stimulus-induced activity (see Part IV for details). That, however, remains to be investigated.

Finally, results from sparse coding are based on investigations in different species. Hence, sparse coding is not an encoding strategy specific to humans. Instead, it seems to occur across different species, and so is difference-based coding, as I suggest. This may incline one to suggest that sparse coding and difference-based coding characterize the encoding strategy of brains in general across different species.

Difference-based coding and sparse coding may then be regarded as intrinsic features of the brain that define the brain *qua* brain. We will return to the brain and its intrinsic features in the phenomenal context of consciousness in Volume II, where I will propose the brain's intrinsic features, like its encoding strategy, that is, difference-based coding, to predispose consciousness.

Coming back to the purely neuronal context in this volume, one would like to investigate how the different species' biophysical-computational spectrum of their neurons determines the possible degrees of sparse coding and its neural balance with local and dense coding, and how, in turn, that predicts the subsequent behavioral capabilities of the respective species, including their differences from humans. That, however, remains to be investigated.

CHAPTER 2
Sparse Coding and Neural Inhibition

Summary

So far, I have discussed the neuronal mechanisms of sparse coding and how it presupposes difference-based coding on the level of single neurons and a population of neurons. However, I left open the question of the exact physiological and biochemical mechanisms; that is, neural excitation as mediated by glutamate, and neural inhibition related predominantly to GABA. The focus of this chapter is on discussing how difference-based coding and consequently sparse coding are related to neural inhibition and excitation. The findings suggest that GABA and glutamate act in conjunction, thereby constituting what is called the "excitation-inhibition balance" (EIB). Despite their conjunction in the EIB, the empirical findings suggest distinct roles for neural inhibition and excitation in yielding difference-based coding. Glutamate seems to be central in constituting early neuronal excitation, whereas GABA yields delayed neural inhibition, which reduces and suppresses the former. As such, GABAergic-mediated neural inhibition may be crucially involved in temporally and spatially sparsening stimulus-induced activity, as can be demonstrated by the example of the olfactory system. How is the action of GABA and glutamate related to difference-based coding? Based on various empirical findings in (especially) the olfactory system of insects, rats, and other species, I propose that the distinct but co-exerted contributions of GABA and glutamate are central in constituting spatial and temporal differences between different stimuli across their different discrete points in physical time and space. Therefore, GABA and glutamate and consequently the EIB may be central in making possible difference-based coding and ultimately sparse coding on a cellular and population level of neural activity.

Key Concepts and Topics Covered

Sparse coding, neural inhibition, neural excitation, GABA, glutamate, single cells, population of neurons, excitation-inhibition balance, different species

Neuroempirical background: difference-based coding and the brain's neural organization

In addition to the visual cortex (see Chapter 1), strong evidence for sparse coding also comes from the insect's olfactory system, which is well investigated in detail and can therefore be regarded as a model system for studying the neural code (see Theunissen 2003; Laurent 2002; Papadopoulou et al. 2011; Assisi et al. 2007). This will provide a more detailed view of the neuronal, and especially neurophysiological, mechanisms underlying sparse coding.

I postulate that this will be highly relevant for understanding how the spatial and temporal differences signifying difference-based coding are encoded into neural activity. By showing the underlying neurophysiological and biochemical mechanisms, I ultimately aim to demonstrate why the neurons and the brain in general cannot avoid and are thus predisposed to encode spatial and temporal differences, i.e., difference-based coding, rather than the stimulus itself, i.e., stimulus-based coding.

More generally, I postulate that difference-based coding (and ultimately sparse coding) is a necessary and unavoidable characteristic of the brain's neural organization and thus an intrinsic, i.e., defining, feature of the brain. While sounding rather abstract and lofty at this point, this will turn out to be important when it comes to consciousness, as will be detailed in Volume II.

Now, however, we need to understand the neurophysiological and biochemical mechanisms themselves that realize and implement difference-based coding and sparse coding. For that, I will turn to the olfactory system of the insect as paradigmatic example of the brain in general.

Neuronal findings IA: "spatialization" and "temporalization" in the insect's olfactory cortex

The insect's olfactory system's antenna contains about 90,000 olfactory receptors, where many neurons respond at once to a particular odour. This organization of the receptors biases them toward spatial distribution and dense coding, with a one-to-many relationship between stimuli and receptors. One and the same olfactory input, or stimulus, is received and processed by several receptors at the same time which occupy different positions in space.

What does this anatomical organization imply for the encoding of the olfactory stimuli? The encoding of the olfactory stimulus and its single discrete point in the physical space of the environment implies the spatial distribution of the stimulus in the neural activity of various receptors that are located in different discrete points in physical space. One may therefore want to speak of what I describe as "spatialization" of the olfactory stimulus during its encoding into the receptors' neural activity.

The spatially distributed signals related to the olfactory receptors are then further processed to the antennal lobe in insects, which in humans corresponds to the olfactory bulb. The antennal lobe contains about 830 projection neurons that receive excitatory input from the olfactory receptors and inhibitory input from interneurons.

Olfactory input leads to a modulation of the neuron's mean firing rate with the activity being synchronized across different neurons with 20–30 Hz oscillations as measured in local field potentials. The olfactory input is thus put into temporal space by means of synchronizing temporally distinct inputs in the antennal lobe neurons' activity.

This means that the initial olfactory stimulus and its single discrete point in the physical time of the environment are distributed across different discrete points in physical time namely those covered by the 20-30Hz synchronization operating across the different neurons (and their respective time scales). In other terms, the olfactory stimulus becomes 'temporalized' during its encoding into the antennal lobe neurons' activity.

What does such temporalization and spatialization of the stimulus in neural activity imply for the relationship between the actual stimulus and the different neurons? The odour identity of the stimulus no longer corresponds one to one to the mean firing rate of a single neuron but rather to the integrated activity and synchronization of many neurons. This means that the representation of the stimuli in the neural activity of the receptors and the antennal lobe neurons', the "representational space," is no longer identical, that is, one to one, with the space of the stimuli, the "stimulus space."

Neuronal findings IB: "stimulus space" and "representational space" in the insect's olfactory cortex

What exactly is meant by the terms "representational space" and "stimulus space"? The concept of "stimulus space" describes the chemical combinations of the odour itself, independent of any neural activity. In contrast, the term "representational space" pertains to the spatiotemporal patterns during the encoding of the stimulus into neural activity, such as, for instance, into the receptors' and the antennal lobe neurons' activity.

The lack of one-to-one correspondence between chemical combinations, for example, the stimulus space, and the spatiotemporal activity patterns, the representational space, entails that the former are decorrelated and processed as independent variables in the antennal lobe neurons's activity. Such decorrelation entails that the number of neurons representing the respective odour may be larger than the number of chemical dimensions present in the odour.

One may now propose that the encoding of the stimulus by such large number of neurons, that is receptors and antennal lobe neurons, may be essential for putting the olfactory stimulus and its single discrete point in physical time and space, the stimulus space, into a larger spatial and temporal context in the encoded neural activity, the representational space.

The anatomical organization with the high number of receptors and the temporally synchronizing antennal lobe neurons' seem to make such spatialization and temporalization of the olfactory stimulus in the encoded neural activity almost necessary and thus unavoidable. In other words, the anatomical organization seems to predispose spatiotemporal coding with subsequent spatialization and temporalization, during the encoding of the olfactory stimuli into neural activity.

Neuronal findings Ic: From spatiotemporal coding to sparse coding in the *insect's* olfactory cortex

What are the next steps in the neural processing in the insect's olfactory system? The spatiotemporal coding of the antennal lobe and its projection neurons, the described spatialization and temporalization, is transformed into a sparse code in the next relay station, the Kenyan cells in the mushroom bodies. Theunissen (2003) suggests three processes to be at work that allow for the transformation of the antennal lobe's spatiotemporal code into the sparse code of the Kenyan cells (Fig. 2-1).

First, there is high divergence in the number of cells between the antennal lobe and the mushroom body. One projection neuron from the antennal lobe corresponds to about 500 Kenyan cells in the mushroom body. This means that when receiving inputs from the projection neuron, many of the Kenyan cells are not activated, entailing sparse coding. Hence, the number of Kenyan cells active or recruited is rather low when compared to their total number, which predisposes them for sparse coding.

Second, the Kenyan cells react particularly strongly to simultaneously arriving inputs from the projection neurons. This favours integration of different inputs, including their nonlinear interaction. Such nonlinearity implies that the activity elicited by simultaneously arriving inputs is much stronger (or weaker) when compared to the addition of their activities when arriving sequentially. We already discussed in Chapter 1 an analogous instance of non-linearity in the context of the visual system where it was central in allowing for sparse coding (see Olshausen and Fields 1996, 1997). We will see later that the non-linearity in the case of the insects' olfactory system and its Kenyan cells is equally central in allowing for sparse coding.

Third, neural inhibition plays a major role in synchronizing the different neurons' activity in the antennal lobe as well as in inhibiting Kenyan cells in the mushroom bodies (via the lateral horn). Such inhibition may turn off cells before or after the detection of excitatory synchronized input from the projection neurons of the antennal lobe.

Taken together, all three processes, divergence, non-linearity, and inhibition, entail that only a small number of Kenyan cells respond to each odour identity with few temporally precise spikes. The spatiotemporal patterns from the antennal lobe are thus integrated and sparsened by the Kenyan cells in the mushroom body into few and specifically active neurons without though losing any of the associated information. Accordingly, the Kenyan cells sparsen neural activity in both spatial and temporal respects. This means that the initial spatiotemporal code as encoded into the receptors and the antennal lobe projection neurons is now transformed into a sparse code; the initially encoded "spatialization" and "temporalization" is thus not lost but sparsened.

Neuronal findings Id: Mechanisms of sparsening neural activity in the insect's olfactory cortex

In order to better understand what exactly happens during the sparsening of the initial spatiotemporal code, we need to better understand how the projection neurons in the antennal lobe

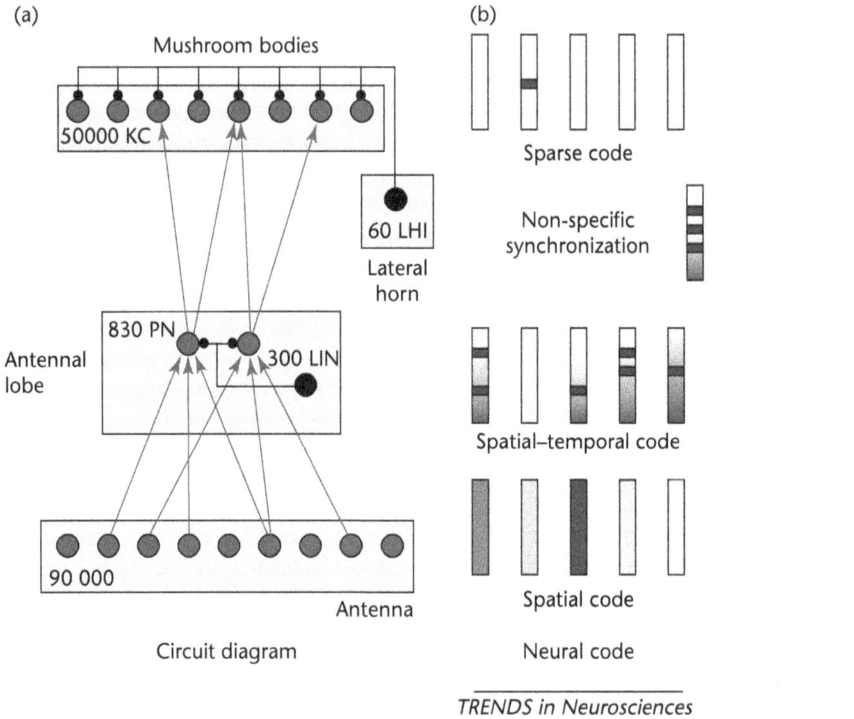

Figure 2.1 Neural organization and processing in olfactory cortex. Circuitry of the ascending olfactory circuit in the locust and the neural code found at each level of processing. (*a*) In the circuit diagram, the arrows and circles represent excitatory connections and the black circles represent inhibitory neurons and inhibitory connections. Approximate numbers of each type of cell are given. The input to the inhibitory neurons is not shown [the local inhibitory neurons of the antennal lobe (LIN) receive input from both the projection neurons of the antennal lobe (PN) and the olfactory receptors (OR). The lateral horn inhibitory neurons (LHI) receive extensive converging input from the PN]. (*b*) In the neural code diagram, the responses of sample neurons from each level of the circuit are schematized with a vertical rectangle in which the vertical dimension represents time. The dark areas show epochs of synchronized spiking activity. *Abbreviation*: KC, Kenyon cells. (Reprinted with permission of Elsevier, from Theunissen FE. From synchrony to sparseness. *Trends Neurosci.* 2003 Feb;26(2):61–4.)

are connected to the Kenyan cells in the mushroom body. Many projection neurons contact and converge onto one and the same Kenyan cell, with each Kenyan cell receiving direct input from about half of the projection neurons (see Jortner et al. 2007). This yields the following question: How can such massively convergent input from so many projection neurons lead to the sparse and highly selective responses as observed in the Kenyan cells (see also Stopfer 2007)?

Following Jortner et al. (2007), three different mechanisms may need to be considered. First, the antennal lobe projection neurons react to odour not only with neural excitation but also with inhibition. This means that only some of the activated projection neurons provide an excitatory input to the Kenyan cell while others relay rather an inhibitory input with the subsequent inhibition of the Kenyan cells. There are thus both excitatory and inhibitory projection neurons which exert opposite effects on their respectively connected Kenyan cells. That reduces the effect of the high number of the projection neurons on the Kenyan cells considerably.

Second, many of the excitatory postsynaptic currents (EPSCs) triggered in Kenyan cells by the excitatory projection neurons are rather small so that they do not reach the threshold necessary to elicit action potentials and thus neural activity. Such subthreshold activity reduces the effect of the excitatory projection neurons on the Kenyan cells considerably. Finally, and third, oscillatory output from the projection neurons prohibits Kenyan cells from firing during that oscillatory cycle which reduces the effects of the excitatory projection neurons even further.

Taken together, there may be three different neuronal mechanisms at work in order to reduce and thus sparsen the effects of the high number of antennal lobe projection neurons onto the much lower number of Kenyan cells. These mechanisms include inhibitory projection neurons as well as subthreshold and oscillatory activity in projection neurons which all three prevent the Kenyan cells from being activated by the projection neurons.

Neuronal findings Ie: different mechanisms of sparsening neural activity in different species

Why are these mechanisms of reducing and thus sparsening the effects of the projection neurons onto the Kenyan cells are so important? Due to the high number of projection neurons and the lower number of Kenyan cells, there is a vast number of possible combinations between projection neurons' activity and the Kenyon cells' activity pattern. Such a high number of possible combinations can optimize and thus sharpen and therefore decorrelate the differences between different sensory inputs received by the projection neurons and the signals relayed by the Kenyan cells. This means that ultimately each olfactory input can lead to an extremely selective or decorrelated and sparse representation in the neural activity as encoded in the Kenyan cells. This holds for insects and their olfactory system.

Do the same mechanisms of sparsening neural activity also apply to species other than insects, however? Stopfer (2007), in his commentary to the study by Jortner et al. (2007), remarks that the fruit fly and the rat show a different organization in their olfactory cortex. According to him, this makes it rather unlikely that sparseness of neural activity is achieved in these species through the same mechanisms like inhibitory neurons, subthreshold activity, and oscillatory activity as in the insect. He therefore proposes that different mechanisms of sparsening neural activity may be at work in different species. We therefore shift our focus now to rats and their olfactory cortex.

Neuronal findings IIa: sparse coding in the rat's olfactory cortex

I demonstrated that neural inhibition is central in mediating the sparsening of neural activity in the insect's olfactory cortex. More specifically, there seem to be inhibitory projection neurons that inhibit rather than excite the Kenyan cells. This suggests a central role of neural inhibition in mediating sparsening effects and thus sparse coding in olfactory cortex. Does the central role of neural inhibition also apply to species other than the insects? For that I now turn to rats, and more specifically to a study by Poo and Isaacson (2009).

Poo and Isaacson (2009) (see also Poo and Isaacson 2011) undertook electrophysiological studies of the pyramidal cells and interneurons in the rat's anterior piriform cortex, which is related to olfaction. They used in vivo cell-attached recording and whole-cell recording to measure these neurons' action potentials (APs) and synaptic currents, for example, excitatory postsynaptic current (EPSC) and inhibitory postsynaptic current (IPSC) while, at the same time, stimulating them with four different monomolecular odours.

Let's start with the APs. They observed a low spontaneous firing rate of all pyramidal cells and only a sparse number of them (10%), when compared to the total number of neurons, showed APs during odour stimulation. Mostly, APs were induced only by one single odour so that different odours elicited APs in different cells. Hence, each odour induced APs in only approximately 10% of the total number of cells with different cells being recruited by different odours. Moreover, the intensity in firing rate was rather low with an average increase of 2.01 +/– 0.04 Hz in the recruited neurons. Stronger responses (>5 Hz/ >10 Hz) were only observed in 19%/6% of the recruited neurons.

How do these results stand in relation to sparseness? This activity pattern implies a high degree of sparseness both temporally and spatially. Temporal sparseness can be expressed by "lifetime sparseness" (see also Chapter 1), the response pattern of an individual cell to multiple stimuli across time; this yielded a value of 0.88, indicating that cells responded highly selectively to the different odours at different discrete points in time.

Analogous results can be observed in the spatial domain. Spatial sparseness is expressed by "population sparseness" (see Chapter 1 for details) that measures how an individual stimulus is represented in the activity pattern of different cells; this also yielded a high value, 0.93 that mirrors a rather sparse representation of the odours in the activity of different neurons. Taken together, these data show that induction of APs in pyramidal cells of the rat's piriform cortex show a temporally and spatially sparse activity pattern when exposed to different odours.

Neuronal findings IIb: Neural excitation and inhibition in the rat's olfactory cortex

In addition to APs, Poo and Isaacson (2009) also investigated the EPSCs and IPSCs. EPSCs (22.7%) were observed more often than APs (8.3%) across cells. Both EPSC and AP were thus relatively rare compared to the IPSC, which were found much more often: namely, in half of all cells investigated (51%). There is thus sparseness in the overall occurrence of both APs and EPSCs, while there seems to be no sparseness in IPSCs. Interestingly, the same pattern can be observed with regard to odour selectivity. Similar to the APs, EPSCs were highly selective, being induced only by one particular odour rather than by all odours, meaning that 60% of all cells showed EPSCs in response to only one particular odour. This distinguished them from IPSCs, where 66% of all cells showed inhibition in response to 3–4 odours. Hence, excitation seems to be related to odours in a highly selective and thus sparse way whereas this is not the case in inhibition that seems to be induced by various odours in a rather non-selective and non-sparse way.

In addition to different odours, Poo and Isaacson (2009) also investigated the effects of different odour concentrations. Higher concentrations of the preferred odour led to higher EPSCs, thus showing a graded response pattern. In contrast, IPSC responses remained largely independent of odour concentration with already low concentrations of both preferred and nonpreferred odours inducing high IPSCs.

These results show that neural excitation, i.e., EPSCs, is directly dependent upon the odour concentration whereas neural inhibition, i.e.,IPSCs, is not. Neural inhibition thus seems to show an all-or-nothing response pattern whereas the one of neural excitation is characterized rather by a more-or-less pattern.

Taken together, neural inhibition, i.e., IPSCs, seem to remain rather unspecific with regard to the kind of odour and the odour concentration. Unlike neural excitation, i.e., EPSCs, neural inhibition seems to be neither tuned to specific odour nor to varying odour concentrations. Such unspecific response pattern let Poo and Isaacson (2009) speak of "global inhibition" that describes the unspecific nature of neural inhibition with regard to the eliciting stimuli.

Neuronal findings IIc: Anatomo-structural organization of interneurons and pyramidal cells in the rat's olfactory cortex

Where does such global inhibition come from? One would propose that it comes from interneurons that are characterized by predominant inhibition (see Buzsaki 2006 for details). The interneurons themselves must receive some excitatory input, however, in order to get activated and to consecutively exert neural inhibition. Poo and Isaacson (2009) (see also Poo and Isaacson 2011) therefore investigated both pyramidal cells and interneurons separately with regard to their excitation pattern. They demonstrated that odours evoked excitation in a much larger number of interneurons (50% +/– 3.9%) than in pyramidal cells (11% +/– 2.3%). This suggests non-selective response and thus unspecificity with regard to the interneurons that are excited.

Furthermore, unlike in pyramidal cells, the response in interneurons was also nonselective with regard to the odour with different odours inducing excitation in the same interneurons. Hence, excitation in interneurons seems to be widespread and broadly tuned so that its remains unspecific with regard to both odour and cells. This distinguishes the interneurons from pyramidal cells where excitation is more specific in terms of both odours and cells.

Why do the interneurons receive excitation in such unspecific way than the pyramidal cells? Conducting further experiments, the authors could show that the increased number of excitation in interneurons may originate from increased convergence of olfactory bulb cells (M/T cells) onto interneurons when compared to pyramidal cells. Hence, interneurons simply seem to receive more excitatory input from the olfactory bulb than pyramidal cells. This means that the interneurons have a much higher likelihood of getting excited than pyramidal cells, which in turn explains their higher degree of excitation. Such increased likelihood of excitatory input predisposes the interneurons to show a rather non-selective and thus unspecific response pattern with regard to both odours and cells as it is observed in the data.

Accordingly, the high degree of neural excitation of interneurons may ultimately be traced back to an anatomical-structural feature, that is, the connectivity pattern between olfactory bulb cells and interneurons. Due to the much higher degree of convergence onto interneurons, neural inhibition as relayed by interneurons seems to predominate in terms of pure quantity over the degree of neural excitation in pyramidal cells. Such predominance of neural inhibition over neural excitation, that is, global inhibition as described earlier, may then lead to increased sparsening of subsequent neural activity.

Based on these considerations, one can postulate that the mismatch between the number of pyramidal cells and the one of interneurons and the consecutive dysbalance between neural excitation and inhibition makes unavoidable and thus predisposes the possible temporal and spatial sparsening of neural activity in pyramidal cells. In short, the sparsening of neural activity and thus sparse coding may ultimately be predisposed by anatomo-structural organization of the olfactory cortex.

Neuronal findings IId: temporal sparsening of neural activity in the rat's olfactory cortex

Poo and Isaacson (2009) also investigated how the recruitment of single cells relates to the oscillatory patterns of the whole network of cells and population of cells. Let me first describe the rather complicated physiological processes before interpreting the data. Thereby we will consider both insects and rats together.

Measuring local field potentials, prominent odour-evoked beta-frequency oscillations (18 Hz) were observed in similar ways for the different odours. APs were phase-locked to the onset of the beta oscillations: APs in different cells were not coupled to the same phase of the beta oscillations. Instead, APs in each individual cell were preferentially linked to specific and thus different phases of the beta oscillation as being specific for each odour (see below for details).

This indicates a precise relationship between the timing of individual APs and the phases of the synchronized network oscillations. There is thus, as the authors themselves remark, temporal sparsening of neural activity during the encoding of odours. How can describe such temporal sparsening in further detail? Temporal sparsening may be signified by the temporal relation in the occurrence of IPSCs, EPSCs, and AP's which was also investigated by Poo and Isaascson (2009).

They observed that EPSCs almost always preceded IPSCs by a short time period of around 10 ms (9 +/- 0.3 ms). Odour-evoked APs occurred largely (67% +/- 11%) within this short time window between the EPSCs and the IPSCs within the same cells, for example, between the onset of EPSCs and the onset/rise of IPSCs. In contrast to these earlier AP's, much fewer APs were observed in later time periods as during the onset and rise of IPSCs. Interestingly, IPSCs and EPSCs were always coupled to different phases of the beta oscillation in each cell; this is consistent with the specific coupling between APs and beta oscillation phases described earlier. These phase differences between IPSCs and EPSCs with regard to the phases of the beta-oscillation may further enforce the precise spike time and phase coupling of APs in olfactory cortex.

What do these rather intricate physiological processes imply for the neural coding of odours in the olfactory system? Based on their findings, Poo and Isaacson (2009) postulate that the rat's olfactory cortex, for example, the anterior piriform cortex, can be characterized by sparse coding both temporally and spatially. Such sparseness may be driven by both selective excitation of specific pyramidal cells in response to specific odours and global (and unspecific) inhibition of interneurons. Thereby the temporal difference in the occurrence between EPSCs and IPSCs, for example, 10 ms, may provide the time window for APs to be generated. The occurrence of such specific rather short time window for the generation of the AP's may promote the AP's selectiveness and specificity with regard to both cells and odour and thus (a high degree of) sparse coding.

Neuronal hypothesis Ia: presence of neural inhibition in different species

How can we, on the basis of these data, generate a sound neuronal hypothesis that applies to sparse coding in general? The presented data were obtained in insects and rats. The development of a neural coding hypothesis about the brain in general is thus confronted with the question of whether these findings are species-specific or apply to the brain in general across different species. In order to address this question in our case of the olfactory system, we discuss the similarities between insects and rats.

Poo and Isaacson (2009) point out the similarity of their results in rats with the ones from the insect's mushroom body and the Kenyan cells. In both insects and rats, lifetime and population sparseness of cell responses can be observed. And there is a low response firing rate in both species with a specific and direct excitatory drive. Most important, broadly tuned and unspecific neural inhibition is present in both species. This stems from different sources: for example, interneurons in the rats' piriform cortex and the insect's neurons in the lateral horn in the mushroom body. Finally, both species (rats, insects) show stimulus-triggered bursts of beta oscillations and the phase delay of inhibition relative to excitation. This suggests that both the rat's piriform cortex and the insect's mushroom body seem to function in analogous if not similar ways.

Most prominent in both species is the central role of neural inhibition, which, as provided by the interneurons (or the neurons of the lateral horn), may be central in promoting sparseness (see also Papadopoulou et al. 2011). While inhibition remains nonsparse by itself and therefore unspecific with regard to both cells and odours (and therefore "global" as described by the authors), inhibition may nonetheless prove essential in enabling sparseness of neural excitation and consecutively of APs in pyramidal cells.

Neuronal hypothesis Ib: neural inhibition predisposes sparse coding

Based on the cross-species similarities, one may propose that global inhibition is a necessary condition for sparseness of neuronal excitation. This amounts to the following hypothesis as applicable to different species: the higher the degree of possible neural inhibition provided by inhibitory interneurons, the higher the degree to which neural activity, that is, neural excitation in pyramidal cells, can be spatially and temporally sparsened. Hence, to say it more simply, the degree of neural inhibition may predispose the possible degree of sparse coding in different species (Fig. 2-2).

The nonexpert may be slightly puzzled now. Everybody knows about the major differences between insects and rats, especially in the summer when being bitten by the various insects flying around. Both insects and rats show completely different behavioural capacities and obviously their brains are also quite different. How then is it possible that both species seem to rely on similar neural mechanisms underlying and driving sparse coding in their olfactory system?

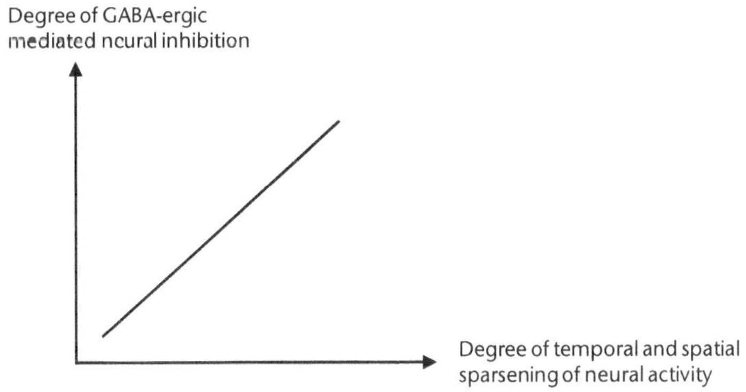

Figure 2-2 Neural inhibition and sparse coding. The figure shows the relationship between the degree of GABAergic-mediated neural inhibition and the degree of sparse coding in both temporal and spatial domains. The higher the degree of GABAergic-mediated neural inhibition, the higher the degree of spatial and temporal sparsening of neural activity.

One key to answer this question may be found in evolution. The olfactory system is a phylogenetically old system whose functional principles may be preserved across different species. Most important, the cross-species similarities point to the central role of neural inhibition in the neural coding of stimuli, that is, olfactory stimuli, that may be preserved throughout the different stages of evolutionary history.

Accordingly, neural inhibition and consequently sparse coding may have evolutionary roots and origins. This, however, is a rather daring and speculative hypothesis at this point. Therefore, let's return to the much safer ground of the empirical findings in yet another species: the cat.

Neuronal findings III: neural inhibition and sparse coding in the cat's visual cortex

We so far focused exclusively on the olfactory cortex. There we demonstrated sparse coding to hold true and to be predisposed by the possible degree of neural inhibition. Does such global inhibition as observed in olfactory cortex also apply in the same way to other sensory cortices? In his commentary on Poo and Isaacson (2009), Schoppa (2009a and 2009b) denies this.

Following Schoppa et al. (2009), neurons in sensory cortices other than the olfactory cortex are ordered according to their functional cell type; this means that, unlike in olfactory cortex, similarly but non-identically responding neurons are not direct, but only near and thus indirect, neighbors. Unlike in olfactory cortex, there is thus a lack of direct connection between different cell types; that is, between pyramidal cells and interneurons, in other sensory cortex. This entails that neuronal inhibition must function according to different principles than in olfactory cortex, where it is based on direct contact, or connectivity.

How can we test this assumption? For that, we may need to switch our sensory allegiance from the olfactory cortex to another sensory cortex like the visual cortex and thereby also from rats to cats. Hence, we are now moving not only to yet another species, from insects and rats to cats, but also to another sensory modality, from olfactory to visual cortex. This leads us a study on cats conducted by Haider et al. (2010) who investigated the cat's primary visual cortex, where they measured IPSPs in interneurons and EPSPs in pyramidal cells in classical and non-classical receptive fields.

How about their results? They observed that the sparseness, reliability, and temporal precision of spiking and membrane potential in the EPSPs of pyramidal neurons depended on the degree of the IPSP in the interneurons: the higher the degree of inhibition and thus the interneurons' IPSP, the more sparse, selective, and temporally precise the EPSP in the pyramidal neurons. These findings further support our earlier developed neuronal hypothesis in yet another species, the cat, that the degree of neural inhibition predisposes the degree of subsequent neural excitation and its associated degree of sparseness.

This was observed in the classical receptive field. How about the relationship between EPSPs and IPSPs in the non-classical receptive field? Interestingly, the interneurons' IPSP increased nonlinearly during stimulation in the nonclassical receptive field. Most important, this was accompanied by significant increases in the pyramidal cells' EPSP's selectivity, sparseness, and temporal precision.

Accordingly, unlike stimuli in the classical receptive field, stimulation in the nonclassical receptive field activates a higher number of interneurons. This, in turn, increases neural inhibition in a nonlinear way with subsequent increase in the degree of sparseness of pyramidal neural excitation (Fig. 2-3).

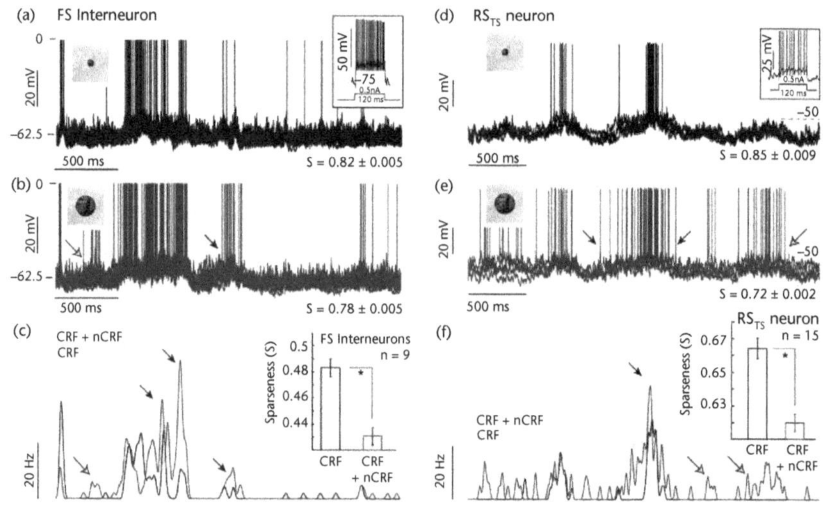

Figure 2-3a Neural excitation and inhibition in visual cortex. Fast-spiking interneurons and thin-spike regular-spiking neurons become more active and less sparse during CRF + nCRF stimulation. (*a*) Intracellular responses of an electrophysiologically identified FS interneuron (inset, shows sustained firing rate >300 Hz in response to current pulse) during ten trials of CRF stimulation (black). (*b*) CRF + nCRF stimulation (red) elicits larger responses, compared with the CRF configuration (closed arrows). (*c*) PSTHs from 15 repeated trials of CRF (black) and CRF + nCRF presentations (grey) reveal elevated PSTH peaks (closed arrows), and the appearance of new peaks (open arrow) during wide-field stimulation. FS interneuron population (n = 5 intracellular, n = 4 extracellular) significantly decreased response sparseness (12%) with CRF + nCRF stimulation ($S_{CRF} = 0.48 \pm 0.007$; $S_{CRF+nCRF} = 0.43 \pm 0.007$; $p < 0.01$). Values are mean ± SEM. (*d*) Intracellular response of an RSTS neuron (inset, adapting firing pattern to current pulse, rate ~100 Hz, spike width at half height 0.25 ms) during five trials of CRF stimulation (black). (*e*) Response of same neuron to five trials of CRF + nCRF stimulation (gray). Note increased action potential response (closed arrows) and addition of new responses (open arrow). (*f*) PSTH across 15 trials of CRF stimulation (black) and CRF + nCRF stimulation (grey) reveals elevated PSTH peaks (closed arrow), along with addition of peaks (open arrows) during wide-field stimulation. Inset, RSTS neuron population (n = 12 intracellular, 3 juxtacellular) significantly decreased sparseness (7% average decrease; $S_{CRF} = 0.66 \pm 0.006$; $S_{CRF+nCRF} = 0.62 \pm 0.005$; $p < 0.01$) during CRF + nCRF stimulation. Values are mean ± SEM. (Reprinted with permission of Cell Press from Haider B, Krause MR, Duque A, Yu Y, Touryan J, Mazer JA, McCormick DA. Synaptic and network mechanisms of sparse and reliable visual cortical activity during nonclassical receptive field stimulation. *Neuron.* 2010 Jan 14;65(1):107–21.)

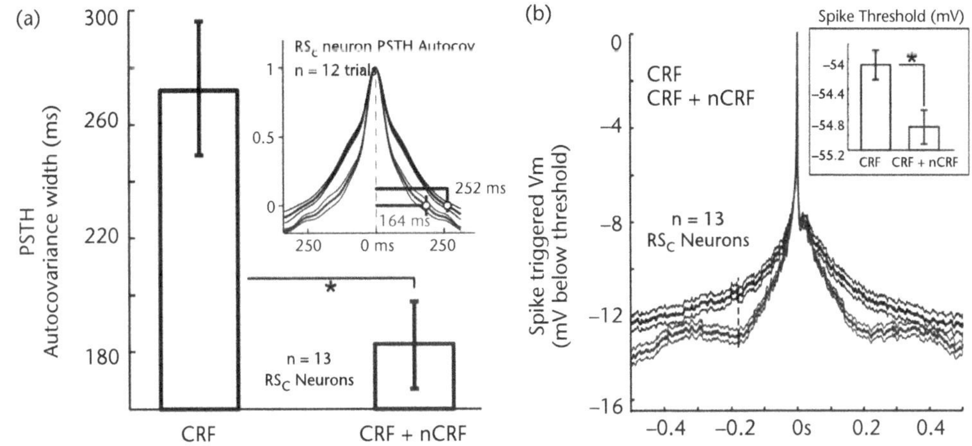

Figure 2-3b **Neural excitation and inhibition in visual cortex. Temporal precision of spike responses in RS_C neurons increases with CRF + nCRF stimulation and is associated with narrowing of the underlying synaptic events. (*a*) Width of the autocovariance function of a representative RS_C neuron's PSTH is significantly (35%) narrower with combined CRF + nCRF stimulation (grey) compared with CRF alone stimulation (black). Across the population of RS_C neurons (n = 13), there was a significant narrowing (by 33%) of the average event in the PSTH with combined CRF + nCRF stimulation (181.6 ± 15.6 ms, grey bar) compared with CRF alone stimulation (272.4 ± 23.9 ms, black bar; $p < 0.01$). Values are mean ± SEM. (*b*) Spike-triggered average of Vm in these same neurons reveals a narrower synaptic potential underlying spikes, and more rapid prespike trajectory (from −179 ms to threshold) with CRF + nCRF stimulation compared with CRF alone stimulation ($dV/dt_{CRF} = 0.062 \pm 0.002$ mV/ms; $dV/dt_{CRF+nCRF} = 0.073 \pm 0.002$ mV/ms; $p < 0.01$). Traces aligned at spike threshold voltage before averaging (0 on ordinate). Inset shows that spike threshold is also significantly lower with wide-field stimulation ($\text{Threshold}_{CRF+nCRF} = -55.1 \pm 0.2$ mV; $\text{Threshold}_{CRF} = -54.2 \pm 0.2$ mV; $p < 0.01$). All data for n = 13 RS_C neurons (mean ± SEM). (Reprinted with permission of Cell Press from Haider B, Krause MR, Duque A, Yu Y, Touryan J, Mazer JA, McCormick DA. Synaptic and network mechanisms of sparse and reliable visual cortical activity during nonclassical receptive field stimulation. *Neuron*. 2010 Jan 14;65(1):107–21.)**

Neuronal hypothesis IIA: neural inhibition and the brain's entrance gates in sensory cortex

These findings further support our hypothesis that the degree of neural inhibition in interneurons predicts and thus predisposes the degree of sparseness during subsequent neural excitation in pyramidal cells. Moreover, by distinguishing between classical and non-classical receptive fields, the relevance of non-linear increases in neural inhibition was observed. This suggests that non-linearity and neural inhibition are closely tied together in yet-unclear ways.

Do the same mechanism that is neural inhibition driving sparseness and non-linearity driving neural inhibition, also operate in sensory cortices other than the visual cortex? The authors of our study, Haider et al. (2010, pp. 119), remark that the same principles can also be observed in somatosensory and auditory cortex. Hence one may propose that the suggested relationship between non-linearity, degree of neural inhibition, and sparseness of neural excitation also applies to other sensory cortex (and possibly also to the cortex in general including the non-sensory cortical regions which however remains to be demonstrated).

How can we better illustrate the central role of neural inhibition for sparse coding? For that I turn to a metaphorical example of the zoo and compare it (figuratively) to our various findings in different species and sensory cortices. Our imaginary (and figurative) zoo of different

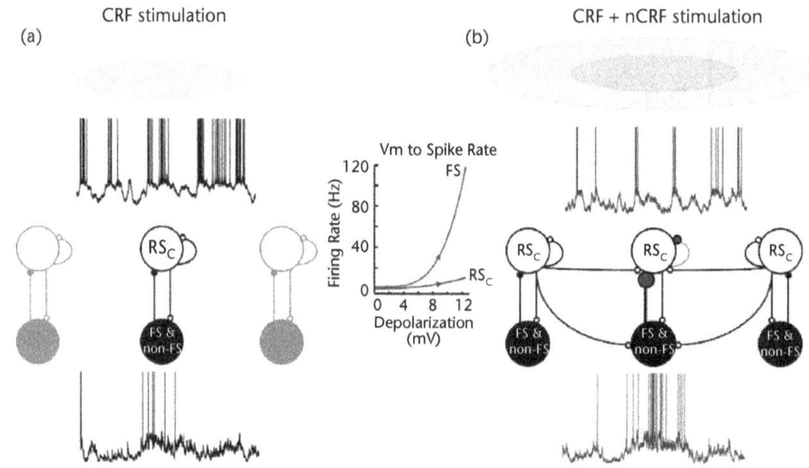

Figure 2-3c **Neural excitation and inhibition in visual cortex. Schematic diagram of the excitatory-inhibitory interactions during wide-field visual stimulation. (*a*) Local cortical networks composed of excitatory (white) and inhibitory (black) neurons form interconnections with each other, with the great majority of connectivity occurring among excitatory neurons. During CRF stimulation, both excitatory and inhibitory cell types are driven, with RS_C neurons and FS neurons generating elevated and temporally varying responses (traces). (*b*) Upon simultaneous engagement of the CRF and nCRF, inhibitory interneurons become strongly activated by increased excitatory drive arising from a larger spatial distribution of inputs. The increased depolarization and enhanced synaptic fluctuations in interneurons are nonlinearly transformed into greater numbers of spikes compared with excitatory neurons (inset at center). This causes RS_C neurons to receive enhanced inhibitory synaptic barrages at specific time points, which leads to increased sparseness and precision of visually evoked spike responses in RS_C neurons. These sparser but less variable spikes are amplified through the recurrent excitatory connections among RS_C neurons in the local network (grey synapse), which leads to more reliable and precise sensory encoding across the ensemble of pyramidal neurons (grey trace). (Reprinted with permission of Cell Press from Haider B, Krause MR, Duque A, Yu Y, Touryan J, Mazer JA, McCormick DA. Synaptic and network mechanisms of sparse and reliable visual cortical activity during nonclassical receptive field stimulation. *Neuron*. 2010 Jan 14;65(1):107–21.)**

species and distinct sensory cortices seems to be framed and surrounded by a fence, corresponding to neural inhibition. While from the outside of the fence there seem to be many gates, that is, channels for neural excitation, only a few of these seem to lead to and reach the inside of the zoo. Once the outside gates of neural excitation are open, another adjacent subsequent gate, the inhibition gate, seems to slide in and close the entrance to the inside of the zoo. Hence, unlike in a real zoo, visitors bringing in excitation are sparsened right at the entrance gates in our imaginary zoo of different species and sensory cortices.

Why is all that important? First and foremost it describes the neuronal mechanisms including the central role of neural inhibition which predisposes sparse coding. This seems to hold across different species and different sensory cortices as the entrance gates of our brain and its neural processing. We can thus see that there is high selectivity with a high degree of sparse coding already at work at the entrance gates of our brain.

Neuronal hypothesis IIb: neural inhibition and consciousness

This is how the brain functions, or better, is predisposed to function. What if, for instance, the brain's "entrance doors," its sensory cortices, break down or shut down? In that case, one would expect abnormal alterations in the degree of neural inhibition that may be either too low or too high, which should then, if our hypothesis is correct, entail abnormal changes in the degree of sparse coding.

Is there any empirical evidence for such scenarios? Despite rather patchy empirical evidence, the psychiatric disorders of schizophrenia and depression may be considered examples of abnormal entrance gates like sensory cortex. Schizophrenia can be characterized by various abnormalities in the early sensory processing in sensory cortex like auditory and visual cortex with seemingly decreased degrees of GABA-ergic mediated neural inhibition (see Chapters 17 and 22 for details). This signifies decreased levels of neural inhibition which, as I postulate, leads to abnormally low degrees of sparse coding in the brain of these patients (see Chapters 22 and 23 for details).

How about the opposite, abnormal shut-down rather than abnormal opening of the brain's entrance doors, its sensory cortices? This may be the case in major depressive disorder where patients feel disconnected from the environment and show abnormally negative emotions. The imaging findings show indeed abnormalities in both sensory cortices and GABA-ergic-mediated neural inhibition (see Chapters 17 and 27 for details). Whether that leads to abnormally high degrees of sparse coding remains open at this point however.

Since the neural abnormalities in psychiatric disorders like depression and schizophrenia, are associated with phenomenal abnormalities, i.e., abnormal contents in consciousness, I describe them in full detail in volume II. This makes it clear, that there here described neuronal mechanisms of global and unspecific neural inhibition, non-linearity, and sparseness of neural excitation are not only neuronally relevant but also phenomenally that is for consciousness.

However to fully grasp their phenomenal relevance, we first need to understand their neuronal relevance and thus the respective neuronal mechanisms underlying sparse coding in full detail by themselves, that is independent of consciousness. This and especially the relationship between difference-based coding and sparse coding shall be discussed in the final sections of this chapter.

Neuronal hypothesis IIIa: Difference-based coding and sparse coding

Thus far, I have pointed out the central role of neural inhibition in driving sparse coding. However, it is not inhibition alone that promotes sparseness. Instead, the specific spatial and temporal relationship of neural inhibition to neural excitation may be central in determining the degree of sparseness. This needs to be pointed out in further detail. What is encoded in the resulting distributed and sparse spatiotemporal neural activity may correspond to the integral of the spatiotemporal difference value between neural inhibition and excitation, or the excitation-inhibition balance (EIB). And it is this integral, the spatiotemporal difference value between neural inhibition and excitation, that may be the crucial variable in determining the degree of sparse coding and its reciprocal balance with the degree of dense or local coding (see Chapter 1 for that balance).

Let me be more specific. We recall that Poo and Isaacson (2009) showed that the EPSCs precede the IPSCs by around 9–10 ms. The larger this time window between EPSCs and IPSCs, the larger the probability of excitation being preserved and channelled through the gates or front of the interneurons and their neural inhibition. The degree of subsequent excitation and action potentials thus depends on the length of the time window between excitation and inhibition.

Occurrence and distribution of neural excitation and action potentials must be considered a function of the temporal difference or integral between neural excitation and inhibition: The degree of sparseness of neural excitation thus depends on the degree of the temporal difference between neural excitation and inhibition. This means that sparse recruitment of excitation and action potentials presupposes difference-based coding temporally. An analogous case can be made with regard to the spatial distribution of inhibition and excitation with the resulting sparse excitation and action potentials of only a few neurons presupposing difference-based coding spatially.

Neuronal hypothesis IIIb: Neural inhibition and sparse coding

How exactly is neural inhibition involved in constituting spatial and temporal differences in neural activity? Let's conduct another thought experiment. Imagine the complete absence of any interneurons, and consecutively of neural inhibition, altogether. There is nothing but pyramidal cells and neural excitation. In such a case, there would be no neural inhibition, meaning that no neural difference between excitation and inhibition can be yielded at all.

Since sparse coding is based on and (necessarily and unavoidably; see earlier) presupposes neural inhibition, both spatial and temporal sparsening of neural excitation would remain impossible in such a case. This means that sparse coding and its many-to-one relationship between stimuli and neuron would be replaced by another code as, for instance, local or dense coding, that is, one-to-one or one-to-many relationships (see Chapter 1 for details).

Most important, in such a case, difference-based coding would remain impossible, too. Neural differences both spatially and temporally could simply no longer be generated. Difference-based coding would consecutively be replaced by stimulus-based coding, the encoding of the single stimulus itself independent of other stimuli (as described in the introduction).

Taken together, I postulate that neural inhibition as mediated by interneurons is a necessary (but nonsufficient) condition, that is, a neural predisposition (see introduction in volume I and especially the introduction in volume II for an exact definition), of (possible) difference-based coding and consecutively of sparse coding. In other words, the implementation and realization of neural inhibition into the brain's neural processing makes the introduction of difference-based coding as the brain's encoding strategy almost necessary and thus unavoidable. Shortly put, neural inhibition predisposes possible difference-based coding rather than stimulus-based coding.

However, neural inhibition by itself may not be sufficient to yield a neuronal difference and thus difference-based coding. For that it needs (on both logical and natural grounds) an accompanying neural excitation. As the aforementioned empirical findings show, it is the difference between neural inhibition and excitation that determines the degree of subsequent sparsening of neural activity. Therefore, one may regard the relation between neural inhibition and excitation, the excitation-inhibition balance (EIB), as sufficient neural condition of both difference-based coding and sparse coding (Fig. 2-4a).

One may consequently hypothesize that the EIB predicts the degree of sparse coding during stimulus-induced activity in single neurons and a population of neurons: the larger the difference between neural inhibition and excitation coded in the EIB, the higher the degree of sparseness, that is, sparse coding, in the subsequent neural activity of single cells and a population of neurons. While this hypothesis is strongly supported by the findings discussed earlier, it nevertheless warrants stronger empirical support with regard to especially the neural difference values encoded in the EIB (see later for details) during sparse coding.

Neuronal hypothesis IIIc: Neural inhibition and temporal differences

So far, I have hypothesized that the conjunction of neural inhibition and excitation constitutes differences in neural activity that can thus be characterized by difference-based coding and sparse coding. How exactly are the alleged differences constituted? One central dimension is the temporal one.

Wehr and Zador (2003) conducted single-cell recording in vivo in single neurons of rats' auditory cortex while exposing them to auditory stimuli. As in the earlier mentioned study in cats, they too observed a precise and stereotyped temporal sequence of neural inhibition and excitation: there was a rapid initial excitatory input followed by temporally slightly delayed neural inhibition, which in turn truncated and thus sparsened the spiking rate related to neural excitation within 1–4 ms. This means that the onset of the interneurons' IPSPs is slightly delayed when compared to the one of the pyramidal cells' EPSPs (see Buzsaki 2006, 62–66 for details).

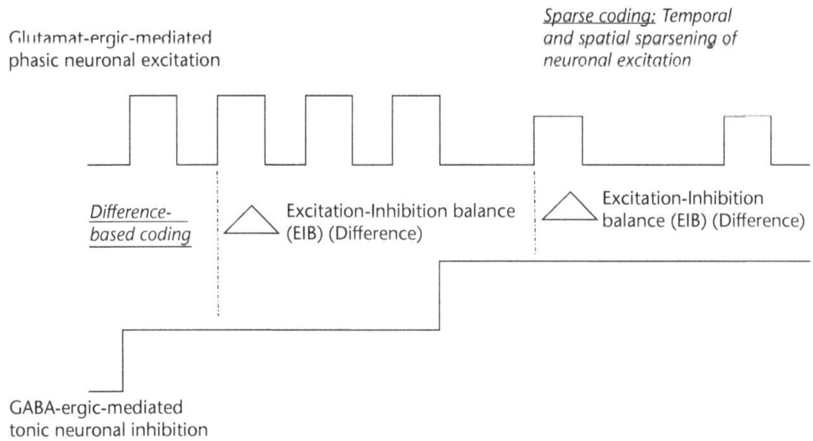

Figure 2-4a Excitation-Inhibition balance and sparse coding. The figure shows the more phasically operating glutamatergic-mediated neural excitation in the *left upper* part as indicated by the *bars* (as if it would operate independently of neural inhibition). Below, *lower left*, is the more tonically operating neural inhibition (as if it would operate independently of neural excitation). What is actually encoded into neural activity is the difference between neural excitation and inhibition and thus what is called the "excitation-inhibition balance" (*middle left/middle*). This is reflected on the *right*, where the observable neural activity results from the integral or difference value between neural excitation and inhibition, reflecting the sparsening of glutamatergic-mediated neural excitation by neural inhibition.

These data suggest that neural inhibition is central for the timing of neural excitation, that is, its temporal precision (see also Haider et al. 2010 as earlier). This is possible on the basis of an exact temporal sequence between neural excitation and inhibition, an "excitation-inhibition sequence," as Priebe and Ferster (2008, 493–494) say, Such "excitation-inhibition sequence," may be evoked in all sensory cortex though its exact timing, i.e., the temporal delay between the initial neural excitation and the subsequent neural inhibition, may be different in the different sensory cortices.

Let us describe the functional implications of the "excitation-inhibition sequence," in more detail. The temporal delay in the onset of neural inhibition provides a temporal window of opportunity for neural excitation to spread to different cells and other population of neurons (see Buzsaki 2006, 62–66). That spread of neural excitation may however come to an end with the onset of neural inhibition which sparsens the already initiated neural excitation.

Accordingly, the temporal difference between the onset of neural excitation and the consecutive one of neural inhibition may determine the degree of possible temporal and spatial sparsening of neural excitation, that is, APs: the longer that temporal difference, the more likely subsequent neural excitation and APs can be temporally and spatially sparsened.

Neuronal hypothesis IIId: non-linearity and consciousness

Why is all that important? We will see later, in Volume II, that the degree of neural differences encoded into neural activity may be central in associating the purely neuronal stimulus-induced activity with consciousness: the larger the spatial and temporal differences encoded into neural activity, the more likely the respective stimulus and its associated stimulus-induced activity can be associated with consciousness (see Chapters 28 and 29). Since I here demonstrated the degree of difference-based coding to predispose the possible degree of sparse coding, the latter may also be relevant for consciousness as we will be discussed in volume II.

Let me explicate the relationship to consciousness in slightly more detail. The dependence of the degree of sparse coding on the amount of the temporal difference between neural excitation and inhibition further underlines the dependence of sparse coding on difference-based coding, as postulated above. In other words, the degree of the temporal difference between neural excitation and inhibition may be proposed to predict the degree of subsequent spatial and temporal sparsening.

Thereby, a certain degree of temporal difference between neural excitation and inhibition may set in motion a non-linear increase in the degree of sparsening of the neural excitation. Hence difference-based coding may be closely aligned with non-linear mechanisms and their sparsening of neural activity, that is sparse coding (see Fig. 2-4b, c). This as well as the exact neural mechanisms of such non-linear increase in the degree of sparsening remain to be shown in the future, however.

We will see later in volume II that such linkage between difference-based coding and non-linearity may prove essential in allowing to associate a phenomenal state, that is consciousness, to a purely neuronal state as for instance during stimulus-induced activity. Accordingly, the apparently close and seemingly inevitable relationship between difference-based coding, non-linearity, and sparse coding may be centrally involved in making possible consciousness.

This linkage may, for instance, be abnormally altered in patients in a vegetative state (VS). These patients may show reduced degrees of difference-based coding, which may make any non-linear increase in the degree of sparse coding impossible. And that in turn may prevent the association of consciousness with the otherwise purely neuronal stimulus-induced activity (see Chapters 28 and 29 in Volume II). In short, the linkage between difference-based coding, non-linearity, and sparse coding may be central for inducing consciousness, as will be discussed in further detail in Volume II (see Chapters 28 and 29).

Neuronal hypothesis IVa: Difference-based coding of GABA and glutamate

One may want to go even one step further, however. Buzsaki et al. (2007) show that both neural inhibition and excitation are mutually and constitutively dependent on each other. On one hand, release of Na+ ions to induce depolarization will increase in glutamatergic neurons when GABA-A receptor-mediated neural inhibition is present; this leads ultimately to an increase in the degree of neural excitation. On the other hand, increase in GABA-A receptor-mediated neural inhibition leads to a decrease in depolarization in the excitatory neurons and hence decreases their overall degree of neural excitation. The same, however, in a converse way also holds for the GABAergic interneurons. Cl– influx will increase in GABAergic interneurons in the presence of glutamatergic-mediated neural excitation. This makes, as Buzsaki et al. (2007, pp. 776–777) argue, an isolated consideration of neural inhibition and excitation and hence of GABA and glutamate impossible.

Why is such isolated consideration of neural inhibition and excitation impossible? I hypothesize that this is due to the fact that the release of Na^+ and Cl^- in glutamatergic and GABAergic neurons is encoded in mutual relationship and thus difference to each other. In short, I hypothesize difference-based coding of neural inhibition and excitation and thus of GABA and glutamate.

The assumption of difference-based coding of neural inhibition and excitation and consecutively of GABA and glutamate is strongly supported by the earlier described observation of their mutual dependence on each other. Most important, one may propose such interaction between GABA and glutamate, and thus between neural inhibition and excitation, to be non-linear rather than linear. If for instance the degree of neural excitation surpasses a certain level, neural inhibition will increase in a disproportionate, or non-linear way. This is, for instance, supported by the findings of a disproportionate and non-linear increase of neural inhibition in relation to neural excitation in the rats' somatosensory cortex (see Kapfer et al. 2007).

Neuronal hypothesis IVb: Excitation-inhibition balance as difference-based signal

Taken together, this leads me to postulate that difference-based coding also applies to the

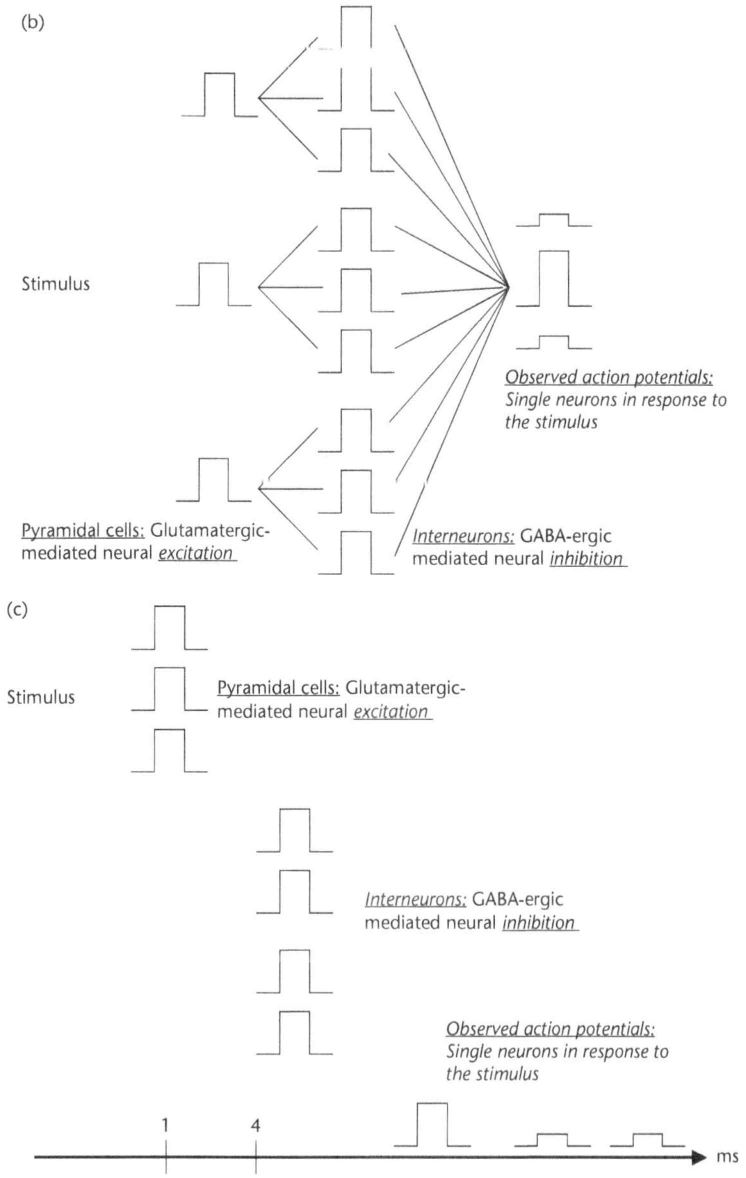

Figure 2-4b and c **(*b*) Neural inhibition and sparse coding in the spatial domain. The figure shows how neural activity is sparsened in the spatial domain by neural inhibition. The stimulus (*left part*) activates three excitatory pyramidal neurons (*left-middle part*), which in turn are connected to multiple interneurons (*right-middle part*) that are excited by the former. However, the excitation of the interneurons leads to increased neural inhibition and subsequently to the sparsening of the initially excited pyramidal neurons, only one of which remains active (*right part*). (*c*) Neural inhibition and sparse coding in the temporal domain. The figure illustrates the mechanisms shown in (*b*) in the temporal domain. The three glutamatergic excitatory pyramidal neurons are activated first (*right part*), followed by the delayed recruitment and activation of the interneurons (*middle part*). This, in turn, sparsens the pyramidal cells' activity to one cell subsequently, as depicted on the right.**

biochemical level of GABA and glutamate and thus neural inhibition and excitation: glutamatergic-mediated neural excitation can only be (and is thus necessarily and unavoidably, i.e., by default) constituted relative to the level of GABAergic-mediated neural inhibition; the same obviously holds true for GABAergic-mediated neural inhibition that is encoded relative to glutamate-ergic mediated neural excitation. What does this entail for the characterization of the excitation-inhibition balance (EIB)? The excitation-inhibition balance (EIB) is based on the encoding of two relative differences, the one of GABA-ergic mediated neural inhibition relative to glutamatergic-mediated neural excitation and the latter being encoded relative to the former. In short, the excitation-inhibition balance is based on difference-based coding. This means that, for instance, any neural inhibition we observe always already reflects the result of prior encoding of some degree of neural excitation against or relative to neural inhibition.

Accordingly, what we as observers describe as "neural inhibition" or "excitation" must be taken in a relative rather than an absolute sense, i.e., as the result of prior difference-based coding. This implies that what we describe as EIB does not reflect the mere subtraction or addition between neural inhibition and excitation in an absolute sense. Instead, the EIB signifies an integrated and thus relative value, i.e., a difference-based value, where the deciphering of absolute degrees of neural inhibition and excitation remains impossible by default.

Neuro-Metaphorical Excursion: *Yin* and *Yang* and the Excitation-Inhibition Balance

Let me conclude by comparing the relationship between neural excitation and inhibition to the famous relationship between the life forces of *yin* and *yang* in Chinese philosophy. Yin and yang always go together, which mirrors the situation with neural inhibition and excitation. And in the same way that yin and yang stand opposite each other do neural excitation and inhibition show equally contrasting differences. As in the case of yin and yang, the contrast is as stark as black and white. Whether the black corresponds to neural inhibition and the white to neural excitation, I leave for the reader to decide.

Most important, in the same way as yin and yang are intrinsically connected, neural inhibition and excitation seem to be intrinsically linked to each other; one cannot do without the other. In the same way as yin would not exist without yang, neural inhibition would remain impossible without prior neural excitation. If there were no prior neural excitation, the inhibitory interneurons would not be excited and could consequently not exert their inhibitory effects. Conversely, the subsequent sparsened neural excitation would remain impossible without the preceding neural inhibition. Hence the mutual dependence between neural excitation and inhibition signifies an intrinsic relationship which mirrors the one between yin and yang.

There is one important difference, however. Yin and yang occupy the same amount of space with both sharing equally the available space. This is different in the case of neural inhibition and excitation. As shown by the reported data, neural inhibition is much more widespread temporally and distributed spatially than neural excitation, which is temporally more precise and spatially more localized. Hence, literally and figuratively, neural excitation takes less space (and less time since it occurs in a shorter interval) than neural inhibition.

Neural excitation and inhibition in the EIB are thus not as equally well balanced spatially and temporally as yin and yang. This difference, however, is crucial for yielding difference-based coding and consequently sparse coding. If, in contrast, neural inhibition and excitation would correspond completely to yin and yang and would be as equally balanced both spatially and temporally, difference-based coding and sparse coding would probably remain impossible. Hence, sometimes it may be rather beneficial for us, at least for our brain, to not follow the example of yin and yang.

Open Questions

This chapter focused on neural inhibition in relation to sparse coding on the cellular and population level. One issue that was left open was how neural inhibition is related to the encoding of the stimuli's natural statistics; for example, their statistical frequency distribution across time and space. Encoding of the stimuli's natural statistics presupposes the encoding of spatial and temporal differences, that is, difference-based coding.

Based on the findings, one may now postulate that neural inhibition is central for inducing and generating neural differences. If so, one would postulate that these neural differences in spatial and temporal regard conform more or less to the statistical frequency distribution of the stimuli across different discrete points in physical time and space.

The spatiotemporal pattern of, for instance, neural inhibition (in relation to neural excitation) should then mirror the spatiotemporal pattern of the statistical frequency distribution, or the natural statistics, of the stimuli. In other words, the neuronal statistics of neural inhibition (in relation to neural excitation) including its spatiotemporal pattern should conform to the stimuli's natural statistics and their spatiotemporal pattern. While this is a rather daring hypothesis, it is at least experimentally amenable and testable.

Besides the empirical relevance, there is a philosophical-epistemological implication to be considered. I postulate that neural inhibition does generate a particular spatiotemporal pattern that allows to encode the stimuli's spatiotemporal pattern. If so, the difference between both spatiotemporal patterns, the one of the stimuli and the other of neural inhibition, may signal the difference between the way we think of the world (as empirically related to the spatiotemporal pattern of neural inhibition) and the world itself as it is independent of our cognition (as related to the spatiotemporal pattern of the stimuli). That, however, means that we may never be able to think of and perceive the world in a completely objective way; i.e., independently of our own brain's spatiotemporal pattern of neural inhibition.

Would thus a brain without any neural inhibition allow us to cognize the world as it is by itself, that is independent of our cognition, in a purely objective way? The answer to that question would be *yes* if conceived in a purely logical way, since the absence of neural inhibition would remove the obstacle standing in the way of a purely objective cognition of the world.

However, empirical and epistemological reality may not conform to logical reality. Why? In the absence of neural inhibition, there would be no longer difference-based coding, but rather stimulus-based coding. That however, as detailed in Volume II, would make consciousness as the necessary basis for any possible cognition and knowledge of the world impossible.

Accordingly, the absence of consciousness entails the absence of cognition and knowledge of the world. In the case of absent neural inhibition, we would thus no longer cognize and know anything at all, so that the question of objective cognition and knowledge could not be raised at all. This however dents deeply into basic epistemological issues, which will not be discussed further in either of these volumes (but see Northoff 2004, 2011).

CHAPTER 3
Sparse Coding on a Regional Level

Summary

So far, I have discussed sparse coding as the brain's coding strategy on the cellular and population level, where it describes the relationship between stimuli and neurons as well as between neurons and neurons. This raises the question of whether sparse coding also applies to the regional level of neural activity—the relationship between stimulus and regions—as well as to the relationship between different regions, the region–region interaction. I first show that sparse coding applies, not only to the visual and the olfactory cortex, but also to other sensory and non-sensory regions. The occurrence of sparse coding in cellular and population activity throughout the whole brain leads me to hypothesize that sparse coding also holds on the regional level of the brain. My hypothesis will be illustrated empirically by recent findings from imaging studies on perceptual decision-making as a paradigmatic example. These studies show that already lower-order sensory regions like the fusiform face area and closely related neighboring regions encode differences between different stimuli into their neural activity rather than the stimuli themselves. This entails a many-to-one relationship between stimuli and region, which is indicative of sparse coding on a regional level of neural activity. Furthermore, the data demonstrate that neural activity in higher-order cognitive regions like the dorsolateral and the ventromedial prefrontal cortex result from the integral, or difference value, between the neural activities of different lower-order sensory regions. This means also that different sensory regions' neural activities are encoded in a sparse way into the neural activity of higher-order cognitive regions. Taken together, these findings clearly indicate that both stimuli and lower-order regions' activities are encoded into lower-order; such as sensory, and higher-order; such as cognitive, regions' neural activities in a difference-based and consequently in a sparse way. Therefore, these findings, although limited to the paradigmatic example of perceptual decision-making, provide direct empirical evidence in favor of difference-based coding and sparse coding on the regional level of neural activity.

Key Concepts and Topics Covered

Sparse coding, level of regions, perceptual decision-making, lower-order sensory regions, difference-based coding, higher-order cognitive regions, amplification and condensation hypothesis

Neuroempirical background IA: sparse coding in sensory cortex

The previous chapters showed that sparse coding holds on the level of the neural activity of single neurons and a population of neurons. This was demonstrated mainly for the visual cortex and the olfactory cortex. However, such sparse coding remains to be shown for neurons in regions other than sensory regions like the prefrontal cortex.

One would therefore postulate that sparse coding reflects a principal, basic encoding strategy of the brain's neuronal activity in response to stimuli from the environment. Before we can make such a strong statement, we need to show that sparse coding on the cellular and population level of neural activity also holds in regions other than the olfactory and visual cortex—for which there is indeed abundant empirical evidence.

As detailed in the preceding chapters, several studies provide strong evidence of sparse coding in primary visual cortex (see Brenner et al. 2000; Vinje and Gallant 2000, 2002; Wolfe et al. 2010; Willmore et al. 2011; see Chapter 1 for details). Beyond the primary visual cortex, higher regions in the visual system such as the inferotemporal cortex do also seem to show sparse coding (Young and Yamane 1992; see also Rolls and Tovee 1995).

Besides the visual system, sparse coding has also been demonstrated in the cellular and population activity of auditory cortex and the sensorimotor cortex (see Simmons and van Stevenivck 2010; Jadhav et al. 2009; Wolfe et al. 2010; Terashima and Hosoya 2009; Greene et al. 2009; Crochet et al. 2011; Rolls and Treves 2011). This suggests that sparse coding is not limited to visual cortex but seems to be the encoding strategy of how the sensory cortex in general encodes stimuli into neural activity.

Let's go into a little more detail with regard to sparse coding in the auditory cortex. DeWeese et al. (2003) demonstrated that neurons in auditory cortex generate only a single spike during exposure to a sound that, due to its complex physical features, should instead elicit multiple spikes. The overall probability of spiking is consequently rather low in auditory cortical cells, thus reflecting sparse encoding of the sound, with a many-to-one relationship between the sounds' physical features and the firing neurons.

This is consistent with the results obtained by Hromádka et al. (2008), who investigated representations of sounds in the nonanesthetized auditory cortex of awake rats. They observed that auditory stimuli elicit high firing rates in less than 5% of neurons at any instant; this reflects sparse scheme rather than local or dense coding of the stimuli in auditory cortical activity.

Neuroempirical background IB: encoding of natural statistics in sensory cortex

How about the encoding of the statistical frequency distribution of the auditory stimuli into single cells and the activity of populations of neurons in auditory cortex? As in visual and olfactory cortex, the encoding of the stimuli's statistical frequency distribution across different discrete points in physical time and space—that is, their natural statistics—also holds true for the auditory cortex. Using natural sounds as experimental stimuli, Rieke et al. (1995) showed that the frog's neurons in the early stages of auditory processing encode the statistical structure of the natural vocalizations of the animal rather than the single stimuli and their respective physical features.

Correspondingly, naturalistic stimuli induced a higher rate of information transmission in the cat's auditory midbrain neurons when compared to non-naturalistic ones (Schreiner and Langner 1997). Since naturalistic stimuli occur more often, these results presuppose the encoding of the stimuli's frequency distribution across different discrete points in physical time rather, than the stimuli themselves at their discrete point in physical time. If the auditory cortical neurons do indeed encode the stimuli's statistical frequency distribution, one would expect changes in the neurons' activities when being exposed to changes in the stimuli's frequency distribution. This has indeed been observed in a simulation study by Lewicki (2002).

Lewicki showed that the activity of auditory cortical neurons adapts to different auditory environments, as tested for by two different sets of stimuli: animal vocalizations and non-biological environmental sounds (see also Olshausen and O'Connor 2002 for a commentary): increased frequencies in the presentation of both biological animal vocalization and non-biological environmental sounds induced increased firing rates in the simulation model. This strongly suggests that the auditory cortical neurons' encoding is based on the stimuli's statistical frequency distribution rather than the stimuli themselves and their respective biological or non-biological features.

Taken together, these data suggest that the auditory cortical neurons' activities are primarily tuned to, and thus encode, the stimuli's statistical frequency distribution rather than the stimuli themselves and their respective physical features. That, though, as demonstrated in Chapters 1 and

2, is possible only by presupposing the encoding of spatial and temporal differences between different stimuli and their respective, different, discrete points in physical time and space.

Accordingly, as in visual and olfactory cortex, there is strong empirical support for the claim that difference-based coding and sparse coding hold true in auditory cortex, too. This makes it rather likely that the remaining sensory cortices' neural activities, like the one in somatosensory cortex (see Jadhav et al. 2009), are also encoded in a difference-based and thus sparse way.

Neuroempirical background Ic: sparse coding in other non-sensory regions of the brain

Does sparse coding apply to regions other than the sensory cortex? Sparse coding has indeed been shown for non-sensory regions like the motor cortex. For instance, specific neurons in layer 6 of the motor cortex in rabbits generate only one single spike during locomotion (Beloozerova et al. 2003). Moreover, stimulation of single motor-cortical neurons in rats may be sufficient to generate movements as complex as whisker movements (Brecht et al. 2004). Even the bird's rapid learning of a song that requires complex movements is closely tied to rather sparse neural activity patterns in the bird's premotor cortex (see Fiete et al. 2004). This brief (rather sparse!) overview already suggests that neurons and populations of neurons in motor and premotor cortex may encode movements and actions into their neural activity in a rather sparse way when compared to the various and complex physical features of the respective output, the actual movement or action.

How about sparse coding in regions other than sensory and motor cortex? Beyond the sensory and motor cortex, sparse coding has also been demonstrated in the hippocampus. This is suggested by observations in the rat and macaque hippocampus and medial temporal lobe that show rather low overall firing rates during stimulation; functionally, such sparse pattern in the hippocampus has been proposed to be related to the observation of face-specific neurons (Quiroga et al. 2007, see also Freiwald et al. 2009). Finally, a study by Bach et al. (2011) showed that neural activity in an area adjacent to the hippocampus, the amygdala, also shows a rather sparse neural activity pattern during fear-conditioning (see Bach et al. 2011; see also Rolls and Treves 2011 for a general overview).

Though tentative, these data suggest that sparse coding holds true for cellular and population levels of neural activity in regions other than the sensory cortex, like the motor and premotor cortex, as well as the hippocampus and amygdala in the medial temporal lobe. This suggests that sparse coding may not be specific to the sensory cortex but may also apply to other regions in the brain. If this can be demonstrated in the future, one may consider sparse coding as the basic and principal encoding strategy the brain applies to encode sensory input and motor output into neural activity on a cellular and a population level.

Neuronal hypothesis Ia: difference-based coding versus origin-based coding

We have to be careful, however. So far, we have considered predominantly only lower-order regions like sensory and motor regions. In contrast, no results for sparse coding in higher-order regions like the prefrontal cortex or the default-mode network (comprising cortical midline structures and the lateral parietal cortex) are yet available. This is especially relevant given that these higher-order regions neither receive direct sensory input like the sensory regions, nor mediate direct motor output like the motor regions. Instead, they receive input from other lower-order regions, like the sensory cortex, while they send their outputs either to other higher-order regions or back to lower-order sensory regions. This means that input and output are neuronal rather than sensory and motor.

What does this imply for sparse coding? If sparse coding holds true as the basic and principal encoding strategy of the whole brain's cellular and population activity, one would expect that it applies to any kind of input or output, regardless of its origin as either sensory, motor, or neuronal.

The neurons (and the population) would then encode the spatial and temporal differences between different inputs and outputs; i.e., difference-based coding, rather than the stimuli themselves and their respective origins; i.e., stimulus-based coding as "origin-based coding" if one wants to say so (see Chapter 25 in Volume II for an extensive discussion of such origin-based coding). The stimuli's origin may thus be not encoded into neural activity in difference-based coding and consequently in sparse coding. Therefore, difference-based coding and sparse coding can be applied to any kind of input and output throughout the whole brain regardless of their origin in either brain, body, or environment.

In sum, I hypothesize that the encoding of neural activity on a cellular and a population level may be difference-based and thus sparse, rather than origin-based and thus dense or local. This makes possible the application of difference-based coding and consequently sparse coding throughout the whole brain and its various regions, including lower- and higher-order regions and their different inputs and outputs.

However, I am well aware that the characterization of difference-based coding and sparse coding in such a way—i.e., as independent of the origin of the stimuli or inputs and outputs—is at best a tentative hypothesis at this point, while, at worst, it may be regarded as pure speculation. What is clear, though, is that any kind of "origin-based coding" that would amount to stimulus-based coding rather than difference-based coding is not supported by the data. Instead of origin-based coding, the data favor a statistically based coding, as is suggested by the encoding of the stimuli's natural statistics in sparse coding.

Neuronal hypothesis IB: experimental testing and relevance of difference-based coding

What can we do? This hypothesis can be tested experimentally in the future. One could, for instance, experimentally create the same spatial and temporal differences—the same statistical frequency distribution or natural statistics—between stimuli of different origins such as from the body or the environment. If my hypothesis holds, one would expect the degree of the neurons' cellular neural activity to be a function of the degree of spatial and temporal difference between the stimuli, regardless of their origin. In other words, differences in neural activity levels should be related to differences in the stimuli's spatial and temporal differences rather than to differences in their origins.

Why is such difference- rather than origin-based encoding relevant? First and foremost, it is relevant in order to better understand how the brain works in a purely neuronal way on the cellular and population (and possibly also the regional) levels of neural activity. There is thus what one may want to describe as "neuronal relevance."

In addition, difference- rather than origin-based encoding of neural activity may also be relevant for consciousness and its contents, thus showing "phenomenal relevance": Contents in consciousness can originate either from the brain's resting-state activity itself (as in dreams) or from the environment (as in the awake state). As we will see in Volume II, this can only be accounted for by difference- rather than origin-based encoding of neural activity (see Chapters 25 and 26).

Neuronal hypothesis IIA: sparse coding on the regional level of neural activity

We demonstrated that sparse coding seems to hold on the cellular and population level of neural activity in different regions of the brain. As such, sparse coding describes how the brain encodes stimuli into neural activity on the level of single neurons and a population of neurons. The neural activity level of the single neurons and the population of neurons in turn determines the neural activity of a single region in unknown ways (see Logothetis 2008).

Since the regional level of neural activity is based on the cellular and population level, one may propose that sparse coding may also apply to the encoding of neural activity on a regional level. In short, I hypothesize sparse coding and its principles to also apply to the encoding of neural activity on a regional level of the brain.

How about empirical evidence for sparse coding on the regional level of neural activity? First, preliminary attempts have been undertaken in this direction that aim to develop methods to modeling especially the encoding (as distinguished from decoding) of neural activity on the level of regions, as, for example, in fMRI (see Park et al. 2012a and 2012b; Kay et al. 2008, Lee et al. 2011, Guillen et al. 2011, and Naselaris et al. 2009, 2011, for first steps in this direction, especially concerning the encoding of the stimuli's natural statistics while they though do not explicitly test for sparse coding). A particular focus of recent investigations is the brain's resting state, whose activity and functional connectivity patterns across different regions may indeed by determined by sparse coding (see Lloyd 2011, Wang et al. 2009). Since they concern the resting state activity and thus the brain's intrinsic activity, we will describe these results in full detail in the second part of Chapter 6.

How can we extend and apply sparse coding from the microscopic level of cells and populations to the more macroscopic level of regions? Does, for instance, sparse coding hold for the activity pattern of area V1 of the visual cortex as a whole, as distinguished from other areas like V2-5 in visual cortex?

While these questions may not even arise for neuroscientists who are using single- and multiple-cell recordings, they may nevertheless be highly relevant for the neuroscientists who use imaging techniques like functional magnetic resonance imaging (fMRI) and positron emission tomography (PET), which visualize the neuronal activity of whole regions and networks. Hence, we now need to shift our focus from the single and population neuron level to the level of single regions and their relationships when forming neural networks.

Neuronal hypothesis IIb: principles of sparse coding

We may want to briefly recall from the previous chapters what sparse coding is all about. Sparse coding is a neuronal hypothesis about the relationship between the neural activity of single cells or populations of cells on one hand, and the number of stimuli or inputs, including their physical features, on the other. Barlow (2001, 2009), for instance, associates sparse coding with the neuronal activity pattern of the single cell across different discrete points in physical time and space, which, he proposes, integrate several inputs by encoding them in a sparse way.

The term "sparse" means that the number of stimuli/inputs, including their respective physical features, exceeds the number of neurons that are recruited during the encoding of the former into the latter's neural activity. Since this amounts to a many-to-one relationship between the number of stimuli and the number of activated neurons, one can speak of a sparse encoding of the stimuli into the neurons' neural activity.

Sparse coding in this sense must be distinguished from both dense and local coding. As detailed in Chapter 1, dense coding implies the reverse relationship—that is, one-to-many—between the number of stimuli and the number of active/recruited neurons. This means that one stimulus "recruits" many neurons. Sparse coding is also different from the local coding model, which assumes a one-to-one relationship between the number of stimuli and the number of recruited neurons; in this case, one specific stimulus activates one particular neuron.

How can we characterize sparse coding in further detail? It is important to note that the frame of reference of sparseness is the number of recruited or active neurons compared to the total number of (possibly available) neurons. One hallmark of sparse coding is that the total number of neurons far exceeds the number of active and recruited neurons (see also Barlow 2001, 250). This accounts for the many-to-one relationship between the number of stimuli and the number of active neurons, which distinguishes sparse coding from both local and dense coding.

Sparse coding is consequently not only a neuronal hypothesis about the relationship between stimuli and neurons, but also an assumption (most often rather tacit or implicit) about the relationship between active and inactive neurons: The higher the number of inactive neurons relative to the number of active neurons at a particular point in time, the higher the degree of sparseness.

NEURONAL HYPOTHESIS IIC: STIMULUS–REGION RELATIONSHIP AND SPARSE CODING

How can we now apply these principles of sparse coding to the level of regions? Rather than relating the stimuli to single neurons and populations of neurons, we now have to consider the relationship between the number of stimuli and the number of recruited or active regions, as well as the one between the actually and possibly activated regions. Taking both relationships, between stimulus–region and between actual region–possible region, may lead to different scenarios and thus different ways of encoding neural activity on a regional level. These different encoding strategies shall briefly be discussed in the following.

Different stimuli may induce neural activity in one and the same region, leading to a many-to-one relationship between stimuli and regions. Furthermore, the number of actual regions activated by the stimulus must remain small compared to the number of regions that could possibly be recruited. For instance, regions x and y may be recruited, while regions a, b, c, and d may remain inactive and thus silent. Hence, one would propose that only a sparse number of regions may be active, compared to the number of regions that could possibly be recruited by the stimulus. If both conditions are met—a many-to-one relationship between stimulus and regions and a low number of activated regions relative to all possible regions—one may speak of sparse coding as holding true on the regional level of neural activity.

Such sparse coding with a many-to-one relationship between stimuli and regions must be distinguished from the one-to-one relationships where one stimulus activates only one region. Furthermore, the different stimuli may activate different regions, so that the number of activated regions relative to the number of possibly activated regions is rather high when considering all possible stimuli. This may consequently be described as "local coding" on the regional level of neural activity.

Finally, as on the cellular and population level, there may also be dense coding on the regional level of neural activity. In this case, one stimulus recruits several regions, implying a one-to-many relationship between stimulus and regions. That goes along with an extremely high number of active regions relative to the number of non-activated regions, thus yielding a scenario that stands diametrically opposite to the one of sparse coding (Fig. 3-1).

In sum, I postulate that sparse coding holds, not only on the microscopic level of single cells and populations of neurons, but also on the more macroscopic level of regions. This means that the number of regions recruited by a stimulus remains lower and thus sparse when compared to the number of stimuli and their physical features. Moreover, this implies that the number of active regions is rather low when compared to the number of regions that could possibly be recruited by the stimulus.

NEUROEMPIRICAL BACKGROUND IIA: PERCEPTUAL DECISION-MAKING AS A PARADIGMATIC EXAMPLE OF SPARSE CODING ON THE REGIONAL LEVEL

How can we illustrate such sparse coding of neural activity on the regional level in further detail? For that, I now turn to the case of perceptual decision-making, where imaging studies do indeed lend substantial empirical support to sparse coding holding on the regional level (see Tamir and Mitchell 2011 for another example in the domain of mentalizing). Perceptual decision-making thus serves as a paradigm that supports the assumption that sparse coding holds on the regional level during the encoding of stimulus-induced activity. The same, i.e., sparse coding on a regional level, also applies to the brain's resting-state activity as will be discussed in Chapter 6 (and see Lloyd et al. 2011, Wang et al. 2009, Nishimoto et al. 2011).

To better understand what perceptual decision-making is about, let's imagine the following scenario. You are driving your car through the streets. Suddenly you see somebody walking on the sidewalk, and you suspect that it may be your child walking home from school. What

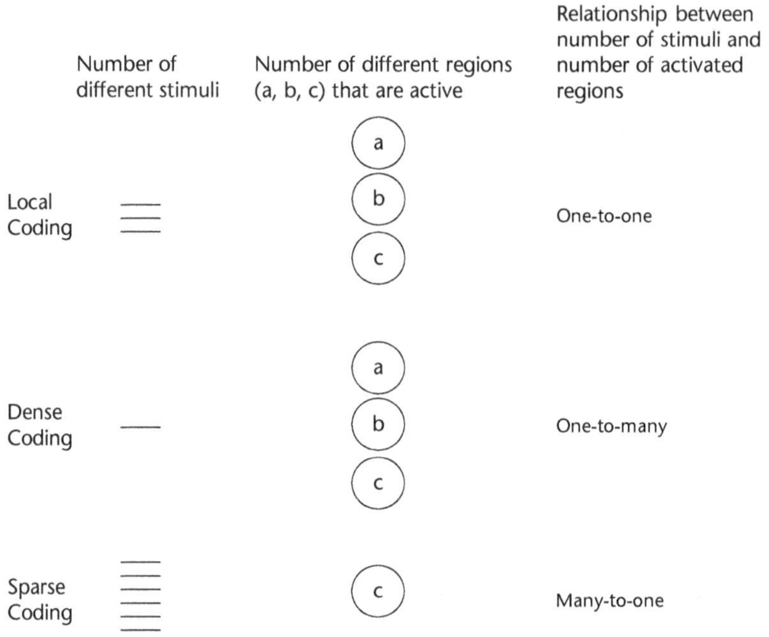

Figure 3-1 Different forms of neural coding on the regional level of neural activity. The figure shows the different forms of encoding strategies on a regional level of neural activity depending on the relationship between stimulus types and the number of activated regions (or networks). (*a*) If the number of stimulus types is the same as the number of regions, one speaks of local coding. This means that for each stimulus type, one particular region (or network) is activated. (*b*) If the number of stimulus types is lower than the number of regions/networks, one could speak of dense coding. In that case, one stimulus type is encoded in the neural activity of more than one region/network. (*c*) If the number of stimulus types is higher than the number of regions/networks, there is sparse coding. In that case, the same regions/network may encode more than one stimulus type with the former thus participating in the neural processing of more than one stimulus type.

do you do? Will you stop the car and ask your child to join you? That will probably happen if you are sure that it is your child. Imagine, however, that you are not sure whether it is your child. Since it starts getting dark early, you can barely distinguish the person you suspect to be your child from two other children. How can you make a decision whether to stop based on your perceptions? This is what is called "perceptual decision-making," and there has been much research on it recently.

One of the questions perceptual decision-making is dealing with is how sensory information can be assembled to make a decision (see Deco et al. 2012). In our example with the child, this concerns the possibly conflicting sensory information, which is unclear, considering the darkness and the other children you see. There is, however, more to perceptual decision-making than mere sensory information. More cognitive functions like attention, task difficulty, prior probability of the occurrence of the event, and the outcome need to be considered, too. Imagine the street is narrow and full of cars. That will considerably distract your attention from the child you see and suspect to be your own.

Imagine also that you know that your child has a soccer lesson at this time of the day at the other end of town; this will make it rather unlikely that the person you suspect to be your child will in fact be your child. This concerns what is called "prior probability" of the occurring event. And finally, imagine that you will not be able to stop right away on the street because it is not allowed. Hence, you would need to think about how and where to stop to pick up your child. And even more important, you would need to let her or him know that you are around but cannot park your car right away.

Neuroempirical background IIb: different components in perceptual decision-making

One of the pivotal researchers in the domain of perceptual decision-making is Hauke Heekeren. Originally from Germany, Heekeren spent time in the United States at the National Institutes of Health, where he conducted excellent studies on perceptual decision-making. He later returned to Berlin, Germany, to continue his work.

In the following, I will rely predominantly on his studies (while neglecting many others in the broad and complex field of perceptual decision-making), which go deeply into the mechanisms and coding of neural activity on a regional level (see also his recent study, Park et al. 2012b, which we will not be able to describe in full detail here). Such a focus is justified by the fact that this chapter is not about perceptual decision-making itself, which would require a full and extensive account. Instead, I here consider perceptual decision-making only as an example for demonstrating sparse coding of neural activity on a regional level.

Given the complexity of the various factors influencing perceptual decision-making as illustrated by our example with the child, Heekeren et al. (2008) distinguish four components of perceptual decision-making. The first concerns the accumulation of sensory evidence. This is well reflected in our example, where it consists of the different sensory inputs you receive in the situation.

The second component of decision-making targets perceptual uncertainty or difficulty that will, in turn, lead to the recruitment of additional attentional resources. In our example, such perceptual uncertainty consists of the conflicting sensory inputs from the different children in the darkness, so that you do not know which of the children you should direct your attention to.

Following Heekeren et al. (2008), the third component represents decision variables like the predictability of the outcome, and includes also a motor component to implement the action accompanied by your decision. You see your child and want to stop and park your car in order to pick your child up. Finally, the fourth component focuses on performance-monitoring of the actual decision in order to adjust the decision during, for instance, changing circumstances if necessary. In our example, this corresponds to the situation where you cannot find a spot to park the car while at the same time signaling to your child that you are there. In the following sections, I will discuss the neural mechanisms underlying the different components of perceptual decision-making.

Neuronal findings Ia: single-cell activity in sensory cortex during perceptual decision-making in animals

Let's start with the first component of decision-making: the involvement of the sensory system in decision-making. I first demonstrate results from the cellular level of neural activity and later, in the next section, results from the regional level, with both suggesting sparse coding of neural activity.

Romo et al. (1998, 2000) undertook single-cell recordings in the somatosensory cortex of monkeys who had to perform a vibrotactile task in which they, as behavioral choice, had to decide the frequency of oscillations of two sequentially presented flutter stimuli. This requires not only perception but also decision-making, and thus may be regarded as a typical perception decision-making task. Interestingly, the electrophysiological trial-to-trial fluctuations in the firing rates of the cells in the somatosensory cortex (S1) predicted the subsequent behavioral choice of the monkey. However, the averaging of somatosensory firing rates according to the trials themselves—that is, trial-based—did not yield any correlation with the behavioral choices. This suggests that the actual decision is already somehow related to neural activity in a lower-order sensory region like S1, and particularly to the variability; i.e., the fluctuations, in its neural activity level.

We saw that the fluctuations in S1 are related to the behavioral choices. How, though, do they stand in relation to the stimuli as presented during the experiment? Interestingly, the degree of fluctuations in the firing rate (in somatosensory cortical neurons) depended on the stimulus's presentation frequency. If the stimulus's oscillation frequency increased, the S1 neurons' firing rate also increased in a monotonic way. This suggests that the firing rate and its fluctuations in S1 do indeed encode the statistical frequency distribution of the stimulus—that is, its natural statistics—rather than each stimulus by itself. Such encoding of the stimulus' natural statistics suggests sparse coding rather than local or dense coding as the main and predominant encoding strategy.

Taken together, these results clearly demonstrate the relevance and direct involvement of the somatosensory cortex in perceptual decision-making, with its trial-to-trial fluctuations predicting subsequent behavioral choices. Moreover, the results suggest sparse encoding of the stimuli into the neural activity of the somatosensory cortex during perceptual decision-making.

Can we lend further support to the direct involvement of sensory cortex in the behavioral choices one is confronted with during perceptual decision-making? In another single-cell recording study in monkeys, Newsome and colleagues (Newsome et al. 1989, see also Rorie et al. 2010 and Cohen and Newsome 2008) recorded from neurons in the motion area (MT) as a higher part of the visual cortex that is involved in visual motion) while the monkeys had to make decisions in a direction-of-motion discrimination task.

The monkeys had to decide whether a noisy field of dots was moving in one direction or another (i.e., upward or downward). They could indicate their decision by a quick eye movement to a target on the respective side. The recorded activity of some of the neurons in MT correlated well with the subsequent behavior of the monkey; for example, its decision about the direction of the moving dots. Analogous results were also obtained by microstimulation of MT, underlining the relevance of neurons in this sensory region for perceptual decision-making.

What can we learn from these studies? Both studies provide evidence for the central role of sensory cortex; i.e., S1 and area MT, in predicting the behavioral choices during perceptual decision-making in monkeys. Most important, they lend evidence to the assumption that neural activity in sensory cortex is encoded in a sparse way on a cellular level during perceptual decision-making (see below for more details). This is well reflected in the encoding of the stimuli's statistical frequency distribution; that is, their natural statistics, as hallmark feature of sparse coding (see below for details).

Neuronal findings IB: Regional activity in sensory cortex during perceptual decision-making in humans

How about corresponding evidence on the regional level of neural activity in humans? Heekeren et al. (2004) used a house–face discrimination task in fMRI to test for the involvement of the sensory regions in perceptual decision-making. Faces are known to preferably activate the fusiform face area (FFA), while houses are more associated with neural activity in the parahippocampal place area (PPA).

Subjects now had to decide in their behavioral choices whether they saw a face or a house; the authors then compared all correct trials with those where subjects made the wrong or incorrect decision. The experimenters further promoted the generation of mistakes by presenting stimuli in either a supra-threshold (high number of correct trials) or a peri-threshold (high number of incorrect trials) way.

During correct trials where subjects made the right decision about their perceptions (house or face), activity in both regions (i.e., FFA and PPA) was significantly higher than in incorrect trials, where they misperceived the house as a face and the face as a house. Accordingly, the level of neural activity in early sensory regions like the FFA and the PPA already predicts the kind of perception and the subsequent behavioral choice. These results clearly indicate that sensory regions like

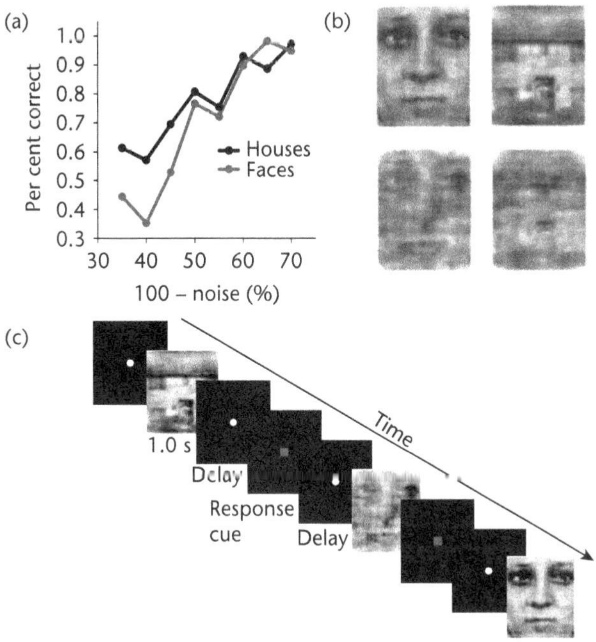

Figure 3-2a Neural processing in perceptual regions during perceptual decision making. Experimental task. Subjects decided whether an image presented on a screen was a face or a house. By adding noise, the amount of sensory evidence in the stimuli was varied parametrically. (*a*) Results of behavioural study to assess the amount of noise to add to the images. Thresholds (82% correct) were about 45% noise for both faces and houses. (*b*) In the fMRI experiment, we used images of faces and houses that were either easy (95% correct, suprathreshold, B top) or difficult (82% correct, perithreshold, B bottom). (*c*) Rapid event-related fMRI design. Stimuli were presented for 1 s, subjects responded with a button press after a forced delay (response cue shown for 300 ms, delay 1–5 s).

the PPA and the FFA are directly involved in making decisions and thus are behaviorally relevant (see Fig. 3-2).

The same group around Hauke Heekeren used the face–house categorization task and combined it with a probabilistic delivery of a reward, thus introducing a value component in perceptual decision-making (Philiastides et al. 2010a and 2010b, 2011). Rather than on sensory evidence, as in the first study, the focus here was more on probabilistic evidence related to reward.

While sensory evidence is related to the processing of houses and faces in the FFA and the PPA, the probabilistic evidence associated with reward was more related to neural activity in neighboring regions; for example, the posterior fusiform gyrus (PFG) and the parahippocampal gyrus (PHG). The authors observed neural activity in PFG and PHG specifically related to face and house, respectively. However, activity changes in both regions were induced not only by the respective target stimulus (face or house) but also by the other stimulus, the *non*-target stimulus: Both regions decreased their activity (relative to baseline) in response to the respective other stimulus—the alternative option or the non-target stimulus. More specifically, the PFG increases its activity in response to faces, while the presentation of houses leads to a decrease in neural activity in the same region. The converse pattern was observed in the PHG, where houses increased and faces decreased the level of neural activity (see Fig. 3-2c).

The authors conclude that both regions' neural activity not only encodes the preferred stimuli, the target stimulus (such as house or face) but also the other stimulus, the non-preferred one, the non-target stimulus (see also Lemus

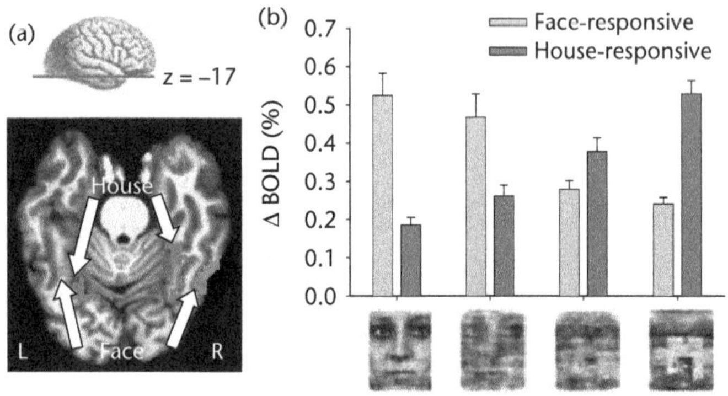

Figure 3-2b **Neural processing in perceptual regions during perceptual decision making. FMRI data illustrating representation of sensory evidence in maximally face- and house-responsive voxels. (*a*) Maximally face- (Face, orange) and house-responsive (House, green) voxels in one subject. (*b*) BOLD change corresponds to perceptual evidence for respective classes of stimuli. Mean responses (n = 12, error bars represent standard error of the mean) in face- and house-selective voxels to the four different conditions (from left to right: suprathreshold face (~10% noise), perithreshold face (~45%), perithreshold house (~53%), suprathreshold house (~10%)). For the respective preferred category, both face- and house-selective regions responded more to suprathreshold than to perithreshold images (face-selective: $P < 0.041$, paired t-test one-tailed; houseselective: $P < 0.001$) while the opposite was true for the non-preferred category (faceselective: $P < 0.013$; house-selective: $P < 0.002$). For face-responsive: suprathreshold face. perithreshold face > perithreshold house > suprathreshold house (analysis of variance, linear contrast, $P < 0.001$); for house-responsive: opposite pattern ($P < 0.001$).**

et al. 2010 for further support showing multimodal involvement of sensory cortex in perceptual decision-making). The resulting and observable stimulus-induced activity in each region can then be traced back to the integral or difference value in activities elicited by both stimuli in isolation. The authors themselves do therefore propose that both regions' neural activity encodes not only the preferred stimulus but also the non-preferred one during perceptual decision-making.

These and other studies (see Heekeren et al. 2008 for review) clearly demonstrate the direct relevance of visual and other (auditory, somatosensory) sensory regions in perceptual decision-making. Sensory regions do seem to encode both sensory and probabilistic evidence on which subsequent behavioral choices and thus decision-making are based. By encoding sensory and probabilistic evidence of the respective stimuli into the neural activity of the sensory cortex, the latter seems to directly participate in shaping the actual behavioral choice and thus the decision.

Neuronal hypothesis IIIa: Difference-based coding of cellular activity in sensory cortex

The first main finding in the various studies is the involvement and relevance of the sensory cortex in perceptual decision-making. Studies observed that the trial-to-trial fluctuation in, for instance, the activity of the somatosensory cortical neurons predicted the subsequent behavioral performance in the decision-making task (see above). What kind of neuronal mechanisms, or more specifically, coding strategy must be presupposed to exist in sensory cortex in order to make such prediction possible?

Let's consider the first monkey example from Romo et al. (1998, 2000), where trial-to-trial fluctuations in somatosensory cortex predicted subsequent behavioral choices (see above). What correlated with behavioral performance were the trial-to-trial fluctuations rather than the (averaged) trials themselves. The authors directly compared fluctuation-based and trial-based

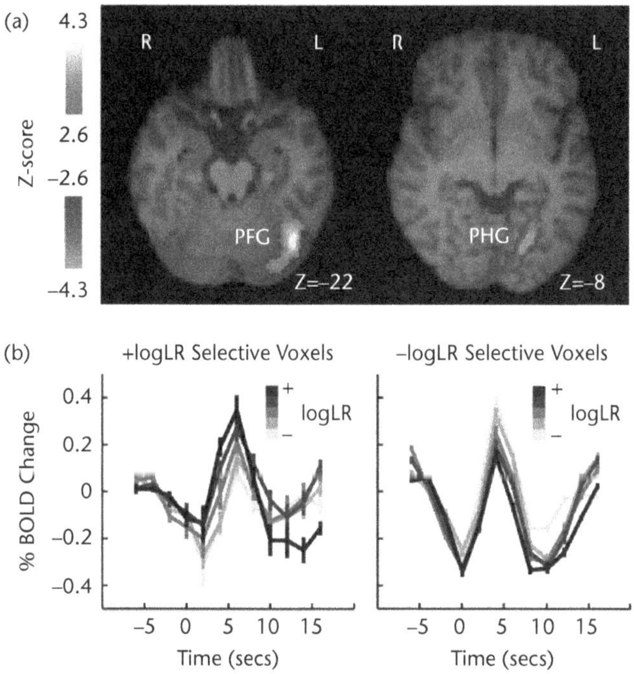

Figure 3-2c Neural processing in perceptual regions during perceptual decision making. Representation of probabilistic evidence in ventral temporal cortex. (*a*) A region in the left PFG [(x −40, y −70, z −20), Z = 4.13, peak Montreal Neurological Institute (MNI)] correlated positively with logLR (+logLR selective voxels), whereas a region in the left PHG [(x −20, y −74, z − 8), Z = 4.28, peak MNI] correlated negatively with logLR (−logLR selective voxels). Activity in corresponding voxels in the right hemisphere showed a similar pattern but ultimately failed to survive our stringent significance tests. For visualization purposes, images are thresholded at $Z > 2.6$ and $Z < -2.6$, respectively (uncorrected). Images are radiological convention. (*b*) Event-related BOLD signal averages (Eq. 10) for five different logLR levels, from each of the two regions shown in Figure 3-2a. Traces are aligned to the onset of visual stimulation at 0 s. The statistical contrast used to identify the regions (logLR) predetermined the shape of these plots, which are shown for illustrative purposes. Error bars represent SE across subjects. Reprinted with permission of Nature Publishing Group, from Heekeren HR, Marrett S, Bandettini PA, Ungerleider LG. A general mechanism for perceptual decision-making in the human brain. *Nature*. 2004 Oct 14;431(7010):859–62; and from Proceedings of the National Academy of Sciences, Philiastides MG, Biele G, Heekeren HR. A mechanistic account of value computation in the human brain. *Proc Natl Acad Sci USA*. 2010 May 18;107(20):9430–5.

analyses of data and observed that only the former (but not the latter) predicted behavioral choices. Behavioral performance is thus encoded into somatosensory cortical neural activity—not in the amplitudes of the single trials themselves but rather in the fluctuations across or between trials.

What does such encoding into the fluctuations across or between trials imply for the encoding of neural activity? This means that the single stimulus itself and its induction of neural activity in a single trial do not encode any information about the subsequent behavioral choice. Instead, behavioral choices are rather encoded in the differences between the different stimuli as neuronally reflected in the fluctuations between different trials.

More generally, this means that the behavioral choices are encoded in the neural differences between the different trials; i.e., the fluctuations. Since it is based on the differences between the different trials; i.e., the fluctuations, the encoding of the behavioral choices in somatosensory cortex presupposes difference-based coding rather than stimulus-based coding.

The study by Romo et al. (1998, 2000) lends indirect support to difference-based coding during the encoding of behavioral choices in somatosensory cortical activity. How can we gain more direct support? There is another study on decision-making that lends further and more direct support to the assumption of the difference-based encoding of behavioral choices in the sensory cortex. This will be the focus in the next section.

Neuronal hypothesis IIIb: behavioral relevance of difference-based coding of cellular activity in sensory cortex

Selezneva et al. (2006) recorded electrophysiological single-cell activity in auditory cortex in monkeys. The monkeys had to perform a categorical decision-making task in which they had to recognize and decide about tone sequences and obtained a reward for the correct behavioral choice. Most important, the investigators analyzed the data in two alternative ways. Either the single-cell recordings were grouped and averaged according to the respective responses, thus presupposing a trial-based analysis. Or the single recordings were set in relation to each other by calculating the ratios between the actual trial and the (respectively) preceding trial. One may want to speak of "ratio-based analysis" rather than "trial-based analysis." The hypothesis was here that the monkey may perform serial comparisons between the subsequent tones in order to make its behavioral choice. If so, the ratio-based analysis should serve and thus predict the subsequent behavioral choice much better than the trial-based analysis.

Which analysis, trial-based or ratio-based, predicted the behavioral choices and thus the rewarding effects of the tones? Only the neural activity in auditory cortex as related to ratio-based analysis predicted the behavioral choices; i.e., the rewarding effects of tones. In contrast, auditory cortical activity, as analyzed in a trial-based way, did not predict any behavioral choices.

What does this mean with regard to the behavioral effects, more specifically the assignment of value, or reward, to the tones? It means that value or reward is constituted on the basis of differences, more specifically the difference between the actual tone and the preceding tone. Accordingly, value is thus not generated on the basis of neural activity related to a single stimulus alone but rather by the relationship between the neural activities associated with the actual and the preceding stimulus. In short, value is based on difference-based coding rather than stimulus-based coding.

These results favor the assumption that difference-based coding holds true on the level of single cells in sensory cortex. Difference-based coding allows for the integration and comparison between different stimuli in sensory cortex, which in turn serves to make decisions; i.e., behavioral choices. Accordingly, difference-based coding on the cellular level is not only neuronally relevant but also behaviorally relevant in that it makes possible the encoding of behavioral choices as early as in sensory cortical activity. As we will see later in Volume II, both neuronal and behavioral relevance of difference-based coding will be complemented by the phenomenal relevance of difference-based coding for consciousness (see Fig. 3-3).

Let us here remain, though, at the neuronal and behavioral levels of neuronal activity. One would now suggest that what holds true at the level of single cells may also apply to the regions as a whole. Hence, one would hypothesize that difference-based coding also holds on the regional level of neural activity in the various sensory regions like visual and auditory cortex. This is clearly a tentative hypothesis at this point; it will be discussed in the next section.

Neuronal hypothesis IVa: difference-based coding of regional activity in sensory cortex

Let's briefly recapitulate the described findings within the context of our child example. You are able to clearly discern your child. Your beloved child wears a colorful red jacket, which clearly distinguishes her from the other two children, who wear black and brown coats. Your sensory input can thus yield clear and large enough differences for you to distinguish them from each

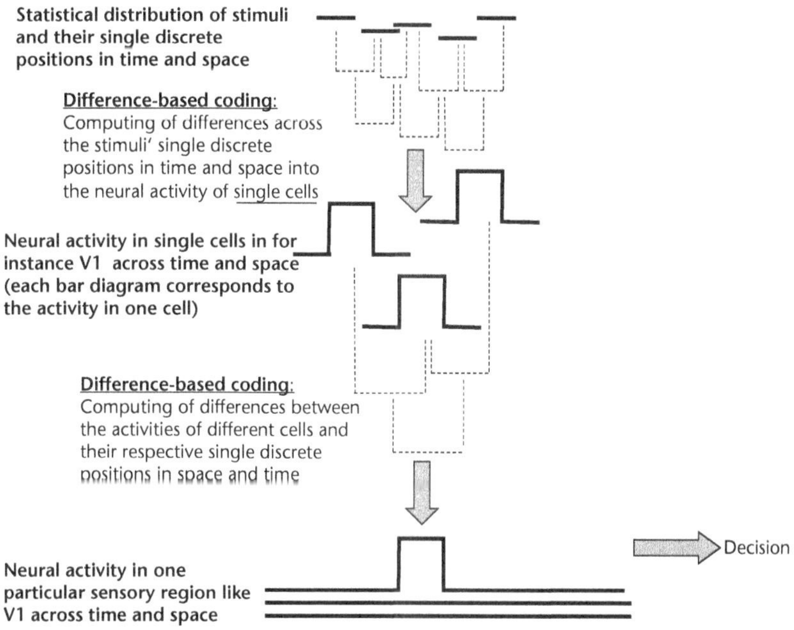

Figure 3-3 **Difference-based coding in sensory cortex. The figure shows the relationship between difference-based coding on a cellular level and a regional level of neural activity and how that ultimately results in decision-making. The upper part illustrates the distribution of the stimulus across different discrete points in physical time and space and how it is encoded into the neural activity of a few sparse cells in, for instance, primary visual cortex (V1); this presupposes different-based coding as indicated by the middle part. If the number of recruited neurons is sufficient, this, in turn, will lead to sparse activation of one particular region like V1 as a whole as indicated in the lower part; that is supposed to reflect (and predict) the resulting behavior; that is, the decision in our case. Hence, I suppose difference-based and sparse coding to be central in mediating the transition from the single-cell level over the regional/network level to the behavioral level.**

other in your perception and to guide your subsequent behavioral choices.

The situation is different, however, if the two other children also wear the color red, though a slightly darker red. Despite the fact that your child wears the same jacket, you will no longer discern her as easily. Why? Because your perception is based on differences. And the differences are rather small now, with all three children wearing red.

Since it is based on the differences between different stimuli, your sensory cortical activity may be rather low due to the small degree of differences in the three children's red jackets. Your sensory cortical activity will thus convey rather conflicting perceptual evidence and will consecutively no longer be able to provide you with a clear signal on how to make your subsequent behavioral choice.

Our example seems to presuppose that difference-based coding and behavioral prediction hold true on the regional level of neural activity of the sensory cortex. This goes well with my assumption that difference-based coding holds in sensory cortex on the cellular level of neural activity. However, my assumption seems to oppose the often rather tacitly assumed regional specialization of sensory regions like V1–5.

NEURONAL HYPOTHESIS IVB: DIFFERENCE-BASED CODING VERSUS REGIONAL SPECIALIZATION IN FFA AND PPA

In our specific case of perceptual decision-making, the assumption of difference-based coding seems to be incompatible with the specialization of FFA and PPA. The FFA is specialized for processing faces, while the PPA prefers houses. Hence, these regions' neural activity seems to be specifically tied to one particular stimulus (i.e., houses or faces). One would consequently propose that each trial by itself, rather than the difference between different trials, would predict the subsequent perception. This is much more compatible with stimulus-based coding than difference-based coding on a regional level of neural activity.

Do we thus have to assume that the regional level of neural activity is characterized by stimulus-based coding rather than difference-based coding? While both FFA and PPA are certainly specialized in processing specific stimuli (i.e., faces and houses), this specialization is not absolute. Other stimuli are processed in these regions, too, though to either a much weaker degree or in a different way. This is shown, for instance, in the aforementioned study by Philiastides et al. (2010), who investigated the face–house discrimination task in the context of reward. While they observed strong positive signal changes in both PFG and PHG in response to their preferred stimuli (i.e., faces and houses), they also observed negative signal changes in each region in response to the respectively non-preferred stimulus. Faces yielded positive signal changes in the PFG and negative signal changes in the PHG, whereas for houses the reverse pattern could be observed.

What do these data tell us? The data demonstrate that neither region's activity exclusively and completely codes one particular stimulus alone (faces or houses). Even the respectively non-preferred stimulus, the non-target stimulus, is well able to induce signal changes in both PFG and PHG. This suggests that there is no "absolute stimulus specificity" in these regions' neural activity during the encoding of the stimuli's probabilistic evidence. Instead, there may only be "relative stimulus-specificity" as manifested in the encoding of the one stimulus relative to the other into the regions' neural activity.

How, then, can we describe such relative stimulus-specificity in further detail? Rather than encoding one particular stimulus alone, these regions' neural activity does seem to encode the difference between the preferred and the non-preferred stimulus, between target and non-target stimulus. Even if the non-preferred stimulus remains absent, the degree of signal change elicited by the preferred one may most likely still be tuned by a difference, the virtual difference between the (present) preferred and the (absent) non-preferred stimulus

This leads me to suggest the following, admittedly rather speculative, hypothesis. I hypothesize that even the sensory regions that are seemingly strongly specialized for one particular stimulus (or stimulus feature) may encode their neural activity on the basis of differences between different (i.e., preferred or specific and non-specific or non-preferred) stimuli (or stimulus features) rather than the specific, i.e., preferred stimulus (or stimulus feature) alone.

Neuronal hypothesis IVc: Encoding of minimal differences and regional specialization in FFA and PPA

One may now want to object that difference-based coding in this sense may hold for PFG and PHG during probabilistic processing, but it may not apply to FFA and PPA and their purely sensory processing (see earlier for the description of probabilistic and sensory evidence). In contrast to PFG and PHG, FFA and PPA seem to process only the preferred stimulus; i.e., face and house, but not the non-preferred one. Therefore, one may propose stimulus- rather than difference-based coding in the case of the FFA and the PPA. This seems to suggest that PFG/PHG and FFA/PPA use different coding strategies: stimulus-based coding and difference-based coding. If so, stimulus- and difference-based coding are not mutually exclusive but can exist apparently side by side in different regions.

Is such parallelism between different encoding strategies empirically plausible? Perhaps what looks like difference-based coding in PFG and PHG is in reality stimulus-based coding. Then one would suggest that stimulus-based coding holds for both FFA/PPA and PFG/PHG. This, however, conflicts with the empirical data of a difference-based signal in the latter regions in the PFG and PHG. Alternatively, one could also argue for the reverse case by assuming that stimulus-based coding in FFA and PPA is, in fact, difference-based coding. In short, what looks as stimulus-based coding may result from difference-based coding.

More specifically, one may suggest that what we describe as stimulus-based coding may result from the encoding of minimal spatial and/or temporal differences between different stimuli into neural activity. The alleged stimulus-based coding in FFA and PPA may then reflect one extreme end of the continuum of different degrees of spatial and temporal differences that can possibly be encoded into the neurons' neural activity on the basis of difference-based coding. And that continuum of possible differences in turn may be traced back to the neurons' and the regions' biophysical-computational spectrum as discussed in Chapter 1.

Why is all that relevant? It provides an understanding of the neural mechanisms and processes that may underlie the kind of signal changes we observe on the regional level of neural activity. There is thus neuronal relevance. We will see later, in Volume II, that such neuronal relevance translates into phenomenal relevance; i.e., for consciousness. The degree of spatial and temporal differences as they are encoded into neural activity on the basis of difference-based coding may decide and thus predict whether the purely neuronal stimulus-induced activity can be associated with consciousness: If the encoded spatial and temporal differences are too small, the resulting stimulus-induced activity will be less likely associated with consciousness. This may, for instance, be the case in disorders of consciousness like vegetative state (see Chapters 28 and 29). In contrast, the encoding of larger spatial and temporal differences into neural activity will make the latter's association with consciousness more likely (see Chapters 28 and 29). Accordingly, the degree of differences encoded into neural activity may turn out to be what these days is described as a "neural correlate of consciousness" (see Volume II for details).

NEURONAL HYPOTHESIS IVD: BEHAVIORAL RELEVANCE OF DIFFERENCE-BASED CODING ON THE REGIONAL LEVEL

Another even more direct way to lend empirical support to my assumption of difference-based coding holding on the regional level is the prediction of behavioral data. We saw in the study by Selezneva et al. (2006) that the differences in single-cell activities between the actual and the respectively preceding trials predicted subsequent behavior; that is, reward. One could do the same now on the regional level. For that, the behavioral relevance of the signal difference between houses and faces in each region alone and thus in FFA/PFG and PPA/PHG would need to be shown.

Unfortunately, as I understood, this analysis was neither performed by Philiastides et al. (2010) nor by Heekeren et al. (2004). I would hypothesize that the difference value in the signals between house and face within the FFA/PFG rather than the signals related to the face alone predicts subsequent behavioral choices related to the face. The same may hold true with regard to the house for the PPA/PHG whose difference-based signals between house and face may, analogously, predict subsequent behavioral choices related to the house.

What would this tell us about the encoding strategy of seemingly specialized regions like the FFA and the PPA? It would tell us that what is behaviorally relevant is predicted by neural differences related to different stimuli rather than by the neural activity based on one stimulus alone in isolation independent of the others. If so, difference-based coding must be proposed to hold to be behaviorally relevant also on the regional level of activity.

NEURONAL HYPOTHESIS IVE: DIFFERENCE-BASED CODING AS BRIDGE BETWEEN CELLULAR AND REGIONAL LEVELS OF NEURAL ACTIVITY

The assumption of difference-based coding on the regional level is well in accordance with the aforementioned results by Selezneva et al. (2006) and Romo et al. (1998, 2000) that show the behavioral relevance of difference-based coding on the level of single cells. Such correspondence between single cell and regional level with regard to behavioral relevance is possible only, as I suggest, if both cellular and regional levels of activity are encoded in the same way.

In other words, cellular and regional levels of neural activity must use the same encoding strategy for both to allow for behavioral prediction in the same way. Let me explain this in further detail. Cellular and regional levels of neural activity show different outputs; action potentials/spikes signify the cellular level while local field potentials and frequency fluctuations dominate the regional level. When considering the major differences in their outputs, one would wonder how it is possible for both cellular and regional levels of neural activity to predict subsequent behavioral choices.. One way for this to be possible may consist in using the same encoding strategy;i.e.,difference-based coding and sparse coding.

More precisely, I propose difference-based coding to be such a common encoding strategy that is shared between cellular and regional (and possibly other) levels of neural activities in the sensory cortex. That, in turn, could account for the orientation and tuning of both cellular and regional activities in sensory cortex toward behavior, thus accounting for what we as investigators measure and frame as prediction of behavioral choices.

Finally, in addition to the prediction of behavioral performance, difference-based coding as common coding between regional and cellular levels may also make possible their direct interaction. Single- and population-cell activities are suggested to account for the neural activities of whole regions (see Logothetis 2008). The exact mechanisms providing such a transition from the cellular/population to the regional level of neural activity remain unclear, however.

I propose that, for the interaction between cellular and regional levels of neural activities to be possible, both need to apply the same format and thus the same encoding strategy, which I hold to be difference-based coding and sparse coding. Most importantly, the degree of difference-based coding and sparse coding may determine the degree of possible interaction between cellular and regional levels of neural activity. Therefore, I for instance hypothesize that the degree of neural activity on the regional level may be predicted by the degrees of difference-based coding and sparse coding on the cellular or population level of neural activity.

Neuronal findings IIa: Higher-order non-sensory regions and perceptual decision-making

So far, we have focused only on the sensory cortex. However, other regions of the brain also participate in perceptual decision-making. Results from single-cell recordings in monkeys show that regions downstream of the sensory cortex are centrally involved in forming a decision. This concerns regions like the dorsolateral prefrontal cortex (DLPFC), the frontal eye field, the lateral parietal cortex, the medial premotor, and the ventral premotor cortex (see Heekeren et al. 2008; Shadlen and Newsome 2001; Kim and Shadlen 1999; Philiastides et al. 2010a and b, 2011).

Most important, the involvement of these regions in perceptual decision-making seems to be based upon computing the difference values from different inputs stemming from lower-order regions such as the sensory cortex. There must thus be some comparison or matching process in the higher-order region between inputs from the different lower-order regions. And the outcome of this comparison or matching process may correspond to the subsequent behavioral choices.

Let me be more specific with regard to the comparison process in humans. Applying the earlier described face-house discrimination task, Heekeren et al. (2004) required two criteria to allow for such a comparison or matching process in humans on a regional level of neural activity. First, the region had to show greatest activity during those stimuli that were most clearly presented and thus predisposed unequivocal perceptual decision.

And second, the region's activity had to correlate with the difference value in neural activity in those regions that processed faces and houses; for example, FFA and PPA. To test the second criterion, they first obtained the signal changes in each region, FFA and PPA, during the perceptual decisions involving faces and houses. This allowed them to compute their difference values in neural activity, which they then correlated with the signal changes in the whole brain and its various regions during the perceptual decision-making task.

Neuronal findings IIb: prefrontal cortex in perceptual decision-making

One region fulfilled both criteria: the left DLPFC. The neural activity in the left DLPFC may thus signify such comparison or matching process; that is the computing of difference values stemming from lower-order sensory regions like the FFA and PPA. Let us the specify this in the following.

The left DLPFC showed several interesting findings. First, the left DLPFC showed higher activity during clearly presented face and house stimuli on a suprathreshold level when compared to degraded; for example, perithreshold stimulus presentation. Second, neural activity in the left DLPFC predicted behavioral performance in the categorization task. Third, neural activity in the left DLPFC also correlated with the difference values from the signal changes in FFA and PPA during the presentation of faces and houses.

Most important, DLPFC signal changes could neither be explained by the neural activity in FFA or PPA alone nor by mere task difficulty. This means that the left DLPFC actively compares and computes differences in neural activity from sensory regions like FFA and PPA. Finally, the difference value of FFA and PPA signal changes in DLPFC predicted the subsequent behavioral choices (see also Philiastides et al. 2011 for further support of the causal role of the DLPFC in perceptual decision-making). In contrast, signal changes in FFA and PPA alone did not predict behavioral choices (or to a much lesser degree) (see also Philiastides et al. 2011).

Taken together, this suggests that the left DLPFC's neural activity stems from computing differences; i.e., difference values, in neural activity from lower-order sensory regions; that is, FFA and PPA. This suggests the neuronal relevance of difference-based coding even in a higher-order regions like the left DLPFC. Also, only the difference-based signal in left DLPFC but not the region-based signal (i.e., from either FFA or PPA alone) predicted behavioral preferences. This underlines the behavioral relevance of difference-based coding in the case of a higher-order region like the left DLPFC.

Is the neural processing and computation of difference-based signals from other lower-order regions specific to the left DLPFC as distinguished from other regions? The group around Heekeren applied the same methodological procedure when combining their face-house categorization task with reward as described earlier in the probability-reward task (Philiastides et al. 2010a and 2010b). They now computed the difference value between the here involved lower-order sensory regions; that is, PFG and PHG (see earlier), and correlated them with signal changes in the rest of the brain. This showed that the difference value between PFG and PHG correlated with and thus predicted the neural activity in the ventromedial prefrontal cortex (VMPFC), a region centrally implicated in reward (see Part III for details; also see Fig. 3-4).

Importantly, neural activity in the VMPFC could neither be explained by changes in PFG and PHG alone nor from regions encoding only house and face themselves; for example, FFA and PPA. Hence, in the context of value and reward, neural processing and computation of difference value from the signal changes of other regions can also be observed, though not in the left DLPFC but in the VMPFC (see also Tamir and Mitchell 2011 for the demonstration of an analogous difference-based signal in the VMPFC in the context of mentalizing of others with respect to the own self).

Neuronal hypothesis Va: difference-based coding in prefrontal cortex

These results show that the neural activity in higher regions like the DLPFC and the VMPFC seems to result from the neural processing and computing the difference values in neural activity from lower sensory regions. In humans, for instance, the neural activity in the DLPFC could only be explained by the integral or difference value of the signal changes in FFA and PPA rather than by each region's (i.e., FFA and PPA) neural activity alone (or the task difficulty). The same holds for neural activity in VMPFC that could only be explained by the difference-based signal between PFG and PHG (see also Tamir and Mitchell for an analogous result with a difference-based signal in the VMPFC during mentalizing).

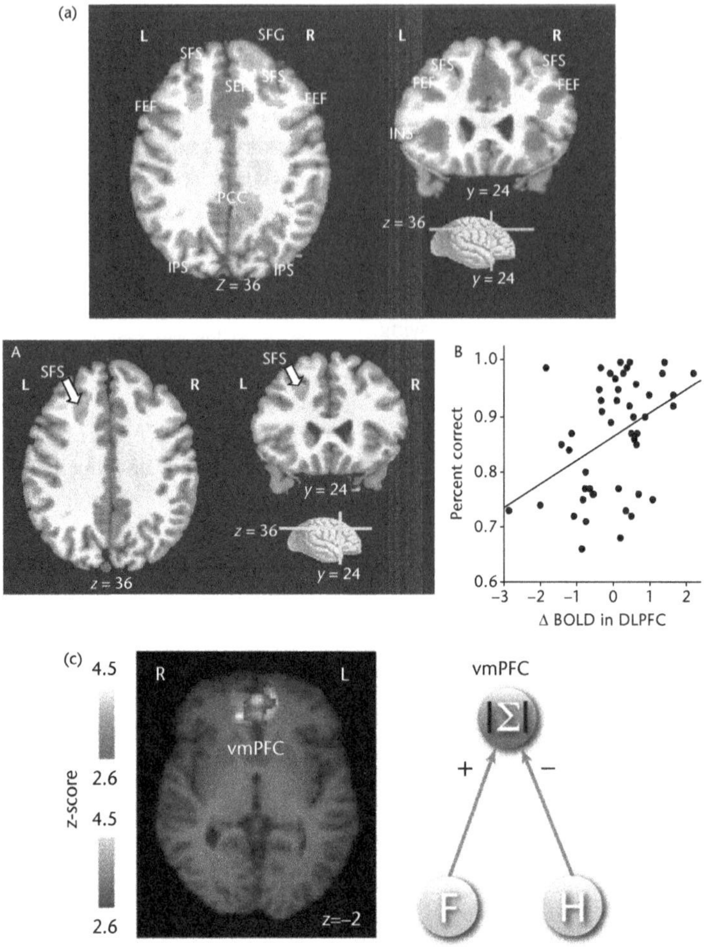

Figure 3.4a–c Neural processing in prefrontal regions during perceptual decision making. (*a*) Brain regions showing a main effect of task difficulty: grey: easier (low noise proportion) > harder (high noise proportion); dark: harder > easier. Abbreviations: FEF, frontal eye field; INS, insula; IPS, intraparietal sulcus; PCC, posterior cingulate cortex; SEF, supplementary eye field; SFG, superior frontal gyrus; SFS, superior frontal sulcus. (*b*) Perceptual decision-making in posterior DLPFC. (A) Region in the depth of the left SFS, showing both a higher response to suprathreshold images of faces and houses relative to perithreshold images, and a correlation with |Face(t) – House(t)| suggesting that this brain region integrates sensory evidence from sensory processing areas to make a perceptual decision (BA8/9, easier > harder: x = 224/y = 24/z = 36, z_{max} = 4.20; correlation with |Face(t) > House(t)|: x = 222/y = 26/z = 36, z_{max} = 3.66, coordinates in MNI system refer to local cluster maxima, and z_{max} to the corresponding z-value). (B) Signal changes in the posterior portion of the DLPFC predicted task performance (r = 0.413, P = 0.004). Points represent average BOLD change and performance for each condition (suprathreshold face, perithreshold face, perithreshold house, and suprathreshold house) and subject. (*c*) Value signal computation in vmPFC. A region of the vmPFC covaried both with |logLR| [(x −6, y 50, z −2), Z = 4.07, peak MNI] and |PFG(t) – PHG(t)| [(x −2, y 52, z −2), Z = 4.45, peak MNI], providing strong evidence that this region is involved in computing a value signal by combining the weight of evidence for face (F) and house (H) by using a difference-based comparator operation. For visualization purposes, images are thresholded at Z > 2.6 (uncorrected). Images are radiological convention. Reprinted with permission of Proceedings of the National Academy of Sciences, Philiastides MG, Biele G, Heekeren HR. A mechanistic account of value computation in the human brain. *Proc Natl Acad Sci USA*. 2010 May 18;107(20):9430–5; and from Nature Publishing Group, from Heekeren HR, Marrett S, Bandettini PA, Ungerleider LG. A general mechanism for perceptual decision-making in the human brain. *Nature*. 2004 Oct 14;431(7010):859–62.

This means that the activity in VMPFC and DLPFC is based on the neural processing and computing (and comparing) neural differences, the ones between FFA/PFG and PPA/PHG. One must consequently postulate difference-based coding to encode the neural activity in DLPFC and VMPFC on a regional level. Accordingly difference-based coding must be considered neuronally relevant in that it guides and predicts neural activity in higher-order regions.

In contrast, neural activity in DLPFC and VMPFC cannot be explained on the basis of neural activity changes in a single lower-order region alone. The findings by Heekeren's group clearly exclude such scenarios when showing that neither FFA/PFG nor PPA/PHG signal changes alone can account for neural activity in VMPFC and DLPFC. This means that stimulus-based coding of neural activity in DLPFC and VMPFC is rather unlikely to determine the encoding in these higher-order regions.

The assumption of difference-based coding in DLPFC and VMPFC is further supported by the behavioral data. Neural activity in both regions, DLPFC and VMPFC, predicted the subsequent behavioral choices and thus decisions. This means that a difference-based signal predicts behavioral choices and preferences. Hence, difference-based coding is not only neuronally relevant but also behaviorally as mirrored in the prediction of decision preferences by difference-based signals.

Let's go back briefly to our initial example with the child. It is due to your difference-based activity in the DLPFC that you are able to make a decision about whether the child is yours. If, however, the differences generated in your sensory cortex, your FFA and your PPA, are too small to convey a signal that is large enough to induce proper neural activity in your left DLPFC, they may not provide you with a sufficiently distinct difference value to signal and predict a clear behavioral choice.

This is, for instance, the case when you are not sure anymore whether the child in question is your child. You are then unable to make a clear decision about how to proceed: do you leave your car window open to shout your child's name, or do you decide to silently pass by?

NEURONAL HYPOTHESIS VB: SPARSE CODING IN PREFRONTAL CORTEX

What about sparse coding on the regional level? While these findings support the assumption of difference-based coding on the regional level of neural activity, they themselves do not tell us anything about sparse coding. However, we saw that difference-based coding is closely tied to sparse coding on the single-cell and population level of neural activity (see Chapters 1 and 2). Since difference-based coding seems to clearly apply to the regional level of neural activity, one would postulate that sparse coding also holds on the level of regions.

Let's recall from the beginning of this chapter. In our initial empirical reflections, we characterized sparse coding by specific stimulus-to-region and region-to-region relationships. Many stimuli may recruit one particular region yielding many-to-one and thus sparse relationship between stimuli and regions. This may apply to lower-order sensory regions since they are directly exposed to stimuli, but it may not hold for higher-order regions like VMPFC and DLPFC that do not receive direct stimulus input. However, their stimulus input comes from other regions such as the FFA and the PPA. Hence, in their case the region-to-region relationship may be of central relevance.

The region-to-region relationship may be characterized in sparse coding by two features. First, as in the case of the stimulus-to-region relationship, there may be a many-to-one relationship. Many active lower-order sensory regions may, for instance, go along with a lower number of active higher-order cognitive regions such as the VMPFC and the DLPFC. This is indeed the case. In the studies by Heekeren, the activity in sensory regions such as the FFA/PFG and PPA/PHG converged in the activity of a single higher-order region, the DLPFC or the VMPFC. One may consecutively speak of a many-to-one relationship characterizing region-to-region relationship.

Second, sparse coding on the regional level also implies that only a low number of higher-order regions may be active when compared to the total number of regions that could possibly be activated. In our example, that means that the FFA alone could recruit a number of higher-order regions, including the DLPFC and many others (like the various regions in parietal, temporal, or prefrontal cortex). The same holds for the PPA as well as for the PFG and the PHG.

Neuronal hypothesis Vc: Temporal and spatial sparsening of neural activity on a regional level

How is such difference-based coding across different regions possible? One may postulate that this is possible because all these regions show structural connections with various regions throughout the whole cortex. In principle, the lower-order regions like FFA and PPA could possibly recruit a high number of available higher-order cognitive regions.

This, however, is apparently not the case because difference-based coding holds on a regional level of neural activity. Instead of recruiting many higher-order regions, the lower-order regions recruit only one higher-order region, the DLPFC or the VMPFC. Thus, the number of active higher-order regions is rather low when compared to the number of higher-order regions that could possibly be activated.

In sum, both criteria for sparse coding on a regional level, many-to-one relationship and low number of actually recruited regions, are fulfilled. One may consequently be inclined to speak of sparse coding on the regional level. This, however, must be considered a tentative hypothesis. One would need to apply quantitative measures of sparseness to the neural activities observed on the regional level. While this has been done on the level of single cells and population of cells (see Chapters 1 and 2), it remains to be investigated on the regional level of neural activity (see Wang et al. 2009 and Lee et al. 2011 for first steps in this direction).

More specifically, one would like to measure temporal and spatial sparsening. Temporal sparsening can be accounted for by the degree of "lifetime sparseness," the recruitment of a region across different discrete points in physical time (by the same and different stimuli). While spatial sparsening may be measured by the degree of "population sparseness," on the regional level, this may better be called "region sparseness" describing the relationship between active and total number of regions.

Besides applying quantitative measures of sparseness, one may also need to investigate different functions. I here demonstrated difference-based coding and sparse coding in the context of perceptual decision-making taking it as paradigmatic example. This, however, is only one function of many others such as attention, reward, perception, working memory, and so on. Hence, future studies may pool the imaging data from different functions and investigate their general regional activation pattern. I would suggest that the same kind of organizational principle; for example, sparse coding, predicts the various regional activation pattern across both the different regions/networks and the different functions.

Neuronal hypothesis VIa: Sparse coding on a regional level—"amplification hypothesis"

I provided evidence for both difference-based coding and sparse coding on the regional level of neural activity. The question now is how both are related to each other. We remember that on the single cell and population level, difference-based coding was postulated to be a necessary condition that first and foremost makes possible the spatial and temporal sparsening of neural activity, that is sparse coding. If so, one would suggest the same to hold on the regional level of neural activity too; that is, difference-based coding enables and drives sparse coding.

If sparse coding on the regional level does indeed presuppose difference-based coding, one would expect the following relationship: the higher for instance the degree of difference-based coding between lower-order sensory and higher-order cognitive regions, the lower number of higher-order regions like the DLPFC are recruited entailing higher degrees of sparseness. This suggests that the degree of spatial and temporal differences encoded into the regions neural activity via difference-based coding drives and predicts the degree of sparseness and thus the number of actually recruited regions. That is a clear hypothesis that can be tested experimentally in the future.

What are the neuronal mechanisms that link difference-based coding to sparse coding? We must consider the continuously ongoing generation of spatial and temporal differences in neural activity within and across the different regions. For instance, as we saw earlier, neural activity in the PHG and the PFG may most likely stem from the difference value between the positive signal changes related to the preferred stimulus and the negative signal changes associated with the non-preferred stimulus. This neuronal differences in PHG and PFG are then relayed to other regions such as the VMPFC: the difference constituting neuronal activity in PFG is compared and matched with the difference constituting neuronal activity in the PHG.

Such matching and comparison between different neuronal differences results in a novel neuronal difference that is manifest in the degree of neuronal activity change in the VMPFC. Accordingly, neuronal activity in the VMPFC is based on the neuronal difference (PHG-PFG) between the stimulus-based differences (face–house) in each region alone; that is, PFG and PHG, thus amounting to an integral of different difference values; for example, ([PHG (House–Face])—[PFG (Face–House]).

Since both stimulus-based and neuronal differences are not only relayed to other regions but apparently also amplified, I here propose what I describe as the "amplification hypothesis." The amplification hypothesis describes the continuous generation of novel neuronal differences between neural activities from different regions whose signals themselves are based on either stimulus-based or other neuronal differences. In short, I postulate continuous amplification of neuronal differences on the basis of stimulus-based and neuronal differences.

Neuronal hypothesis VB: Sparse coding on a regional level—Behavioral and phenomenal relevance of the "amplification hypothesis"

The amplification of neural activity across different regions throughout the whole brain is relevant in different ways. The amplification hypothesis is neuronally relevant because it describes the neuronal mechanisms how the regions' neural activity is generated. Moreover, as we have seen in the earlier described results, such amplification of neuronal and stimulus-based differences to other regions like the DLPFC or the VMPFC is essential for making proper behavioral choices and thus perceptually guided decisions. The amplification hypothesis is thus not only neuronally relevant but also behaviorally relevant.

Finally, the amplification hypothesis of neural activity may prove central for consciousness and thus be phenomenally relevant. The global distribution of neural activity is often considered central for consciousness, as is well reflected in the global workspace theories by Baars (2005, 2007) and Dehaene (Dehaene and Changeux 2011; also see Introduction I as well as Chapters 18 and 19 in Volume II for details).

Why, though, is such globalization of neural activity so central for consciousness? The degree of neuronal differences as suggested in the amplification hypothesis may predict the degree of consciousness that can be associated to the otherwise purely neuronal activity: the more neuronal differences are computed and processed throughout the whole brain in a globalized way, the higher the likelihood that sufficiently large neuronal differences are generated to associate consciousness with the newly resulting neuronal activity (see Chapters 28 and 29 for details).

Neuronal hypothesis VC: Sparse coding on a regional level—"condensation hypothesis"

What I describe as "amplification hypothesis" is based upon difference-based coding. Without the neural coding of stimulus-based or neuronal differences, the amplification of neural differences across different regions would be impossible. How though does the amplification of neuronal differences enable and promote the sparse recruitment of the regions' neural activity? For that we may need to complement the "amplification hypothesis" by yet another hypothesis, the "condensation hypothesis" as I call it.

The "condensation hypothesis" describes the concentration or condensation of neural activity in a few regions. By for instance processing and computing the difference value in neural activity between FFA and PPA, the DLPFC concentrates and ultimately condenses the neural activity of two regions into one region. Sparse recruitment of higher regions may thus be possible on the basis of condensing the neural activity from different lower-order regions (see also appendix 2 for the discussion of localizationism and holism).

Most important, such condensation of neural activity does not go along with a loss of information. Due to the generation and amplification of stimulus-based and neuronal differences, the information from the lower-order sensory regions is conveyed to and preserved in the neural activity of the higher-order cognitive region. The sparse recruitment of higher-order regions thus goes along with a maximum of preserved information. As on the level of single cells (see Chapter 1), one may therefore characterize sparse coding on the regional level as "economic or efficient coding."

This is well reflected in our example with the child. All the incoming sensory information about your child and his or her relation to the others is well preserved. If their sensory-based contrast and thus difference between the different children is large enough, you will be well able to make a decision as most likely predicted by the activity level of your left DLPFC.

In contrast, the activity level of your left DLPFC may be lower in the case of conflicting sensory evidence as it may be related to smaller stimulus-based differences in the lower sensory regions (Fig. 3-5. This is indeed empirically

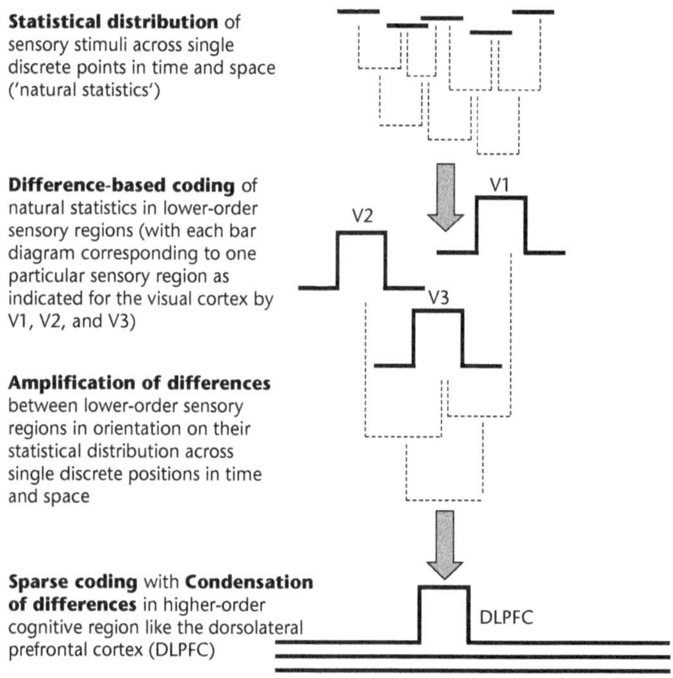

Figure 3-5 **Amplification and condensation hypothesis. The figure shows the relationship between lower and higher-order regions in decision-making. Based on its "natural statistics," that is, its statistical frequency distribution across different discrete points in physical time and space (*upper part*), the stimulus, based on difference-based coding, leads to stimulus-based differences with the subsequent activation in various sensory regions (*upper middle part*). The involvement of various sensory regions like V1, V2, and V3, in turn, implies the amplification of their stimulus-based and neuronal differences in the neural processing from lower-order sensory to higher-order cognitive regions (*lower middle part*). This results in the sparsening of neural activity; that is, condensation, in one particular higher-order region like the dorsolateral prefrontal cortex (DLPFC), while the other higher-order cognitive regions are not recruited (*lower part*). Hence, difference-based coding goes along with both amplification and condensation of stimulus-based and neuronal differences in the neural processing from lower to higher-order regions. This is what I describe as the "amplification and condensation hypothesis."**

supported by the data from Heekeren et al. (2004) in their perithreshold condition with low contrasts between the different sensory stimuli that were barely visible (see earlier).

Neuronal hypothesis Vd: Sparse coding on a regional level—behavioral and phenomenal relevance of the "condensation hypothesis"

Why is the condensation hypothesis relevant? I demonstrated the neuronal relevance of the condensation hypothesis in that condensation and thus sparsening of neural activity seems to determine the neural activity, in especially higher-order regions. And since these regions activities also predicted the subjects' behavioral choices, the condensation hypothesis must be assumed to be also behaviorally relevant.

Finally, like the amplification hypothesis, the condensation hypothesis may also turn out to be phenomenally relevant; that is for consciousness. For instance, patients with neuropsychiatric disorders like depression and schizophrenia show abnormal linkages between the different contents in their consciousness (see Chapters 22 and 27). How is such abnormal linkage between different contents in their consciousness possible? I postulate that it may, in part, be related to the abnormally increased or decreased condensation of stimulus-based and neuronal differences throughout the whole brain.

For instance, patients with schizophrenia show neuronally severe hypoactivity in left DLPFC, while behaviorally they can be characterized by high ambiguities in their decision-making. Based on the earlier described data by Heekeren and our condensation hypothesis, one may now hypothesize that the left DLPFC hypoactivity may in part be due to the inability of properly condensing stimulus-based and neuronal differences from lower-order sensory regions.

If the stimulus-based and neuronal differences from other regions can no longer be properly compared and matched with each other as to yield a novel neuronal difference, the activity level in left DLPFC will not change anymore. The resulting hypoactivity in left DLPFC may then prevent the subjects from proper decision-making as it is behaviorally manifested in their extreme ambiguity, while neuronally they seem to remain unable to condense neural activity.

Neuronal hypothesis Ve: Sparse coding on a regional level—local and dense neural coding as alternative options

Finally, one may also want to compare sparse coding on the regional level of neural activity with alternative forms of neural coding: dense coding and local coding (see Chapter 1). Let us imagine first how dense coding would like on the regional level of neural activity.

In the case of dense coding, one would propose a one-to-many relationship between lower-order sensory and higher-order cognitive regions, which would entail a rather high number of recruited higher-order regions. Neural activity in FFA and PPA should have been accompanied by the recruitment of many higher-order regions as in prefrontal, temporal, and parietal cortex. The empirical data showed the opposite, however, with activity changes occurring only in the left DLPFC as described earlier. Hence, the relationship between different regions may be characterized by sparse coding rather than dense coding.

How about local coding on the regional level of neural activity? Local coding implies a one-to-one relationship between lower-order sensory and higher-order cognitive regions. In such a case, the FFA should have been related to neural activity in one higher-order region, while the PPA would have been linked to another one.

This, again, was not the case in the empirical data since the neural activities of both regions converged in and predicted the activity level in the left DLPFC. Taken together, the empirical findings presented here make both dense coding and local coding unlikely candidates for the encoding of neural activity on a regional level.

Open Questions

> The first question pertains to the encoding of natural statistics as a central hallmark feature of sparse coding. Sparse coding on the cellular and population level focuses on the sensory cortex

and demonstrates the encoding of the statistical frequency distribution of the stimulus across different discrete points in physical time and space. If sparse coding holds on the level of regions, including non-sensory regions like the DLPFC and the VMPFC, the question for the encoding of statistical frequency distributions from other regions' neural activity; i.e., their regional or neuronal statistics as one may want to say, arises.

Alternatively, one could also propose that the encoding of the stimuli's natural statistics in sensory cortex is conveyed to the higher regions' neural activities which then would encode the lower-order regions' regional or neuronal statistics (and hence ultimately; that is, indirectly, the stimuli's natural statistics). Or one may deny altogether that the higher regions encode any statistical frequency distributions at all. In that case, one would suggest either local or dense coding rather than sparse coding, and possibly stimulus-based coding rather than difference-based coding. This, however, as we have seen earlier is empirically rather implausible. The second question focuses on neural inhibition. I demonstrated in Chapter 2 the central role of neural inhibition and GABAergic modulation in implementing sparse coding on a cellular and population level of neural activity. If now sparse coding is supposed to apply to the regional level of neural activity, too, one would postulate GABAergic-mediated neural inhibition to play a central role here. There is, however, not much human data available on the macroscopic effects of GABA on the regional distribution of neural activity (see Chapters 6 and 12 for more detailed discussion of the effects on GABA on regional activity levels).

This is even more important since psychiatric disorders like schizophrenia and depression show alterations in GABA-ergic mediated neural inhibition. Most interestingly, schizophrenic and depressed patients' symptoms can be alleviated almost immediately by the application of GABAergic agonists drugs like lorazepam (though only transiently) or glutamatergic antagonists drugs like ketamine. This suggests that GABAergic and glutamatergic mechanisms, and thus the excitation-inhibition balance, may indeed be central in yielding regional activation pattern as it is predicted by the assumption of sparse coding holding true on the regional level of neural activity.

PART II
Encoding Intrinsic Activity

General Background

Part I introduced sparse coding, which occurs when stimuli recruit and activate a lower number of neurons/regions (when compared to the number of stimuli and the total number of available neurons/regions) in the brain, entailing a many-to-one relationship between stimuli and neuron/regions. This distinguished sparse coding from other forms of neural coding like dense coding and local coding, where there is a one-to-many and one-to-one relationship between stimuli and neurons, respectively.

Such sparse coding allows for encoding the stimuli's statistical frequency distribution across time and space; that is, their natural statistics. This is possible only, as I hypothesize, if the neural activity encodes spatial and temporal differences between stimuli across their different discrete points in physical time and space rather than the stimuli themselves—what I describe as "difference-based coding" (as distinguished from "stimulus-based coding"). Difference-based coding and, consequently, sparse coding should hold true on the cellular and population levels as well as on the regional level of neural activity, where both forms of encoding may determine the distribution of neural activity across different regions in a sparse way.

Why does the brain employ difference-based coding (rather than stimulus-based coding) and, consequently, sparse coding (rather than dense or local coding) to encode the extrinsic stimuli from the environment (and body) into its neural activity? The employment of difference-based coding and sparse coding requires active involvement of the brain itself: The brain does not passively receive extrinsic stimuli from the environment (and body) and encode and process them in a one-to-one way, as proposed in stimulus-based coding and local coding. Instead, it actively "scans" the spatial and temporal differences between the different stimuli; that is, their statistical frequency distribution across the different discrete points in physical time and space, which are then encoded into cellular and regional levels of neural activity.

How can the brain actively "scan" and account for the spatial and temporal differences between the different stimuli at their different discrete points in physical space and time? The brain itself must possess some kind of intrinsic spatial and temporal measure against which it can compare and match the spatial and temporal differences between the different extrinsic stimuli from its environment (and body). In other words, there must be some kind of intrinsic spatial and temporal template in the brain itself.

Such an intrinsic spatial and temporal template may allow the brain to encode the extrinsic stimuli in terms of spatial and temporal differences rather than encoding the extrinsic stimuli themselves, including their different discrete points in physical time and space. Accordingly, the brain's intrinsic spatial and temporal template or grid may predispose the brain to employ difference-based coding (rather than stimulus-based coding) and sparse coding (rather than local or dense coding) during the encoding of extrinsic stimuli. Where does such an intrinsic spatial and temporal template or grid come from? The famous German philosopher Immanuel Kant proposed in the eighteenth century that such an intrinsic spatial and temporal grid for the processing of extrinsic stimuli is constructed by our mind and its cognitive capacities, like reason and understanding (see Kant 1998, as well as Appendix 3 herein, Appendix 3 in Volume II, and Northoff 2012a and 2012b). Since then, there has been much discussion and speculation in philosophy and psychology about the existence of some kind of mind and how it operates and processes extrinsic stimuli. This is well reflected in the current disciplines of philosophy of mind and cognitive psychology/sciences.

Nowadays, however, we know better. What the earlier (and also current) philosophers attributed to the mind may rather be related to the brain. We may thus need to search for the spatial and temporal "template" or "grid" in the brain itself (rather than outside the brain in some kind of "mind"). More specifically, the spatial and temporal template or grid may be an intrinsic feature of the brain itself.

What is an "intrinsic feature"? An intrinsic feature defines and determines the brain *qua* brain by making possible its neural activity and the various functions of the brain. Most importantly, such intrinsic features distinguish the brain from other organs of the body (like the heart, kidney, pancreas, etc.) (see Epilog in this volume as well as Introductions I and II in Volume II for further determination of extrinsic versus intrinsic features of the brain). Withholding further conceptual discussion, I now suggest that the brain's spatial and temporal template is such an intrinsic feature, without which the brain would encode and generate its neural activity in a completely different way.

How can the brain itself generate such spatial and temporal template or grid? To find the answer, we need to consider the brain's intrinsic activity, the neural activity that the brain generates by itself. Such intrinsic activity, which is also called "resting-state activity" (see the beginning of Chapter 4 for conceptual clarification), must be distinguished from extrinsic activity, stimulus-induced activity, which is induced in the brain by extrinsic stimuli from outside the brain, i.e., from environment and body. To understand why and how the brain's employs difference-based coding and sparse coding to achieve the encoding of its own neural activity, we must therefore understand the brain's intrinsic activity and how it encodes changes in its own activity level during either spontaneous resting-state changes or extrinsic stimuli.

The aim of Part II is to understand the brain's intrinsic activity; that, its resting-state activity, and how it constructs its own intrinsic spatial and temporal template or grid. Most importantly, we want to reveal the exact neuronal details of that intrinsic spatial and temporal template or grid in order to understand how it predisposes the brain to employ difference-based coding (rather than stimulus-based coding) and sparse coding (rather than dense or local coding) during the encoding and generation of its neural activity. In a nutshell, I propose that the brain's intrinsic activity and its spatial and temporal template predispose it to use difference-based coding and consequently sparse coding.

General Overview

Chapter 4 discusses the basic anatomical structure of the brain and investigates how that translates into function, and ultimately into the brain's intrinsic activity. I demonstrate that such a structure–function transition is possible only by applying difference-based coding to the brain's own intrinsic activity. This means that difference-based coding may apply not only to the encoding of extrinsic stimuli into neural activity, but also to the encoding of the brain's own activity, its intrinsic activity. Such difference-based coding in turn is supposed to make possible the construction of a particular spatial structure that operates across and thus supersedes the brain's anatomical structures.

Chapter 5 investigates the temporal features of the brain's intrinsic activity. Here we will consider neuronal measures of neural activity like functional connectivity and frequency fluctuations, which, as I demonstrate, are inherently temporal. Presupposing again the encoding of the brain's intrinsic activity in terms of difference-based coding, these neuronal measures constitute a particular temporal structure that supersedes and operates across the physical time constraints given by the neurons' and the regions' biophysical-computational features.

Finally, Chapter 6 discusses how neural inhibition as mediated by GABA is central for enabling difference-based coding of the brain's intrinsic activity. This, in turn, provides the means for the brain's intrinsic activity to encode its own intrinsic activity and its rest–rest interactions in a sparse way, resulting in sparse coding of the brain's intrinsic activity itself.

In sum, I postulate that difference-based coding and sparse coding already apply to the brain's intrinsic activity itself. The use of difference-based coding and sparse coding predisposes the brain's intrinsic activity to construct a spatial and temporal structure that supersedes and operates across its anatomical and biophysical-computational features. We will see later that this spatial and temporal structure of the brain's intrinsic activity will prove central in encoding extrinsic stimuli into neural activity (see Chapters 11 and 12).

In other words, the construction of such spatial and temporal structure has major ramifications for any kind of subsequent neuronal processing and encoding, including the generation of stimulus-induced activity. This will be the focus in parts III and IV in this volume where we will demonstrate the neuronal and behavioral relevance of the spatial and temporal structure of the brain's intrinsic activity.

In addition to its neuronal and behavioral relevance, I will argue that the spatial and temporal structure of the brain's intrinsic activity is central also for consciousness with phenomenal relevance. By applying difference-based coding and sparse coding, I propose that the intrinsic activity and its spatial and temporal structure makes possible and necessary the association of consciousness and its phenomenal features to the otherwise purely neuronal activity during either the resting-state (as in dreams; see Chapters 25 and 26) or stimulus-induced activity (see Chapters 28 and 29) (see also Northoff 2013).

Finally, it will turn out that the brain's intrinsic activity and its spatial and temporal structure may be abnormally altered and thus dysfunctional in psychiatric disorders like schizophrenia and depression (see Chapters 22 and 27). Recent findings in these disorders indicate abnormal resting-state activity whose spatial and temporal structure may therefore be dysfunctional by providing the "wrong" kind of spatial and temporal template or grid for the subsequent encoding of extrinsic stimuli from environment and body. We will see in Volume II that such a hypothesis is indeed supported by both the neuronal findings and the observed psychopathological symptoms (see Chapters 22 and 27). Accordingly, taken together, these findings indicate that the intrinsic activity and its spatial and temporal structure are not only neuronally and behaviorally relevant, as discussed in this volume, but also phenomenally and psychiatrically relevant, as will be revealed in Volume II.

CHAPTER 4
Spatial Structure of Intrinsic Activity

Summary

We now switch from the brain's extrinsic activity, i.e., stimulus-induced activity, as discussed in the first part on sparse coding, to the brain's intrinsic activity, the activity that the brain generates by itself and that stems from inside the brain. The brain's intrinsic activity is very much based on its anatomical structure. As an alternative to the traditional medial-lateral and subcortical-cortical distinction, I here, based on neuroanatomical data, suggest a threefold anatomical structure. This threefold anatomical structure has three rings—inner, middle, and outer—that extend and span from the subcortical to the cortical regions. The inner ring (limbic and paralimbic ring) is characterized by continuous interoceptive input from the body, while the outer ring (lateral cortical and sensorimotor regions) receives continuously unspecific exteroceptive inputs. Based on their different inputs, I associate different levels of resting-state activity with inner and outer rings and speak consequently of an "interoceptive baseline" (inner ring, interoceptive) and "exteroceptive baseline" (outer ring, exteroceptive). How about the third ring, the middle ring? The middle ring (subcortical and cortical midline regions) does not receive direct inputs from outside the brain (from either the body or its environment) and may therefore mirror the brain's intrinsic activity the most closely; that is, the neural stimuli, so that, analogous to the other two baselines, I here speak of a "neural baseline." How are these three anatomical-structurally defined rings related to each other on the functional level of the resting-state activity? Rather than operating in a parallel and segregated fashion, I suggest that the different baselines directly interact and balance each other on the functional level of neural activity in an interactive-integrative way. This is possible, however, I propose, only on the basis of difference-based coding that allows the encoding of the neural differences between the three rings and their respective levels of resting-state activity. Such a difference-based coding of the brain's intrinsic activity leads, in turn, to the constitution of a spatial structure on the functional level of the resting-state activity that supersedes and operates across the underlying anatomical structures; that is, the three rings.

Key Concepts and Topics Covered

Anatomical structure, medial-lateral, subcortical-cortical, three rings, resting-state, baseline, intrinsic activity, default-mode network, midline regions, difference-based coding, spatial structure

NEUROEMPIRICAL BACKGROUND I: BRAIN-BASED ACCOUNT OF THE SPATIAL AND TEMPORAL TEMPLATE

Part I focused on the encoding of extrinsic stimuli into neural activity by the brain. I proposed the brain to encode extrinsic stimuli from the environment (and the body) into its neural activity in a sparse way, which implies a many-to-one relationship between stimuli and neural activity. Such sparse coding, however, is possible only on the basis of difference-based coding as distinguished from stimulus-based coding. In other words, sparse coding presupposes difference-based coding.

One may now want back up one more step and raise the following question: How and why does the brain employ difference-based coding rather than stimulus-based coding in its encoding of extrinsic stimuli into neural activity? We saw in Part I that difference-based coding can be described by the encoding of spatial and temporal differences between the different discrete points in physical space and time associated with the extrinsic stimuli. This means that the stimuli themselves and their respective discrete points in physical time and space are not encoded into neural activity in an isolated and independent way, as would be the case in stimulus-based coding.

How is it possible that the brain itself extracts and encodes temporal and spatial differences between different stimuli rather than the stimuli themselves and their respective discrete points in physical time and space? For that, I hypothesize, the brain must itself provide some kind of intrinsic spatial and temporal template or grid against which the spatial and temporal differences of the extrinsic stimuli can be measured, extracted, computed, and encoded into neural activity.

Where can we find such a spatial and temporal template? Philosophers such as Immanuel Kant long assumed such a spatial and temporal template to be "located" in some kind of "mind." One may want to speak here of a "mind-based account." This, however, has changed in the last 30 or 40 years, when cognitive functions have been explored which are now suggested to provide the kind of spatial and temporal blueprint we are looking for. Such a cognition-based account is the predominant view of many, if not most, of the current philosophers, psychologists, and neuroscientists.

I deviate from both mind- and cognition-based accounts when I postulate that the brain itself and its intrinsic activity themselves construct the spatial and temporal template. Rather than embracing either a mind- or cognition-based account of the spatial and temporal template, I here opt for a brain-based account (see Appendix 3 for details of such a brain-based account). This shifts the empirical focus from the encoding of extrinsic stimuli into the brain's neural activity, as dealt with in Part I, to the brain itself and its intrinsic activity. This is our focus next.

Neuroconceptual prelude Ia: concept of "intrinsic activity"

Before going ahead with the detailed empirical findings, we need to make some conceptual clarification about the terms "intrinsic activity," "resting-state," and "baseline." Therefore I start this chapter with three short neuroconceptual remarks.

Let's start with the concept of intrinsic activity. Intrinsic activity must be distinguished from extrinsic activity; the concept of *intrinsic* refers to the brain itself as distinguished from the body and environment, which are *extrinsic* to the brain. Hence, when describing the brain by its intrinsic activity, we refer to the origin of the activity that is to be traced back to the brain itself. Accordingly, the concept of intrinsic activity refers only and exclusively to the origin of the stimuli and thus to the brain itself.

Such a neural origin of the brain's neural activity must be distinguished from the bodily or environmental origins of the brain's neural activity during the neural processing of intero- and exteroceptive stimuli. If the origin of neural activity in the brain stems from outside the brain; that is, from the body and environment, one may speak of "extrinsic activity" (see Fig. 4-1).

One may now want to argue that there is no purely intrinsic activity in the brain. This may be so since any activity is always already confounded by the unspecific intero- and exteroceptive inputs from body and environment that can never be shut off completely. One may thus propose that the brain's intrinsic activity is not purely intrinsic, but represents rather a mixture of both intrinsic and extrinsic activity.

This, however, should not deter us from searching for approximations where the brain's neural activity comes closest to a state of pure intrinsic activity. As we will see later, the default-mode network (DMN) may be an instance where there seems to be a high degree of intrinsic activity while the degree of extrinsic activity seems to be rather low.

Accordingly, when we speak of "intrinsic" activity, we refer to a certain balance between

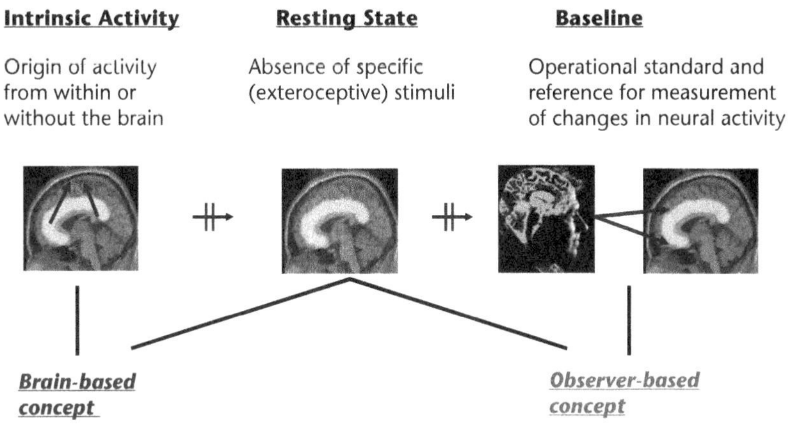

Figure 4-1 **Concepts of intrinsic activity, resting-state, and baseline. The figure illustrates the three concepts of intrinsic activity, resting-state activity, and baseline. The concept of intrinsic activity regards the origin of neural activity in the brain that may stem from either inside of the brain (i.e., intrinsic) or outside the brain (i.e., extrinsic). The concept of the resting-state refers to the absence of specific exteroceptive stimuli, as this proposes the brain to be in rest with regard to exteroceptive stimuli. This concept is somehow paradoxical since there is no real "rest" in the brain, which shows ongoing and continuous activity even in the supposedly resting-state. The resting-state is tested experimentally by closing the eyes, indicating the absence of visual stimuli. The concept of the baseline describes a standard for measuring neural activity changes in the brain as, for instance, induced by stimuli. As such, the concept of baseline is a purely operational concept used for experimental purposes. That implies that it is strongly related to the observer and his or her way of experimental measurement rather than the brain itself for which the concept of intrinsic activity seems to be more paradigmatic.**

neural activities stemming from sources both intrinsic and extrinsic to the brain. This is the way I understand and use the concept of intrinsic activity in the following discussion.

Neuroconceptual prelude Ib: concept of "resting state"

While the concept of intrinsic activity describes the origin of neural activity within the brain, the term *resting-state activity* refers to the (presence or) absence of specific stimuli. Specific bodily (i.e., interoceptive) and environmental (i.e., exteroceptive) stimuli may be either present, in which case one speaks of stimulus-induced activity, or any specific stimuli may be absent, in which case, at least operationally, one speaks of resting-state activity (see Northoff et al. 2010a and b, Logothetis et al. 2009, Duncan and Northoff 2012). Experimentally, resting-state activity in this sense is probed by measuring neural activity while the subject's eyes are closed.

The concept of resting-state activity suggests by its very definition that the brain is at rest. That, however, is not true. There is the brain's intrinsic activity, which is continuously present as sketched above. And there is the continuous unspecific intero- and exteroceptive input from both body and environment that cannot be eliminated completely, even with eyes closed. Neither the continuous interoceptive input from the body nor the continuous unspecific exteroceptive input from the senses (other than the visual) that remain "open" (the auditory and all other senses) can be shut off completely in the resting state.

On whole, this implies that the term "resting state" is somewhat paradoxical. The concept of "rest" implies that the brain does not do anything and is completely inactive. That however, as shown, is not true. The opposite holds; namely, that the brain is continuously active and is continuously encoding changes into its own neural activity with the changes being related either to the intrinsic or to the extrinsic activity.

The brain itself, and its continuous encoding and generation of neural activity changes, thus seems to defy the concept of resting-state that we observers apply to experimentally investigate its different forms of neural activity. We should be careful, however. The term "resting state" makes more sense once we consider it in the context of our observation. All we can do experimentally is to eliminate specific sensory inputs so that, from our experimental perspective as observers, the state of the brain comes maximally close to a pure and real resting-state. The term "resting state" thus stands between the brain itself and our observation of it; it may therefore be regarded as both a brain- and an observer-based concept.

Neuroconceptual prelude Ic: concept of "baseline"

Finally, both concepts, intrinsic activity and resting-state activity, need to be distinguished from that of "the baseline." The concept of the baseline refers neither to a specific origin (like the concepts of intrinsic and extrinsic activity) nor to the absence or presence of specific stimuli (like the concept of resting-state). Instead, the term "baseline" pertains very much to the way we as observers can observe and investigate the brain's intrinsic activity or resting-state activity.

We conduct our experiments by applying specific stimuli or tasks and investigating their effects (i.e., stimulus-induced or task-related activity). To calculate the degree of activity change the stimuli or task elicit in the brain, we need to set them against a specific standard or measure. This standard or measure is the brain's *baseline*, which often is cancelled out and neglected in the analysis of imaging data (see Raichle et al. 2001; Raichle 2010; Morcom and Fletcher 2007a and 2007b).

Accordingly, the term "baseline" refers to a standard or reference for our measurement of neural activity changes. As such, it is related only to the observer and thus to us, rather than to the brain itself, independent of any observers. I consequently characterize the term "baseline" as an *observer-based* concept (as distinguished from a *brain-based* concept).

After shedding some light on the concepts of "intrinsic activity," "resting state," and "baseline," we are now ready to further investigate how the brain encodes and generates its own intrinsic activity and thereby constitutes a spatial template.

Neuroanatomical background Ia: medial-lateral distinction versus radial-concentric organization

The brain can be characterized by different regions, such as, for instance, the cortical and subcortical regions, which are also connected to each other by various tracts and fibers. This is the anatomy of the brain; its anatomical structure. The anatomical structure describes the organization of regions and connections across the whole physical space of the brain; that is, its different regions and their connections. Any intrinsic activity in the brain, i.e., its resting-state activity, can only arise on the basis of the brain's anatomical structure. In short, function is based on structure. Before considering the brain's intrinsic activity by itself, its resting-state activity, we will therefore discuss the brain's anatomical structure.

How can one describe the anatomical structure of the brain? Traditionally, the brain is divided into medial and lateral parts as well as into subcortical and cortical regions. Such a medial-lateral and subcortical-cortical distinction is mainly based on how the observer considers the brain from the outside as he views its anatomical structure. From the outside of the brain, as observed by us, the brain can be divided into medial and lateral parts as well as into subcortical and cortical regions. This led to the medial-lateral and subcortical-cortical distinctions as they are commonly employed in neuroanatomy in particular and neuroscience in general.

However, the traditional subcortical-cortical distinction especially has been called into doubt by the Dutch neuroanatomist Nieuwenhuys, who suggested integrated subcortical-cortical systems. And he also refined the medial-lateral distinction into a threefold ring-like (inner, middle, outer) distinction. Rather than distinguishing between medial and lateral parts of the brain, he characterizes the brain anatomically by three different rings that, like the different layers of an onion, form a radial-concentric organization.

How is such a radial-concentric organization of the brain's anatomy related to its intrinsic activity and its spatial pattern? I suggest that the spatial organization of the brain's intrinsic activity follows the radial-concentric organization of its underlying anatomy. Accordingly, in order to understand the spatial patterns of the brain's intrinsic activity, we need to shed some light on the radial-concentric organization of its anatomy. This is the focus in the next sections.

Neuroanatomical background Ib: radial-concentric organization on the subcortical level

Let's start with the subcortical regions. Nieuwenhuys proposed a radial-concentric organization in subcortical regions; these are located concentrically or radially around the aqueduct and extend progressively from medial to lateral locations (Nieuwenhuys 1996, 1999; Nieuwenhuys et al. 1988/1989). Based on various features (see below), he distinguished the subcortical regions into three distinct territories: core, paracore (including median and lateral paracore territories), and lateral regions, which, despite being closely interconnected, can be distinguished from each other on anatomical-structural grounds.

How can we assign such a radial-concentric organization to concrete anatomical regions and nuclei in subcortical regions? "Core subcortical regions" refers to the regions that are located in direct proximity to the aqueduct (third ventricle) and may thus be described as "paraventricular" or "periaqueductal." These subcortical regions include the periaquaductal gray (PAG), the pontine central gray, the medial hypothalamus, the septum, the parabrachial nuclei, and the dorsal vagal complex.

How about the middle ring, the paracore, on the subcortical level? The subcortical paracore regions are located directly adjacent to the core regions, where one may distinguish between median and lateral paracore regions. Subcortical median paracore regions include the raphe nuclei, the lateral hypothalamus, and the bed nucleus of the stria terminalis. These are closely connected to the bilateral paracore regions that include the ventral tegmental area (VTA), the locus coeruleus, the substantia nigra, and the nucleus reticularis.

How about the third ring in the subcortical territory? There is a subcortical territory lateral to the paracore and its median and lateral regions. This most lateral territory is described by Nieuwenhuys as "lateral regions"; these include mainly the ascending and descending sensory and motor tracts. In addition to its anatomical-structural features, the subcortical radial-concentric organization can also be characterized by biochemical and functional features that distinguish the three rings (core, paracore, lateral) in analogous ways. The inner and middle rings (core and paracore regions) can be distinguished from the outer (lateral-peripheral) ring with respect to their fibers (myelinated or unmyelinated); biogenic amines (serotonin, noradrenaline/adrenaline, dopamine, histamine); circumventricular organs, gonado-steroid receptors, and coherent behavior (as induced by localized electrical stimulation of the brain) (see Nieuwenhuys 1996, pp. 560–567; Feinberg 2009; for details).

How can we distinguish the three subcortical divisions in functional terms; for example, by the stimuli they process? According to Niewenhuys and coworkers, the core and paracore regions are functionally characterized by their predominant involvement in processing interoceptive stimuli and regulating the body's homeostatic milieu, vegetative-autonomic functions, and a variety of specific emotional and motivational processes. In contrast, the most lateral or peripheral subcortical ring is rather involved in the processing of exteroceptive and sensorimotor stimuli (see also Northoff et al. 2011, and Feinberg 2009 and 2011 for more details).

Neuroanatomical background Ic: inner and outer rings in the radial-concentric organization on the cortical level

How is such a radial-concentric organization of the subcortical regions into three rings related to higher regions and ultimately the cortex? Taking MacLean's and Nauta's concept of the limbic system (and midline system) as a starting point, Nieuwenhuys (1996, 2011, 2012) proposes the subcortical core-paracore system to extend into the mesencephalon and diencephalon, where it is closely connected to the hypothalamus and various regions in the forebrain, including the amygdala, septum, hippocampus, and parahippocampal gyrus.

This led to the concept of the "greater, distributed or extended limbic system" (de Olmos and Heimer 1999; Heimer 2003; Morgane et al. 2005; Morgane and Mokler 2006). Todd Feinberg (2009, 2011) takes this one step further, and proposes the radial-concentric organization to also hold on the level of the cortex; he consecutively suggests the three subcortical rings to extend and continue to the cortex, where he distinguishes three corresponding cortical rings.

The first cortical ring is the inner ring at the most medial location directly adjacent to the first and second ventricle. The cortical inner ring includes paralimbic areas that comprise the lower parts of the orbitofrontal cortex, the perigenual and supragenual anterior cingulate cortex (PACC, SACC), the posterior cingulate cortex (PCC), the retrosplenial cortex (RSC), the temporal pole, and the insula (see Nieuwenhuys 2012 for a recent paper specifically on the anatomy of the insula). The inner ring on the cortical level must be considered an extension of the subcortical inner ring and its core regions, as described earlier.

Both cortical and subcortical inner ring regions are closely connected to each other and can thus be proposed to form some kind of functional unity (see below). More specifically, the cortical regions of the inner ring, like the anterior cingulate (PACC, SACC, PCC), the caudal orbitofrontal cortex, the temporal poles, and the insula, are characterized by strong inputs from especially the subcortical core regions like the PAG (see Nieuwenhuys 1996, 573). Due to their tight and close connections, he postulates the cortical inner ring regions to continue and extend the predominant processing of interoceptive stimuli from the body as conveyed from the subcortical core regions.

Another cortical ring is the outer ring that is located most laterally at the outer surface of the brain. This includes the sensory cortex, the motor cortex, and lateral cortical regions like the lateral prefrontal, parietal, and occipital cortex. Such an outer ring on the cortical level must be considered an extension of the lateral regions subcortically. Hence, both subcortical and cortical outer rings do predominantly process exteroceptive stimuli from and to the environment, thus concerning the diverse sensory and motor stimuli.

Neuroanatomical background Id: Middle ring in the radial-concentric organization on the cortical level

Finally, there is also a middle ring on the cortical level that is sandwiched between inner and outer rings and must be considered an extension from the subcortical median and lateral paracore regions. The middle ring includes regions like the medial orbitofrontal cortex, the ventromedial and dorsomedial prefrontal cortex (VMPFC, DMPFC), and the medial parietal cortex (MPC), which have recently been subsumed under the concept of *cortical midline structures* (CMSs) (Northoff and Bermpohl 2004 Northoff et al. 2006).The VMPFC and the DMPFC receive, for instance, strong input from especially the raphe nuclei as median paracore regions, and the locus coeruleus as lateral paracore regions (Morgane et al. 2005; Nieuwenhuys 1996). Therefore, subcortical and cortical middle rings are closely linked and must therefore be considered a functional unity.

In contrast to the inner and outer rings, the middle ring does not receive any direct input from either the body or the environment and may therefore predominantly integrate intero- and exteroceptive stimuli as processed in the other two rings. For instance, Feinberg (2009) proposes the middle ring to account for intero-exteroceptive integration, which ultimately constitutes what he describes as "integrative self-system" (see Volume II, Part VII, for the discussion of the self in the context of the cortical midline structures).

Taken together, the traditional medial-lateral twofold anatomical dichotomy is here challenged by a threefold anatomical distinction between three different concentric rings, inner, middle, and outer, that extend from subcortical to cortical regions. On the cortical level, these three rings can be characterized as paralimbic (inner ring), heteromodal/CMS midline (middle ring), and exterosensorimotor/lateral association (outer ring).

Subcortically, the three rings correspond to the distinction between core, median/lateral paracore, and lateral subcortical regions. Due to the strong connections between subcortical and cortical regions within each ring, inner, middle, and outer rings must be considered to be three distinct anatomical-structural and functional unities (see Fig. 4-2).

The question now is how this anatomical structure translates into the brain's resting-state activity and its pattern and distribution across the different regions and rings of the brain, thereby constituting the resting-state's spatial structure. For that, I now consider recent findings from the imaging of the brain's resting-state; that is, its intrinsic activity (see below for conceptual clarification of both terms).

Neuronal Findings IA: Neural Activity in the Resting State during Eyes Closed and Open—Initial Findings

How does the radial-concentric anatomical-structural organization translate into the brain's intrinsic activity? For that answer, we may need to investigate the brain in what is called the

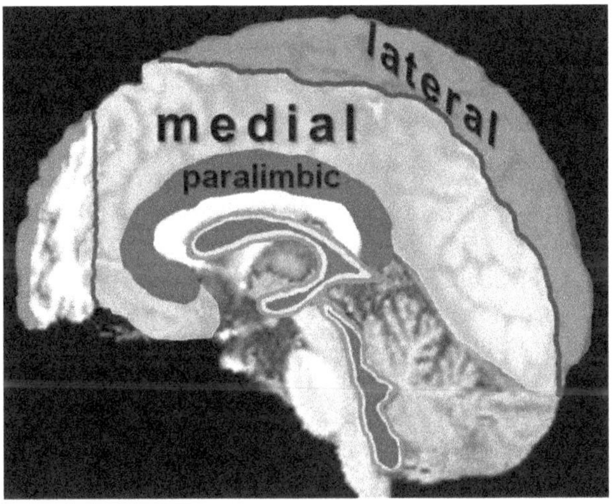

Figure 4-2 Radial concentric anatomo-spatial organization in subcortical and cortical regions. The figure illustrates the three different rings in the anatomical organization of subcortical and cortical regions. The inner ring is marked in grey and describes the core-paralimbic system located adjacent to the ventricles (marked in dark grey) on both levels subcortical and cortical. The middle ring is marked in dark white (and signed as medial on the cortical level) and describes the paracore-midline system located adjacent to the inner ring on both subcortical and cortical levels. Finally, the outer ring concerns the most lateral regions (lateral-lateral system) and is marked in lighter grey (and signed by lateral on the cortical level) on both levels subcortical and cortical. The threefold ring-based radial anatomical organization is supposed to replace the twofold medial-lateral dichotomy, which concerns only the cortex rather than, as the former, integrating subcortical and cortical regions into an anatomical continuum. The exact assignment of the different subcortical and cortical regions to the three different rings is discussed in the text.

"resting state," the absence of any specific stimuli from the environment (see below for more detailed conceptual clarification). The standard and operationalized way of doing this experimentally is to close your eyes and to compare that neural activity with what you can observe when opening your eyes (see also Logothetis et al. 2009, as well as Duncan and Northoff 2012). I therefore describe some (of the many) recent imaging results on the neural effects of closing and opening the eyes while the subjects are otherwise at rest.

Marx et al. (2004) compared the fixation of a light-emitting diode with eyes closed. Open eyes with fixation yielded increased signal changes in the lateral orbitofrontal cortex, the lateral and medial prefrontal cortex, the inferior parietal lobule, the dorsal thalamus, the putamen, the caudate, and the globus pallidus, when compared to closed eyes. However, decreased signal changes were observed in visual (that is, primary, secondary, and tertiary), somatosensory, acoustic, and vestibular areas, meaning that signal changes in the regions were reduced when opening the eyes and fixating on the stimulus (i.e., the light-emitting diode). The authors also investigated two further conditions, eyes open in a dark room and eyes open in an illuminated room while no fixation was required. These two conditions led to signal changes in predominantly visual areas when compared to each other, as well as to eyes open with fixation, and eyes closed.

Another study by McAvoy et al. (2008) also compared the neuronal differences between eyes open and closed in functional magnetic resonance imaging (fMRI). They observed that the BOLD spectral density and thus the BOLD oscillations were mostly modulated in visual (primary, secondary, and tertiary), auditory, sensory-motor, and retrosplenial cortex when switching from eyes closed to eyes open. Using a 7 Tesla scanner,, Bianciardi et al. (2009) observed that spontaneous activity (as distinct from evoked activity) in visual areas was significantly reduced (that is, up to 44% in amplitude and 25% in coherence) in the eyes-open and fixating condition, compared to the eyes-closed condition.

Neuronal findings Ib: neural activity in the resting state during eyes closed and open—recent findings

A study in our group (Qin et al. 2013) also investigated the change in activation pattern during the transition from eyes closed to eyes open. In addition to the visual cortex, the bilateral auditory cortex was also activated more strongly during eyes open when compared to eyes closed. Hence, the unspecific visual input during eyes open exerted also a cross-modal effect on the auditory cortex and its specific resting-state activity level.

The involvement of the auditory cortex was also confirmed in another study by Qin et al. (2013). He compared auditory cortical activity during the presence and absence of the fMRI noise using a special acquisition technique called "sparse sampling." This allowed him to observe the auditory cortex in a true resting state; that is, absence of "scanner noise," even in fMRI.

In a next step, he investigated how such a resting-state activity in the auditory cortex is modulated by opening and closing the eyes: eyes open leads to considerable activity increases in the auditory cortical activity and concurrent changes in visual-auditory cortical connectivity. These data further support the assumption of cross-modal effects between, for instance, visual and auditory cortex being already present in the resting-state.

Another recent study by Jao et al. (2013) observed a decrease in various dynamic measures of brain function during eyes open in different regions, including the visual cortex, other sensory cortices, medial and lateral cortical regions, and subcortical regions like the thalamus. For instance, the degrees of functional connectivity, signal variability, and amplitude of low frequency fluctuations decreased during eyes open when compared to eyes closed.

Taken together, these results (and others not detailed here, also using EEG in addition to fMRI; see Chapter 5 for the EEG results) show clear neuronal differences between eyes open and eyes closed. As expected, the data show neural activity differences, mainly in the visual cortex, but also in various other subcortical and cortical regions, which, following the results, concerned especially lateral prefrontal and parietal regions in the outer ring (see later for discussion of the inner and middle rings' regions during eyes open and closed).

NEURONAL HYPOTHESIS IA: SHIFT FROM EYES CLOSED TO EYES OPEN AS SHIFT FROM INNER TO OUTER RING

I distinguished three different subcortical-cortical rings on neuroanatomical grounds. Thereby the outer ring on the cortical level concerned especially sensorimotor and lateral frontal and parietal regions, whereas the inner ring concerned mainly cortical midline and limbic regions. The question now is whether, and if so, how, such a radial-concentric anatomical structure is mirrored on the functional level of the brain's intrinsic activity; that is, its resting-state activity.

Since it concerns exteroceptive input, one would expect the difference between eyes open and closed to induce neural activity changes, predominantly in the regions of the outer ring like the sensory cortex and the lateral frontal cortex. This was indeed the case in various neuronal measures like signal variability, functional connectivity, and amplitude of low frequency fluctuations, as the aforementioned results show.

The sensory regions included not only the visual cortex but also other sensory regions such a as the auditory and somatosensory cortex. In addition, lateral cortical regions like the lateral prefrontal and parietal cortices also changed their neural activity during the transition from eyes closed to eyes open (see the next section for the involvement of midline regions in eyes closed and open).

The observed activity pattern during the transition from eyes closed to open is well in accordance with the neuroanatomical assumption of an outer ring. The regions activated during the shift from eyes closed to open, the sensory cortices and the lateral cortical regions (as well as the lateral subcortical regions), conform (more or less) to the regions that form the outer ring on anatomical-structural grounds. This means that there seems to be some kind of relationship between the anatomical-structural organization and the functional level of the resting state activity.

NEURONAL HYPOTHESIS IB: "INTERO- AND EXTEROCEPTIVE STATES" DURING EYES CLOSED AND OPEN

How can we specify the link between anatomical-structural organization and the functional level of the resting-state activity? On the basis of their results (see earlier), Marx et al. (2004) propose an "interoceptive state" of the brain when the eyes are closed and the person is at rest. Closing the eyes means that the visual (and in an ideal case, all sensory and thus exteroceptive) inputs are prevented from entering and modulating the brain's activity.

The only input the brain receives here is the interoceptive input from the body. Hence, if we subtract the neural activity induced by the external or exteroceptive sensory input during eyes open from the one during eyes closed, the brain's activity related to interoceptive stimuli may surface in the "interoceptive state" of the brain (see also Chang et al. 2013 for a recent study on the dependence of the resting-state functional connectivity on the heart rate variability, thus further supporting the assumption of an interoceptive state in resting-state activity).

How can we characterize such an "interoceptive state" during the brain's resting-state activity? The "interoceptive state" of the brain can be characterized functionally by the predominance of interoceptive input into the neural activity of the brain. This is operationalized and tested experimentally by closing the eyes. Accordingly, we seem to tap into a predominant "interoceptive state" when we measure neural activity during eyes closed.

If, in contrast, the exteroceptive input dominates the neural activity of the brain during the supposed resting-state as it does during eyes open, one may speak, analogously, of an "exteroceptive state." Note that the person is still at rest (by definition) since the person does not need to process specific stimuli or tasks (see earlier for more detailed explanation of the concept of "resting-state"). In a nutshell, I suppose eyes closed to reflect an "interoceptive state" while eyes open leads to an "exteroceptive state."

Neuronal hypothesis Ic: outer ring and the "exteroceptive baseline" of the resting-state activity

How can we now further specify both "intero- and exteroceptive states of the brain"? These are states of the brain when the person is at rest, meaning that the subject does not need to do anything actively by himself, such as processing particular stimuli or performing specific tasks (motor, sensory, cognitive, social). If during such a resting state, i.e., the absence of specific stimuli or tasks, the unspecific interoceptive input (from the body) dominates, one can speak of an "interoceptive state of the brain." If, in contrast, the exteroceptive input (from the environment) predominates, the brain is rather in an "exteroceptive state" with only unspecific but no specific exteroceptive input.

What is the functional role of such a "exteroceptive state of the brain" and its unspecific exteroceptive input? Barry et al. (2007) propose that the processing of such a unspecific visual input (as during eyes open) prepares and activates the visual cortex (and other sensory cortices) for the subsequent processing of more specific visual (and other sensory) inputs. Thereby the unspecific visual input sets a baseline neural activity into motion that serves as threshold for the subsequent processing of the more specific visual stimuli.

Barry et al. (2007) consequently speak of what they describe as an "activation baseline." The concept of the "activation baseline" describes the recruitment of neural activity especially in sensory cortex by unspecific exteroceptive; that is, sensory, stimuli that activate the respective regions. This is the level of activation in especially the sensory cortical regions that more specific sensory stimuli encounter and must surpass in order to be processed and induce stimulus-induced activity.

The "activation baseline" is constituted of exteroceptive stimuli and operates as threshold for any subsequent neural processing of more specific exteroceptive stimuli. Due to the shaping of the activation baseline by exteroceptive stimuli, I prefer to speak of an "exteroceptive baseline" (rather than an activation baseline). The term *exteroceptive baseline* better indicates the kind of stimuli that set the threshold or level of baseline for any subsequent neural processing.

In addition to such a conceptual refinement, I also suggest neuroanatomical extension is in play. Rather than being limited to the sensory cortex (and especially the visual cortex) as the concept of the activation baseline implies, I consider the exteroceptive baseline to apply to other regions, too. The earlier described findings during the shift from eyes closed to open indicate that various regions to change their activity level, mostly those in the outer ring. Therefore, I hypothesize the "exteroceptive baseline" to signify resting-state activity, especially in the regions of the outer subcortical-cortical ring.

Neuronal hypothesis Id: inner ring and the "interoceptive baseline" of the resting-state activity

How about the resting-state activity in the subcortical and cortical regions of the inner ring? As detailed earlier, the inner ring is characterized by the predominant processing of interoceptive stimuli. This may be best visible when closing the eyes, thereby coming into what Marx et al. (2004) described as "interoceptive state." Barry et al. (2007) refer to such interoceptive state as the "arousal baseline," which describes an unspecific state of arousal related to the predominantly interoceptive input.

However, as in the case of the "activation baseline," I prefer to specify the kind of stimuli that set the resting-state activity level. I therefore speak of "interoceptive baseline" that, as I suggest, characterizes the resting-state activity level in the inner ring. I hence postulate that the "interoceptive baseline" is most prevalent in regions like the anterior and posterior cingulate cortex as well as in the insula as the inner ring's core regions (see Fig. 4-3).

I here distinguish between "intero- and exteroceptive baselines" that are supposed to characterize the resting-state activity in inner and outer rings, respectively. Thereby, both

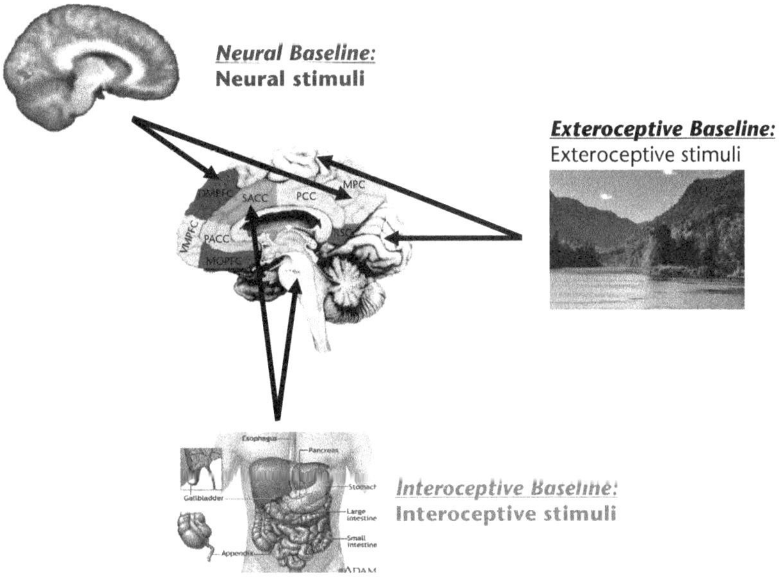

Figure 4-3 **Different baselines in the brain. The figure shows the three different kinds of baselines I hypothesize to be present in the brain and their relation to the basic anatomy. The "neural baseline" describes the resting-state activity of the brain that is generated within the brain itself as distinguished from being traced back to stimuli from outside the brain. The neural baseline is best visible in the midline structures and thus the middle ring (see Fig. 4-1), which do not receive direct intero- or exteroceptive input. The "interoceptive baseline" describes the resting-state activity in the brain that can be traced back to the interoceptive input from the body that the brain receives continuously. Since interoceptive stimuli enter the brain through its inner ring, the region adjacent to the ventricles, I marked the interoceptive baseline accordingly. Finally, one may also want to speak of an "exteroceptive baseline" that describes the resting-state activity that can be traced back to the continuous exteroceptive input through the senses (except for the visual sense, all four other senses still process exteroceptive stimuli during rest). Since they are processed mostly in lateral regions of the outer ring, I marked the exteroceptive baseline accordingly.**

baselines describe the resting-state activity level that as an operational term refers to the brain's intrinsic activity (see earlier discussion). I propose that the brain's intrinsic activity in the inner and outer ring is maintained predominantly by the neural processing of the continuous input of unspecific intero- and exteroceptive stimuli.

In contrast to the specific intero- and exteroceptive inputs, the continuous input of unspecific intero- and exteroceptive stimuli can never be completely shut off and thus prevented from entering the brain. Due to the continuous input of such extrinsic stimuli, i.e., intero- and exteroceptive, the brain's resting-state activity is *not* as purely intrinsic as the term suggests; there is always already some extrinsic ingredient as related to the unspecific intero- and exteroceptive input.

Neuronal findings IIa: Resting-state activity in midline regions – signal changes

So far, I have considered mainly the regions of the outer ring when discussing the results from eyes open and eyes closed. This, however, neglects the fact that the middle and inner rings' midline regions, like the VMPFC, the PACC, the DMPFC, and the PCC, do also change their level of neural activity during the transition from eyes closed to eyes open. We could also see in the earlier described results by Marx and McAvoy as well as others, the involvement of these regions. This has been further substantiated in a more recent study by Qin et al. (2012a) from our group and others (see later, as well as Jao et al. 2013).

Comparing blocks of 20s with eyes open with blocks of 20s with eyes closed, Qin et al. (2012a) showed that eyes open induced significantly stronger signal changes in various midline regions when compared to eyes closed (see Fig. 4-4a). This concerned regions from both inner and middle rings like PACC and PCC, as well as VMPFC, DMPFC, and the precuneus. Hence, the regions of the inner and middle ring seem to change and modulate their neural activity in response to changes in the visual input during the transition from eyes closed to open (see Fig. 4-4a).

How can we gather further empirical support for the possible involvement of the midline regions in the brain's resting-state activity? For that, we now focus on neuronal measures other than mere signal changes; these include functional connectivity, signal variability, and amplitude of low frequency fluctuations and how they change during the transition from eyes closed to open. To do that in fMRI, one has to investigate longer periods like 5–6 minutes of either eyes closed or open. Let's now look into whether opening the eyes changes functional connectivity (and the other neuronal measures) between the various midline regions within, for instance, inner and middle rings.

Neuronal findings IIb: resting-state activity in midline regions – functional connectivity

Yan et al. (2009) investigated and compared different resting-state conditions with each other: eyes closed, eyes open without fixation cross, and eyes open with fixation cross. Using fMRI, they measured functional connectivity by constructing connectivity maps for the target regions as well as low-frequency oscillation amplitude (0.01–1 Hz). They focused in particular on the default-mode network (DMN) (see later for more details about the DMN), and more specifically on the CMSs, while neglecting the other regions of the brain.

They observed that generally the functional connectivity between anterior (PACC, VMPFC) and posterior (PCC, precuneus) midline regions

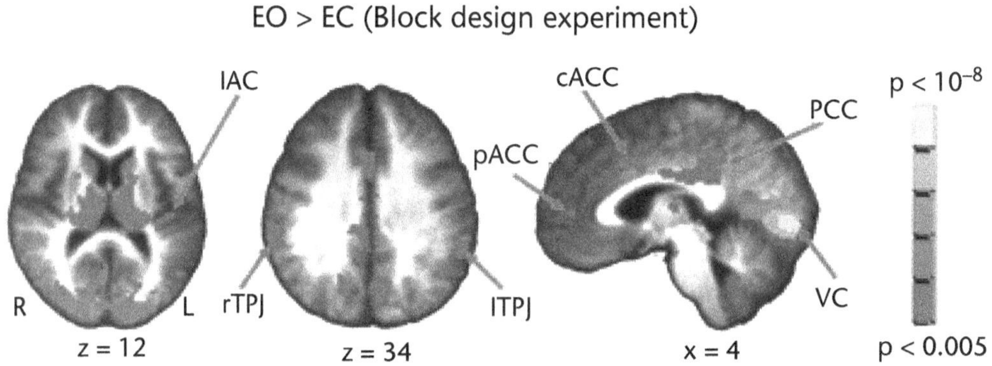

Figure 4-4a Resting-state activity in inner and middle ring. Activated brain areas based on the contrast Eyes open (EO) > Eyes closed (EC) from a block-design experiment (20sec eyes open, 20 eyes closed with multiple blocks). The results were significant at $p < 0.05$ (FWE corrected). For display purposes, the results are exhibited with a threshold of $p < 0.005$ uncorrected. Note the predominant involvement of cortical midline regions which cover the inner and middle ring.PCC, posterior cingulate cortex; rTPJ, right temporoparietal junction; lTPJ, left temporoparietal junction; cACC, caudal cingulate cortex; pACC, perigenual anterior cingulate cortex; VC, visual cortex; lAC, left auditory cortex.

changed significantly during the transition from eyes closed to both-eyes-open conditions (see also Jao et al. 2012). Interestingly, the eyes-open condition with fixation cross showed even higher degrees of functional connectivity between these regions when compared to eyes open without fixation cross.

The changes—i.e., increase in the degree of functional connectivity between anterior and posterior midline regions during eyes open with and without fixation cross—seem to go along with changes in entropy, signal variability, and amplitude of low-frequency fluctuations (see Chapter 5 for details about low-frequency fluctuations) in the same regions (see also Jao et al. 2013 and Duncan et al. 2013).

Taken together, these findings demonstrate neural activity changes in the inner and middle rings' midline regions during the transition from eyes closed to open. This is exemplified by changes in neuronal measures like functional connectivity, low frequency fluctuations, entropy, and signal variability. Most important, the regional occurrence of these changes seems to more or less conform to the anatomical-structural boundaries as related to the inner and middle rings and their respective regions.

Neuronal findings IIc: structure and function in posterior midline regions

Do the changes in resting-state activity really remain within the anatomical-structural boundaries of the three rings and their respective regions? For that answer, I turn to the young neuroscientist Daniel Margulies, originally from New York and now works in Berlin.

Margulies et al. (2009) investigated the functional connectivity of the precuneus and the posterior cingulate in the resting state of both humans (eyes open) and monkeys, using fMRI. Based on their resting-states' functional connectivity to other regions in the brain, he distinguished different parts (central, posterior, anterior) within the precuneus (cognitive: connecting to prefrontal regions; visual: connecting to visual cortex; sensorimotor: connecting to sensorimotor cortex).

Most important in the present context is his finding that the resting state's functional connectivity pattern of the PCC differed very much from that of the adjacently located precuneus, with both regions showing almost no overlap. Unlike the precuneus (and its distinct parts), the PCC mainly connected to limbic and paralimbic regions in medial prefrontal and temporal cortex (anterior cingulate cortex, hippocampus, ventro- and dorsomedial prefrontal cortex).

How do these findings relate to the three anatomical-structural rings postulated here? The resting state's functional connectivity of the PCC unfolded mainly along the inner (and in part middle) ring, while that of the precuneus was instead associated with regions in the middle (and in part outer) ring. This is further supported by the observed correspondence between human and monkey data in the Margulies et al. (2009 study as well as by similarities between their functional findings and early tracer studies showing anatomical–structural connections.

Neuronal findings IId: function conforms to the radial-concentric structure of the three rings

What do these data tell us? They show that, to some degree, functional connectivity in the resting state preserves the structural divisions of the anatomical-structurally defined three radial-concentric rings. This means that changes in neural activity during the resting state, as during the transition from eyes closed to open, occur along the anatomical-structural boundaries of the three rings: inner, middle, and outer.

There may thus be a certain degree of correspondence between anatomical structures, i.e., the three rings, and functional activity, i.e., resting state, with the latter being structured and organized along the lines of the former (see Chapter 5 for extensive discussion of the relationship between structure and function in the brain).

How about the functional connectivity between the different rings? Zou et al. (2009) observed that the visual cortex showed negative correlations with the thalamus, especially the dorsomedial thalamus and the ventrolateral nuclei of the thalamus, during eyes closed,

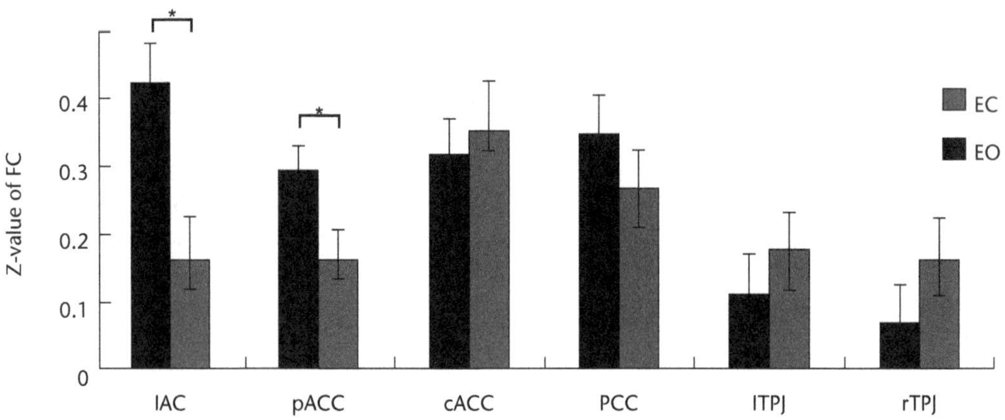

Figure 4-4b Functional connectivity of visual cortex with auditory cortex and other cortical regions. Histogram of Z-values for the functional connectivity between visual cortex and activated regions from contrast [EO > EC] (block design experiment) during EC and EO. FC, Functional connectivity.. indicates $p < 0.05$ uncorrected. Compared with EC, FC between the visual and auditory cortices was significantly reduced during EO ($t = 2.87$, $p = 0.01$ uncorrected), as was FC between visual cortex and pACC ($t = 2.46$, $p = 0.024$ uncorrected). Note the reduction of functional connectivity between midline regions and the visual cortex from eyes closed (EC) to eyes open (EO) ($p < 0.05$, FWE corrected). Visual cortex was taken as seed region, the functional connectivity between visual cortex and the default-mode network (DMN) was significantly reduced, as well as the functional connectivity between visual and auditory cortex. MPFC, medial prefrontal cortex; rAC, right auditory cortex; lAC, left auditory cortex; rTPJ, right temporoparietal junction; lTPJ, left temporoparietal junction; PL, paracentral lobule (own nonpublished data).

which was significantly weakened when opening the eyes.

An analogous finding of a weakening of functional connectivity between regions from different rings was also observed by Qin et al. (2012a). They showed that the transition from eyes closed to eyes open is accompanied by a decrease in the strength of functional connectivity between visual cortex and midline regions like the PCC, PACC, and DMPFC (see Fig. 4-4b).

Taken together, the findings demonstrate the involvement of midline regions from inner and middle ring during the transition from eyes closed to eyes open. Thereby, functional connectivity seems to rather increase between regions within the inner/middle rings, while it apparently decreases between regions from different rings.

More generally, this lends further empirical support to the assumption that the functional level of resting-state activity seems to be structured and organized along the boundaries of the three rings as defined on anatomical-structural grounds. In other words, there seems to be some degree of correspondence between anatomical-structural and functional levels, which will be discussed and supported further in the next sections (see also Chapter 5 for extensive discussion on the relationship between structure and function).

Neuronal findings IIIa: Resting-state activity in the default-mode network

Why do I emphasize the regions of the middle (and inner) ring so much? The regions of the inner and middle ring form the core regions of the DMN. Early studies in humans using positron emission tomography (PET) identified high oxygen and glucose consumption in the resting state in a particular set of regions, including anterior and posterior cortical midline regions like the VMPFC, the DMPFC, the different parts (sub-, pre-, and supragenual) of the ACC, the PCC, and the precuneus, as well as other regions like the lateral parietal cortex and the hippocampus (see Raichle et al. 2001; Simpson et al. 2001; Greicius et al. 2004).

These regions have consequently been subsumed under the concept of the DMN that includes the cortical midline structure as their core regions (Raichle et al. 2001; see Buckner et al. 2008 and Broyd et al. 2009 for recent reviews; see Morcom and Fletcher 2007a and 2007b for a critical view; and Northoff et al. 2010, Buckner et al. 2008, Raichle 2009, 2010). Since then there have been numerous investigations that established the DMN well in both humans (for excellent reviews, see Buckner et al. 2008; Raichle 2009, 2010) and animals (see Vincent et al. 2007; Lu et al. 2012; Mantini et al. 2011). Furthermore, there is also a strong developmental aspect to the DMN that is left out completely here (see Power et al. 2010 for a review).

Complementing the early PET investigations, the DMN was also observed in fMRI. During presentation of external stimuli like, for instance, emotional or cognitive tasks, these regions show predominantly negative signal changes in fMRI, deactivation, or negative BOLD response (NBR) in their neural activity (Simpson et al. 2001; Wicker et al. 2003, Grimm et al. 2009). The regions showing such a deactivation or NBR during stimulation must be distinguished from those that show activation or positive BOLD responses (PBR) in fMRI. This has led to the distinction between task-positive regions and task-negative regions. Task-negative regions are regarded as "typical" resting-state regions where negative signal changes, i.e., deactivation, are elicited in fMRI during specific tasks like cognitive tasks. In contrast, the concept of task-positive regions refers to the regions that show positive signal changes, i.e., activation in fMRI during cognitive (or other) tasks (see also Northoff et al. 2010).

While being deactivated during stimulus- or task-induced activity, the regions of the DMN show high activity and a high degree of intrinsic functional connectivity in the resting state (Damoiseaux et al. 2006; Fox et al. 2005; Greicius et al. 2004; Buckner et al. 2008; Beckmann et al. 2005; Fransson 2005). At the same time, the task-negative regions of the DMN a are negatively correlated; for example, anticorrelated with the task-positive regions during the resting state.

This means that higher functional connectivity within the DMN and its task-negative regions is accompanied by lower degrees in functional connectivity in the task-positive network and its more lateral regions. Accordingly, task-positive and task-negative regions are not only anatomical-structurally but also functionally distinguished; that is, in their resting-state activity, i.e., in BOLD responses (positive versus negative) and functional connectivity (opposite or anticorrelating changes).

Neuronal findings IIIb: default-mode network and the brain's intrinsic activity

Based on these findings, the DMN has been characterized as a resting-state network that typically shows high neural activity especially in the resting-state. The DMN is therefore associated with the brain's resting-state activity, as distinguished from its stimulus-induced activity, which is supposed to be mediated by other regions. Such an anatomical distinction between resting-state and stimulus-induced activity contradicts, however, the observation of spontaneous activity that is resting-state activity in basically all regions and networks of the brain.

While the DMN may be unique in several of its neuronal features, it is clear that the occurrence of certain levels of activity during the resting state is not confined to the DMN. All regions in the brain, inside and outside the DMN, show intrinsic activity, including sensory regions, lateral cortical areas, and subcortical regions (see Freeman 2003; Shulman et al. 2004, 2009; Buckner et al. 2008; Wang et al. 2007; Hunter et al. 2006).

There is thus what has been described as *spontaneous activity* throughout the whole brain and its various regions and networks. Further support for spontaneous resting-state activity across the whole brain comes from electrophysiological studies that show spontaneous neuronal oscillations and synchronizations in various parts of the brain, including the hippocampus and the visual cortex (Buzsáki 2006; Buzsaki and Draguhn 2004; Arieli et al. 1996; Llinas 1988; Singer 1999, 2009; Fries et al. 2001, 2007).

Stepping from the regional to the network level, other networks besides the DMN can be distinguished, with all networks showing resting-state activity. For instance, Menon (2011) distinguished the central executive network (lateral parietal and prefrontal cortex) from the salience network (insula, dorsal anterior cingulate cortex, amygdala, ST/VTA) within the task-positive regions. The salience network seems to include regions from especially the inner ring, while the central executive network predominantly implicates the outer ring's regions. Both salience and central executive networks are distinguished from the DMN, the resting-state network.

In sum, the whole brain, including all its regions and networks, shows neural activity in the resting-state. The brain's intrinsic activity thus seems to be everywhere in the brain, excluding neither regions nor networks. Therefore, while the DMN may have a special yet unclear role, it cannot be considered unique in showing resting-state activity. What is clear nevertheless is that the DMN's level and features of its resting-state activity are different from that of other regions and networks.

Neuronal hypothesis IIa: "neural stimuli" and "neural baseline" in the middle ring

So far, I have characterized the inner and outer rings' resting-state activity—that is, their intrinsic activity—by the terms "interoceptive baseline" and "exteroceptive baseline." But this left the exact characterization of the middle ring's resting-state activity open. The earlier described data show that the middle ring's midline regions are subsumed under the concept of the DMN that shows particularly high levels of resting-state activity and other neuronal features that distinguish it from other regions and networks in the brain.

How is such a high resting-state activity in the regions of the middle ring possible? Unlike in the inner and outer rings' regions, the regions of the middle ring do not receive any direct input; that is, intero- or exteroceptive stimuli, from body and environment (see earlier for details).

Where, then, does their high degree of resting-state activity stem from? The middle ring's regions' high resting-state activity level cannot have its origin in the stimuli from either the body or its environment, since they do not receive any direct intero- or exteroceptive input. The source of its high resting-state activity can only be the brain itself; for example, the spontaneous activity in the midline regions of the middle ring.

How can we characterize the high spontaneous activity in the midline regions of the middle ring? As said, it does not stem from either intero- or exteroceptive stimuli in the body or environment. Instead, it must originate from within the brain itself, within the midline regions of the middle ring, and has therefore been described as "spontaneous."

Rather than of intero- and exteroceptive stimuli, one may therefore want to speak of "neural stimuli": the concept of "neural stimuli" means that the stimuli generating the high resting-state activity in the midline regions originate and thus stem from within the brain itself, rather than from body and environment as intero- and exteroceptive stimuli.

This leads me to propose what I call the "neural baseline." The concept of "neural baseline" describes the predominance of neural stimuli (as distinguished from intero- and exteroceptive stimuli) that originate from within the brain itself and determine the resting-state activity in the middle ring and its midline regions. Therefore, as in the cases of the "intero- and exteroceptive baselines" of the inner and outer rings, the concept of "neural baseline" determines the origin of the resting-state activity in the middle ring.

On a whole, I characterize the resting-state activities in the three different rings in different ways, based on the origins of the predominant stimuli. The inner ring can be characterized by strong input from interoceptive stimuli, which signifies its resting-state activity as "interoceptive baseline." In contrast, the outer ring shows rather strong exteroceptive input, implying that its resting-state activity may be described as "exteroceptive baseline."

Finally, the middle ring shows neither direct interoceptive nor exteroceptive input, so that the input from within the brain itself, the neural stimuli, dominate here; the corresponding resting-state activity may therefore be designated as "neural baseline." We will see later, in Volume II, that the balance between the three rings' resting-state activity level is central, as it can be altered in psychiatric disorders like depression or schizophrenia (see Chapters 22 and 27).

Neuronal hypothesis IIb: Intero- and exteroceptive stimuli lower the resting-state activity level in inner and outer rings

Do the neural stimuli originate exclusively in the midline regions of the middle ring? This would be rather contradictory to the above described observation that spontaneous activity is observed throughout the whole brain, including the regions from all three rings, inner, middle, and outer. Since spontaneous activity is generated in and by the brain itself, one would assume that neural stimuli are present in all regions of the brain. This means that all three rings and their respective regions can be characterized by neural stimuli from within the brain itself as input to its own resting-state activity.

If the neural stimuli originate throughout the whole brain their corresponding resting-state activity, and thus the "neural baseline" should hold in all regions of the brain. This means that the neural baseline cannot be limited to the midline regions of the middle ring but should extend to both the inner and outer ring. That however is to neglect the strong intero- and exteroceptive input the regions of the inner and outer ring receive from body and environment.

The continuous intero- and exteroceptive inputs in the regions of the inner and outer ring supersede their neural input and thus the neural baseline. What we described earlier as the "intero- and exteroceptive baselines" that characterize the resting-state activity in inner and outer rings may thus be specified now. One may therefore suggest interaction between neural and interoceptive stimuli in the inner ring, while in the outer ring, the neural stimuli may interact with the exteroceptive stimuli.

The respective baselines in inner and outer rings, intero- and exteroceptive baselines, may thus result from the interaction between neural and intero- or exteroceptive stimuli. Therefore, based on the earlier described findings, one may tentatively propose that the increased intero- and exteroceptive input lowers or decreases the resting-state activity level in inner and outer rings (when compared to the middle ring and its default-mode network).

Neuronal hypothesis IIc: Less disruption of resting-state activity in middle ring by extrinsic stimuli

Such a interaction of neural stimuli with other stimuli from outside the brain, i.e., intero- and exteroceptive stimuli from body and environment, is apparently minimized in the midline regions of the middle ring. Why? Unlike the inner and outer regions, the regions in the middle ring do not receive any direct input from outside the brain, or intero- and exteroceptive stimuli.

The spontaneous activity in the midline regions of the middle ring as generated by the neural stimuli themselves is less confounded by intero- and exteroceptive stimuli than the inner and outer ring regions' resting-state activity. The resulting level of resting-state activity in the middle rings' midline regions is consequently closer to the original spontaneous activity level than in the inner and outer rings.

Since it less interrupted by other stimuli from outside the brain, or intero- and exteroceptive stimuli, the level of resting-state activity may be higher in the middle ring, compared to that in the inner and outer ring. This is exactly what the data show, as described earlier in the high levels of resting-state activity in the DMN.

That inclines me to suggest the following hypothesis. I postulate that the higher levels of resting-state activity in the midline regions of the middle ring as the central part of the DMN is related to the absence of any direct input from outside the brain, i.e., intero- and exteroceptive stimuli from body and environment:

Why is all that relevant? By introducing the concepts of the different baselines—neural, intero- and exteroceptive—in relation to the three rings, inner, middle, and outer, I aim to link the anatomical-structural level of the brain to its functional level of resting-state activity. The findings do indeed suggest there is a certain degree of correspondence between anatomical-structural and functional levels in that the resting-state activity levels and its three baselines (intero- and exteroceptive and neural) seem to be structured and organized along the lines and boundaries of the three radial-concentric rings.

There is thus what I describe as *neuronal relevance* to our characterization of the three baselines in that they allow us to establish anatomical-structural-functional correspondence. And that correspondence may in turn be central in structuring and organizing the resting-state activity in spatial terms, amounting to what I later describe as "spatial structure." To understand that, however, we need to first investigate how the three baselines from the three rings interact with each other: this will be focus in the next sections.

Neuronal hypothesis IIIa: parallel-segregated versus interactive-integrative coding between the three rings' resting-state activities

How can the brain encode the relationship between the three different resting-state activities? One can suggest different models of how the interaction between the resting-state activity levels of the different rings and their respective networks could possibly take place. In other terms, one could describe different possible encoding strategies on the network level, which I will do in the following discussion.

One encoding strategy is that the three rings and their networks may act largely in a parallel and segregated way; their particular resting-state activity levels may then be constituted and determined independent of each other, due to the different origins of the respectively dominating stimuli and their baselines.

This encoding strategy may be described as "parallel-segregated coding." Since it is very much based on the stimuli generated and processed in each of the three rings, the parallel-segregated coding may be considered the extension of stimulus-based coding on the level of neural networks (see Fig. 4-5a).

How does such a parallel-segregated coding relate to the earlier described empirical findings? One would expect the increase in exteroceptive input during eyes open to yield neural activity changes predominantly in the regions of the outer ring, and more specifically in visual cortex and other sensory regions. While this can indeed be observed, there are also changes in the midline regions and thus in inner and outer rings' regions that should not occur if parallel-segregated coding holds. Hence, the empirical findings do not support the assumption of parallel-segregated coding in the neural processing of the three different rings' resting-state activities.

Alternatively to parallel-segregated coding, one may propose what I refer to as "interactive-integrative coding." "Interactive-integrative coding" means that the encoding of stimuli in the one ring is constitutively dependent on what happens in the other rings. In that case, any change in, for instance, the outer ring's resting-state activity level should go along with changes in the inner and middle ring, and vice versa. This means that the resting-state activity levels in each of the three rings are constituted in balance and adjustment to the ones of the respective others.

More specifically, the intrinsic activity in the outer ring is encoded relative to the ones of the inner and middle rings (and vice versa). This is possible only if there is interaction and subsequent integration between the three rings' resting-state activities in the gestalt of difference. "Interactive-integrative coding" may consequently be regarded as the extension of difference-based coding on the level of neural networks (see Fig. 4-5b).

How does such "interactive-integrative coding" stand in relation to the empirical data? Changes in resting-state activity in the outer ring, as during eyes open, go along with changes in the inner and middle rings' resting-state

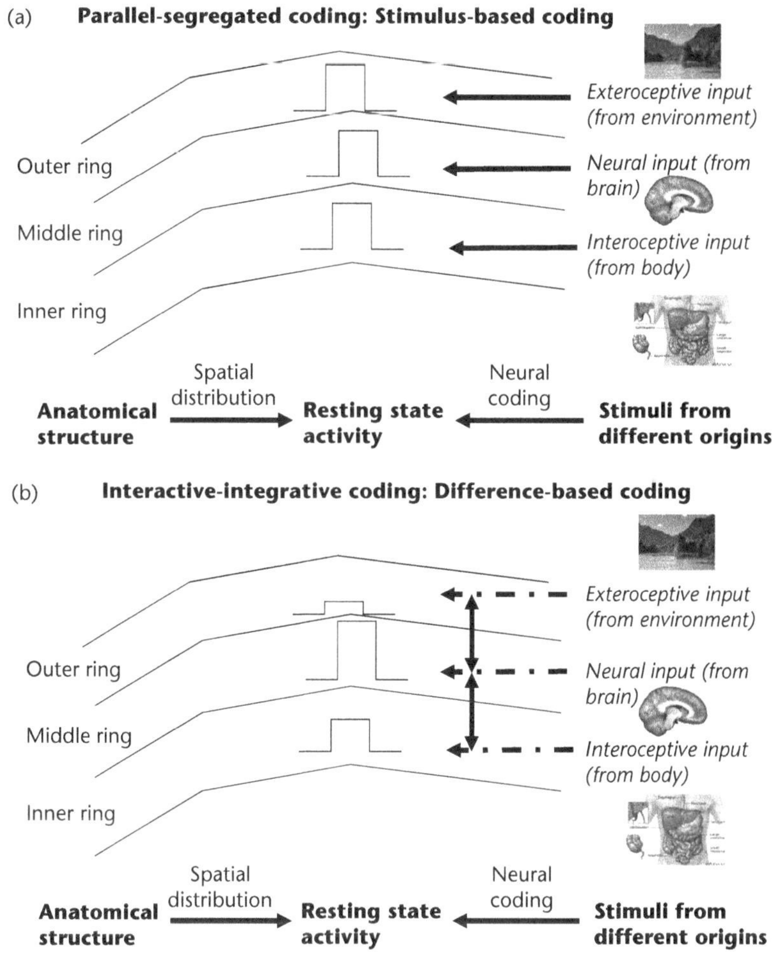

Figure 4-5 Different encoding strategies in the relationship between the three rings. The figures show the relationship between the three rings and different kinds of neural coding on the level of neural networks and their intrinsic activity. (*a*) In the case of stimulus-based coding, neural activity in the three rings is processed largely in parallel and segregated from each other. This implies clear-cut segregation between the three different baselines (exteroceptive, interoceptive, neural) in their respective rings (outer, inner, middle) with not much interaction between them. This amounts to stimulus-based coding of the brain's resting-state activity on a network level. (*b*) In the case of difference-based coding, neural activity in the three rings is processed largely through dependence on each other, which presupposes integration and interaction between each ring. This implies interaction between the three different baselines (exteroceptive, interoceptive, neural) and their respective rings (outer, inner, middle), making segregation impossible. This amounts to difference-based coding of the brain's resting-state activity.

activity and connectivity. There is thus interdependence between the different rings' intrinsic activities.

This is further supported by the observed anti-correlation in functional connectivity between task-positive and task-negative regions, as described earlier. Accordingly, I postulate the interactive-integrative coding strategy to be more empirically plausible than parallel-segregated coding of resting-state activity in different neural networks like the three rings.

Neuronal hypothesis IIIb: Difference-based coding between the three rings' resting-state activities

How can we now specify such a interactive-integrative coding? I suggest that interactive-integrative coding presupposes difference-based coding on the level of neural networks and thus the three rings. To explicate that, let us first go back to the empirical findings.

There were two main findings reported earlier with regard to functional connectivity. First, there is a remarkable surfacing of the anatomical structure and its three rings in the results on resting-state functional connectivity during eyes closed. The changes in resting-state functional connectivity during eyes closed and the transition to eyes open seem to more or less conform to the anatomical-structurally defined boundaries of the three rings. There is thus quite a high degree of correspondence between anatomical structure and the functional level of resting-state activity.

The second main finding shows that a purely exteroceptive stimulus—that is, opening the eyes—that is predominantly processed in the regions of the outer ring leads to neural activity and functional connectivity changes within the regions of the inner and the middle ring. This means that there must be some kind of interaction between outer and inner/middle rings and their respective resting-state activity levels, which is also reflected in the observation of decreased functional connectivity between rings (see earlier).

What kind of neuronal mechanisms underlie and make possible the interaction between the three rings and their levels of resting-state activity? This is the question of how the relationship between the three rings' resting-state activities is encoded into neural activity. More generally put, we are asking how the relationship between different neural networks is encoded into neural activity.

Let us recall the discussion from the first Part: There we proposed difference-based coding to hold during the encoding of extrinsic stimuli into stimulus-induced activity on both cellular and regional levels of neural activity. Rather than encoding the single stimulus itself into neural activity (as suggested in stimulus-based coding), difference-based coding suggests that the temporal and spatial differences between different stimuli are encoded into neural activity.

How does that stand in relation to the relationship between the three rings and their resting-state activities? I suggest that the brain uses exactly the same strategy when encoding the relationship between the three rings' resting-state activities that constitute their different baselines. Rather than the encoding the resting-state activity of each ring by itself in an isolated and independent way, the relationship between the resting-state activity levels of the three different rings is encoded into their neural activity.

In a nutshell, I postulate difference-based coding (rather than stimulus-based coding) to determine the encoding of the three rings' resting-state activities. This means that the resting-state activity level in for instance the inner ring is encoded relative to and thus in difference to the ones in middle and outer rings (and vice versa).

The interaction between the different rings' resting-state activity is thus built-in by the encoding of differences into the resting-state activity level of each ring. Such a mutual dependence in the encoding of their resting-state activity is well compatible with the observed anti-correlation between task-negative and -positive networks that reflect mainly middle and outer rings. In contrast, this anticorrelation between task-negative and -positive networks remains incompatible with stimulus-based coding where no such a anti-correlation would be possible. This will become even more clear in the next section.

Neuronal hypothesis IIIc: Difference-based coding and the anti-correlation between inner/middle and outer rings' resting-state activities

I propose that what is encoded in each of the ring's baselines; that is, inner, outer, middle rings' resting-state activity levels, is not so much the degree of the respectively dominating stimuli; that is, interoceptive, exteroceptive, and neural, by themselves in isolation and independent of each other. Instead, the neural activity level of the one ring's baseline is always already encoded relative and thus in difference to the ones of the respective others (and vice versa). What we observe as resting-state activity level in one ring may be the result of its prior interaction and integration with the ones of the respective other rings.

Accordingly, the resting-state activity levels in the three rings, that is their respective baselines, must be considered to be difference-based (i.e., between the three different rings or networks) rather than stimulus- or network-based. Each rings' or networks' resting-state activity level thus reflects an integral or difference value between the three different rings/networks and thus a relative value rather than an absolute value that would be exclusively and completely related to the respective ring or network alone.

How does the assumption of difference-based coding between the three rings' baselines stand in relation to the empirical data? Based on the data described earlier, one must postulate that the functional connectivity between outer and inner/middle ring is stronger during eyes closed than eyes open (see Qin et al. 2012, Jiao et al. 2012).

A high degree of functional connectivity means that the regions of the outer and inner/middle rings' activity is more synchronized during eyes closed when compared to eyes open. Such a increase in neuronal synchronization implies that their difference in resting-state activity levels must be rather low. This, however, changes once one opens the eyes. This changes neural activity in visual cortex and thus the outer ring, which in turn introduces a larger difference between outer and inner/middle rings' resting-state activity.

How now do the regions' of the inner/middle ring react to that? They also change their level of resting-state activity, meaning they increase it in order to keep the difference to the visual cortex and the other regions of the outer ring as small as possible. Such an increase in the inner/middle regions' activity level is possible only if they detach themselves from the functional constraints; that is, their functional connectivity, of the outer ring. This means that the inner/middle regions' must decrease their functional connectivity to the regions of the outer ring which is exactly what the data suggest.

At the same time the inner/middle rings' regions have to increase their functional connectivity among themselves; this elevates the resting-state activity level in the whole middle ring and keeps their difference to the outer ring's resting-state activity level and its decreasing functional connectivity as low as possible. This is exactly what the earlier described data show with the well established anti-correlation between task-negative and task-positive networks (that more or less correspond to the distinction between inner/middle and outer rings).

Neuronal hypothesis IIId: Difference-based coding of resting-state functional connectivity and the intentionality of consciousness

How does the functional connectivity between different regions and networks stand in relation to difference-based coding on the network level?

I suggest that functional connectivity between different regions or networks presupposes difference-based coding and its encoding of relative or difference values between the resting-state activity levels in the different regions or networks: This implies that the degree of functional connectivity between different regions or networks can be predicted by the degree of neural difference values, e.g., continuum between small and large, between the different regions' or networks' resting-state activity levels (see Chapter 25 for more extensive discussion of this point).

The encoding of the networks' resting-state activity levels and their functional connectivity is not only relevant in neuronal regard but also phenomenally. If the resting-state activities' difference values tend towards the inner/middle regions' resting-state activity level, the latter is relatively stronger than the one in the outer ring. This may direct our consciousness toward contents related to the own body and the own mental states as they stem originally from the interoceptive and the neural stimulus inputs into inner and middle rings. That may for instance be the case in mind wandering (see Chapter 26 for details).

If, in contrast, the resting-states' difference values tend toward the outer ring's resting-state activity level, the latter is relatively stronger than the one in the inner/middle rings. This may direct our consciousness toward contents related to the external environment as they stem originally from the strong exteroceptive stimulus input into the outer ring (see Chapter 25 for detailed discussion of such a directedness).

Accordingly, the direction of the relative difference value between the resting-state activity levels of the different rings may be central in directing consciousness toward either internal, i.e., mental and bodily, or external, i.e., environmental, contents. The difference-based coding on the network level of the brain's resting-state activity is consequently not only neuronally relevant but also phenomenally that is, for the directedness that is, intentionality of consciousness. This will be discussed in further neuronal and especially neurophenomenal detail in Chapters 25 and 26 in Volume II.

Neuronal hypothesis IVa: The brain's intrinsic activity constructs a virtual statistically-based spatial structure in its neural activity

Let me briefly recapitulate where we stand now. I propose that difference-based coding operates also on the network level of the brain's intrinsic activity. More specifically, I postulate that the different baselines (that is, intero- and exteroceptive and neural baselines) and thus presumably the intrinsic activities of the three rings are determined and encoded in relation and thus in relative difference to each other.

Most important, such a difference-based coding between the three rings operates and supersedes the given anatomical structures and divisions. This means that the functional level of resting-state activity; that is, intrinsic activity, does not mirror one to one the underlying anatomical structures and its three rings. Despite the earlier mentioned correspondence, there may nevertheless be some discrepancies between the anatomical structure and the functional level of resting-state activity. This, as I suggest, may be due to the determination of each of the rings' resting-state activity levels in terms of integrals or relative difference values as based on the direct comparison between all three rings.

Accordingly, I propose difference-based coding on the network level of the brain's intrinsic activity to be central in making possible or predispose structural-functional dissociation (see Chapter 5 for empirical and conceptual details on structural-functional dissociation).

What does this mean? By encoding differences between the three rings' resting-state activities, a novel spatial structure is constituted on the functional level of the brain's intrinsic activity. Such a spatial structure must be characterized as functional since it stems from and is based on the brain's intrinsic activity or resting-state activity. Such a spatial structure on the functional level of neural activity must be distinguished from the anatomical spatial structure of the brain (see Figure 4-6).

The assumption of such a spatial structure is well reflected in a recent quote taken from Leopold and Maier (2012, 2198): "To summarize this section on the spatial nature of the spontaneous neural activity, correlation and coherence measurements in humans and animals demonstrate a high degree of spatial organization over the cortical surface and across cortical laminae. In addition, a significant component of the global fMRI signal appears to be driven by neural activity fluctuations that are themselves coordinated over large regions of the cerebral cortex."

Neuronal hypothesis IVb: Difference-based coding allows for the differentiation between "physical space" and "neuronal space"

How are both anatomical and functional spatial structure related to each other? The spatial structure on the functional level of the resting-state activity supersedes the anatomical structure like the three rings so that both can possibly differ from each other. This accounts for the above mentioned structural-functional dissociation which will be discussed in further detail in the subsequent chapter, Chapter 5.

At the same time, the spatial structure on the functional level of the resting-state activity

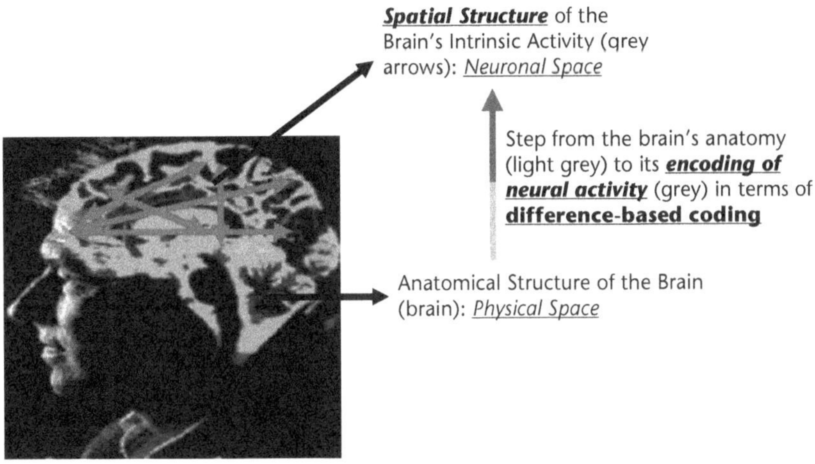

Figure 4-6 Constitution of Spatial Structure by the Brain's Intrinsic Activity. The figure illustrates schematically that the brain's intrinsic activity constitutes in its neural activity a spatial structure (grey arrows within the brain symbolize functional connectivity) that supersedes and operates across the anatomical structure (the brain). The physical space of the brain's anatomical structure is thus superseded by the neuronal space of the brain's intrinsic activity that operates across the former. That is made possible by encoding neural activity in terms of difference-based coding as it is indicated on the right with the arrow from the anatomical structures and their physical space to the intrinsic activity's spatial structure and its neuronal space.

is based on the underlying anatomical structure. Since it is based on; that is, predisposed by, the anatomical structure, the three rings and their radial-concentric organization, the intrinsic activities' spatial structure may still bear many remnants of the former. This is, for instance, apparent in the distinction between the task-positive and task-negative regions within the context of the DMN that (more or less) parallels the distinction between outer and middle/inner rings.

I propose that the brain's intrinsic activity constructs a spatial structure in its neural activity that supersedes the brain's anatomical structure. We should be aware however that we here presuppose two different concepts of space, physical space and neuronal space. The concept of a purely physical space is presupposed by the anatomical structure of the brain; that is for instance manifest in the radial-concentric organization of the three rings as described earlier. Such a anatomical space as purely physical space is superseded by the construction of the spatial structure on the functional level of the brain's intrinsic activity.

What do I mean by "superseding"? "Superseding" means that the intrinsic activity's spatial structure operates across the anatomical-structural boundaries set up by the different cortical and subcortical networks and regions. The resulting neuronal space of the brain's intrinsic activity thus differs and differentiates itself from the physical space of the underlying brain and its anatomical structures.

How is such a differentiation between the physical space of the brain's anatomical structure and the neuronal space of its intrinsic activity possible? I suggest that this is possible by the encoding of integrals and thus relative difference values between the resting-state activity levels in the different regions or networks. Accordingly, I postulate that difference-based coding is a necessary condition of the differentiation between physical and neuronal space.

If, in contrast, the resting-state's neural activity were encoded in terms of stimulus-based coding, the neuronal space could not supersede and thus operate across the physical space of the different regions and networks. Stimulus-based coding would thus not allow for any differentiation between physical and neuronal space and consequently for the construction of a spatial structure by the brain's intrinsic activity across its merely physical features.

Neuronal hypothesis IVc: From the spatial structure of the brain's intrinsic activity to the experience of space in consciousness

One may now be slightly puzzled. I postulated that the brain's intrinsic activity constitutes a spatial structure in its neural activity. The spatial structure is supposed to supersede and operate across the brain's anatomical structure which, as I postulate, is made possible by difference-based coding. In contrast, I left open the exact spatial features of the intrinsic activity's spatial structure.

The intrinsic activity's spatial structure can be characterized by different neural networks that more or less conform to the three concentric-radial rings as outlined earlier. These networks are negatively or reciprocally related to each other as observed in their anti-correlation. In addition to such spatial features, one may also describe the spatial structure by particular temporal features as we will discuss it in detail in the next chapter. Apart from that we however do not really know the exact features of the intrinsic activity's spatial structure at this point in time. This is left to future research.

How however can we know more about the intrinsic activity's spatial structure? Besides direct empirical investigation, one may also take a more indirect methodological strategy for generating hypotheses. That leads me again to the phenomenal realm of consciousness. I postulate that the way our subjective experience and thus consciousness are spatially structured and organized may be based on and thus predisposed by the brain's intrinsic activity and its spatial structure.

The phenomenal features of our subjective experience of space in consciousness, may then give us some hint or clue about how the intrinsic activity's spatial structure must be structured and organized in order to make possible such a "inner space consciousness" (see Chapter 16). One may thus infer from the phenomenal realm of consciousness to how the neuronal realm of the brain's intrinsic activity and its spatial structure must look like. This will generate novel purely neuronal hypotheses about possible features of the intrinsic activity's spatial structure which can be tested experimentally.

Open Questions

The first question pertains to the exact neuronal mechanisms that allow for the transition from anatomical structure to the functional level of intrinsic activity. Metabolism and energy may be central here, shedding some light on the neurometabolic coupling as, for instance, investigated by R. Shulman. It may indeed be the case that the metabolism and the degree of energy provided by the body to the brain may set up a very basic baseline, a "metabolic or physiological baseline," as one may say.

Such a "metabolic or physiological baseline" may provide the baseline upon which the three other neuronal baselines postulated here, intero- and exteroceptive and neural baselines, can operate. It would be interesting to see in the future how the continuous intero- and exteroceptive input in inner and outer rings affect the interaction with the neurometabolic activity. Based on the many investigations in the context of the DMN, one may propose that the continuous intero- and exteroceptive input may lower the degree of neurometabolic coupling and hence the intrinsic activity level in the respective rings. This, however, is rather speculative at this point.

The second question pertains to the function and purpose of the intrinsic activity's spatial structure. As I will discuss in the next chapter in more detail, others like Fingelkurts et al. (2010a and b, Fingelkurts and Fingelkurts 2011) also suggest a spatial (and temporal) structure to be constituted in the brain's resting-state which they call "operational space and time." However, they neglect its particular structure and organization and also do not clearly delineate the mechanisms, processes, and encoding strategies that underlie the constitution of such a spatial structure by the brain's intrinsic activity.

Fingelkurts and Fingelskurts (2011) consider the intrinsic activity's spatial and temporal structure to be essential for consciousness; this is so because they propose the phenomenal space of consciousness to be isomorphic to and thus already ingrained in the spatial structure of the brain's intrinsic activity. This amounts to what one may want to call "neuro-phenomenal isomorphism" which however needs to be distinguished from the concept of neural predisposition as I use here and in Volume II (see also Northoff 2013). I propose that the intrinsic activity's spatial structure predisposes consciousness rather than being isomorphic to it. For that, refer to Volume II.

The assumption of such a "neuro-phenomenal isomorphism" is however problematic. This is nicely illustrated by a recent study by Huth et al. (2012). They measured neural activity during the exposure to natural movies in fMRI and then used voxelwise models to search for the encoding of the 1.705 object and action categories in the movie. By generating a semantic space as related to the objects, they were able to compare it directly with the neuronal activation space over visual and nonvisual cortex. Unfortunately, they did not include the brain's intrinsic activity so that the neuronal space refers to stimulus-induced activity rather than resting-state activity.

What are their results? Rather than each object category being associated with one particular compartment of the brain's neuronal space, the results showed smooth gradients in neuronal space between the different objects/action categories. Such a shared neuronal space with its neuronal continuum between the different semantic categories was observed and shared across different individuals.

What do these results imply for the assumption of isomorphism in general? These results show that one cannot assume one-to-one relationship between semantic categories and the brain's neuronal space. The brain's neural activity seems to operate on the basis of a neuronal continuum by means of which it provides a shared neuronal space that commonly underlies the different semantic categories. Hence, rather than being isomorphic to the semantic space and its different categories, the brain's neuronal space provides a predisposition and thus, put metaphorically, the underlying ground or floor upon which the different kinds of furniture, the objects, stand on.

We have to be careful however, Our empirical example is about neuro-semantic isomorphism rather than neuro-phenomenal isomorphism which shall be discussed in Volume II in detail.

CHAPTER 5
Temporal Structure of Intrinsic Activity

Summary

Chapter 4 focused on the spatial structure of the brain's intrinsic activity. This neglected the temporal dimension, which is the focus of this chapter. Recent findings show that while structural and functional connectivity are often aligned with each other, they may also dissociate from each other. This means that there may be functional connectivity without underlying structural connectivity. How is that possible? Functional connectivity describes the correlation between two (or more) regions' activity levels across different discrete points in physical time and thus how their respective fluctuations in activity are temporally aligned; that is, synchronized to each other. If now functional connectivity dissociates from its underlying structural connectivity, it means that the temporal correlations between the two regions' activity no longer adhere to the biophysical-computational conduction delays as predisposed by structural connectivity. This means that functional connectivity operates across and thus supersedes structural connectivity and its predisposed conduction delays. Such operation across the biophysical-computational conduction delays makes it possible for functional connectivity to link, coordinate and integrate different discrete points in physical time. This is well manifest in the relationship between fluctuations in different frequency domains in the brain's resting state activity as shown in recent data: low-frequency fluctuations in the resting state's neural activity (0.0001–0.1 Hz) align and coordinate, that is, entrain, the high-frequency fluctuations (1–60 Hz) to themselves, or the onsets of their phases. Such integration of different time windows is, as I suppose, only possible on the basis of the encoding of temporal differences (rather than discrete points in physical time) into neural activity; i.e., difference-based coding (rather than stimulus-based coding). Difference-based coding allows the brain's intrinsic activity to construct a web of neural differences across the different discrete points in physical time that are associated with the biophysical-computational features of the underlying neurons. This leads to the construction of a virtual statistically-based temporal structure that as such supersedes and operates upon the biophysical-computational predispositions; that is, the conduction delays. In addition to the spatial structure as discussed in the previous chapter, I therefore propose the constitution of a temporal structure by the brain's intrinsic activity, which, as indicated, is not only neuronally but also behaviorally and especially phenomenally relevant; that is, for consciousness.

Key Concepts and Topics Covered

Structural connectivity, functional connectivity, structure-function dissociation, structure-function predisposition, low- and high-frequency fluctuations, neuronal statistics, sparse coding, difference-based coding, temporal structure

Neuroempirical background IA: Definitions of the concepts of "structure" and "structural connectivity"

I discussed the resting state's spatial structure in the previous chapter. The question arises now whether there is an analogous temporal structure in the resting state. I will argue that the constitution of the resting state's temporal structure starts with the spatial structure; i.e., the anatomical structure of the brain, including its various regions and networks. More specifically, the data will show that functional connectivity allows for the constitution of virtual statistically-based temporal relationships between the different anatomical regions/networks.

The temporal relationships as established on the basis of functional connectivity may supersede and operate across the different anatomical structures; i.e., the regions and networks. This makes possible the divergence and dissociation of the functional connectivity from the underlying anatomical-structural connectivity. This leads to what I describe as "structural-functional dissociation."

Before going into empirical details, we need to briefly describe the concepts of "structure" and "function." The brain can be characterized by anatomical structures that may be organized in a certain way, as discussed in the previous chapter.

The term "structure" refers here to "the spatial and topological arrangement of connections between neuronal elements" (Honey et al. 2010, 767). The different anatomical structures may also be connected to each other via tracts running in the white matter of the brain; these are "structural connections" that can, for instance, be measured in diffusion tensor imaging tractography (see Hagmann et al. 2008; Sporns 2011).

Neuroempirical background IB: Definition of the concepts of "function" and "rest–rest interaction"

While the determination of the terms "structure" and "structural connectivity" is relatively easy, the terms "function" and "functional connectivity" are harder to track down. The concept of "function" may refer to, for instance, behavioral and psychological functions (i.e., affective, cognitive, social, etc.); this, however, is not the way the term is used in the present context. Instead, I here reserve the term "function" to describe neuronal processes that operate across and thereby supersede the anatomical structures and their given biophysical-computational temporal and spatial constraints. The concept of "function" as used here describes neuronal processes that operate across and therefore supersede the anatomical structures. I consequently distinguish the functional level of neural activity, such as the brain's intrinsic activity, from the brain's anatomical structures and its biophysical-computational constraints. This makes possible the dissociation of the functional level of neural activity during the resting state from both the biophysical-computational constraints of the neurons themselves and the anatomical-structural level. When talking about "structural-functional dissociation" I therefore refer to this dissociation between neuronal activity on the one side and biophysical-computational constraints and anatomical structure on the other.

What exactly happens on the level of neural activity? There may be various interactions between the different neural activity levels in the different regions and networks. Since as demonstrated in the previous chapter, different regions and networks may show different levels of resting state activity, there may already be plenty of interaction between different regions/networks in the resting state itself. One can consequently speak of what I describe as "rest–rest interaction."

The concept of "rest–rest interaction" describes the linkage, coordination, and mutual adjustment between different activity levels in different regions and networks. As implied by the term "function" (see earlier), such rest–rest interaction operates both spatially and temporally by superseding the spatial and temporal constraints related to the neurons' biophysical-computational features (and their anatomo-structural constraints). In other words, rest–rest interaction describes what happens on the functional level of neural activity.

The neural activity may also be modulated by specific stimuli or tasks. In that case a particular stimulus or task encounters the brain's intrinsic activity, its resting state activity. This implies interaction between the resting state and the stimulus/task which I describe as rest–stimulus interaction which in turn leads to what is described as stimulus-induced or task-related activity. Since this chapter focuses on the brain's intrinsic activity by itself, I discuss here only rest–rest interaction while the exact neuronal mechanisms underlying rest–stimulus interaction will be discussed later in Part IV.

Neuroempirical background Ic: Definition of the concept of "functional connectivity"

How is rest–rest interaction manifest in the neural activity of the resting state? One hallmark feature of the brain's intrinsic activity is its functional connectivity as already discussed in the previous chapter. This raises the question of what exactly is referred to when we use the term "functional connectivity." The concept of "functional connectivity" is usually taken to describe the purely statistical correlation between the time series of signal changes associated with two or more different regions' activities (see later for more empirical details).

This highlights two hallmark features of the concept of functional connectivity. First, describing a correlation between different regions' neural activities, functional connectivity is understood in a purely statistical way. Such statistically based understanding does not yet imply any physiological mechanisms that may mediate and underlie the observed purely statistical correlations between the different regions' neural activities (see also Fingelkurts et al. 2004a–c; Leopold and Maier 2012; and Friston 2010, for a good discussion of this point).

That also means that the term functional connectivity does not describe any causal mechanisms operating between the two regions' neural activities; this is rather captured by the concept of "effective connectivity," which refers to the causal impact of one region's activity on another one. In the following I will focus predominantly on functional connectivity and how it operates across and supersedes the anatomical structure's spatial and temporal constraints.

The second hallmark feature of the concept of functional connectivity is its temporal dimension. By signifying the correlation between the time series of two (or more) regions' neural activities, it operates not only across different discrete points in physical space; i.e., the different regions, but also across different discrete points in physical time as associated with the neural activities of the different regions.

For instance, increases in functional connectivity between two regions mean that the temporal courses of their neural activities—i.e., the time series of signal changes—are integrated and coordinated, and thus synchronized. In contrast, decreases in functional connectivity indicate lower degrees of temporal coordination and integration, i.e., synchronization, between the temporal courses of the regions' neural activities.

In sum, "functional connectivity" describes the spatial and temporal coordination and integration between the neural activities of different regions or networks. Most important, such spatial and temporal integration and coordination operate across and thus supersede the spatial and temporal constraints as related to the neurons' biophysical-computational features and their anatomical structure.

This makes it possible for the brain's intrinsic activity to constitute a virtual statistically-based spatial and temporal structure on the functional level of neural activity. The spatial structure of the brain's intrinsic activity, as discussed in the preceding chapter, is thus complemented by a particular temporal structure on the functional level of the brain's neural activity. This temporal structure and how it is constituted is the focus in the present chapter.

Neuroempirical background Id: The resting state's spatiotemporal structure and the phenomenal features of consciousness

Why do I put such strong focus on the constitution of a virtual statistically-based spatial and temporal structure by the brain's intrinsic activity? I claim that the resting state's spatial and temporal structure is both neuronally and phenomenally relevant (See also Northoff 2013).

The constitution of the intrinsic' activity's spatial and temporal structure makes it possible for the brain to operate across and supersede its biophysical-computational constraints and to establish its own neuronal level of activity as distinguished from the merely physical level of its anatomical structure. This makes the spatial and temporal structure neuronally and thus functionally relevant (as distinguished from mere anatomical and structural relevance).

In addition, the spatial and temporal structure is also phenomenally relevant; that is, for consciousness. As we will see in Volume II, the spatial and temporal structure of the brain's intrinsic activity makes possible and thus predisposes the association of certain phenomenal features of consciousness with the otherwise purely neuronal neural activity; this can occur during any kind of neural activity including both resting state itself (as in dreams; see Chapters 25 and 26) and stimulus-induced activity (as in the consciousness of for instance objects and events in the environment; see Chapters 28–30). For now, however, we restrict ourselves to the neuronal relevance of the resting state's temporal structure in order to understand the neuronal mechanisms that allow and predispose its constitution. This is the focus in the present chapter.

Neuronal findings Ia: structural connectivity predicts functional connectivity

How are structural and functional connectivity related to each other? For that, I focus on the groundbreaking work by Honey and Sporns, who conducted several paradigmatic studies on the relationship between structural and functional connectivity.

Honey et al. (2009) investigated structural connectivity (SC) in the whole brain using diffusion spectrum imaging (DSI) while the same subjects also underwent functional magnetic resonance imaging (fMRI) in the resting state to determine functional connectivity (FC) throughout the brain. This allowed them to construct SC maps based on tractography, which reveals the various tracts in the white matter that link and connect different regions throughout the brain.

FC in the resting state was determined on the basis of correlations between the time series of signal changes from different regions during the resting state. Thereby both maps were constructed on the basis of the same regions of interests, which allowed them to directly link SC and resting state FC. How is FC linked to SC? Honey et al. (2009) observed positive correlation between structural and functional connectivity maps: the higher the degree of structural connectivity, the higher the degree of functional connectivity in the resting state. When they took out missing structural data for the structural connections between particular regions, the degree of structural-functional correlation increased even further.

This strongly suggests that structural connectivity predicts and thus predisposes functional connectivity in the resting state. Such prediction means that functional connectivity in the resting state will more likely be constituted between those regions where there is already some structural connectivity. Since these findings were confirmed in subsequent studies, one would postulate that SC predisposes and therefore predicts FC in the resting state (see Fig. 5-1).

Neuronal findings Ib: "structure-function predisposition"

This amounts to what I call "structure-function predisposition" in the following. The term "structure-function predisposition" indicates that a particular organization on the structural level of the brain's anatomy, like its structural connections, makes possible and more likely a corresponding organization of neural activity on the functional level; as, for instance, in the functional connectivity of the resting state. Such structure-function predisposition not only applies to the brain as a whole, as investigated by Honey et al. (2009) and others (see Honey et al. 2010 for a review as well as Sporns 2011 for an excellent book) but also for particular networks like the default-mode network (DMN). Van den Heuvel et al. (2009) started with the investigation of resting state functional connectivity in especially the DMN and revealed high correlation of the time series in the signal changes between its different regions (PCC, PACC, VMPFC, precuneus, SACC, medial temporal, bilateral parietal). Based on the regions showing functional connectivity in the resting state, that is, statistical correlation in the time course of their signal changes, they analyzed whether their resting state FC

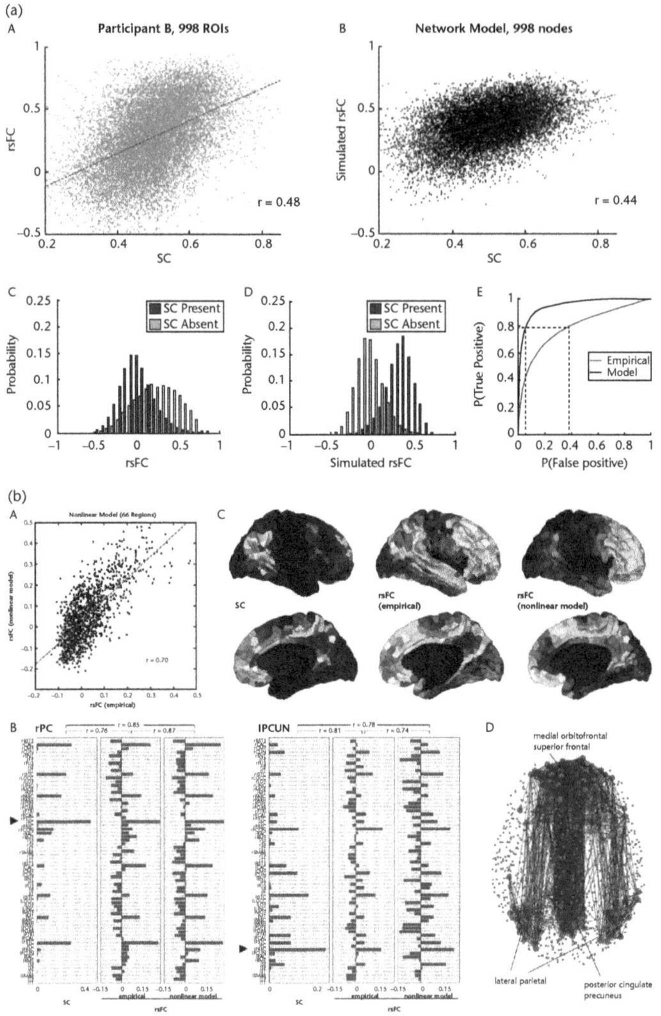

Figure 5-1 Relationship between structural and functional connectivity. (*a*) Overall SC–rsFC relationships. (A) Scatter plot (single acquisition, 20 min) of rsFC against SC at high resolution for participant B, showing edges with nonzero SC. (B) Scatter plot (single run, 16 min) of simulated rsFC against SC (from participant B) at high resolution, showing edges with nonzero SC. (C) The probability densities of rsFC values between structurally connected and unconnected region pairs, data for participant B at the high resolution. (D) Same as (C), but for simulated rsFC. (E) ROC curves, indicating the signal detection performance when inferring SC by thresholding empirical (*grey*) and simulated (*black*) rsFC maps at the high resolution. (*b*) Computational model of functional connectivity. (A) Scatter plot of empirical rsFC versus simulated rsFC obtained from the nonlinear model, down-sampled to the low resolution. (B) Comparison of SC, rsFC (empirical), and rsFC (nonlinear model) for 2 single-seed regions, the posterior cingulate in the right hemisphere (rPC) and the precuneus in the left hemisphere (lPCUN). The plot displays SC and rsFC values for the seed regions in relation to all 66 regions within the corresponding low-resolution matrices. (C) Mapping of SC, rsFC (empirical), and rsFC (modeled) within the DMN. Lighter grey colors indicate stronger SC and rsFC. Within the posterior cingulated/precuneus, medial orbitofrontal cortex, and lateral parietal cortex in both hemispheres we selected a cluster of 5 ROIs at positions that most closely matched the coordinates of peak foci of the DMN. These 30 ROIs served as the seeds from which SC and rsFC were determined. (D) Structural connectivity within the DMN. We selected the top 200 most correlated ROIs within the DMN and plotted all structural connections among them. (Reprinted with permission of *Proceedings of the National Academy of Sciences* from Honey CJ, Sporns O, Cammoun L, Gigandet X, Thiran JP, Meuli R, Hagmann P. Predicting human resting-state functional connectivity from structural connectivity. *Proc Natl Acad Sci USA*. 2009 Feb 10;106(6):2035–40.)

corresponds to specific white matter tracts and thus SC. They could demonstrate that the cingulum tract corresponds on the structural side to the resting state functional connectivity between anterior and posterior cingulate cortical regions, whereas the resting state functional connectivity between right and left anterior DMN (medial prefrontal cortex) was structurally mediated by the genu of the corpus callosum.

Finally, the left and right frontal-occipital fasciculus correlation corresponds structurally to the resting state functional connectivity between the medial prefrontal cortex and the bilateral parietal cortex. Since these regions are core regions of the DMN (see Chapter 4), they support the assumption that the DMN can be characterized not only in functional—that is, neuronal (and also metabolic), terms as for instance reflected in high degrees of resting state functional connectivity,—but also anatomically and thus structurally (see Honey et al. 2009; Hagmann et al. 2008; Sporns 2011).

Taken together, these findings demonstrate that functional connectivity in the resting state is often based on and aligns itself with the underlying structural connectivity. This means that structural connectivity predisposes and predicts functional connectivity in the resting state, which I describe as "structure-function predisposition."

Neuronal findings Ic: "structure-function dissociation"

Does the prediction and predisposition of functional connectivity in the resting state by structural connectivity mean that there is a one-to-one relationship between structure and function? We should be careful here. There may be functional connectivity in the resting state where there is no corresponding structural connectivity.

For instance, as shown in both imaging data and simulation studies, resting state functional connectivity may be high between two regions that are not connected structurally in a direct way but, if at all, only indirectly (see Honey et al. 2009). Moreover, FC may even be present when there is no SC at all, whether direct or indirect. These data imply that the reverse inference from functional to structural connectivity remains impossible: SC can predict resting state FC, while the reverse with resting state FC predicting SC does not hold.

Resting state FC may thus dissociate from SC by connecting regions functionally and thus neurally with each other that are neither directly nor indirectly connected anatomically by structural connections. In short, function may dissociate from structure, which I describe by the term "structure-function dissociation" in the following. The term "structure-function dissociation" indicates that the functional level of the brain's neural activity in (for instance) the resting state and its functional connectivity does not completely conform and align to the structural level of the brain's anatomy; i.e., its regions and networks; in a one-to-one way.

How can the two terms "structure-function predisposition" and "structure-function dissociation" be compared with each other? The first, "structure-function predisposition," emphasizes the dependence of FC on SC, whereas the second, "structure-function dissociation," focuses more on the independence of FC from SC.

Neuronal findings Id: intra-individual variability of functional connectivity in the resting state

How can such independence of FC from SC be further characterized? In addition to constitution of FC in the absence of SC, FC also shows a much higher degree of variability than SC. Honey et al. (2009) investigated resting-state FC in the same subjects twice on separate days, which allowed them to correlate the two different FC maps from the two days.

Interestingly, the FC maps obtained on different days in the same subject did not show a high correlation with reliability coefficients ranging only from $r = 0.39$ to $r = .61$ in the different individual subjects. This was further confirmed by their simulation model of functional connectivity that showed more or less equally low reliability coefficients. These data suggest quite a high degree of intra-individual variability in resting state FC; this is rather remarkable given that the anatomical structure—structural connectivity (SC)—did not obviously change between the different days when resting state FC was measured.

The observation of intra-individual variability in resting state FC is thus possible only if FC remains somehow independent of SC which entails a certain degree of structure-function dissociation. In short, the observation of intra-individual variability of resting state FC further supports the assumption of structure-function dissociation. Taken together, the findings demonstrate that while structural connectivity predicts the resting state's functional connectivity, the latter may also deviate and thus dissociate from the former. This means that what I described as "structure-function predisposition" goes along with "structure-function dissociation" with both being apparently compatible and complementary rather than being contradictory.

Neurometaphorical excursion: established and non-established paths

How can we better illustrate the relationship between structure and function in the brain? For that I turn to an imaginary example, a "neurometaphorical comparison," as I describe it.

If there is a well-established path from your house to the supermarket, you usually take that path. The established and regular path predisposes the route you actually take, thus corresponding to "structure-function predisposition." Now, however, the supermarket is about to close in five minutes. Hence, you do not want to take the established 1-km path to the supermarket, because it takes at least about 10 minutes if you are walking.

How, now, can you get to the supermarket within maximum five minutes? You could take the car. That, however, is not an option, because your car broke down and is in for repairs. Or you could run rather than walk the established path; that should bring you there in less than the 10 minutes which it usually takes to walk. This is not an option either, however, because you recently strained your leg muscles while playing soccer; this makes running impossible. The only way for you to get to the supermarket in time is thus to take a shorter, more direct path.

There is no established and regular path, however besides the one that takes 10 minutes. What do you do? You take a more direct though non-established way that leads through the corn field and brings you in about maximal 3 minutes to the supermarket. You thus deviate from the regular and established path by taking a non-established way.

This is what also happens in the brain when the functional connectivity takes a rather non-established way: in this case the functional connectivity deviates and dissociates from the underlying structural connectivity, entailing "structure-function dissociation." One may consequently say that sometimes our brain's intrinsic activity takes a rather direct and fast though non-established path when it wants to adjust, coordinate, impact, and modulate the different resting state activity levels between different regions.

In the same way as you take the more direct though non-established way through the corn field to the supermarket, the brain's intrinsic activity and its functional connectivity sometimes also prefer the direct route to another region, independent of the underlying anatomical-structural paths and their constraints. Accordingly, in the same way you want to go shopping in time, the brain's intrinsic activity in one particular region may also want to "shop" in another region's activity in time, since otherwise, as in the case of the supermarket, it may be too late.

Neuronal hypothesis Ia: structural connectivity is neither necessary nor sufficient for functional connectivity

How is the here-described structure-function dissociation possible? Let me first characterize it in more detail. "Structure-function dissociation" indicates that FC can occur without SC. The assumption is that SC is not necessary for FC, since otherwise any FC would presuppose SC. However, we need to distinguish the suggestion that SC is not a *necessary* condition from the one that it may nevertheless *predispose* subsequent FC.

Let's go back to our supermarket example. The established and regular path "predisposes" you to take it on your way to the supermarket. However, the established path is not *necessary* for you to get to the supermarket because other ways like the one through the corn field also lead you there. Moreover, the presence of the established path does not by itself lead you to the supermarket. You still have to walk it. Hence, the existence of the path itself (independent of your walking) is not sufficient by itself for you to get to the supermarket. The necessary condition, the established path, may thus be present while the sufficient one, you walking that path, remains absent.

This corresponds in the brain to the observation that SC can also occur without subsequent FC, as demonstrated by Honey et al. (2009, 2010). This means that SC is not sufficient for FC because otherwise SC would always occur in conjunction with FC. How is it possible that SC is neither necessary nor sufficient for FC? This suggests that the neuronal mechanisms underlying the constitution of FC must remain somehow independent of the anatomical-structural features that characterize SC.

Let us specify that and go back to what FC exactly means. As pointed out at the beginning of this chapter, FC describes a mere statistical correlation between the time series of the different regions' neural activities. The case of structure-function dissociation implies that such statistical correlation between different time series of the regions' neural activities can occur in the absence of any SC.

Neuronal hypothesis IB: "functional freedom" of the brain's intrinsic activity and consciousness

This raises the question for the neuronal (or physiological) mechanism (see also Fingelkurts et al. 2004; Friston 2011; Leopold and Maier 2012 for a good discussion of the concept of functional connectivity) that makes such statistical correlation between the different regions' time series and thus FC possible in the absence of SC. The neuronal mechanism underlying such statistical correlation must remain independent to some degree of the anatomical-structural features of SC. Therefore, the neuronal mechanism in question must operate across and supersede the anatomical and structural features of the brain.

Why do I emphasize the independence of the neuronal mechanism in question from the underlying anatomical and structural features of the brain? By operating across and thus superseding the brain's anatomical-structural features, the intrinsic activity can construct its own spatial and temporal structure on the basis of the neuronal mechanism in question.

By remaining independent of the anatomo-structural level, the functional level of the brain's intrinsic activity, figuratively put, "gains a certain degree of functional freedom from the brain's anatomical structure." Such "functional freedom" may allow the brain's intrinsic activity to diverge and dissociate from the brain's anatomical structure to which it no longer conforms and aligns. This is well reflected in the earlier described "structure-function dissociation" that signifies the independence and thus the "functional freedom" of the brain's intrinsic activity.

How is such "functional freedom" manifest in the brain's intrinsic activity? I argue that it is manifest in the construction of a statistically based and virtual spatial and temporal structure that supersedes and operates across the anatomo-structural features of the brain. Most importantly, I postulate that the constitution of such spatiotemporal structure is not only neuronally relevant but also phenomenally; that is, for consciousness. Let me briefly indicate this point.

How is the resting state's spatial and temporal structure related to consciousness? By showing "functional freedom" and remaining (more or less) independent of the brain's anatomical-structural features, the functional level of the brain's intrinsic activity can constitute novel spatial and temporal features (see below and Chapter 4 for details). These novel spatial and temporal features predispose the association of the phenomenal features of consciousness to the otherwise purely neuronal activity changes during either resting state or stimulus-induced activity. This will be the main focus in Volume II (parts V–VII).

Neuronal hypothesis IIa: neuronal mechanisms of functional connectivity

Let us return to the more specific neuronal mechanisms themselves, and particularly those that underlie the constitution of functional connectivity. What kind of neuronal mechanisms could underlie the statistical correlation between two regions' neuronal activities as observed in FC? Possible suggestions are so-called traveling waves, shared innervation, and intrinsic local oscillations or fluctuations (see Hagmann et al. 2010; Deco et al. 2011; Murphy et al. 2009; Cabral et al. 2011). I will here briefly discuss the first two neuronal mechanisms—traveling waves and shared innervation—while leaving the third one, intrinsic local oscillations or fluctuations, for later discussion.

The term "traveling waves" describes bouts or waves of neuronal excitation that move across different regions that may connect them and account for the statistical correlation of their neural activities across different discrete points in physical time, that is, FC. It seems, however, that such traveling waves may be more the result of a prior neuronal mechanism that links the two regions' neural activities rather than being the neuronal mechanism itself. Hence, traveling waves may correspond on the neuronal side to what we describe statistically as FC.

The traveling waves may consequently be considered a possible neuronal correlate of the purely statistical FC. However, the traveling waves do not reveal the neuronal mechanisms; that is, the neural predisposition, that drives and thus makes necessary and possible the constitution of FC and thus its underlying traveling waves.

How about the "shared innervation"? The assumption of "shared innervation" refers to a common cortical source for both regions' neural activities as, for instance, a third region that feeds both regions. What does such a relation to a third region look like? Despite not being connected directly with each other via SC, two regions may nevertheless both be structurally connected to a third region that is then shared between the two regions. Such a shared third region may make it possible to constitute FC between the two regions, even though they show no direct SC with each other. Accordingly, even though direct SC can remain absent, shared innervation presupposes at least some indirect SC between the regions showing FC. This, however, is not compatible with the empirical findings that show FC in the absence of any SC whether direct or indirect (see earlier discussion). This makes the suggestion of shared innervation rather implausible.

Taken together, different neuronal mechanisms like traveling waves and shared innervation (and local oscillations) have been discussed as underlying the constitution of functional connectivity. However, the suggested neuronal mechanisms turn out to be problematic, given the empirical data.

Neuronal hypothesis IIb: difference-based coding and functional connectivity

Both suggested neuronal mechanisms, traveling waves and shared innervation, seem to be insufficient to account for the neuronal mechanisms that constitute FC. I propose that the constitution of FC independent of SC makes necessary the assumption of a particular neural mechanism that remains independent of the underlying anatomical and structural features. More specifically, I suggest that difference-based coding is the neural mechanism that drives and makes necessary the constitution of FC.

Let me be more specific and sketch the following scenario. Region a's neural activity occurs at the time point x, while region b's neural activity happens slightly later at time point $x + 1$. How now can both regions' neural activities be linked such that they can statistically correlate with each other as observed in FC? I postulate that region a's neural activity at time point x is encoded relative and thus in difference to the one of region b at time point $x + 1$. And obviously the converse holds for region b whose neural activity at $x + 1$ is coded relative and thus in difference to the one of region a at time point x.

If now the two points, x and $x + 1$, are not too far, that is, temporally distant, from each other, their respective regions' neural activities, that is,

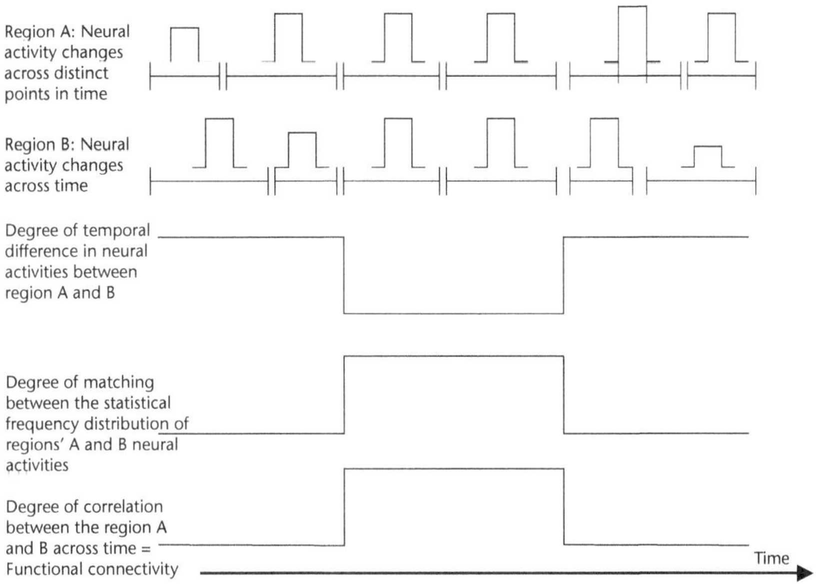

Figure 5-2 Difference-based coding and functional connectivity. The figure shows the relationship between functional connectivity and difference-based coding. Two regions (*upper part*) show changes in their neural activity across time, as indicated by the bars. While their activity may initially and finally be temporally out of tune (right and left side of upper part), it may synchronize transiently (in between), as indicated in the middle side of the upper part. Here they show similar onsets and heights in their neural activity. This means that now the degree of neural differences between their respective neural activities across different discrete points in physical time and space decreases as indicated in the upper middle part. Such decrease in neural differences across time and space goes along with an increase in the degree of the statistically based comparison and matching of the regions' neural activities, as indicated in the lower middle part. That, in turn, implies an increase in the degree of functional connectivity (*lower part*). Hence, the degree of functional connectivity may be directly and inversely proportional to the degree of spatiotemporal differences between two regions' neural activities: the lower the spatiotemporal differences in neural activities between two (or more) regions' neural activities, the higher their respective degree of functional connectivity.

regions a and b, can be linked and synchronized to each other. Such linkage may then, in turn, result in what we observe as statistical correlation between the time series of signal changes from the neural activities of different regions; i.e., functional connectivity. If, in contrast, the two time points, x and $x + 1$, are temporally too distant from each other, the two regions' neural activities cannot be linked and thus correlate with each other, resulting in the absence of FC (see Fig. 5-2).

Difference-based coding in this sense operates across distinct discrete points in physical time such as x and $x + 1$. This, in turn, makes it possible to link and integrate distinct discrete points in physical time, which we observe as statistical correlation between the time series of the signal changes from the two regions' neural activities. Let us describe this in further detail by focusing on increases and decreases in FC.

Neuronal hypothesis IIc: Encoding of spatial and temporal differences during changes in functional connectivity

Increase in FC may then reflect the successful encoding of one coherent temporal difference between the distinct discrete points in physical time of the two regions' neural activities. Since such neural difference spans between the two regions and the discrete time points of their neural activities, we observe statistical correlation between the time series of the regions' signal changes. Difference-based coding in this context may then be characterized by the encoding of spatial and temporal differences between different regions' neural activities, which in turn makes possible the construction of what we describe as FC. How about decreases in FC? Decrease in FC may indicate that the temporal difference between the distinct discrete time points may either be too large or too small (i.e., beyond the neurons' spatial and temporal capacities that they can possibly process on the basis of their biophysical-computational features; see later) to be linked and integrated into one coherent neural difference. That means that the degree of difference-based coding, the encoding of spatial and temporal differences, also decreases.

The two regions' neural activities and thus the time series of their signal changes consecutively no longer correlate with each other in our statistical analysis indicating a decrease in or even absence of FC. Accordingly, decrease or even absence of FC means that the degree of difference-based coding decreased due to the impossible encoding of the (too large or too small) temporal and spatial differences between the different regions' neural activities.

Taken together, I here suggest difference-based coding to be a candidate for the neuronal mechanism that allows to constitute FC during both presence and absence of SC. I consequently suggest that difference-based coding is at work during both "structure-function predisposition" and "structure-function dissociation." This makes it clear that difference-based coding operates on the functional level of neural activity and therefore supersedes the spatial and temporal constraints of the anatomical-structural level of the brain and its biophysical-computational constraints.

Neuronal findings IIa: functional connectivity in different ranges of frequency fluctuations

"Functional connectivity" describes the coordination between the temporal fluctuations from different regions' neural activities (see also Cabral et al. 2011). Resting-state activity in different regions may now fluctuate in different frequencies of their fluctuations (see later for details).

One may now question the relationship between functional connectivity and the different frequency domains in the neural activities' fluctuations. This leads us to the few available studies that directly test and measure the relationship between frequency fluctuations and functional connectivity (see, however, the simulation study by Cabral et al. 2011).

Using functional near infrared spectroscopy (fNIRS), Sasai et al. (2011) demonstrated that inter- and intrahemispheric connectivity (as operationalized by the temporal correlation of continuous oxy-HB signals as measured in fNIRS) operate in different frequency domains. Interhemispheric connectivity as, for instance, between homologous right and left occipital and frontal regions was high within a wide frequency range, 0.009–0.1 Hz. This contrasted with intrahemispheric connectivity as between frontal and posterior regions, where the frequency range of high functional connectivity was restricted to 0.04–0.1 Hz. In sum, these results show that the degree of functional connectivity and the frequency domain of the fluctuations are closely related to each other.

Further empirical support comes from Shmuel and Leopold (2008). They investigated the right and left visual cortex (V1) in monkeys in fMRI and electrophysiology and how both regions' neural activities are related to each other. This is of particular interest since there are no direct structural connections between right V1 and left V1. They observed FC between right V1 and left V1 which can thus be considered an instance of structure-function dissociation.

Neuronal findings IIb: relationship between functional connectivity and frequency fluctuations

How about the relationship between fluctuations and FC? Their results showed that neural activity in the right V1 (as measured with fMRI) was correlated with activity fluctuations in the lower frequency range (around 0.1 Hz) in the left V1 (see also Vincent et al. 2007 for an analogous finding). This means that right V1 and left V1 showed functional connectivity despite there being no direct interhemispheric structural connections between them. Furthermore, these results point out that functional connectivity is linked to a particular frequency domain in the fluctuations of the regions' neural activities across time.

Another investigation by Nir et al. (2008a and 2008b) provides some evidence in the same direction from human subjects on whom they performed intracranial recordings in bilateral auditory cortex during rest and sleep. Based on the local field potentials (LFP) as recorded intracranially, they observed that right and left auditory cortical LFPs correlated especially strongly with each other in lower frequency ranges (<0.01 Hz), while this correlation was weaker in higher frequencies (>0.01 Hz). Interestingly, an analogous observation was made in another group of subjects that underwent fMRI; these data showed that (fMRI-based) signal changes in right and left auditory cortical activities correlated with each other; that is, showing FC, especially in the low-frequency fluctuations (<0.1 Hz).

Taken together, these results show that FC may be linked to particular frequency ranges or domains in the fluctuations of the regions' neural activities. Thereby it seems that especially low-frequency fluctuations (around and lower than 0.1 Hz) seem to be of special relevance in constituting FC.

Neuronal hypothesis IIIa: Functional connectivity and fluctuations of neural activity

The data show that the FC is closely linked to particular frequency domains in the fluctuations of the regions' neural activities. The question now is how these observations relate to difference-based coding as sketched earlier. For that, we need to describe what exactly the concept of "frequency fluctuations" refers to. Frequency fluctuations describe the changes of neural activity across different discrete points in physical time.

Such changes may occur in short time intervals in which case higher frequency fluctuations are yielded (as, for instance, >1 Hz). Or the changes in neural activity may take longer to occur, thus presupposing longer time intervals and thereby yielding low-frequency fluctuations (as for instance < 0,1Hz). Taken together, frequency fluctuations describe time intervals, that is, temporal differences, between changes in neural activity.

How does that relate to functional connectivity and its constitution by difference-based coding? Difference-based coding implies that functional connectivity is constituted by computing (and thus encoding) the temporal differences between two regions' neural activities into one coherent neural difference. How can we now characterize the temporal patterns of each region's neural activity in a more specific way? Very simple. Each region's neural activity fluctuates in certain frequencies which means that its activity changes are determined by neural differences and more specifically by the temporal differences of the respective frequency range.

If now the neural differences—that is, the temporal differences and thus the respective frequency ranges—are similar between two different regions, their respective neural activities correlate with each other, thus showing FC. If, in contrast, their neural differences and thus their temporal differences differ grossly from each other, their respective neural activities cannot correlate with each other, meaning that there this is no FC.

I consequently hypothesize that difference-based coding of functional connectivity is closely linked to the frequency fluctuations of neural activity. Frequency fluctuations describe temporal differences in neural activity changes across different discrete points in physical time. The neural activity changes ultimately reflect the statistical frequency distribution of the regions' neural activity across time; i.e., their "neuronal statistics" if one wants to say so (see below for detailed explanation).

Neuronal hypothesis IIIb: Encoding of "neuronal statistics" and functional connectivity

What does this imply for the interaction between the different regions' neural activities? The interaction between two regions' neural activities amounts then to a comparison and matching between the statistical frequency distributions of their neural activity changes; i.e., their neuronal statistics:

If the regions' neuronal statistics match well with each other and operate thus in the same frequency range, their neural activities correlate and yield FC. If, in contrast, the regions' neuronal statistics do not match with each other, meaning that they fluctuate in different frequency ranges, their neural activities will not correlate and therefore yield no FC (see Fig. 5-3).

This means that, ultimately, FC can be traced back to the comparison and matching between different statistical frequency distribution; i.e., neuronal statistics, the statistics of the frequency fluctuations of the two regions' neural activities across different discrete points in physical time.

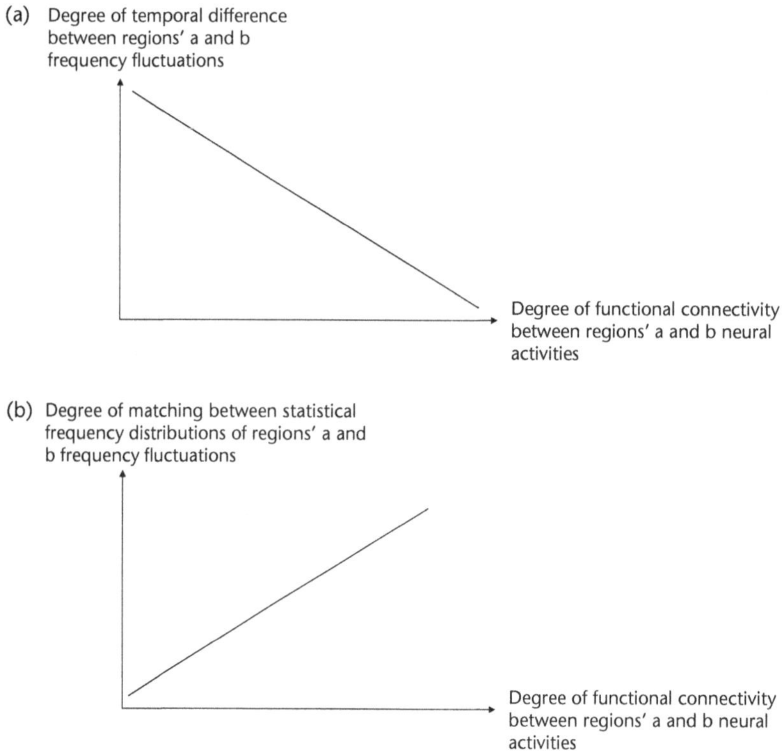

Figure 5-3 Frequency fluctuations and functional connectivity. The figure shows the relationship between functional connectivity and the frequency fluctuations as characterized by their phase durations. (*a*) The figure shows the inverse relationship between the regions' degree of frequency fluctuations and their degree of functional connectivity: the higher the degree of frequency fluctuations within each of the regions, the higher the temporal difference between the phase durations of their respective frequency fluctuations, the less likely temporal synchronization can occur between them, and the lower their subsequent degree of functional connectivity. Hence, the degree of functional connectivity between regions as spatial measure may be directly dependent on the regions' temporal relationship, that is, the temporal differences between the phase duration of their frequency fluctuations. (*b*) The figure describes the relation of functional connectivity to its underlying process, the comparison and matching of the statistical frequency distributions between the two (or more) regions' neural activities. The better the two (or more) regions' neural activities—that is, the phase durations of their frequency fluctuations—match across time, the better their neural activity is matched across space as well, resulting in increased functional connectivity.

Since such statistical frequency distribution concerns the regions' intrinsic neural activity, I here speak of "neuronal statistics." The concept of neuronal statistics describes the statistical frequency distribution of the changes in the brain's intrinsic activity levels across different discrete points in physical time (and space, that is, in different regions). The concept of neuronal statistics must be distinguished from the one of "natural statistics" that, as introduced in Part I, refers to the statistical frequency distribution of sensory stimuli (rather than to changes in the intrinsic neural activity levels).

Based on these considerations,, I propose that difference-based coding can be specified as the matching and comparison between the temporal differences of different regions' changes in their resting state activity levels. This implies that FC is constituted by the comparison and matching between different neuronal statistics as associated with the changes in the different regions' intrinsic activity levels. In short, resting state FC must be regarded a statistically based feature of the brain's intrinsic activity.

Neuronal hypothesis IIIc: Predisposition of functional connectivity by the brain's conduction delays

I postulate that resting state FC is constituted by matching and comparing the different temporal differences and thus the neuronal statistics of the changes in the different regions' resting state activity levels. Such matching and comparison between the regions' different statistical frequency distributions is purely functional. Accordingly, the introduction of both difference-based coding and the matching between different neuronal statistics allows one to tentatively account for the independence of FC from the anatomical-structural features of the brain; i.e., SC. This accounts well for the functional level of neural activity and what we described earlier as structure-function dissociation and "functional freedom."

We left open, however, how its "sibling," that is called "structure-function predisposition," stands in relation to the neural mechanisms of difference-based coding and the matching between different neuronal statistics. This is the focus in the present section.

How is the matching between the regions' neuronal statistics compatible with the predisposition of FC by SC? SC describes structural connectivity and that, in turn, implies certain conduction delays between different regions. Based on the biophysical-computational constraints of the neurons and regions, their structural connections limit the speed of the information transfer between the two regions' neural activities. Such conduction delay signifies by itself a particular temporal difference, the biophysical-computationally based delay in the conduction between two regions' neural activities.

How does the conduction delay's temporal difference stand in relation to the regions' temporal differences in their neural activity changes, that is, their neuronal statistics? One may first specify the respective temporal differences. The temporal difference of the conduction delay is biophysical and computationally based, whereas the one in the case of the neuronal statistics is neuronal and statistically based.

How now does the biophysical, computationally based temporal difference and thus the conduction delay, impact the other, the statistically based difference, as the matching between the two regions' neuronal statistics (of their intrinsic activity)? This leads me to sketch different possible scenarios in the relationship between biophysical-computational conduction delays and the regions' neuronal statistics. In a first scenario, the actual statistically based temporal difference of the two regions' neuronal statistics may be (more or less) similar to the biophysical, computationally based temporal difference of the conduction delay. In this case one would expect that functional connectivity builds on existing structural connectivity, with the latter thus predisposing the former.

I consequently hypothesize the following. The closer biophysical, computationally based and statistically based temporal differences, the more likely structural and functional connectivity will correspond and thus conform to each other. More generally, this means that the assumption of structure-function predisposition may well hold for instances of similarity between biophysical, computationally based and statistically based temporal differences.

Neuronal hypothesis IIId: structure-function dissociation and consciousness

Now let's turn to the second scenario that is opposite to the first. Such structure-function predisposition may no longer hold in those instances where biophysical, computationally based and statistically based temporal differences diverge from each other. More specifically, I hypothesize the following: the more biophysical, computationally based and statistically based temporal differences diverge from each other, the less likely functional connectivity will follow structural connectivity and its specific conduction delays.

Instead, functional connectivity will dissociate from structural connectivity by establishing functional connections with temporal differences that are either higher or lower than the biophysical, computationally based ones from the conduction delays: the higher the disparity or difference between biophysical, computationally based and statistically based temporal differences, the higher the likelihood of structure-function dissociation (see Fig. 5-4). Empirically, such a case is, for example, given when two regions' neural activities such as right and left V1 are synchronized with zero delay, as reported by the aforementioned study from Shmuel and Leopold (2008).

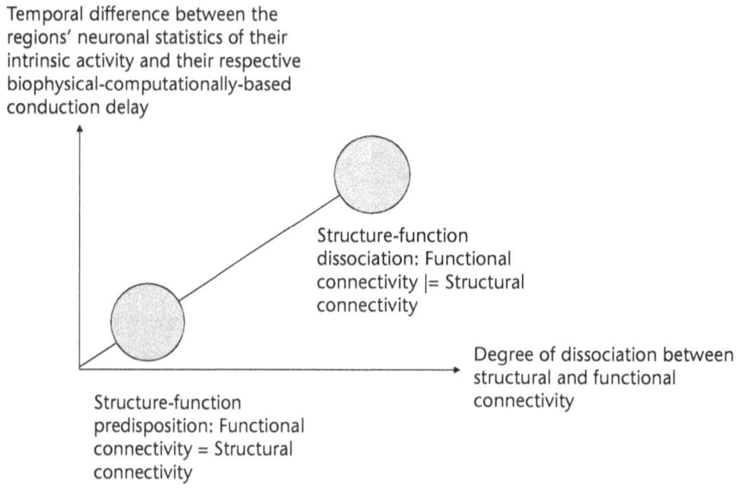

Figure 5-4 Structure–function relationship and conduction delays. The figure shows the relationship between the degree of structure-function dissociation on one hand and the conduction delays on the other. The y-axis stands for the subtraction of the two (or more) regions' conduction delays from the temporal difference in their neural activities (as resulting from the matching of their respective neuronal statistics across time and space). The x-axis describes the degree of dissociation between structural and functional connectivity as measured in the actual data. I now propose a linear relationship between the two variables on the x- and y-axis: the higher the subtraction value (between temporal difference values and conduction values of the two regions), the more the two (or more) regions' structural and functional connectivity will dissociate from each other. If the subtraction value on the y-axis tends toward zero, structural and functional connectivity will not much dissociate from each other (blue circle on the left). If, in contrast, the subtraction value deviates from zero and gets higher with the temporal difference in the regions' activity level being larger than the regions' difference in conduction delays, their respective functional connectivity will deviate significantly from their structural connectivity (see blue circle on the right).

Taken together, the relationship between the neuron's biophysical-computational conduction delays and the functional level of the temporal differences signaling changes in the brain's intrinsic activity levels can vary on a spectrum between maximal and minimal degrees of convergence. If there is maximal convergence, structure-function predisposition predominates; whereas in the opposite in case of minimal convergence, structure-function dissociation is more likely. This makes it clear that both structure-function predisposition and dissociation reflect different degrees of convergence (or divergence) between biophysical-computational constraints and functional changes in the brain's resting state activity levels.

This is not only neuronally important but also phenomenally; that is, for consciousness. Due to the strongly decreased metabolic and energy supply, the "functional freedom" of the brain's intrinsic activity (when compared to the biophysical-computational constraints) seems to be rather low or minimal in patients with vegetative state (VS) who have lost consciousness.

These patients' intrinsic activity may thus no longer be able to constitute a proper spatial and temporal structure that remains more or less independent of the anatomical-structural features of the brain (see Chapters 28 and 29 for details). This is well manifested in the observation of reduced functional connectivity in the resting state in these patients (see Chapter 28 for details).

Accordingly, the VS patients may suffer from an abnormal shift of the aforementioned continuum toward the pole of maximal convergence with abnormally high degrees of structure-function predisposition and low degrees of structure-function dissociation. If, finally, there is no structure-function dissociation at all anymore, the patients slip into coma and ultimately into brain death. This further underlines the central importance of the relationship between structure-function predisposition and structure-function dissociation for consciousness, thus signifying phenomenal relevance.

Neuronal findings IIIa: spontaneous fluctuations in the resting state

So far, I have considered the frequency fluctuations of the brain's intrinsic activity only in the context of functional connectivity. Thereby, results showed that FC seems to be predominantly related to low-frequency fluctuations (see earlier), which I have not yet accounted for. We therefore may want to describe in more detail the low-frequency fluctuations themselves and how they are related to high-frequency fluctuations (see also Bullmore and Sporns 2012).

Spontaneous fluctuations of neural activity in the resting state are often observed in especially the DMN, where they are characterized by predominant low frequencies (<0.1 Hz). However, low- (and high-) frequency fluctuations in neural activity can also be observed in regions other than the DMN like sensory cortices, motor cortex, insula, and subcortical regions (like basal ganglia and thalamus) (see Freeman 2003; Shulman et al. 2004, 2009; Buckner et al. 2008; Wang et al. 2007; Hunter et al. 2006; Zuo et al. 2010; Bullmore and Sporns 2012). Further support for spontaneous resting-state activity changes across the whole brain comes from electrophysiological studies showing spontaneous neuronal oscillations and synchronizations in various parts of the brain, including the hippocampus and the visual cortex (Buzsáki 2006; Buzsaki and Draguhn 2004; Arieli et al. 1996; Llinas 1988; Singer 2003; Fries et al. 2001, 2007). This suggests that spontaneous fluctuations in the intrinsic activity levels may be prevalent throughout the whole brain in both humans and animals and are not limited to the DMN.

Neuronal findings IIIb: low-frequency fluctuations in the resting state

Let's be more specific. The spontaneous BOLD fluctuations as observed in fMRI are to be found in lower frequency ranges like infra-slow fluctuations (ISFs) (0.001–0.1 Hz). In fMRI the low-frequency fluctuations can be measured by what recently has been called "amplitude of low frequency fluctuations" (ALFF) that describe the (root means square of the) standard deviation of variability in the resting state activity level across time. The data show that these ALFF do indeed occur in all regions throughout the whole brain.

The slow-frequency fluctuations observed in fMRI have been proposed to correspond to what is measured as slow cortical potentials (SCPs) in electroencephalography (EEG; Khader et al. 2008; He and Raichle 2009a and 2009b; Betzel et al. 2012). The SCPs are not easy to obtain in EEG because they are subject to artifacts caused by sweating, movements, and electrode drift; their measurement therefore requires more direct measurement by direct current (DC) recording. It remains unclear whether what is measured as SCP in EEG corresponds to, is related to, or even identical to the low-frequency fluctuations obtained in fMRI (see also Chapter 14 in Volume II for extensive discussion of the slow cortical potentials).

What is the empirical evidence for such correspondence between the low-frequency fluctuations fMRI signal and the SCPs as measured in EEG? Nagai et al. (2004) conducted a combined fMRI and EEG study focusing on a particular electrophysiological potential, the contingent negative variation (CNV). The CNV is a negative shift in cortical potentials that reflects an SCP; the CNV is induced by expectancy and anticipation of particular stimuli or events and occurs maximally strong over frontal midline electrodes.

How are now low frequency fluctuations related to the slow cortical potentials? Nagai et al. (2004) observed direct relation between the CNV as slow cortical potential as measured in EEG and the fMRI-based low-frequency fluctuations, thus supporting their direct relationship if not identity. Other studies extended these findings by showing that parametric variation of the cognitive load in, for instance, working memory tasks yields corresponding parametric changes in both fMRI-based low frequency fluctuations and EEG-based SCP (for reviews, see He and Raichle 2009; Khader et al. 2008).Taken together, these data provide evidence for the occurrence of low frequency fluctuations in a range lower than 0.1 Hz in the brain's resting state activity. The evidence for such low frequency fluctuations comes from both fMRI, where they are measured in the gestalt of the ALFF, and EEG, where they seem to surface in the SCP.

Neuronal findings IIIc: High-frequency fluctuations in the resting state

In addition to such low-frequency fluctuations, there are also higher frequency fluctuations in the brain's resting-state activity. These fluctuations cover frequencies ranging from 1 Hz and higher, thus including delta (1–4 Hz), theta (4–8 Hz), alpha (8–12 Hz), beta (12–30 Hz), and gamma (>30 Hz) (see Mantini et al. 2007; Sadaghiani et al. 2010).

This raises the question of how low and high frequencies are related to each other in the brain's resting state (see also the recent reviews by Fries 2009; Fell and Axmacher 2011; Canolty and Knight 2010; Sauseng and Klimesch 2008). In the following, I give only a brief overview of the main findings while not discussing all studies in full detail including the phase–phase coupling in specific regions like the hippocampus (see, for instance, Fell and Axmacher 2011). I will give a more detailed account of the relationship between high- and low-frequency fluctuations in Volume II (see Chapters 13, 15, and 20).

Vanhatalo et al. (2004) conducted an EEG study in both healthy and epileptic subjects during sleep and rest, where, using DC-EEG, they were able to record low-frequency oscillations. All subjects showed infraslow oscillations (0.02–0.2 Hz); these were seen widespread over all electrodes and thus the whole brain without showing any specific visually obvious spatial distribution.

Most interestingly, they observed cross-frequency phase-power coupling between the phases of the slow (0.02–0.2 Hz) oscillations and the power/amplitudes of the faster (1–10 Hz) oscillations. The power/amplitudes of the high-frequency oscillations (1–10 Hz) was the highest during the negative deflection phases of the slow-frequency oscillations (0.02–0.2 Hz). Even the higher frequency K-complexes that are characteristic for sleep as well as interictal epileptiform events were phase-locked to the slow-frequency oscillations in that the former occurred preferentially in the negative deflection phases of the latter.

An analogous cross-frequency phase-power coupling can also be described as entrainment of higher by lower frequencies. Such low–high frequency entrainment may not only occur during the resting state as described by the aforementioned study but also during rest–stimulus interaction where it may be central in synchronizing neuronal activity; this will be discussed in detail in Part IV of this volume.

By linking low and high frequencies, such low–high frequency entrainment may allow the brain's intrinsic activity to construct a certain neuronal unity, a spatiotemporal unity, across different discrete points in the physical space (i.e., the regions) and time (i.e., the different frequency fluctuations) in the brain. Such neuronal unity or better spatiotemporal unity in the brain's intrinsic activity may be central in allowing for the constitution of the kind of unity, a phenomenal unity, we experience in consciousness (see Chapters 13, 15, 18, and 20, where I will also go into further detail about the neuronal mechanisms underlying low–high frequency entrainment). Accordingly, low–high frequency entrainment is relevant not only neuronally but also phenomenally.

Neuronal hypothesis IVa: parallel-segregated coding versus interactive-integrative coding

How is it possible that the power or amplitude of high-frequency oscillations can be locked and thus entrained to the phases of low-frequency oscillations? If high- and low-frequency oscillations are coded in parallel and independently, such low–high frequency entrainment would not be possible beyond mere chance. In such a case, each time point and consequently each frequency range and its respective temporal duration would be coded in isolation from the temporal durations of the respective other frequency oscillations.

This would result in what I described in Chapter 4 (in the context of the spatial domain) as "parallel-segregated coding" that may be regarded as an extension of stimulus-based coding. The assumption of such parallel-segregated coding in the temporal domain of low- and high-frequency fluctuations is not empirically plausible, however, given the low–high frequency entrainment described earlier. One may consequently suggest a different coding strategy.

Instead of parallel-segregated coding, one may rather propose interactive-integrative coding (see also Chapter 4, where I applied it in a spatial context) that may be regarded an extension of difference-based coding. Applied to the temporal domain, "interactive-integrative coding" describes the neural coding of the relationship, that is, the temporal differences, between the temporal durations of the fluctuations in the different frequency ranges. More specifically, the temporal differences between neural activity changes are matched and compared with each other: that is, the phase durations in the low-frequency fluctuations are set against the phase durations in the high-frequency fluctuations.

Neuronal hypothesis IVb: difference-based coding and "temporal nestedness"

What does such matching and comparison between the phase durations of low- and high-frequency fluctuations look like? The phase durations of low-frequency fluctuations are obviously longer and do therefore reflect a larger temporal difference than the ones of the high-frequency fluctuations. This means that a larger temporal difference is compared and matched with a smaller one.

How can they be matched and compared with each other? This is possible only by testing whether the smaller temporal difference of the high-frequency fluctuations fits into the larger one of the low-frequency fluctuations. If so, the phase duration of the higher frequency fluctuation becomes integrated into the one of the lower frequency fluctuation, resulting in what has been described as low–high frequency entrainment (see earlier). This is manifested in that the maximal power and amplitude of the high-frequency fluctuation always occur at a particular point within the phase duration of the low-frequency fluctuations, thus reflecting what is described as "cross-frequency phase-power coupling" (for excellent reviews, see Canolty and Knight 2010; Sauseng and Klimesch 2008).

If, in contrast, both larger and smaller temporal differences do not fit together in some way or the other, the high-frequency fluctuation remains independent of the lower. Low–high frequency entrainment remains consecutively impossible. In this case, the amplitude of the high-frequency fluctuation is not tied to a particular point within the phase duration of the low-frequency fluctuations.

Depending on the temporal differences between their phase durations, low- and high-frequency fluctuations may be integrated and linked in different ways. Thereby, due to low–high frequency entrainment, high-frequency fluctuations are nested in the lower frequency fluctuations. One can consecutively speak of "temporal nestedness" (see Canolty and Knight 2010; Sauseng and Klimesch 2008; and Betzel et al. 2012, for empirical support; also see Chapters 13, 15, 18, and 20 in Volume II for more details).

How can we better illustrate such "temporal nestedness"? Let us compare the temporal nestedness between low- and high-frequency fluctuations to the kind of nestedness that can be observed in the case of Russian dolls. As we know, each Russian doll contains a slightly smaller Russian doll, which in turn contains a smaller one, and so forth. The smaller dolls thus nest inside the next-bigger ones, whereas the biggest doll contains the highest number of dolls inside it.

How does the example of the Russian dolls compare to the relationship between low- and high-frequency fluctuations? The biggest doll showing the largest extension (in space) corresponds in our case to the biggest temporal extension—that is, the longest phase durations as the one of low-frequency fluctuations.

The smaller dolls, in contrast, have their equivalent in the shorter phase durations of the higher frequency fluctuations that, analogous to the smaller dolls, are nested within the next bigger one, and so forth. The relation between small and bigger Russian dolls can thus be well compared to the one between the shorter and longer phase durations of high and low frequency fluctuations in the brain. The brain may therefore amount to nothing but a Russian doll, at least in temporal regard.

Neuronal hypothesis Va: The brain's intrinsic activity constructs a temporal structure in its neural activity

By linking and integrating low- and high-frequency fluctuations with the latter's smaller phase durations nesting and residing in the longer ones of the former, the brain's intrinsic activity constructs temporal nestedness. Given the different frequency fluctuations and their different possible constellations, different forms of temporal nestedness can be yielded that ultimately results in the construction of what I describe as "temporal structure."

What do I mean by the concept of "temporal structure"? The term "temporal structure" describes the various kind of possible temporal relationships between low- and high-frequency fluctuations and their respective phase durations and amplitudes. As such, the term "structure" refers here to a particular temporal organization that spans in a virtual way across different discrete points in physical time (and space) (see Fig. 5-5).

How can we now characterize such temporal structure in further detail? Empirically, the temporal structure can be characterized as "highly dynamic" in that it continuously changes. It seems that there are changes within time units of 100–200ms, the so-called *microstates*, as observed in EEG results on resting state activity (see deVille et al. 2010; Britz et al. 2010; Michel and Murray 2012; Hutchinson et al. 2012). However, there are certain "core" microstates that appear more often than others, so that there is a certain structure and organization, a "temporal structure" as I say.

The temporal structure of the brain's intrinsic activity must be considered as truly functional as based on neuronal mechanisms and processes (see beginning of this chapter for the definition of "functional"). Being functional and signifying the level of the brain's intrinsic activity, the concept of temporal structure must be distinguished from the brain's anatomical structure as based on its biophysical-computational features, such as the conduction delays. This makes it clear that the temporal structure of the brain's intrinsic activity is clearly functional rather than structural.

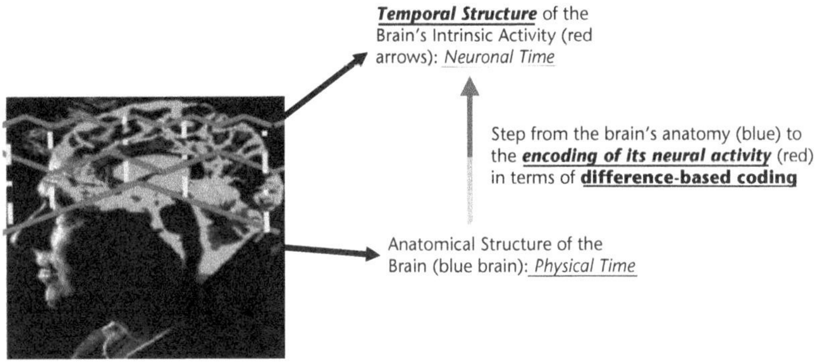

Figure 5-5 Constitution of temporal structure in the neural activity of the brain's intrinsic activity. The figure illustrates schematically that the brain's intrinsic activity constitutes in its neural activity a temporal structure (white horizontal lines symbolize fluctuations in neural activity with the grey vertical lines symbolizing cross frequency coupling) functional connectivity that supersedes and operates across the anatomical structure (brain). The physical time of the brain's anatomical structure is thus superseded by the neuronal time of the brain's intrinsic activity that operates across the former. That is made possible by encoding neural activity in terms of difference-based coding, as is indicated on the right with the arrow from the anatomical structures and their physical time to the intrinsic activity's spatial structure and its neuronal time.

NEURONAL HYPOTHESIS VB: THE TEMPORAL STRUCTURE OF THE BRAIN'S INTRINSIC ACTIVITY IS NEURONAL AS WELL AS DIFFERENCE- AND STATISTICALLY BASED

Moreover, the temporal structure of the brain's intrinsic activity is ultimately based on the matching and comparison between different temporal differences; that is the differences from the phase durations between low- and high-frequency fluctuations.

Therefore, very much like the spatial structure, the brain's temporal structure is statistically based rather than biophysically computationally based. That is what I mean when I characterize both temporal and spatial structure as neuronal rather than as merely physical (see also Chapter 4).

As detailed by the example of structure-function dissociation, the statistically based temporal structure operates across and supersedes the biophysical, computationally based conduction delays and their respective anatomical structure. This means, however, that the statistically based temporal structure is not isomorphic to the biophysical, computationally based temporal structure of the conduction delays.

Accordingly, the temporal structure of the brain's intrinsic activity cannot be identified in a one-to-one way and is thus not isomorphic with the brain's biophysical-computational and anatomical structure (see also Fingelkurts et al. 2010a, 2010b, 2011; for the assumption of a more or less analogous spatial and temporal structure in the resting state when they speak of "operational space-time"; however, they do not detail the mechanisms and processes that are necessary to constitute such "operational space-time"). In other words, there is no isomorphism between anatomical-structural and physiological-functional levels in the brain and thus between its biophysical-computational features and the spatial and temporal structure of the brain's intrinsic activity.

NEURONAL HYPOTHESIS VC: LINKAGE BETWEEN SPACE AND TIME—SPATIOTEMPORAL STRUCTURE

Besides not being isomorphic to the biophysical-computational structure of its underlying anatomy, the intrinsic linkage with the spatial structure must be considered another hallmark feature of the temporal structure. There is, I postulate, an intrinsic integration between spatial and temporal dimensions within one coherent spatiotemporal structure in the brain's intrinsic activity.

Let's be more specific. We already saw earlier that functional connectivity is based upon temporal differences between two regions' neural activities. By coding the temporal difference between the regions' neural activities, the spatial relationship between the two regions also changes by, for instance, increasing or decreasing the degree of functional connectivity. This already establishes an intrinsic link between spatial and temporal dimensions within FC itself.

There is yet another link between temporal and spatial dimensions. Low-frequency fluctuations (<0.1 Hz) show long phase durations that seem to require larger and global spatial extension across different regions of the brain. In contrast, high-frequency fluctuations (like, for instance, gamma >30 Hz) show much shorter phase durations with lower degrees of spatial extension and do therefore operate more locally and regionally (see Canolty and Knight 2010; Singer 1999, 2009).

These observations point toward an intrinsic linkage between spatial and temporal dimensions on the functional level of the brain's intrinsic activity. One may therefore better speak of a "spatiotemporal structure" characterizing the brain's intrinsic activity rather than either spatial or temporal structure.

Such spatiotemporal structure does operate on the functional level of the brain's intrinsic activity as distinguished from its anatomical-structural features. In addition, the spatiotemporal structure is statistically based—that is, based on the encoding of different neuronal statistics and their respective neuronal differences—rather than biophysically computationally based. This is what I mean when I characterize the intrinsic activity's spatiotemporal structure as "neuronal" rather than physical as well as statistically-based.

Open Questions

The first question pertains to the generation of the brain's intrinsic activity itself. I here described how the brain's intrinsic activity generates and constitutes a temporal and spatial structure; that is, a spatiotemporal structure. Thereby I described difference-based coding and matching and comparison between different neuronal statistics (i.e., statistical frequency distribution) as central neuronal mechanisms. While these neuronal mechanisms are supposed to account for the constitution of the spatiotemporal structure by the brain's intrinsic activity, they cannot, however, explain how the intrinsic activity itself is generated. For that, one should turn to simulation models as they have been investigated by Gustavo Deco, a Spanish network modeler (see Deco et al. 2009; Gosh et al. 2008a and 2008b; see also Deco et al. 2011 for an excellent review; see also Mazzoni et al. 2007, 2008). These simulation models aim to show how the brain's intrinsic activity is generated as such, whereas most often they seem to leave open the exact coding strategy the brain itself applies. In the future, one may therefore want to align these simulation models with the here-postulated suggestions of difference-based coding and the matching between different neuronal statistics as the neuronal mechanisms that may underlie the constitution of the spatiotemporal structure of the brain's intrinsic activity.

The second main question concerns a more detailed characterization of the spatiotemporal structure. Neuronally, the spatiotemporal structure of the brain's intrinsic activity is not static and unchanging; instead, it is dynamic and continuously changing, as is well reflected in its variability (see Garrett et al. 2011; McDonnell and Ward 2011). Thereby, it generates what have been described as "microstates" (see van de Ville 2010; Britz et al. 2010; Musso et al. 2010; Lehman et al. 1998, 2010), neuronal assemblies (Fingelkurts et al. 2010a and 2010b, 2011; and many others), or "neuronal transients" (Friston 1995, 1997, 2000), which refer to stable though transient spatiotemporal patterns in the brain's intrinsic activity. It would be interesting for future investigation to determine how such microstates compare to the here-suggested difference-based coding.

Finally, we postulated in the first part that difference-based coding leads to the temporal and spatial sparsening of neural activity on cellular and regional levels. I have so far focused only on difference-based coding while neglecting sparse coding. If difference-based coding is supposed to be central for the constitution of the spatiotemporal structure of the brain's intrinsic activity, one would expect the latter to also show a sparse pattern in its neural activity. In short, the brain's intrinsic activity should be characterized by sparse coding. This will be the focus in the next chapter, Chapter 6.

CHAPTER 6
Sparse Coding of Intrinsic Activity

Summary

Chapter 5 discussed several lines of evidence for the assumption of a statistically based spatiotemporal structure in the resting state. That was supposed to be based on difference-based coding. This raises the question of whether difference-based coding of the brain's intrinsic activity is associated with sparse coding, as we have seen it in the case of stimulus-induced activity on both cellular and regional levels (see Part I). A recent study demonstrates that the actual spatiotemporal activity patterns constrain, that is, sparsen, the possible number of the subsequently following spatiotemporal activity patterns. The actually observed number of spatiotemporal patterns in the intrinsic activity is rather low when compared to the number of possible spatiotemporal constellations. These and other results suggest that the brain's intrinsic activity and, more specifically, its spatiotemporal activity patterns, can be characterized by a high degree of sparse coding and a rather low degree of dense coding. Since sparse coding on the cellular level was shown to be closely related to Glutamate and GABAergic-mediated neural inhibition (see Chapter 2), one would suspect both to be also central in mediating the sparse coding of the brain's intrinsic activity. I hence discuss recent findings on the biochemical mechanisms underlying the constitution of resting-state activity. The findings demonstrate that the resting-state concentration of glutamate is directly related to the degree of resting-state functional connectivity between distal and thus remote regions. However, GABA seems to impact mainly local and thus more proximal neural activity. The imaging findings demonstrate that both GABA and glutamate are related to the differences between different neural activity levels like eyes open and closed rather than being related to one particular activity level by itself. I therefore hypothesize that GABA and glutamate are particularly sensitive and tuned to encode relative neural activity changes—that is, neural differences—rather than absolute values of neural activity by themselves. This suggests that glutamate and GABA encode neural activity in terms of difference-based coding rather than stimulus-based coding. Such difference-based coding may make possible the temporal and spatial sparsening and thus sparse coding of the spatiotemporal patterns of the brain's intrinsic activity. In sum, I hypothesize that the brain's intrinsic activity on a regional level can be characterized by difference-based coding (as distinguished from stimulus-based coding) and sparse coding (as distinguished from dense or local coding) which both seem to be mediated by GABA and glutamate and their excitation-inhibition balance (EIB).

Key Concepts and Topics Covered

Sparse coding, spatiotemporal activity patterns, intrinsic activity, resting state, GABA, glutamate, difference-based coding, excitation-inhibition balance

Neuroempirical background Ia: Sparse coding of the brain's intrinsic activity

The previous chapters in this part (Chapters 4 and 5) described how the brain's intrinsic activity constitutes a statistically based spatiotemporal structure that operates across and supersedes both the anatomical structure and its biophysical-computational constraints. Thereby the term "structure" refers to a particular organization that signifies a statistically based template or grid across the different discrete points in the physical space and time. This, as I suggest, is possible only on the basis of encoding spatial and temporal differences into the brain's intrinsic activity, thus implying difference-based coding rather than stimulus-based coding.

How is the statistically based spatiotemporal structure of the brain's intrinsic activity formatted? We saw so far that it is coded in terms of spatial and temporal differences, that is, difference-based coding, while we left open the formatting of the brain's intrinsic activity.

The concept of format describes the manifestation and thus the result or outcome of the coding process. We saw, for instance, that the resulting neural activity on a cellular level during sensory stimulation was formatted in a sparse way in sensory cortex, which presupposes sparse coding (see Chapters 1 and 2). Analogously, neural activity on a regional level was also spatially and temporally sparsened during perceptual decision making, as we saw in Chapter 3. This suggests sparse formatting and thus sparse coding (as distinguished from dense or local coding) to hold on both cellular and regional levels of stimulus-induced activity.

How about the brain's resting-state activity? We saw that the resting-state activity is not static but rather dynamic when undergoing continuous changes in its level of neural activity (see Chapters 4 and 5). How are these changes in the brain's intrinsic activity formatted and encoded into neural activity? Given the observed sparse coding during stimulus-induced activity, one would suggest sparse coding rather than dense or local coding to also determine the formatting and encoding of the brain's intrinsic activity. This is the focus in the present chapter.

Is the brain's intrinsic activity, as we observe it, indeed the result of sparse coding? If so, the alleged spatiotemporal structure should be constituted on the basis of prior processes of spatial and temporal sparsening. Hence, the first, more specific aim of this chapter is to gather empirical evidence in favor of sparse coding in the brain's intrinsic activity.

Neuroempirical background IB: Neural inhibition and the brain's intrinsic activity

The assumption of sparse coding in the brain's intrinsic activity raises the question of how the processes of spatial and temporal sparsening of neural activity operate and are implemented. In the case of stimulus-induced activity in the sensory cortex (on the cellular and population level), neural inhibition as mediated by GABA was supposed to be central in allowing for spatial and temporal sparsening of neural activity (see Chapter 2). Thereby GABA acted in conjunction with glutamate, which mediates neural excitation. This means that the balance between GABA and glutamate, the excitation-inhibition balance (EIB), is central in determining the degree of spatial and temporal sparsening of stimulus-induced activity.

How about GABA and glutamate and the excitation-inhibition balance (EIB) in the brain's intrinsic activity? One may want to investigate how GABA and glutamate and thus the EIB modulate the resting-state activity within as well as between different regions. In addition, one may want to consider how the EIB drives and predisposes sparse coding of the brain's intrinsic activity and its continuous dynamic changes. This is the second more specific aim of this chapter.

Neuroempirical background IIA: Formal syntactic properties in brain, music, and language

Dan Lloyd was originally a philosopher at the Trinity College in Hartford, Connecticut. Besides philosophizing, he is also very much interested in the mind and more specifically in how the brain yields what we as observers call consciousness and mind. Thus, he is not afraid of tackling empirical issues and approaching them from a sometimes unusual perspective (at least for the neuroscientists, and definitely for philosophers).

Lloyd has raised the question of whether the coding of the brain's neural activity during both resting-state and stimulus-induced activity is similar to the one of music and language (Lloyd 2011). More specifically, he was interested in the formal coding or syntactic properties (see next paragraphs for discussing the term *syntactic* and how it relates to coding) of all three: brain, music, and language.

Similar formal coding or syntactic properties may, for instance, be shared between language and brain, which on the philosophical side would amount to the thesis of a "language of thought": despite their different semantic and thus content features, language and brain may nevertheless share their formal -synaptic features and thus the same kind of coding. Our thoughts arising from the brain would consequently be structured like the language which we use to express them, thus amounting to what is described as "language of thought" in philosophy.

What are formal-syntactic properties? Formal-syntactic properties may, for instance, consist in a particular coding of the different elements and their relationship to each other. The elements may be tones in music, words in language, or activity patterns in the brain.

How are these basic elements related and combined with each other? Certain tones may appear together often, while others hardly ever occur in conjunction. The same holds true for words in language as well as for the spatiotemporal patterns and their constellations in the brain's intrinsic (and extrinsic) activity.

Neuroempirical background IIb: sparse coding of formal-syntactic properties in brain, music, and language

How do the formal-syntactic properties in the different systems—language, music, and brain—stand in relation to sparse coding? If certain constellations between the different elements (tones, words, spatiotemporal activity patterns) occur more often than others, the full range of possible combinations between the different elements (i.e., activity patterns, tones, words) may not be fully exhausted by the respective system; that is, brain, language, or music. Instead, one can observe only a limited number of combinations between the elements to be actually manifest in language, music or the brain's intrinsic activity. In this case one can speak of sparseness and thus sparse coding.

Dan Lloyd aimed to compare the different degrees of sparsening, that is, sparse coding, in the brain's spatiotemporal activity patterns when compared to language and music. For that, he investigated how words are combined in different languages (English, French, Spanish, Finnish, Chinese) and how tones are related and combined in different pieces of music (Schubert, Gershwin, Chinese folk, British folk, African folk).

In addition, he conducted an analysis of different imaging studies during either resting-state activity or stimulus-induced activity (auditory oddball paradigm). For the analysis of the brain imaging studies, he used an independent component analysis that yields different spatiotemporal activity patterns across time and space in the brain; he identified one particular predominating spatiotemporal activity pattern at each point in time, which allowed him to observe the changes in spatiotemporal activity patterns across different points in time.

He was now interested in seeing how the different spatiotemporal activity patterns in the brain are related and combined with each other across time: whether, for instance, certain spatiotemporal activity patterns occurred more often than others and whether the full range of possible spatiotemporal activity patterns was exhausted and actually manifested.

This, as the constellations of tones and words in music and language, was measured with calculations of distinct variants of the standard deviations, that is, the variations across time and space. Since these measures refer to the degree of sparseness in the occurrence of the elements (words, tones, spatiotemporal patterns), they indicate the degree of sparse coding in the respective system (language, music, brain's intrinsic activity).

Neuronal findings Ia: Different degrees of sparseness in the formal-syntactic properties in brain, music, and language

What did Dan Lloyd observe in his results? He observed that music was sparser than language. Certain notes occurred more frequently and others less often, whereas all words in language were actually used quite often. Language thus shows a more dense code, while the one in music is sparser. One would consequently postulate a higher degree of sparse coding in music than in language.

How does now the brain's intrinsic activity stand in relation to this? The results show that certain spatiotemporal activity patterns occurred rather often, while others were rarely or not at all observed. Moreover, the number of actually occurring sequences relative to the number of possible sequences was rather high, so the brain's spatiotemporal activity patterns do not seem to exhaust their full range of possibilities.

This suggests that the brain's spatiotemporal activity patterns exhibited a rather high degree of sparseness that is closer to the one of music than the one of language. The brain's activity patterns across time are thus encoded in a more sparse way than words in language. In contrast, the brain and its sequence of spatiotemporal activity patterns seem to be more or less similar to the formal constellations and sequences as observed between tones in music (Fig. 6-1).

How about the difference between resting-state and stimulus-induced activity with regard to the degree of sparseness? Lloyd observed that the resting-state studies showed a lower degree of sparseness in the distribution of their spatiotemporal activity patterns across time than the stimulus-induced activity studies (that applied an auditory oddball paradigm requiring attention and perception).

Lloyd therefore hypothesizes that the encounter with specific stimuli (as in stimulus-induced activity) or tasks (as in task-related activity) may drive the brain toward increased temporal and spatial sparsening of its own spatiotemporal activity pattern and thus to a higher degree of sparse coding. This is in line with other findings that support both the observation of sparse coding in the brain's intrinsic activity and its changes during stimulus-induced activity (see Wang et al. 2009; Jao et al. 2013; Lee et al. 2011; Zhang et al. 2012; see also Betzel et al. 2012, for the observation of a recruitment of a limited or sparse number of spatiotemporally reoccurring core states in resting-state EEG).

Taken together, Lloyd's study shows that the brain's resting-state and stimulus-induced activity can be characterized by high degrees of spatial and temporal sparseness of its spatiotemporal activity patterns. As such, the brain's intrinsic activity seems to be more similar to the formal activity pattern in music than that of language. Furthermore, resting-state activity seems to show a slightly lower degree of sparseness than stimulus-induced activity. This indicates that the degree of sparse coding is not fixed but can vary across time and space in dependence on the respective neuronal contexts. .

Neuronal findings Ib: "Music of the brain" and its "neuronal melody"

What do these findings imply in more concrete terms? Let's start with the example of music and the structure between the different tones in music. One particular note or tone in music strongly determines and predicts which note will (or must) come next.

The same is true for the brain. Here, the occurrence of one actual spatiotemporal activity pattern seems to determine which spatiotemporal activity pattern will follow (and which ones are less likely to occur, or do not occur at all). The actual spatiotemporal activity pattern limits or sparsens the number of spatiotemporal activity pattern that can possibly follow, thus leading to sparse coding (rather than dense or local coding).

Let us describe the situation in the case of the brain in further detail. The observation of a rather low or sparse number of actual spatiotemporal activity patterns entails that the previous spatiotemporal activity pattern increase the probability of a particular spatiotemporal activity pattern as its possible successor, while

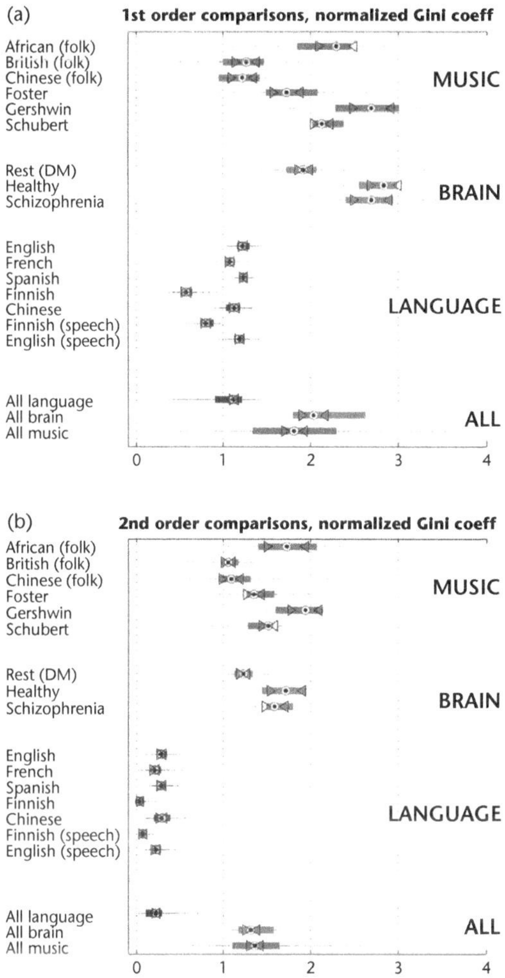

Figure 6-1a Sparse coding in the brain, music, and language. Three-way comparison of music, language, and fMRI data. The bars represent data from 99 subjects in three experiments. Healthy and Schizophrenia subjects both performed an "auditory oddball task," consisting of identifying a target tone in a stream of non-target tones and distracting noises. The largest group comprises 64 subjects in the rest condition (also known as Default Mode). (*a*) 1st-order sparseness; i.e., sparsity/density of single symbols. (*b*) 2nd-order sparseness; i.e., sparsity/density of sequential pairs of symbols. (Reprinted from Lloyd D. Mind as music. *Front Psychol.* 2011;2:63.)

making others less likely. In short, the actual spatiotemporal patterns have a strong say in what will happen next and are therefore predictive. This is different in language. Due to the high number of actually occurring constellations, the use of a particular word does not really predict the following word. Unlike the tones in music and the spatiotemporal activity patterns in the brain, the words in language do not really predict the subsequent words and therefore exert no strong impact on future words and their combinations.

To put it differently: we may be more often caught by surprise by the words in our language than when listening to tones in music and observing the spatiotemporal patterns in our brain's resting state. Accordingly, we are less able to predict the next word in our language

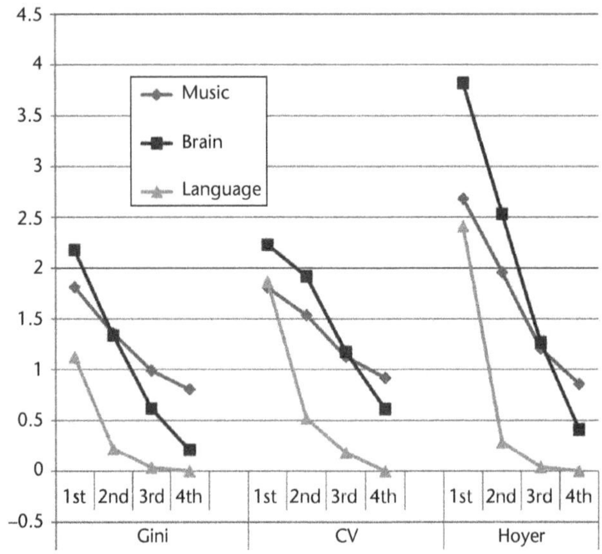

Figure 6-1b **Sparse coding in the brain, music, and language. Normalized sparseness measures for music, brain data, and language (median values). Single symbols (first order), pairs (second), triples, and quadruples, and compared, as calculated with the Gini coefficient, the coefficient of variation, and the Hoyer index. For 10 of the 12 separate observations, the greatest similarity is between brain data and music. In all cases, brain data are more similar to music than they are to language, as measured by Wilcoxon rank sum probabilities. (Reprinted from Lloyd D. Mind as music. *Front Psychol.* 2011;2:63.)**

than the next tone in music or the next spatiotemporal activity pattern in our brain's intrinsic activity.

The similarity between brain and music in the degree of sparse coding inclines Lloyd to speak of a "music of thought" as distinguished from a "language of thought." Since the brain and its spatiotemporal activity pattern mediate our thoughts and show degrees of sparse coding similar to music rather than language, our thoughts may be formatted like music. One can therefore speak, as Lloyd does, of a "music of thought" rather than "language of thought."

One may extend this analogy even further and speak of a "music of the brain." The concept of a "music of the brain" may figuratively indicate the brain's similarity to music with regard to the degree of sparse coding of its formal-syntactic properties, the spatiotemporal activity patterns. Hence, to take this almost literally, the brain may indeed generate some kind of (formal-syntactic) melody during the transitions between its different spatiotemporal activity patterns: a "neuronal melody," if one wants to say so.

Neuronal hypothesis Ia: parallel-segregated coding of the brain's intrinsic spatiotemporal activity patterns

What does the observation of sparse coding in the brain's intrinsic activity imply for the coding of the relationship between the different spatiotemporal activity patterns? Sparseness implies a high degree of predisposition or prediction of one neural activity pattern by the respectively preceding one. How is that possible? This leads us to the question of their coding, the process of how the spatiotemporal activity patterns are generated and how they are related to each other such that one can predict the following one.

Let us discuss different possible options in the encoding of the relationship between the different spatiotemporal activity patterns. One may propose parallel-segregated coding between the different spatiotemporal activity patterns: In this case, the constitution of each of the spatiotemporal activity patterns remains independent of the respective other. This means that the preceding spatiotemporal activity patterns have no direct impact on the constitution of the subsequent ones. The constitution of each spatiotemporal activity patterns depends only and exclusively on the present neural activity levels while remaining independent of the previous ones, the past patterns.

In addition to the neglect of the past patterns, the constitution of the present spatiotemporal activity pattern will also carry no information for the following spatiotemporal activity patterns. Which spatiotemporal pattern will be constituted in the future remains completely independent of the present one which therefore carries no information about future spatiotemporal activity patterns. Accordingly, the different spatiotemporal activity patterns are encoded independent from each other and thus in a parallel and segregated way.

Such independence and segregation in the encoding of different spatiotemporal activity patterns leads naturally to a higher degree of local (one-to-one) or even dense (one-to-many) coding. Following the results by Lloyd, this seems to be the case in language, where one particular word may be followed by many possible words.

Such dense coding is possible only when the different words are coded by themselves independent of and segregated from other words. I consequently postulate a higher degree of parallel and segregated coding in the encoding of words in language.

While such parallel-segregated coding may apply to words and language, it may not, however, apply to the spatiotemporal activity patterns in the brain. This is suggested by the higher degrees of sparse coding of spatiotemporal activity patterns in the brain when compared to the words in language. We therefore have to seek for an alternative coding strategy, one that is different from parallel-segregated coding.

Neuronal hypothesis Ib: Interactive-integrative coding of the brain's intrinsic spatiotemporal activity patterns

What is the alternative to such parallel-segregated coding? As discussed in Chapters 4 and 5, one may consider an interactive-integrative coding strategy. The different spatiotemporal activity patterns in the brain's resting-state activity may then interact with each other; that, in turn, makes possible their integration and the consecutive constitution of a novel activity pattern on the basis of the previous one.

In this case, the previous or past spatiotemporal activity pattern thus predisposes, i.e., predetermines and even predicts the constitution of the actual spatiotemporal activity pattern in the present moment, which, in turn, may predispose the subsequent one and so forth. Let me be more specific. Such interactive-integrative coding strategy allows for the spatiotemporal activity pattern c to be generated in dependence on the previous pattern b, which in turn is dependent on its respective predecessor, pattern a. This means that pattern b is encoded in relation to a, that is (b-a), while the generation of the pattern c depends on b (and so forth) so that the activity pattern c is a function of (b-a), that is (c-(b-a)). And the same applies, of course, to the next activity pattern d that will be based on c, that is (d-((c-b)(b-a))), and so forth.

What does this imply for the characterization of interactive-integrative coding of the brain's spatiotemporal activity patterns? Interactive-integrative coding can be characterized by both interaction and integration: There is interaction between past, present, and future spatiotemporal activity patterns.

Such interaction allows for the integration of information from the past spatiotemporal activity pattern into the present one which then also contains some information about the next future pattern, and so forth. Accordingly, unlike in parallel-segregated coding, past, present, and future spatiotemporal activity patterns transfer their respective information and are therefore closely, that is intrinsically, interwoven and knit together in interactive-integrative coding.

Neuronal hypothesis Ic: Difference-based coding allows for interactive-integrative coding of the brain's intrinsic spatiotemporal activity patterns

How is such interactive-integrative coding possible? The underlying neuronal process must allow for the transfer of spatial and temporal features of the previous spatiotemporal activity pattern into the subsequent one. This means that the previous spatial and temporal features must be somehow encoded into the subsequent spatiotemporal activity pattern and related to its own spatial and temporal features. In other words, past and present spatial and temporal features need to be linked with each other in order to make possible the integration of the past spatiotemporal activity pattern into the present one.

How is such linkage between past and present spatial and temporal features possible? I suggest that this is possible only by encoding the differences between past and present spatial and temporal features into the neural activity related to the present spatiotemporal activity pattern. By encoding spatial and temporal differences, the past spatial and temporal features are preserved and, metaphorically speaking, carried over and transferred to the present spatiotemporal activity pattern.

How can such spatial and temporal differences be encoded into neural activity? That is possible only, as I claim, by encoding spatial and temporal differences between past and present spatial and temporal features into neural activity rather than their respective discrete points in time and space. In other words, I propose difference-based coding (as distinguished from stimulus-based coding) to allow for the linkage between past and present spatial and temporal features in the encoding of the brain's spatiotemporal activity patterns. This implies that the encoded spatial and temporal differences in the present spatiotemporal activity pattern contain some information about the preceding and thus the past pattern.

How about the information about the next, the future spatiotemporal activity pattern? The spatial and temporal differences as encoded into the neural activity underlying the present spatiotemporal activity pattern do constrain the degree of spatial and temporal differences that can possibly be encoded by the next subsequent spatiotemporal activity pattern. This means that the present spatiotemporal activity pattern increases the probability that certain particular spatiotemporal activity patterns will follow, while decreasing the likelihood of others. In other words, the present spatiotemporal activity pattern contains some information about the ones in the future. Taken together, I postulate that interactive-integrative coding of the relationship between the different spatiotemporal activity patterns presupposes difference-based coding rather than stimulus-based coding.

Neuronal hypothesis Id: Difference-based coding of the brain's intrinsic spatiotemporal activity patterns and consciousness

Why are difference-based coding and interactive-integrative coding important? I claim that they are not only neuronally relevant in determining the brain's spatiotemporal activity patterns, but also behaviorally and phenomenally. Let us start with behavioral relevance.

The psychiatric disorder of schizophrenia seems to be characterized by abnormally reduced degrees of difference-based coding in (for instance) the auditory cortex due to abnormally high resting-state activity (see Chapters 22 and 27 for details). Such high auditory cortical resting-state activity leads to auditory hallucinations and subsequently to sometimes rather bizarre behavior in these patients. This signifies the behavioral relevance of difference-based coding and interactive-integrative coding of the brain's intrinsic spatiotemporal activity pattern (see Chapters 22 and 27 for more details).

How about the relevance for consciousness, the phenomenal relevance? Patients in a vegetative state (VS) lost their consciousness and show decreased functional connectivity and low frequency fluctuations in their resting-state activity (see Chapters 28 and 29). The decrease in the resting state's neuronal measures may result from decreased interactive-integrative coding and an abnormally increased parallel-segregated coding of the neural activity.

That, as I will claim, is central for the loss of consciousness as observed in these patients. Accordingly, it seems as if certain degrees of both difference-based coding and interactive-integrative coding are necessary to allow for the association of consciousness with changes in neural activity during either resting-state or stimulus-induced activity.

Neuronal hypothesis IIa: sparse coding of the brain's intrinsic spatiotemporal activity patterns

How does such difference-based coding relate to sparse coding? By encoding a chain of spatial and temporal differences into the neural activity underlying the different spatiotemporal activity patterns), the possible range of the latter becomes constrained. This means that the range of spatiotemporal activity patterns that can possibly be constituted becomes sparsened.

Here, the actual spatiotemporal activity pattern constrains the spatiotemporal configurations the following activity pattern can possibly take. By exerting such a constraining influence, the number of possible candidates for the following spatiotemporal activity pattern is significantly reduced and thus sparsened. Hence, difference-based coding in the constitution of the brain's spatiotemporal activity pattern leads (necessarily or unavoidably) to sparse coding.

Sparse coding, as discussed in Chapters 1 and 2, signifies the encoding of the statistical frequency distribution of stimuli, rather than the stimuli themselves. In the case of the resting-state activity, one may thus suggest that the resting state encodes the statistical frequency distribution of its neural stimuli (see Chapter 4) into its own neural activity. Rather than speaking of natural statistics as in extrinsic stimuli (see Chapters 1 and 2), one may then want to speak of an encoding of "neuronal statistics" in the case of the resting-state activity (see Chapter 9 for details).

How can we support the encoding of the statistical frequency distribution of the neuronal stimuli, the "neuronal statistics," into the neural activity during the resting state? Statistical frequency distribution reflects nothing but variability or standard deviation in the signal changes we observe. If now the resting state signals' statistical frequency distribution is relevant for its encoding of neural activity, its variability (or "standard deviation" in a more operational sense) should contain important information rather than being mere noise.

This is indeed supported by recent data that show the variability in the resting-state activity to encode and predict stimulus-induced activity and the associated behavior (see Duncan et al. 2013; McDonnell and Ward 2011; Garrett et al. 2010, 2011). Though tentatively and indirectly, these data lend further support to the assumption that the resting-state activity is based on sparse coding and its encoding of statistical frequency distribution, i.e., neuronal statistics.

Neuronal hypothesis IIb: different degrees of sparse coding of the brain's intrinsic activity

We have to be careful, though. The results by Lloyd and others show that the degree of sparse coding may differ between resting-state activity and stimulus-induced activity. The degree of sparse coding tends to be higher during the exposure to specific stimuli or particular tasks, and thus during stimulus-induced activity, when compared to resting-state activity (see Lloyd 2011; Zhang et al. 2012; Lee et al. 2011). This means that the degree of sparse coding, the ability to spatially and temporally sparsen neural activity, may be dependent upon the respective neuronal context; that is, on the level of the resting state or stimulus-induced activity.

Therefore, depending on the neuronal context, sparse coding can occur in higher or lower degrees. If, for instance, the degree of sparse coding decreases, the degree local or dense coding may increase. The balance may, in contrast, be shifted on the continuum toward the sparse pole by an incoming stimulus during stimulus-induced activity, as is suggested by the earlier described data. This means that sparse coding and its balance with local/dense coding are relevant not only for the brain's intrinsic activity but also for its transition to stimulus-induced activity, and thus for what we will later describe as "rest–stimulus interaction" and "stimulus–rest interaction." This will be discussed in further detail in Chapter 11 in Part IV of this volume.

Accordingly, sparse coding does not operate in an all-or-nothing way but rather along the lines of a continuum of more-or-less. The degree of sparse coding can change and finds itself in balance to the degree of local or dense coding with both reciprocally modulating each other.

Why is all that this important? We will see in Volume II that the balance between sparse coding and local/dense coding is phenomenally relevant and thus central for consciousness during either resting-state activity (as in dreams; see Chapter 25 and especially Chapter 26) or stimulus-induced activity (as in our consciousness of the environment; see Chapters 28 and 29).

If, for instance, the balance is shifted too strongly toward the pole of local or dense coding at the expense of sparse coding, the association of consciousness with the neural activity during either the resting state or stimulus-induced activity will become impossible. This seems to be the case, for instance, in the vegetative state, under anesthesia, and in NREM-sleep. I consequently propose that a certain degree of sparse coding is necessary in order to make consciousness possible, as will be discussed in full detail in Chapters 28 and 29.

Neuroempirical background III: sparse coding and *GABA* in the brain's intrinsic activity

Lloyd's (and the others') results point out sparse coding of the brain's intrinsic activity, but they do not entail a specific neuronal mechanism that drives the spatial and temporal sparsening of neural activity. We saw in Chapter 2 that, on a cellular and population level of neural activity, the excitation-inhibition balance (EIB) as constituted by GABA and glutamate, is central for mediating difference-based coding and ultimately sparse coding.

This raises the question of whether both GABA and glutamate also mediate the regional level of neural activity and, more specifically, the here-suggested difference-based coding and sparse coding of the brain's intrinsic activity. I now turn, therefore, to recent imaging studies that investigate the modulation of the brain's intrinsic activity by GABA and/or glutamate, while I will report the results on GABA- and glutamate-ergic modulation of stimulus-induced activity in Chapter 12 on rest–stimulus interaction.

Let us start with GABA. I here highlight a study from our group (Qin et al. 2012) that provides direct support for the GABA-ergic modulation of intrinsic activity. More indirect support comes from challenge studies and anesthesia with GABA-ergic agents. Since both challenge studies and anesthesia are accompanied by major changes in consciousness, I will describe these studies in detail in Volume II (see Chapters 17, 28, and 29). Finally, further support comes also from modeling and simulation studies where GABA and glutamate are shown to modulate intrinsic activity (see Deco and Jirsa 2012; Mazzoni et al. 2007).

Neuronal findings IIa: *GABA* modulates the level of resting-state activity in sensory cortex

To investigate the modulation of the brain's intrinsic activity by GABA, Qin et al. (2012) conducted a combined study using fMRI during eyes open and closed and positron emission tomography (PET) for the imaging of GABA-A receptors during rest. Thereby we (Qin et al. 2012a) focused on the sensory cortex, more specifically on visual and auditory cortex (see Chapter 12 for results on GABA and stimulus-induced activity).

As expected, opening the eyes induced neural activity in the visual cortex (Qin et al. 2012a). Due to well-known cross-modal effects (see Chapter 10 for details as well as Kayser et al. 2005, 2008), opening the eyes also increased neural activity in the auditory cortex. Moreover, the functional connectivity between visual and auditory cortex was significantly stronger during eyes closed when compared to eyes open. Hence, opening the eyes weakens the functional connectivity and thus the degree of statistical matching of both regions' neural activity across time; this is consistent with the findings reported in Chapters 4 and 5)

How are these neural activity changes in visual and auditory cortex mediated by GABA-A receptors? For that, we measured the binding potential of the GABA-A receptors (more specifically the benzodiazepine binding site of the GABA-A receptor) using 18F flumazenil PET. We then correlated the density of GABA-A receptor binding in visual and auditory cortex with the neural activity in the very same regions during eyes open and closed as measured with fMRI.

Our results (Qin et al. 2012a) show a direct relationship between GABA-A receptor density and neural activity changes: the higher the density of GABA-A receptors, the larger the difference in signal changes between eyes closed and eyes open. Interestingly, this hold true for both regions visual and auditory cortex. A higher density of GABA-A receptor consequently goes along with a stronger increase in neural activity in visual and auditory cortex when opening the eyes.

This is strongly suggestive of neural inhibition playing a central role in determining the level of the brain's intrinsic activity, that is, during eyes closed, and its subsequent change when opening the eyes. Most important, the density of GABA-A receptors only correlated with the degree of change in neural activity and thus the difference in signal changes between eyes closed and eyes open. In contrast, no correlation was observed with the absolute signal changes during eyes open and closed themselves (Fig. 6-2a).

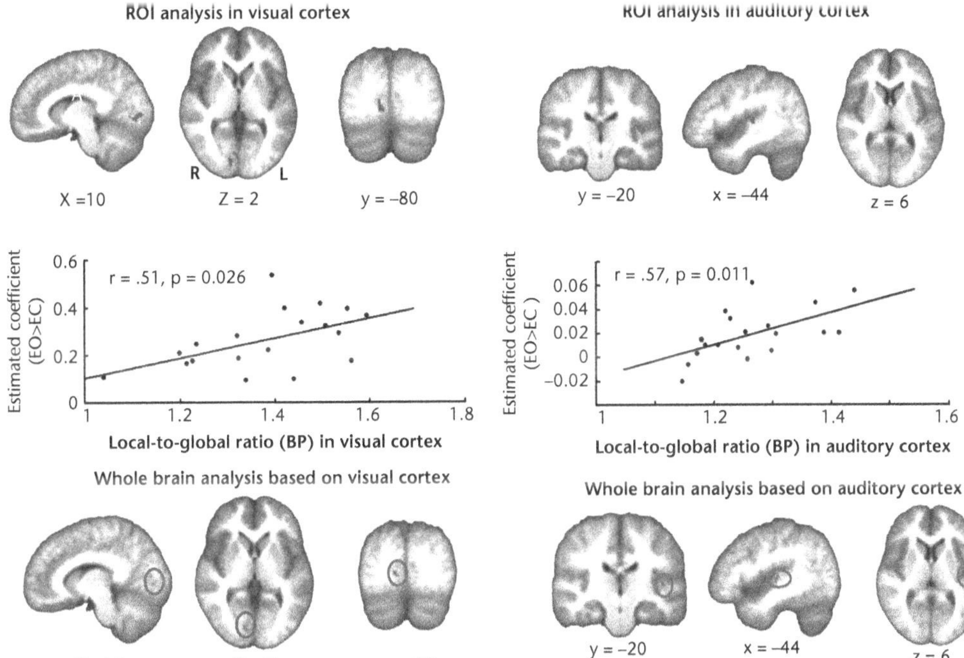

Figure 6-2a **Modulation of resting-state activity by GABA and glutamate Visual cortex:** ***Upper three parts:*** **The activation cluster in visual cortex and the correlation between local-to-global ratio of BP of GABA-A receptor and BOLD signal in the cluster. Upper: the activated regions in visual cortex during eyes open (EO) when compared to eyes closed (EC) (EO > EC, p <.05, FWE corrected) as region of interest (ROI). Middle: the positive correlation between the estimated coefficients of the contrast: EO > EC and the local-to-global ratio of binding potential (BP) of GABA-A receptor in the ROI. Lower: Using the local-to-global ratio of binding potential (BP) of GABA-A receptor in the visual ROI to do the voxel-wised correlation analysis in the whole brain, the activated cluster in visual cortex (p <.05, FWE corrected in visual cortex).** ***Lower three parts:*** **The activation cluster in auditory cortex and the correlation between local-to-global ratio of BP of GABA-A receptor and BOLD signal in the cluster. Upper: the activated regions in left auditory cortex (EO > EC, p <.05, FWE corrected) as ROI. Middle: the positive correlation between the estimated coefficient of the contrast: EO > EC and the local-to-global ratio of BP of GABA-A receptor in the ROI. Lower: Using the local-to-global ratio of binding potential in the ROI to do the voxel-wised correlation analysis in the whole brain, the activated cluster in left auditory cortex (p <.05, FWE corrected in auditory cortex).**

Neuronal findings IIb: *GABA* modulates functional connectivity in sensory cortex during the resting state

If the density of GABA-A receptors predicts the degree of neural activity change during the transition from eyes closed to eyes open in both auditory and visual cortex, one would postulate that their functional connectivity is also modulated by GABA. As said earlier, functional connectivity between visual and auditory cortex decreased when opening the eyes.

Interestingly, this decrease in functional connectivity was directly related to the density of GABA-A receptors in visual cortex: the higher the density of GABA-A receptors in visual cortex, the stronger visual-auditory cortical functional connectivity decreased when opening the eyes. In addition to the auditory cortex, the density of GABA-A receptors in visual cortex also predicted the degree of functional connectivity from the visual cortex to other more distant regions like the precuneus, the temporal cortex, the sensory cortex, and the frontal cortex (see Qin et al. 2013 for details).

Taken together, these results (and the ones from the challenge studies and anesthesia; see Chapters 17, 28, and 29) clearly demonstrate modulation of the brain's intrinsic activity, its signal changes and functional connectivity, in visual and auditory cortex by GABA. Unfortunately Qin et al. [2012a] did not include any measures of glutamate so that we cannot make any assumptions concerning neurochemical specificity with respect to GABA.

Neuronal findings IIc: *GABA* modulates the *temporal* features of intrinsic activity

Fingelkurts et al. (2004) investigated eight healthy subjects in a resting-state condition (eyes closed and open) using EEG and MEG during pharmacological challenge with lorazepam. Lorazepam is a benzodiazepine and acts on the benzodiazepine subunit of the GABA-A receptors being agonists and thus strengthening the degree of neural inhibition. Hence, the application of lorazepam provides an indirect measure of the effects of GABA on resting-state activity.

To assess the influence of lorazepam on EEG, they investigated its effects on delta-, alpha-, and beta-frequency bands. They also calculated an index of synchrony by correlating the electrical activity between different (transregional) electrode pairs as an indicator or measure of functional connectivity (between electrodes and their underlying activity sites).

When compared to placebo, lorazepam increased the degree of synchrony of electrical activity between different (more or less adjacent or proximal) electrode pairs. More specifically, the number of synchronized electrode pairs as well as the strength of synchrony was significantly higher during lorazepam when compared to placebo in the eyes-closed condition. This was especially strong in the alpha- and beta-frequency bands. The same was observed in the eyes-open condition during lorazepam where it concerned especially long-range electrode pairs.

In addition, they also investigated the impact of lorazepam on the global power of different frequency bands. Lorazepam decreased the power in the alpha band (8–12Hz) while it increased the power in the slow rhythms, for example, delta (1–4Hz) and theta (5–8Hz).

Accordingly, lorazepam induced a higher number of EEG segments with slow theta and delta rhythms, while the number of segments with faster frequencies (alpha, fast-theta) decreased. This pattern was observed in more than 65% of the EEG/MEG channels in both eyes open and closed. Finally, lorazepam also changed the dynamic temporal features of the electrical activity as observed in polyrhythmic activity, temporal stabilization, and nonhomogeneity (see Fingelkurts et al. 2004 for details).

Taken both fMRI-PET and EEG-MEG studies together, the findings reported here point out the following features. First, GABA seems to mediate local neural activity levels of the brain's intrinsic activity as suggested by the combined fMRI-PET study. Second, GABA seems to mediate local functional connectivity, that is, functional connectivity between direct and closely connected regions as observed in both studies (as between auditory and visual cortex or between adjacent electrodes pairs). Third, GABA modulates the temporal features of thc brain's intrinsic activity when interfering with the power of its frequency bands and its dynamic temporal features.

Neuronal findings IIIa: Glutamate modulates the level of intrinsic activity

One may now want to raise the question of how glutamate, the main excitatory transmitter, modulates the brain's intrinsic activity. As in the case of GABA, there are not yet many studies on the biochemical modulation of the brain's intrinsic activity on a regional level.

I here highlight two studies from our group (Enzi et al. 2012; Duncan et al. 2013; see also Kapogiannis et al. 2013) that directly addressed the relationship between glutamate and resting-state activity. Further though indirect support for the glutamate-ergic modulation of intrinsic activity comes from challenge studies with ketamine as well as from anesthesia where glutamatergic agents are used. Since both challenge studies and anesthesia are accompanied by major changes in consciousness, they are discussed in Volume II (see especially Chapters 17, 28, and 28).

To investigate the specific association of glutamate with resting-state activity rather than stimulus-induced activity, Bjoern Enzi (Enzi et al. 2012) from our group conducted yet another combined fMRI-MRS study. He investigated whether glutamate modulates local levels of resting-state activity in PACC as distinguished from stimulus-induced activity in the same region.

For that, he applied a reward paradigm to elicit stimulus-induced activity in the PACC using fMRI. He combined the reward task with longer fixation cross periods—that is, resting state—in fMRI, and also measured the resting state concentration of glutamate in the PACC using MRS.

How, now, is glutamate related to resting-state and stimulus-induced activity in the PACC? The resting-state concentration of PACC glutamate correlated significantly with the degree of neural activity in the fixation cross period: the higher the resting-state concentration of glutamate in the PACC, the higher the signal changes during the fixation cross in the same region. In contrast, such correlation did not hold during the stimulus-induced activity in the PACC as elicited by during the reward task (see Fig. 6-2b).

These data suggest that glutamate modulates the level of neural activity in specifically the resting state as distinguished from stimulus-induced activity. This means that glutamate and its neural excitation seem to modulate the resting-state activity levels. Since glutamate is central in mediating cortico-cortical connections, i.e., the connections between the neurons' afferences and efferences, one would postulate that glutamate also modulates the degree of functional connectivity in the resting state.

Neuronal findings IIIb: Glutamate modulates functional connectivity in the resting state

Another study from our group by Niall Duncan (Duncan et al. 2013) focused on the glutamate-ergic modulation of functional connectivity between cortical and subcortical regions (see also Schmaal et al. 2012 for analogous results in the context of stimulus-induced activity that is reward, which therefore will be described in Chapter 12). He measured subcortical-cortical functional connectivity during eyes open and closed using fMRI, as well as the corresponding structural connectivity, using diffusion tensor imaging (DTI) and its anisotropy values as measures of the degree of structural connectivity.

This was complemented by magnetic resonance spectroscopy (MRS) in the same subjects in whom the resting state concentration of glutamate and GABA in the perigenual anterior cingulate cortex (PACC) and the left insula was measured. The PACC is a core region which is closely connected both functionally and structurally with various subcortical regions like the ventral striatum (VS), the thalamus (TH), and the periaqueductal gray (PAG).

He could first observe that the functional connectivity correlated with the structural connectivity: The higher the (anisotropy) values in DTI (and thus the stronger the subcortical-cortical structural connectivity), the stronger the resting-state

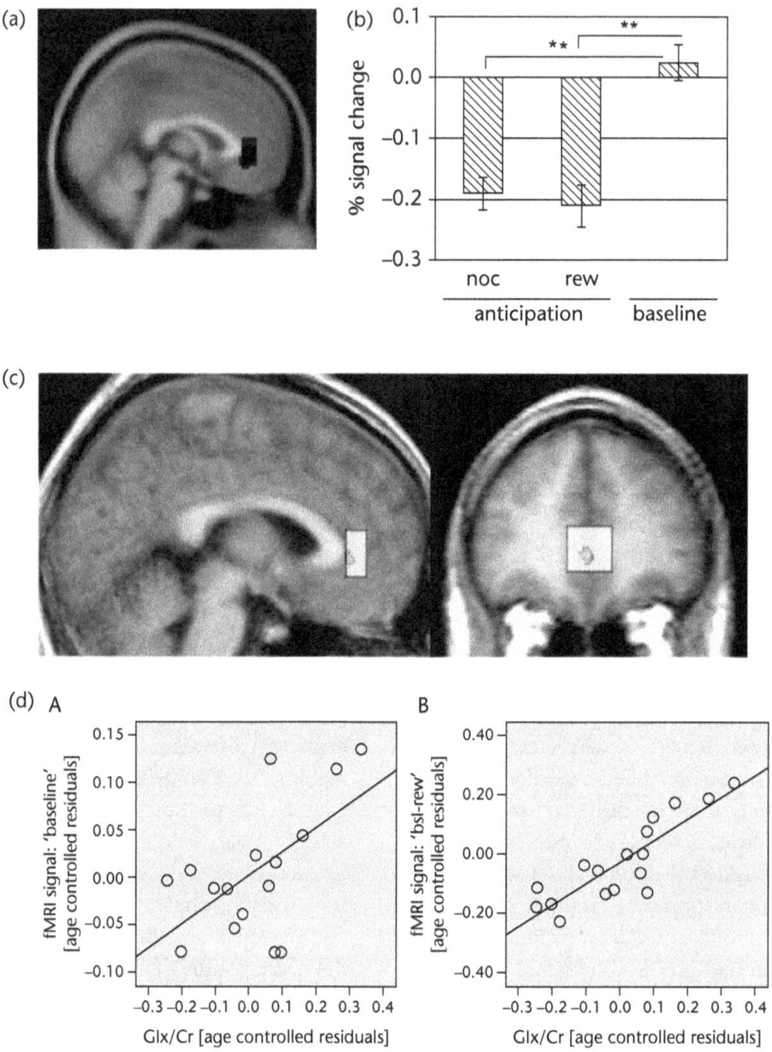

Figure 6-2b **Modulation of resting-state activity by GABA and glutamate Visual cortex. (*a*) Position of the anatomically defined region of interest (ROI) used for percent signal change extraction in relation to the MRS voxel placed in the pregenual anterior cingulate cortex (PACC). (*b*) Percent signal change for the conditions "anticipation of no outcome," "anticipation of reward," and "baseline" derived from the aforementioned anatomically defined ROI placed in the PACC. ** $p < .01$. Error bar represents SEM. (*c*) Contrast "baseline > anticipation of reward" (p[FDR] <.05; k >10) with small volume correction for the MRS voxel placed in the PACC. (*d*) Correlation. Pearson-correlation between the Glx/Cr-ratio derived from the MRS voxel located in the PACC and the fMRI signal for the conditions (A) "baseline," (B) "baseline—anticipation of reward." It should be noted that values can be negative, as they represent residuals after linear correction for age.**

functional connectivity between the same regions during eyes closed (and eyes open). This means that the functional connectivity followed the subcortical-cortical structural connectivity, though this was not always the case, especially during eyes open (when compared to eyes closed).

How about glutamate? Niall Duncan showed that the resting state concentration of glutamate in PACC predicted the degree of functional connectivity from PACC to the VS, TH, and PAG: The higher the resting state concentration of glutamate in PACC, the higher the degree of resting state functional connectivity from PACC to VS, TH, and PAG. This held specifically for PACC glutamate, but it could not be observed for the resting state concentration of glutamate in the left insula.

Analogous results though for another region were reported in a recent study by Kapogiannis et al. (2013). They measured the resting-state concentration of GABA and glutamate in the posterior cingulate cortex (PCC) and resting state functional connectivity using fMRI. Cortico-cortical resting state functional connectivity from the posterior cingulate cortex (PCC) was modulated positively by the concentration of glutamate in the PCC (and negatively correlated to GABA in PCC) (see Kapogiannis et al. 2013).

Coming back to the Duncan study of cortico-subcortical connectivity, most often, PACC glutamate predicted the difference in resting state functional connectivity between eyes closed and open, rather than each alone, eyes open *or* closed. Interestingly, the different subcortical regions, VS, TH, and PAG, showed different modulations of their functional connectivity to PACC during eyes open and closed, x respectively, by glutamate (see Fig. 6-2c).

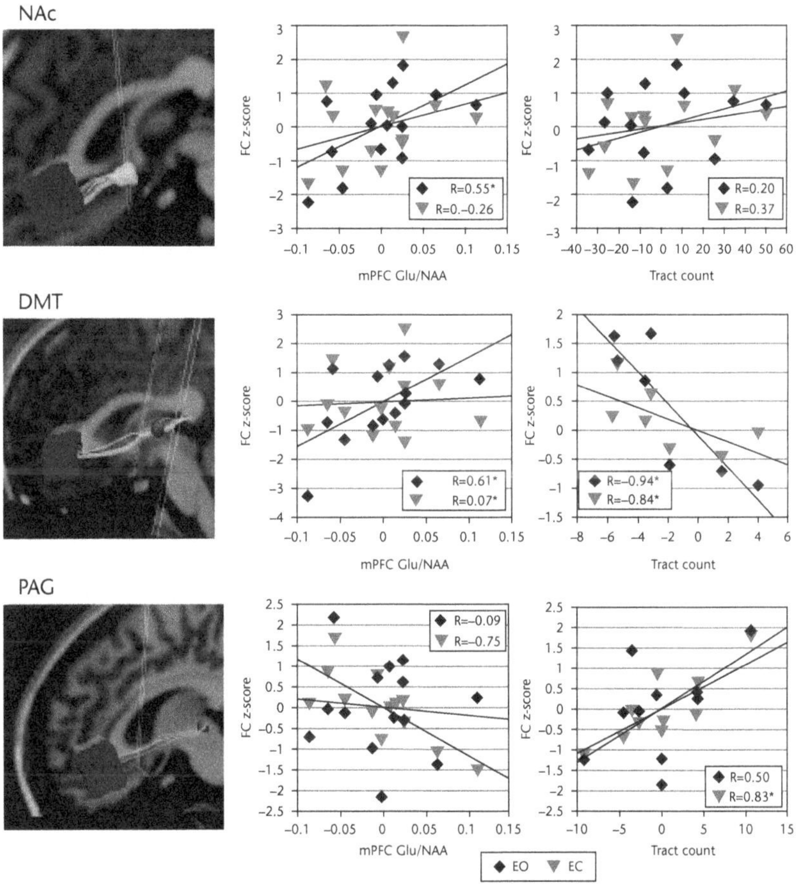

Figure 6-2c **The figure shows the results of a combined fMRI, DTI, and MRS study with placement of the voxel for MRS in medial prefrontal cortex (mPFC). Correlation results between FC, Glu and DTI. Example tracts between the mPFC and each of the target regions are shown along with partial correlation graphs from the right hemisphere. Correlations between FC and Glu are shown, followed by correlations between FC and number of tracts. Note that values represent residuals after confounding variables have been regressed out of the data in the partial correlation. Diamonds = eyes open, triangles = eyes closed. * indicates $p < 0.05$.**

Taken together, these results (and the ones from challenge studies and anesthesia; see Chapters 18, 28, and 29) demonstrate that glutamate modulates neural activity in the resting state, such as, its level of neural activity and its functional connectivity. Unfortunately though there are not many studies at this point in time that specifically address the exact neuronal mechanisms underlying such modulation of resting-state activity by glutamate, which also seems to mediate stimulus-induced activity, as will be discussed later, in Part IV.

Neuronal findings IVa: Glutamate is tied to energetic metabolism

Robert Shulman is a researcher at Yale University in New Haven, Connecticut. As a physicist, he is skeptical about any easy, reductionist account of the brain's function and ultimately of consciousness, as is often implied and postulated in current neuroscience. One of his main arguments is that any neural activity we observe in the brain must be set to a standard or reference, the brain's intrinsic baseline (see Chapter 4 for conceptual determination) since that predisposes the possible degree of change during subsequent stimulus-induced activity.

He thus would probably be equally skeptical about the findings reported earlier. This may be so because we only measured the brain's intrinsic activity indirectly, via the comparison of eyes open and closed. One would instead need a more direct and absolute way of measuring the brain's intrinsic activity. This, however, as he claims, is possible only by including a measure of the brain's metabolism in the resting state that directly signifies its intrinsic activity. Only if we can provide a measure of the brain's metabolism and how that is related to glutamate, could we make the assumption that glutamate modulates the brain's intrinsic activity.

Unfortunately, we did not include such measure (as, for instance, glucose metabolism or the blood flow) in the aforementioned studies. There is, however, strong evidence from the studies by Shulman himself that glutamate is closely related to the brain's energetic metabolism.

The group around Shulman et al. (2003, 2004, 2006, 2007, 2009a and b; Patel et al. 2005; Hyder et al. 2013) investigated the coupling between neural and metabolic activity in various studies. They measured the level of glucose and acetate (as labeled by 13C) and could thereby calculate the dependence of the neuron's firing rate on cerebral energy production rates, that is, the rate of glucose oxidation, and the coupled rates of transmitters like GABA and glutamate. This was done during both resting-state and stimulus-induced activity.

There was a clear relationship between the degree of glucose oxidation indicating energy demand and the change in the concentration of glutamate, with both being coupled to the rate of neuronal firing. Let us describe this in further detail. Glutamate and glutamine were related to about 70%–80% of the energy consumption and transmitter cycling while GABA required about 10%–15% of the total energy (with the remaining 10%–15% of energy metabolism being needed by the glia).

Most important, changes in energy metabolism went along with changes in resting-state activity and glutamate levels: the higher the energy metabolism, that is, glucose oxidation, the higher were the glutamate levels and the subsequent levels of the neurons' firing rate indicating the level of the intrinsic activity. This clearly indicates dependence of both resting-state activity and glutamate on glucose metabolism, entailing what is described as neurometabolic coupling.

Neuronal findings IVb: Intrinsic activity is "energy hungry"

Interestingly, Shulman and his group also showed that about 80% of the brain's total energy metabolism accounts for the maintenance of the brain's resting-state activity. In contrast, only a small fraction, up to 20%, is reserved for stimulus-induced activity, which thus corresponds to a small incremental change (Patel et al. 2005; Shulman et al. 2003, 2004, 2009a and b).

One can therefore say that the brain's intrinsic activity, its resting-state activity, seems to have metabolic and therefore energetic priority over stimulus-induced activity. Let us describe the situation in a slightly different way, in more neurometaphorical terms. Our brain's intrinsic activity is what may be described as "energy hungry." As such, the brain's intrinsic activity may be compared to somebody who wakes up during the night and craves for a chocolate. The only difference is that the brain does crave for energy not only in the night but at any time, day or night.

Most important, glutamate seems to play a major role in mediating the brain's craving for energy, since otherwise it would not require 70%–80% of its energy consumption. The same, however, to a lesser degree, holds true for GABA, which consumes 10%–15% of the energy budget.

While we currently do not know the exact role and mechanisms of glutamate and GABA on the regional level of the brain's intrinsic activity, we can infer from such high energy consumption that both glutamate and GABA must be somehow important. Why does the brain devote so much energy to GABA and glutamate? We currently do not know. What we do know, though, is that GABA and glutamate must be extremely important to the brain and its intrinsic activity.

Just imagine ourselves as persons: Who would devote as much energy to somebody if she or he were not important for one's own well-being? The same seems to hold for the brain, which may thus not be as different from us persons.

Neuronal hypothesis IIIa: biochemical anatomy of the excitation-inhibition balance

What do these findings on GABA and glutamate imply for the coding of the brain's intrinsic activity? I propose that GABA and its interplay with glutamate make possible the encoding of spatial and temporal differences into the neural activity during the resting state. Therefore I suggest GABA and glutamate to be central in making possible difference-based coding of the brain's intrinsic activity.

Before getting started, though, we need to make a quick and rather abbreviated tour of the anatomy of GABA- and glutamat-ergic neurons. Glutamate is closely linked to the pyramidal cells and neural excitation, while GABA is rather related to interneurons and neural inhibition. The pyramidal neurons, being situated mainly in layer 4 of the cortex, receive afferences from other regions and send out long efferences to other regions, with both being mediated by glutamate. This is different in the interneurons that, being strongly present in especially the upper layers of the cortex (like layer 1 and 2), are mainly connected to the pyramidal neurons in the same region.

How are pyramidal cells related to the interneurons? As explicated in Chapter 2, the number of interneurons is much higher than the number of pyramidal cells. Since the pyramidal cells are connected to and activate the interneurons via their neural excitation, the number of interneurons being excited exceeds the number of activated pyramidal cells. This means that, as shown in Chapter 2, the degree of neural inhibition will ultimately predominate over the degree of neural excitation. The initial neural excitation, as promoted by the pyramidal cells, will thus be sparsened by the degree of subsequent neural inhibition of the interneurons (see Fig. 6-3a).

What does this imply for the characterization of the excitation-inhibition balance (EIB)? First and foremost, the resulting EIB is a difference-based signal; that is, it is based on the relative difference between the degree of glutamate-ergic excitation and gaba-ergic inhibition. Such a difference-based signal must be distinguished from a stimulus-based signal, in which case the absolute values of neural inhibition and excitation by themselves, i.e., isolated and independent, would be encoded into the EIB.

Second, most important, the EIB results from the direct interaction between neural excitation and inhibition and their respective cells, the pyramidal cells and the interneurons. Since the balance of the EIB is strongly tilted toward the interneurons, the neural inhibition sparsens the neural excitation, as described in detail in Chapter 2. This means that the EIB itself reflects the result of sparse coding (rather than local or dense coding).

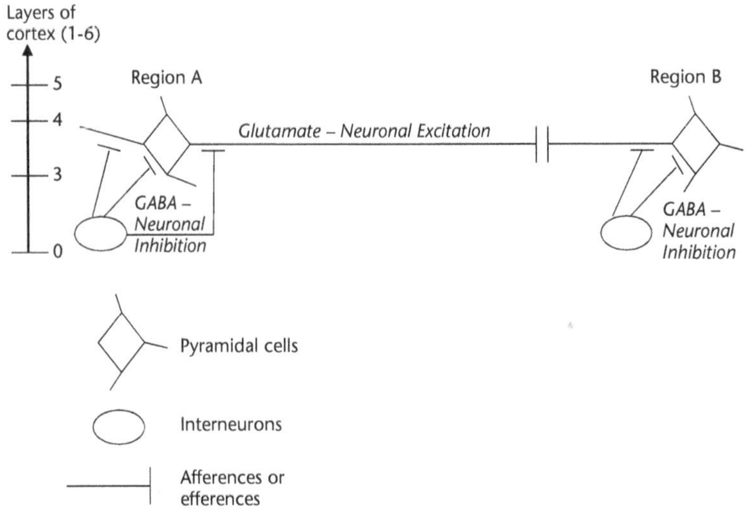

Figure 6-3a The figure shows the relationship between GABA, glutamate, neural inhibition and excitation, and the functional connectivity in the resting state. The figure shows a simplified diagram of the anatomo-structural features of glutamatergic-pyramidal excitatory neurons (in layer 4 predominantly) and GABAergic inhibitory interneurons (in layers 1 and 2 predominantly) and how they connect between two regions via the former's long transregional efferences and afferences. Thereby GABAergic interneurons exhibit an inhibitory impact on glutamatergic excitatory pyramidal cells.

NEURONAL HYPOTHESIS IIIB: DIFFERENCE-BASED CODING OF THE EXCITATION-INHIBITION BALANCE

What does this characterization of the EIB on the cellular level imply for the regional level of neural activity like the brain's intrinsic activity? The earlier described data clearly demonstrate that both GABA and glutamate modulate the level of the brain's intrinsic activity; this is suggested by the effects of GABA and glutamate on the degrees of signal changes, functional connectivity, and neural synchrony in the resting state.

Even though the exact neuronal mechanisms of such GABA- and glutamate-ergic effects remain unclear at this point, these data seem to strongly suggest that GABA and glutamate promote difference-based coding and sparse coding on the regional level of the brain's intrinsic activity. The assumption of difference-based coding holding on the regional level of the intrinsic activity is thus supported by the tentative data described above.

The findings by Qin et al. (2012) clearly demonstrate that the density of the GABA-A receptors only mediated the relative changes in neural activity between eyes closed and open, rather than their absolute levels of activity. Pending future confirmation and extension of these results, this suggests that the GABA-A receptors and GABA in general are attuned and sensitive to specifically detect spatial and temporal differences in neural activity.

The degree of neural inhibition as associated with GABA may specifically encode relative spatial and temporal differences in neural activity—e.g., changes in neural activity—rather than the absolute neural activity levels in isolation by themselves. Accordingly, as on the cellular level of activity (see Chapter 2), I hypothesize that GABA encodes relative difference values rather than absolute activity values.

How about glutamate? The findings by Duncan et al. (2013) show the encoding of differences in functional connectivity between eyes closed and open by glutamate, which, however, was not consistent for all subcortical regions. One could tentatively suggest that glutamate, like GABA, may be particularly sensitive and tuned to detect spatial and temporal differences in neural activity rather than encoding the absolute values by themselves.

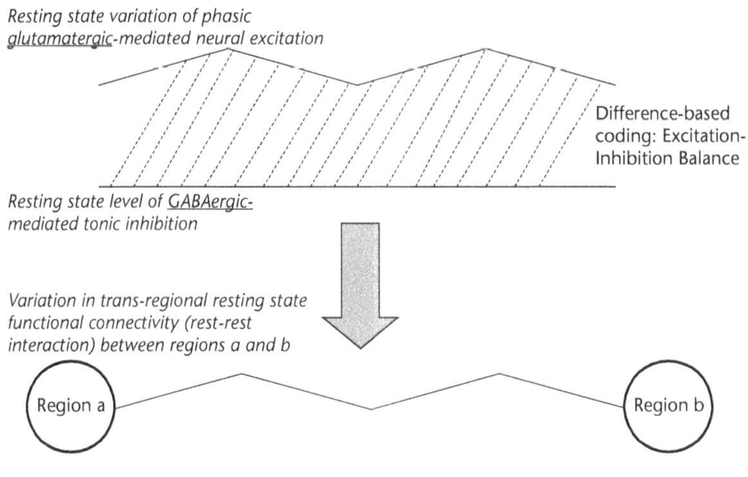

Figure 6-3b **Difference-based coding of the excitation-inhibition balance in the resting state. Based on Figure 6-3a, this figure shows the interplay between the phasic glutamatergic excitatory pyramidal cells and the tonic GABAergic inhibitory interneurons in the resting state. What is encoded in the actual neural activity is the difference between the two, the excitation-inhibition balance (*upper part*) and its fluctuations across time and space (i.e., across the two regions) in the resting state (*upper part*). The excitation-inhibition balance does, in turn, determine the relationship and thus the degree of functional connectivity between the two regions in the resting state (*lower part*).**

What does this imply for the EIB? The EIB may be regarded as a signal that by itself is a difference-based signal that, as such, reflects the encoding of spatial and temporal differences. Let me explain this in detail.

As on the cellular level of neural activity, the EIB on the regional level is first and foremost a difference-based signal that reflects the spatial (that is, different location of pyramidal cells and interneurons) and temporal (that is slightly delayed onset of neural inhibition when compared to neural excitation; see Chapter 2) difference between neural excitation and inhibition. This means that the constitution of the EIB is based on difference-based coding rather than the mere addition of neural excitation and inhibition, as in the case of stimulus-based coding (see Fig. 6-3b).

Neuronal hypothesis IIIc: GABA encodes relative differences rather than absolute levels

What do I mean when I say that GABA and glutamate are "tuned" and "sensitive" to spatial and temporal differences between neural inhibition and excitation? Let us describe in further detail what I mean by such tuning. Take the example of neural inhibition: As said above and in Chapter 2, the resulting degree of neural inhibition depends not only on the level of the phasic or tonic activity of the interneurons by themselves, but also on its relationship to and thus relative difference from the degree of neural excitation. For instance, the degree of neural inhibition may change due to changes in neural excitation, which shifts their relative difference and balance toward the excitatory pole.

GABA may be particularly sensitive and tuned to such relative change in the degree of neural inhibition, i.e., relative to neural excitation. Any relative change in the neural inhibition will consequently lead to changes in the release of GABA with the "aim" of keeping the excitation-inhibition balance (EIB) stable.

How can we better illustrate that? For that, I turn to a thought experiment. Imagine that GABA would not be tuned and sensitive to detect relative differences in the degree of neural inhibition, but could detect only absolute levels. Any change in the level of neural inhibition itself would then go along with a change in the release of GABA, independent of its relative difference from the degree of neural excitation.

Most important, this holds true regardless of whether the EIB changes. Even if the EIB does not change, due to concurrent changes in the degree of neural excitation, GABA, unlike in the empirical reality, will nevertheless be released in order to change the absolute level of neural inhibition. This means that, in our thought experiment, GABA is tuned and sensitive to the absolute level of neural inhibition rather than to its relative difference.

Consider the reverse case within the framework of our thought experiment. The absolute level of neural inhibition does not change by itself, whereas its relative difference from the degree of neural excitation changes due to changes in neural excitation. Since the absolute level of neural inhibition does not change, GABA will not be released in this scenario of our thought experiment. This however is different in empirical reality, where, due to a change of its relative difference from neural excitation, GABA will be released independently of whether the absolute level of neural inhibition is the same.

What does our thought experiment tell us? It demonstrates that whether GABA (and glutamate) are tuned to either absolute levels or relative differences in the degree of neural inhibition (and excitation) makes an empirical difference. This holds in especially those cases with predominantly unilateral changes in the degree of either neural excitation or inhibition. Empirical reality suggests that GABA (and glutamate) are tuned and sensitive to encode relate differences rather than absolute levels (see Chapter 2 for empirical support).

Neuronal hypothesis IVa: Encoding of neuronal statistics by the brain's intrinsic activity

How is such tuning and sensitivity of GABA and glutamate to relative differences possible? The tuning and sensitivity to relative differences imply that the discrete spatial and temporal point of (for instance) neural inhibition is set against the one of the actual (or previous) degree of neural excitation.

And, most important, the change in that relationship between the two (or more) different discrete points, i.e., the spatial and temporal difference, determines whether the level of GABA (or glutamate) changes. This means that GABA and glutamate are tuned and sensitive to changes in spatial and temporal differences.

How can we further describe such changes in temporal and spatial differences? They reflect the statistical frequency distribution of the different discrete points in physical time and space as associated with neural inhibition and excitation. This means that one may want to speak here of what I call the "neuronal statistics" (see Chapter 9 for details) of the EIB. Accordingly, I postulate that the tuning and sensitivity of GABA and glutamate to relative differences in neural inhibition and excitation amounts to an encoding of the neuronal statistics of the EIB.

What do I mean by the term "neuronal statistics"? We recall from Chapter 1 the encoding of extrinsic stimuli—namely exteroceptive stimuli—in the various sensory modalities into the neural activity of the sensory cortex. This revealed that the extrinsic stimuli's statistical frequency distribution rather than the single stimulus itself is encoded into the neural activity of the sensory cortex. Since "the statistical frequency distribution" refers to the occurrence of the extrinsic stimuli in the natural world, the authors also speak of an encoding of "natural statistics" into neural activity.

How do such natural statistics stand in relation to the here-suggested concept of "neuronal statistics"? Analogous to the encoding of the exteroceptive stimuli "natural statistics," I now suggest that the neural activity changes in the intrinsic activity, its "neural stimuli," as I said in Chapter 4, are encoded into the intrinsic activity.

This means that the statistical frequency distribution of the intrinsic activity changes themselves are encoded into the neural activity during the resting state. What is encoded is thus the statistical frequency distribution of the changes in the intrinsic activity. Therefore one may want to say that the brain's intrinsic activity encodes its own "neuronal statistics" into its neural activity (see Chapters 8 and 9 for further details).

This leads me to the following hypothesis. I hypothesize that the intrinsic activity in the brain is based on the encoding of its own neuronal statistics into neural activity. GABA and glutamate are essential in maintaining the EIB that reflects the level of the intrinsic activity. Therefore, I suggest the encoding of the neuronal statistics into the brain's intrinsic activity to be based on GABA and glutamate and their excitation-inhibition balance. Accordingly, I postulate that GABA and glutamate are central in encoding the intrinsic activity's "neuronal statistics" into the excitation-inhibition balance of its own neural activity.

NEURONAL HYPOTHESIS IVB: ENCODING OF "NEURONAL STATISTICS" AND SPARSE CODING OF THE BRAIN'S INTRINSIC ACTIVITY

How can we empirically support the encoding of neuronal statistics into the intrinsic activity? For direct empirical support, we would need to do experiments and analyses analogous to the ones described in the case of the encoding of natural statistics (see Chapters 1 and 2). This remains a task for the future.

How about more indirect empirical support? That is, at least tentatively, provided by the earlier described results by Qin et al. (2012), Duncan et al. (2013), and Fingelkurts et al. (2004), who describe the tuning of GABA and glutamate to relative differences in signal changes, functional connectivity, or frequency bands.

How can we further support the assumption that the brain's intrinsic activity is based on the encoding of its own neuronal statistics? Analogous to the case of the encoding of natural statistics, one would expect the encoding of neuronal statistics to go along with the temporal and spatial sparsening of the neural activity in the resting state. In short, encoding of neuronal statistics should be reflected in sparse coding of the brain's intrinsic activity.

This is exactly what the data initially described in this chapter show; namely, the sparse coding (rather than local or dense coding) of the brain's intrinsic activity. I consequently postulate that the observation of sparse coding supports (though indirectly) my hypothesis that the brain's intrinsic activity is based on the encoding of its own neuronal statistics.

Why is all that relevant? Besides the neuronal relevance, such encoding of the own neuronal statistics may, for instance, be altered in psychiatric disorders like depression and schizophrenia, which show major abnormalities in their resting-state activity as well as in GABA and glutamate (see Chapters 17, 22, and 27).

Based on the here-made assumptions, one would postulate that such resting state abnormalities may lead to abnormal encoding of the intrinsic activity's neuronal statistics into its own neural activity. For instance, abnormalities in GABA or glutamate may lead to the encoding of abnormal degrees of spatial and temporal differences which may therefore no longer reflect the proper neuronal statistics of the brain's intrinsic activity.

NEURONAL HYPOTHESIS IVC: ENCODING OF NEURONAL STATISTICS REQUIRES ENERGY

How is the encoding of the neuronal statistics possible? I suggested that GABA and glutamate are central in allowing for the encoding of the own neuronal statistics into the brain's intrinsic activity. That is the neuronal side of GABA and glutamate. There is, however, also a metabolic-energetic side of GABA and glutamate. As we demonstrated in the data described earlier, glutamate especially is closely related to energetic metabolism, requiring a rather high percentage of the brain's total energy budget even in the resting state.

Why do glutamate (and also GABA) need such an high amount of energy even in the resting state? This remains unclear. Based on the assumptions made so far, I hypothesize the following: GABA and glutamate are supposed to encode the neuronal statistics of the brain's intrinsic activity. This means that GABA and glutamate, as shown earlier, are tuned and sensitive to the encoding of spatial and temporal differences, i.e., relative differences, in neural inhibition and excitation, rather than to their absolute levels.

I now postulate that such encoding of spatial and temporal differences requires energy. The energy is needed to detect the different discrete points in physical time and space as well as to link them by computing their difference value.

I thus propose the following neuroenergetic hypothesis: I postulate that the high energy budget of GABA and glutamate is needed for their computing and encoding of spatial and temporal differences and consequently for the encoding of the own neuronal statistics into the intrinsic activity. Since the encoding of the neuronal statistics goes on continuously, independently of whether resting state or stimulus-induced activity predominates, there is already a high energy demand in the resting state itself. This is quite compatible with the data from the group around Robert G. Shulman as described earlier.

Neuronal hypothesis IVd: Neurometabolic coupling is essential for consciousness

How can I further support my neuroenergetic hypothesis? I postulate a direct relationship between the high energy demand and a particular coding strategy, the encoding of neuronal statistics. There is, as to my knowledge, no direct support for the relationship between energy and coding. We may, however, search for some *indirect* support. That can, for instance, be found in the examples of vegetative state (VS) and anesthesia (see earlier).

In both cases, VS and anesthesia, the global metabolism and energy supply of the brain is highly reduced across all regions by at least 20% if not 40% to 50% (see Hyder et al. 2013; as well as Chapters 28 and 29). How is such reduced metabolic and energy supply manifested in neuronal activity?

The intrinsic activity in both anesthesia and VS is highly reduced, although, especially in VS stimulus-induced activity, it can still be observed (see Chapters 28 and 29). If my neuro-energetic hypothesis holds true, one would now expect the energy reduction in VS and anesthesia to be accompanied by reduced encoding of spatial and temporal differences, that is, the neuronal (and natural) statistics, into neural activity during either resting state (and stimulus-induced activity).

Due to such reduced encoding of spatial and temporal differences into neural activity, the low degree of difference-based coding may be accompanied by a high degree of stimulus-based coding. This is indeed strongly supported by the current data in both anesthesia and VS (see Chapters 28 and 29). Since such an abnormal decrease in difference-based coding goes along with a major decrease in the level of consciousness, as well being visible in VS and anesthesia, I refer the reader to Volume II for further details.

Open Questions

One central question concerns the exact role of GABA and glutamate in constituting sparse coding of the brain's intrinsic activity. While there is some evidence supporting the role of GABA and glutamate in modulating resting-state activity, their function in temporally and spatially sparsening the brain's intrinsic activity remains far from clear (see, Deco and Jirsa 2012; as well as Mazzoni et al. 2007, for recent simulation studies of the intrinsic activity and its relation to GABA and glutamate). One would be tempted to suggest that the same principles of how GABA and glutamate modulate sparse coding also hold in both resting-state and stimulus-induced activity. This though remains to be shown in the future.

Another point in this context is that there are not many data about the role of GABA and glutamate, and especially their direct interaction (see Heinzel et al. 2008) on the regional level of neural activity. This contrasts with the available evidence on the cellular and physiological level (see Chapter 2). Therefore, future studies may need to, not only complement the current lack of data on the regional level, but also bridge the gap between cellular and regional levels. That, in turn, will be crucially relevant for lending further support to the assumption of sparse coding of the brain's intrinsic activity.

The second main issue concerns the question of the purpose of the brain's intrinsic activity. Several suggestions have been made. Some authors argue that the intrinsic activity serves to regulate the brain's metabolic load (see Shulman et al. 2003, 2004, 2009a and b). Others, coming from sleep research, argue that the brain's resting state may serve to clean, maintain, and update synaptic connections, especially during the night (see Nir et al. 2008a and b; and see Chapters 14, 15, and 26 for more details on sleep).

Finally, many authors (Llinas 2002; Raichle and Gusnard 2005; Moshe, 2009a and b; Deco et al. 2009) propose that the main purpose of the brain is making anticipations and predictions of the kind of stimuli that may come. Such anticipations and predictions must be generated during the resting state itself prior to the encounter of a particular stimulus. How is it possible for the resting-state activity to make predictions about particular stimuli in the absence of any such stimuli? This shall be the focus of Part III of this volume, where I will discuss the concept of predictive coding and how it relates to the here-suggested difference-based coding.

PART III
Encoding Predictions

General Background

So far, I have discussed how extrinsic stimuli from the environment are encoded in the neural activity of the brain, thereby focusing on the sensory cortex. As shown in recent data, the sensory cortex encodes into its neural activity the statistical frequency distribution of the extrinsic stimuli: rather than encoding the extrinsic stimuli and their different discrete points in physical time and space, the sensory cortex encodes the spatial and temporal differences between the stimuli's different discrete points in physical time and space.

Such difference-based coding implies that the resulting neural activity does not reflect the extrinsic stimuli in a one-to-one way but that there is instead a many-to-one relationship between the number of stimuli and the number of activated neurons/regions. There is thus what is described as *sparse coding* that holds on both the cellular/population and regional level of neural activity.

By encoding its own neural activity on the basis of applying difference-based coding and sparse coding, the brain actively extracts the spatial and temporal differences between different stimuli and their different discrete points in physical time and space. The extraction must be considered an active process that can only originate in the brain itself and its intrinsic features.

Such active encoding strategy must be distinguished from a more passive form of encoding where each extrinsic stimulus activates one neuron entailing a one-to-one relationship between stimuli and neuron. In that case the stimulus itself and its discrete point in physical time and space would be encoded into neural activity independently of the other stimuli. Such rather passive encoding strategy would lead to stimulus-based coding and local coding rather than difference-based coding and sparse coding.

Where is this active contribution of the brain itself to its own encoding strategy coming from? Based on recent empirical data, I showed in Part II that the brain exhibits an intrinsic activity, a resting-state activity, that is highly dynamic and changes continuously in both its spatial and temporal pattern.

These continuous spatial and temporal changes in the brain's intrinsic activity are apparently also encoded in the same way as extrinsic stimuli; namely, in terms of difference-based coding and sparse coding as distinguished from stimulus-based coding and local coding. This, I hypothesized, leads to the constitution of particular spatial and temporal structure in the intrinsic activity itself as it is empirically reflected in its various spatiotemporal activity patterns.

Where does this leave us? We showed in Part I that extrinsic stimuli are encoded into neural activity in terms of difference-based coding and sparse coding. Such an active encoding strategy is possible only when the brain itself and its intrinsic features make an active contribution.

This led me consider the brain's intrinsic activity, its resting-state activity, that, on the basis of difference-based coding and sparse coding of its own neural activity, constitutes a virtual statistically-based spatial and temporal structure.

How now can the brain's intrinsic actively contribute to the rather active encoding of extrinsic stimuli in terms of difference-based coding and sparse coding? In other words, we need to bridge the gap from the brain's intrinsic activity to the extrinsic stimuli in order to understand how the latter can be encoded in an active rather than passive way by the brain and its intrinsic activity. This bridge from the brain's intrinsic activity to the encoding of extrinsic stimuli into neural activity will be the focus in the remaining two Parts of this volume.

I aim to bridge the gap between the brain's intrinsic activity and the extrinsic stimuli in two steps. First, I will investigate the implications of the brain's intrinsic activity by itself for the encoding of extrinsic stimuli. This leads me to what is described as "predictive coding," the encoding of predictions of extrinsic stimuli into the brain's neural activity. That is the focus in Part III.

Finally, we will investigate the actual manifestation of the extrinsic stimuli in the brain's neural activity, the stimulus-induced activity (or "task-related activity": I will use both in a synonymous way when I speak in the following discussion of stimulus-induced activity). This leads me to investigate how the brain's intrinsic activity interacts with the extrinsic stimuli, i.e., rest–stimulus interaction, as it will be discussed in Part IV of this volume.

General Overview

The goal of Part III is to discuss predictive coding in detail and how it is related to difference-based coding and sparse coding. This means I now pursue the reverse direction when compared to part I. While in Part I, I looked at how the environment affects the brain and how the brain lets itself be affected, I now take the reverse stance and see how the brain aims to affect the environment. More specifically, by anticipating or predicting the possible stimuli coming from the environment, the brain exerts an active impact on the subsequent stimulus-induced activity as associated with the actual stimuli.

Chapter 7 introduces predictive coding predominantly in the context of sensory and motor functions and the mirror neuron system. It elaborates on the mechanisms of predictive coding on the regional level of the brain's neural activity and demonstrates that predictive coding and difference-based coding are compatible with each other. Such predictive coding is made possible by directly comparing and matching the predicted stimulus with the actual stimulus, with their difference yielding what is described as a "prediction error," which in turn is supposed to determine the degree of stimulus-induced activity.

Chapter 8 starts where Chapter 7 ended: the generation of the prediction error as the interaction between predicted and actual stimuli. Taking recent results from studies on reward as a paradigm, it is shown that the prediction error results from the statistically based matching and comparison between different stimuli. This concerns the specific exteroceptive stimulus that is to be valued by reward, the unspecific exteroceptive stimuli from the respective social context, and the interoceptive stimuli from the body. What is encoded into neural activity as the prediction error is the comparison and matching between the statistical-frequency distributions of these different stimuli that is their natural, social, and vegetative statistics, as I call it.

Chapter 9 takes the example of reward further and raises the question of how the prediction of a possibly rewarding stimulus is generated by itself. For that, I consider recent data on the neural overlap between resting-state activity and reward-related activity as a starting point. I consequently postulate that the continuous changes in the resting-state activity themselves, that is their neuronal statistics, may be central in generating the prediction of the extrinsic stimulus as possible reward. Such generation of the predicted stimulus as possible reward by the brain's intrinsic activity itself and its neuronal statistics may be behaviorally manifested in what has been described as "seeking" and "wanting" in the literature on reward.

CHAPTER 7
Predictive Coding and Difference-Based Coding

Summary

Rather than focusing on how the environment and its various stimuli impact the brain's neural activity, I now take the reverse stance and discuss how the brain itself and its intrinsic activity can exert influence on its own neural processing of the extrinsic stimuli from the body and the environment. This leads me from sparse coding to predictive coding. Predictive coding proposes that the neural activity during stimulus-induced activity does not result from the stimulus itself, the actual input, but from its comparison and matching with the anticipation or prediction of that input, the predicted input. The degree to which predicted and actual inputs differ from each other is reflected in what is called "prediction error." Being based on the direct comparison and matching between predicted and actual inputs, the prediction error is supposed to determine the degree of stimulus-induced activity in sensorimotor regions and many other regions of the brain. I here discuss especially sensorimotor examples of predictive coding and their strong empirical support by recent imaging studies. Moreover, I describe how predictive coding can also be applied to functions other than sensorimotor as, for instance, mirroring and empathy. Mirroring and empathy are mediated neuronally by the so-called mirror neurons that allow for the inference of other people's goal orientation on the basis of the observation of their movements. Taking these different examples as starting points, I aim to show that predictive coding and thus the prediction error are possible only on the basis of encoding neural activity in terms of spatial and temporal differences; i.e., difference-based coding. I therefore conclude that predictive coding presupposes difference-based coding rather than stimulus-based coding. To put it differently, predictive coding may be considered one specific instance (e.g., with regard to the comparison between predicted and actual inputs) of difference-based coding that is supposed to apply to any kind of neural activity throughout the whole brain and its various states, including both resting-state and stimulus-induced activity.

Key Concepts and Topics Covered

Predictive coding, visual cortex, motor cortex, actual input, predicted input, common code, mirror neurons, reversed inference, difference-based coding

Empirical Background: Encoding of Natural Statistics and Predictive Coding

We demonstrated in the first part that the brain encodes the statistical frequency distribution of extrinsic stimuli; that is, their natural statistics (see Chapters 1 and 2). That was complemented in the second part by showing the brain's intrinsic activity and its continuous spatial and temporal changes. Due to the encoding of its own activity fluctuations in terms of difference-based coding, the brain's intrinsic activity was proposed to constitute a statistically based spatiotemporal structure (see Chapters 4 and 5).

How, now, are both the encoding of the extrinsic stimuli's natural statistics on the one hand and the brain's intrinsic activity and its spatiotemporal structure on the other related to each other? Due to the fact that the extrinsic stimuli and their natural statistics are encoded into the brain's intrinsic activity, their natural statistics should somehow resurface in the brain's intrinsic activity and its spatiotemporal structure (though possibly in a slightly different way). The intrinsic activity itself and its fluctuations should consecutively somehow reflect and be related to the previous extrinsic stimuli.

Put slightly different, the manifestation of the previous stimuli and their natural statistics in the intrinsic activity should lead to the prediction of the subsequent stimulus that may possibly occur next. Such a prediction on the neuronal level (or anticipation or expectation on a more psychological level) is considered the nucleus of yet another coding strategy, predictive coding. Predictive coding has recently been widely discussed, especially in the context of functional imaging and thus the regional level of neural activity.

What is predictive coding? Briefly, predictive coding proposes that the neural activity related to a particular stimulus results from the comparison between the actual input and the anticipation or prediction of that input. Such a comparison between predicted and actual input yields a difference, the prediction error, that in turn is supposed to determine the degree of the subsequent stimulus-induced activity. The aim of this chapter is to discuss predictive coding including the prediction error and how they stand in relation to difference-based coding.

Neuronal findings Ia: predictive coding in *visual cortex*

One of the most typical examples of predictive coding is the visual cortex (see, e.g., Alink et al. 2010; Spratling 2010, 2012a and b; Langner et al. 2012; Rauss et al. 2011; Egner et al. 2010). We will not be able to discuss all the studies in detail here. Instead, we are only focusing on one earlier simulation study by Rao and Ballard (1999) that showed predictive coding in a paradigmatic way and how it is supported and extended by empirical data in a more recent study by Alink et al. (2010).

In a simulation model of visual processing, Rao and Ballard (1999) (see also Rao 2010 for the extension to decision making) demonstrated that feedback connections from a higher to lower visual area carry predictions of the sensory input, the predicted input, and associated lower visual regions' activities. Feedforward connections from lower to higher visual regions, in contrast, were rather related to the discrepancy or difference, for example, the residual errors, between the predictions and the actual sensory input, for example, the actual lower level activities.

More specifically, effects in nonclassical receptive fields were related to the predicted input from the feedback connections rather than to the actual input transmitted by the feedforward connections. Correspondingly, neurons in the non- or extraclassical receptive fields, especially those in layer 2/3, seem to signal specifically the difference between the actual sensory input and the predicted input transmitted from higher areas.

How can the predicted input be characterized in further detail? Rao and Ballard (1999) postulate that the predicted input itself ultimately reflects the natural statistics of the predicted stimulus. A prediction can only be generated by those stimuli that show a certain frequency of occurrence; otherwise it is rather unlikely that they can be compared and matched with the actual sensory input to keep the subsequent prediction error low.

This means that a low predictable or even unpredictable actual sensory input that deviates from the natural statistics may yield the largest difference between predicted input and actual input and consequently the strongest neural activity. Conversely, one would expect lower or reduced neural activity in the case of a highly predictable sensory input that does not deviate much from the natural statistics and therefore also from the predicted input.

Alink et al. (2010) took the latter assumption as a starting point and compared the neural activity in V1 and hMT/V5 during predictable and nonpredictable visual stimuli using functional magnetic resonance imaging (fMRI). They compared physically identical stimuli whose onset was varied being either predictable or nonpredictable from the trajectory of motion. This yielded significantly reduced signal changes in V1 (but neither in hMT/V5 nor in any other region) during the predicted stimuli when compared to the nonpredictable ones.

They then varied the same stimuli with regard to predictable and nonpredictable motion within the context of apparent motion. Again, the predictable stimulus induced reduced signal changes in V1 (and this time also in hMT/V5). Surprisingly, the predicted stimuli could be behaviorally detected more easily when compared to the nonpredictable ones. Hence, reduced signal changes during predictable stimuli co-occurred with better behavioral detection (see Fig. 7-1).

Based on the model by Rao and Ballard (1999), Alink et al. (2010) propose that the reduced V1 activity during predictable stimuli

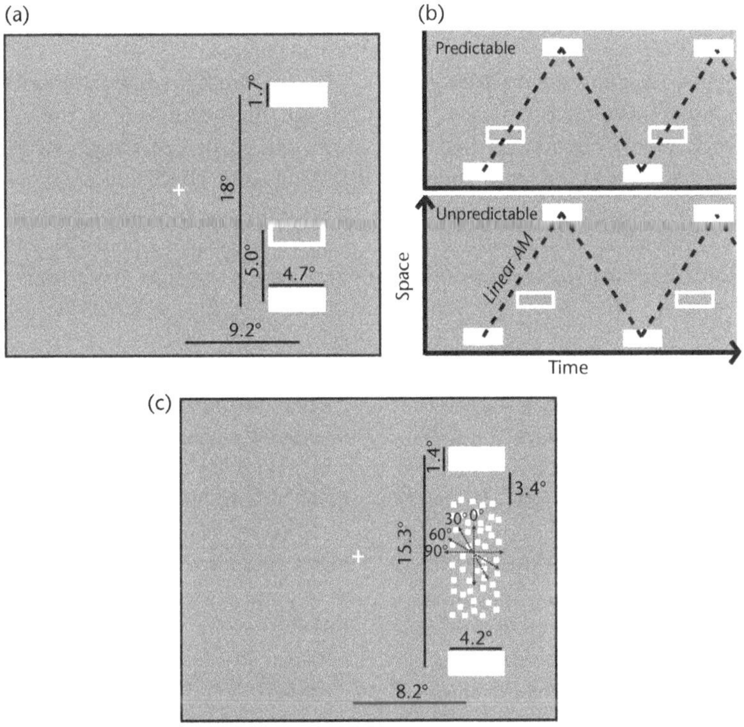

Figure 7-1 **Prediction of stimuli in visual cortex. Stimuli presented during experiments 1 and 2. (*a*) Schematic overview of the spatial layout of the stimuli presented during experiment 1. The top and bottom solid white bars represent the apparent-motion-inducing stimuli that were presented for 200 ms with an interstimulus interval of 150 ms. The empty bar represents the test stimulus that was presented for 16 ms during upward apparent motion, which occurred during the interstimulus interval following the presentation of the lower bar. (*b*) A schematic space–time plot that illustrates the time of presentation of the test bar relative to linear apparent motion during experiment 1. The dotted line represents the trajectory of linear apparent motion between the top and bottom bars. For the predictable condition (top), the test stimulus is presented at the time at which linear apparent motion passes the location of the test bar (41.7 ms after the offset of the lower bar). For the unpredictable condition (bottom), the test bar is presented at the same location but with a greater delay than the predictable test bar (108 ms after the offset of the bottom bar), which corresponds to the time at which linear apparent motion already passed the location of the test bar stimulus. (*c*) A schematic depiction of the stimuli presented during experiment 2. Apparent-motion stimuli were identical to those presented in experiment 1, although they were slightly smaller. During the interstimulus intervals, random-dot motion was presented on the path of apparent motion. The motion direction of these dots was either parallel to the apparent motion or 30°, 60°, or 90° anticlockwise from the apparent-motion direction. (Reprinted with permission of *The Journal of Neuroscience,* from Alink A, Schwiedrzik CM, Kohler A, Singer W, Muckli L Stimulus predictability reduces responses in primary visual cortex. *J Neurosci.* 2010 Feb 24;30(8):2960–6.)**

may stem from top-down influences in higher visual areas (see also Spratling 2010 for further support of predictive coding in V1).

More specifically, the higher visual (and prefrontal) regions may have yielded a prediction about the possible sensory input; this predicted input was then compared and matched to the actual sensory input with the outcome of this matching process determining the degree of activity in V1.

Since the actual stimulus was well predictable, the difference between predicted and actual input, the prediction error, was rather low and therefore induced only small activity changes in V1. In the converse case of nonpredictable stimuli, the prediction error was rather high and induced therefore higher activity changes in V1.

Neuronal findings Ib: generation of prediction error in *prefrontal cortex*

Where is the prediction, the predicted input, generated? In a recent imaging study, Summerfield et al. 2006 applied two different stimuli, houses and faces, matched their physical characteristics, and matched also the stimuli to the individual subjects' thresholds for perception. When comparing face stimuli versus nonface stimuli irrespective of their perceptual sets, they could tap into those regions that were related to the physical features of the stimuli; these stimuli yielded neural activity changes in the fusiform face area, the temporoparietal junction and the inferior occipital cortex.

In addition, their design also allowed them to compare the perceptual sets irrespective of the stimuli's physical features, that is, face sets versus house sets. Comparison between these two sets yielded neural activity changes in the ventro- and dorsomedial prefrontal cortex (VMPFC, DMPFC), which must be related to the perceptual rather than the physical features of the stimuli.

The authors argue that the activity in the frontal regions reflects the generation of some template, a prediction or anticipation. Such prediction as template is supposed to top-down modulate neural activity changes in the visual cortex induced by the stimuli themselves and their physical features.

Accordingly, the prefrontal cortex generates some prediction of possible sensory changes, a template, against which the actually occurring sensory changes are matched and compared. Such matching and comparison between the prefrontal top-down signals, that is, the predicted sensory input, and visual cortical bottom-up signals, that is, the actually occurring sensory input, allows the brain to shape and constitute a visual percept.

One should be careful, however, about associating the generation of the predicted input with the higher order cognitive regions like the VMPFC and DMPFC. Recent studies on early electrophysiological visual potentials in primary visual cortex (like a potential that is called C1) have shown that they may already by themselves reflect some kind of predicted input (see Rauss et al. 2011).

The early visual potential in V1 may then by itself correspond to the rapid comparison between an expected, that is, predicted, and actual input with both being generated in V1. There may thus be preparatory activity early on in visual cortex, that is, in V1, that, when compared with the actual input, yields a prediction error. Following Rauss et al. (2011), this is possible only "when there is an overlap between predictable environmental or task parameters and the given functional characteristics of a given cortical area" (Rauss et al. 2011, 1249).

Taken together, the findings in the visual domain strongly suggest the generation of some kind of predicted visual input that is matched and compared with the actual visual input. The subsequent stimulus-induced activity is then supposed to result from matching and comparing predicted and actual inputs: the larger the discrepancy between actual and predicted inputs, the larger the prediction error, and the greater the degree of the subsequent stimulus-induced activity.

This implicates lower- and higher-order regions like the visual and the prefrontal cortex. Whether there is a strict division of labor with the generation of the predicted input in higher regions and the actual input in lower regions remains unclear at this point.

Neuronal findings IIa: predictive coding in *somatosensory cortex*

Predictive coding has been demonstrated not only in the visual cortex but also in other sensory modalities, such as in the somatosensory system as implicated in tickling. Why are we much more ticklish when tickled by others than by ourselves? Applying a literally ticklish study design, Blakemore et al. (1999a and b) used the same tactile stimulus and allowed it to be applied once by another person and once by the person herself who is being tickled.

As expected, application of the tickling stimulus by another person was experienced as more ticklish and intense than when the person itself applied the same stimulus to itself. Blakemore used brain imaging and demonstrated that neural activity changes in regions like the cerebellum and the somatosensory cortex differed between both conditions, tickling by another person versus tickling by oneself.

How can the difference between the two different applications of tickling be explained? In each case the same physical stimulus was applied so that one would suggest that both stimuli should lead to the same neuronal effects. This, however, was not true since the effects of the stimuli very much depended on the person who applied it.

How is this possible? When applying the ticklish stimulus to oneself, the sensory effects of the self-directed motion and thus the sensory consequences of one's own movements (during one's application of the ticklish stimulus), known as *reafferences*, can be cancelled out because they can be well predicted on the basis of one's own movement; the stimulus is consequently experienced as less ticklish. The generation of the movements during the self-applied stimulus must have thus generated some kind of predicted input, a sensory prediction.

This is well in accordance with the observation that sensory predictions, the predicted input, are generated by linking possible sensory effects to corresponding motor commands (see also Schütz-Bosbach and Prinz 2007a and b, who speak of "prospective coding"). Since the motor commands stem from a different origin, own versus other person, their consequently anticipated sensory effects, the predicted input, are different. These anticipated sensory effects, i.e., the different predicted inputs, are then compared with the actual input, the ticklish stimulus.

Since now the anticipated sensory effects, the predicted inputs, are different, the resulting signal changes in, for instance, the somatosensory cortex and the cerebellum do also differ even though the actual somatosensory stimulus, the tickling stimulus, is the same in both cases. Hence, the difference in neural activity between own and other tickling must stem from the differences in the predicted inputs, and their matching and comparison with the same stimulus, the tickling as the actual input.

Blakemore et al. (1999a and b) also demonstrated that the time delay between motor command and the resulting tickle is crucial. The greater the time delay, the more ticklish the self-applied percept; this entails that sensory effects are more difficult to cancel out with greater time delay between movement and sensory feedback.

This suggests that the sensory feedback during self-application of stimuli can be cancelled out best when being temporally close to the corresponding movement and the respective motor command. If, in contrast, both stimuli are presented in a temporally distant way, sensory effects are more difficult to cancel out, this is so because it is more difficult to generate sensory prediction and thus a proper predicted input without reference to some movement and motor command.

Neuronal findings IIb: predictive coding in *motor cortex*

Besides the sensory system (see also Schütz-Bosbach and Prinz 2007a and b; Noppeney 2008), predictive coding has also been observed in motor function. Wolpert and Miall (1996) and Davidson and Wolpert (2005) demonstrate that the motor system makes a copy from any motor command, a so-called efference copy. On the basis of this efference copy, the motor system can develop what is called a forward model that generates an estimate of the predicted sensory consequences of the executed motor action.

The generation of forward models allows us to predict the sensory consequences of motor action at the very time of its execution.[1] When, for instance, holding an object in a precision grip with the fingers, sufficient grip force must be generated to prevent slip and loss of the object's load force. Increase of the object's load force by a self-generated action, such as moving the arm, is accompanied by a corresponding increase of the grip force with no temporal delay.

This is possible only on the basis of the assumption of a forward model that, at the time of motor execution, estimates and predicts possible sensory consequences. While this remains impossible when assuming mere sensory feedback, that is, reafference, that would introduce some temporal delay in adapting the grip force to the increasing load force.

Neuroanatomically, such a predictive feedforward model has been associated with the cerebellum and the mediodorsal thalamus (see Davidson and Wolpert 2005 for an overview). In addition to forward models predicting sensory consequences, there are also inverse models that predict and estimate the motor consequences and possible motor commands following some sensory input and feedback. Hence, both sensory and motor consequences of ongoing motor action are predicted in the gestalt of forward and inverse models.

Finally, it should be noted that predictive coding is not only present in the sensory and motor domains but also in more cognitive functions like learning and attention (see Sylvester et al. 2007; Spratling 2008), speech (Kotz and Schwartze 2010), mirror neurons (see later section), and reward (see Chapters 8 and 9 for details). It would be beyond the scope of this chapter to show all the details of the literature on predictive coding and cognitive functions. The most important aim at this point is to state that predictive coding seems to determine neuronal activity in different regions ranging from sensory to nonsensory regions.

Neuronal hypothesis Ia: Prediction error and resting-state activity

One central claim of predictive coding is that the observed neural activity in sensory cortex like V1 or somatosensory cortex reflects the prediction error rather than the actual stimulus itself. The prediction error results from the difference between predicted and actual stimulus, and it is this difference that is supposed to determine the degree of subsequent stimulus-induced activity in sensory cortex.

The question is now what kind of neuronal process must occur in order to make the determination of the sensory cortex's activity by the prediction error possible. I hypothesize that the neural coding in terms of differences, that is, difference-based coding, may be central here. This shall be specified and detailed in the following.

How can we describe the prediction error in further detail? The prediction error is supposed to result from the matching and comparison between predicted and actual inputs. Moreover, the predicted input is supposed to temporally and constitutionally precede the actual input and must therefore be related to neuronal activity prior to the occurrence of the actual input.

This raises the question for the kind of neuronal activity that is necessary to generate the predicted input. One may now want to argue that this is the point where cognitive functions come into the picture. Due to cognitive operations, including attention, working memory, reasoning, and so on, the predicted input can be generated. Neuronally, this implies the search for neuronal activity in those regions like the prefrontal cortex that are related to cognitive functions.

The most important question here, however, is not where such neural activity is generated but how it is generated: Where does the neural activity underlying the generation of the predicted input come from, and what are the neuronal mechanisms that generate such neural activity? Since there is still an absence of any specific stimuli, the underlying neuronal activity can only be generated on the basis of the brain's resting-state activity, its intrinsic activity (and its various rest–rest interactions, if one wants to say so), which may be central for yielding the predicted input; see Chapters 4–6).

Neuronal hypothesis Ib: rest–stimulus interaction generates the prediction error

One may consequently hypothesize that the neuronal mechanisms underlying the generation of the prediction error (necessarily) implicate the brain's resting-state activity. Let us specify my assumption by applying them to the aforementioned studies. I hypothesize that Alink's et al. (2010) results of differential activity levels in V1 during predicted and nonpredicted input correspond to different resting-state activity levels in the same region. These different resting-state activity levels may impact stimulus-induced activity during the same actual inputs in different ways; this, in turn, yields different prediction errors going along with different levels of stimulus-induced activity in V1.

The same may hold in the case of tickling and the somatosensory cortex. Depending on whether one tickles oneself or is tickled by another person, one may generate different predicted inputs, which go along with different resting-state activity levels in somatosensory cortex (and other regions like the cerebellum; see earlier). Since different resting-state activity levels entail different modulations of subsequent stimulus-induced activity, different degrees of neural activity are observed during one's own and another's application of the same actual input, the tickling.

Based on these considerations, I hypothesize that, on a purely neuronal level, the interaction between the resting-state activity and the actual stimulus yields the prediction error including the degree of subsequent stimulus-induced activity in sensory cortex. In short, the prediction error can be traced back neuronally to what I call "rest–stimulus interaction" (see Part IV for details).

This implies that the degree of the prediction error may in part be dependent upon the level of resting-state activity level that immediately precedes the arrival of the actual input. One would consequently postulate that the generation of the predicted input must be closely related to the brain's intrinsic activity and the continuous changes in its spatial and temporal patterns. This is a viable hypothesis that shall be developed and discussed in more detail in Chapter 9.

Neuronal hypothesis Ic: prediction error and difference-based coding

Let us for now turn from the resting-state activity itself to its interaction with the actual input, the stimulus, yielding what I describe as "rest–stimulus interaction." How is such rest–stimulus interaction possible? I postulate that such rest–stimulus interaction is possible only on the basis of difference-based coding (see part IV for details).

When the actual stimulus is entering the brain via, for instance, the sensory cortex, it encounters the brain's intrinsic activity, its resting-state activity. The activity that can possibly be induced by the actual stimulus itself is supposed to be dependent on the level of resting-state activity it encounters.

What is encoded into the resulting stimulus-induced activity is thus rather the difference between the resting-state activity level and the (virtual) stimulus-induced activity (if it were independent of the resting-state activity). This means that the resulting stimulus-induced activity is based upon and encoded in terms of a difference-based signal, thus presupposing difference-based coding rather than stimulus-based coding.

How is such difference-based coding related to the prediction error? The prediction error is based on the difference between predicted and actual inputs and thus on the comparison and matching of their respective statistical frequency distributions, their respective statistics (see the earlier assumption by Rao et al. 1999). This means that the prediction error itself reflects a difference-based signal that as such presupposes difference-based coding.

In contrast, the prediction error could not be yielded if there were stimulus-based coding; in such case the predicted input would be coded separately and in parallel to the physical features

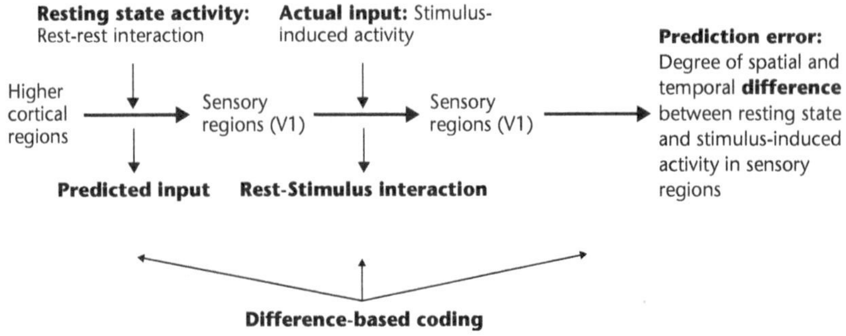

Figure 7.2 Difference-based coding and predictive coding. The figure shows the different stages and their presumed underlying neuronal processes during predictive coding. Predictive coding assumes that the prediction error results from the comparison between the predicted and the actual input (middle and right parts of figure). Such comparison presupposes the matching between the resting state activity and the actual stimulus in sensory cortex, such as in V1 (taken here as paradigmatic example). Such matching is possible only on the basis of difference-based coding. The matching between the sensory cortical resting state activity with the stimulus yields a spatial and temporal difference value, which in turn will determine the degree of activity change and thus the resulting stimulus-induced activity (right part). There is thus rest–stimulus interaction (middle part) (see Part IV for details). Rest–stimulus interaction does in turn rely on the coding of neural difference, thus presupposing difference-based coding. The predicted input is supposed to be generated during the preceding resting state on the basis of rest–rest interaction between higher cortical midline regions and sensory regions (see left part). That, again, is possible only on the basis of coding neural differences; i.e., difference-based coding.

of the actual input. Since such parallel and segregated coding goes along with different codes of predicted and actual inputs, both inputs could no longer be directly compared and matched with each other (see Chapter 8 for more details). This, however, makes the prediction error impossible. I consequently hypothesize that difference-based coding rather than stimulus-based coding must be (necessarily) presupposed in order to make possible and thus to generate the prediction error (see Fig. 7-2).

Neuronal hypothesis Id: predictive coding presupposes difference-based coding

How can we lend further empirical support to my hypothesis of the prediction error presupposing difference-based coding? Let's have another look at the results described so far. Alink et al. (2010) observe that a predictable input yields lower activity changes in V1 than a nonpredictable input in the presence of the same actual input.

How is this possible? The difference between predicted and actual input is larger in the case of a nonpredictable input when compared to the one of a predictable input. Difference-based coding implies that larger differences are accompanied by larger activity changes. This is exactly what Alink et al. (2010) observed. Hence, their results lend strong support to the assumption that predictive coding presupposes difference-based coding.

The same holds for the study by Blakemore et al. (1999a and b) about tickling. Tickling by others is more unpredictable and yields, therefore, a larger prediction error and thus a larger difference when compared to the tickling applied by oneself. Such larger difference should then yield stronger activity changes in, for instance, the somatosensory cortex during tickling by others when compared to tickling by oneself; this is exactly what the authors observed.

Taken together, I hypothesize that the prediction error as the matching and comparison between predicted and actual inputs necessarily and unavoidably presupposes difference-based coding rather than stimulus-based coding. The degree of difference between predicted and actual input in the prediction error determines the degree of the subsequent stimulus-induced activity that can therefore be considered a difference- rather than stimulus-based signal. Accordingly, the prediction error and its associated stimulus-induced activity presuppose difference-based coding rather than stimulus-based coding.

Neuronal findings IIIa: Mirror neurons and simulation

So far I have demonstrated predictive coding to hold for sensory and motor functions. However, recent research applied the concept of predictive coding also to functions other than sensory and motor functions. One such example is the mirror neurons, which have been associated with the ability to infer other people's goal orientation and intentions.

What are the mirror neurons? We are able to infer the intentions and goals of other people's movement as we observe it. On the basis of observing the other's action, we are able to infer her or his intentions and goals. One neural candidate strongly suspected to be involved in this process is the mirror neuron system (MNS) that includes regions like the premotor cortex, the inferior parietal lobule, and the superior temporal sulcus.

The MNS shows activity not only during action observation but also during action execution; regions activated during both action observation and execution include region F5 in the premotor cortex of macaque monkey (which corresponds to the left inferior frontal cortex (Brodmann area 44) in humans) and the inferior parietal lobule (Gallese and Goldman 1998; Rizzolatti and Craighero 2004). Another region, the superior temporal sulcus, has, in contrast, been observed to be active only during action observation, while not being recruited during action execution (see Frith and Frith 1999).

The mirror neuron system was first detected by G. Rizzolatti and V. Gallese in monkeys and later confirmed in humans, too. Both researchers are from Parma, Italy. Parma is well known for its famous ham and other gustatory delicacies. One can thus say that both the excellent ham and the detection of the neuronal underpinnings, that is, the mirror neurons, of our observation of other peoples' enjoyment of that very same ham come from Parma. However, as boastful as the city of Parma may be of its ham display windows, be assured you will not come across any windows displaying mirror neurons.

Let's turn from the display windows of Parma to the windows of science. How can the mirror neurons, that is, the MNS, reconstitute and infer the goals and intentions of the other persons' movements? All that we observe is the other's mere movement while we do not observe her/his intentions and goals associated with that particular movement.

One possible candidate is the MNS and its double involvement in both action execution and observation By recruiting exactly those regions during action observation in other persons that are also active during the execution of the same action in oneself, one is able to infer the intentions and goals associated with the observed movements in the other person from the goals and intentions that guide the execution of the same movement in the observing person himself.

This means that the observing person quasi-simulates his own goals and intentions (which usually guide the execution of his own movements) and associates them now with the movements he observes in the other person. The use of the same neural regions for action observation and execution seems to allow for such simulation of one's own intentions and goals and their subsequent association with the observed movements in the other person (see, e.g., Rizzolatti and Craighero 2004; Gallese and Goldman 1998).

Neuronal findings IIIb: Mirror neurons and reverse inference

The central role of simulation is often complemented by a neuroanatomical "feedforward" recognition model. The observed signal is carried forth neuronally from the visual cortex to the STS and from there to the inferior parietal lobule and ultimately to the highest center, the inferior frontal (premotor) mirror neurons in F5. This goes along functionally with a feedforward movement from the representation of the movement kinematics over the movements to the goals and ultimately the intentions of the observed action.

However, this is where the problem starts, if one follows Karl Friston as one of the main advocates of predictive coding, and his colleague J. M. Kilner (Kilner et al. 2007a and b; Zentgraf et al. 2011; Friston 2010, Neal and Kilner 2010). Kilner laid out the challenges of the simulation and feedforward model of action observation in excellent papers (Kilner et al. 2007a and b), which since has been supplemented by supporting empirical data on both simulation and behavior (Friston 2011; Zentgraf et al. 2011; Neal and Kilner 2010). Let me here concentrate on his critique as so nicely laid out in his 2007 paper.

Following Kilner et al. (2007), the problem starts when assuming the kind of feedforward movement, as discussed earlier. In the case of action execution, the neural constitution of the intentions and goals in the premotor areas (F5) cause the neural activity changes in lower regions like the motor cortex and other regions; these regions' neural activity is then supposed to represent the movements and the kinematics that are necessary to realize the respective goals and intentions.

This, however, is not possible in action observation. Here the scenario is reversed. One can only observe the kinematics and the movements while having no access to the goals and the intentions themselves, as associated with the observed action. The inference is consequently reversed in that one must infer from the observed kinematics and movements to the preceding goals and intentions that caused the former. Hence, the inference in action observation is no longer from the intention or goal to the movement, as in action execution, but follows the reverse direction, from movements to intention or goal.

Such reversed inference is possible if the neuronal processes occurring during action execution can be simply reversed. This is, for instance, possible when the observed sensory input is associated with only one particular cause, that is, intention and goal. However, the observed kinematics and movements can have many underlying possible causes, that is, various goals and intentions, rather than one specific one.

For instance, one observes that somebody raises his hand. What is the intention and goal of that movement? Does the person hail for a taxi, prepare to play the next tone on the piano, or prepare to throw the ball in handball? By just observing the movement and kinematics itself we remain unable to tell.

This makes it rather unlikely that a simple reversal of action execution in the gestalt of a feedforward recognition model can account for the inference of goals and intentions in action observation, as well as for the neural activity in the mirror neuron system during action observation.

Neuronal findings IIIc: mirror neurons and the prediction of inputs

Another argument against the feedforward recognition model is that the monkey premotor cortex in F5 (or in inferior frontal cortex in Brodmann area 44 in humans) becomes not only active when the action of the other can be observed but also when the sight of the other's movement remains hidden (Umiltà et al., 2001). If a simple feedforward recognition model is at work in inferring the intentions and goals of the observed movement, no activity should be observed at all in this region when the movement is hidden. This is so because then there is simply no visual input in lower regions like the visual cortex and the STS that could drive and activate higher regions like the premotor cortex.

The fact that despite the absence of visual input the premotor cortex becomes nevertheless active raises the question for some additional mechanism in inferring the intentions and goals during action observation. Such additional mechanism could consist in the expectation or anticipation of the intentions and goals of the observed action. Before we can even observe the other's action, we apparently generate several models or hypotheses, that is, several predicted inputs, that predict possible intentions and goals by others.

These models or hypotheses and thus the different predicted inputs may have a high or low likelihood given the past and present contexts, thus amounting to what is called either high or low prior probability (this touches upon the Bayesian statistics and its respective concepts, which shall not be pursued in further detail here). The prior probability may, for instance, be raised by also including the movements and kinematics associated with the respective goals and intentions in the respective hypothesis or model.

Why are several predicted inputs generated? The generation of several predicted inputs makes it possible to compare and match the predicted movements and kinematics as generated in the different hypotheses or models, i.e., the predicted inputs, with the actually observed movement and its kinematics. This may lead to different scenarios as sketched in the following.

If the match or correspondence of one particular hypothesis with the observed movement and kinematic is high and thus good, the prediction error is low; the posterior probability is consequently high so that the activation induced by the observed movement is "explained away." In this case, we are well able to infer the intentions and goals of the actually observed movement and kinematics. If, in contrast, the match is low and thus bad, the prediction error is high; the posterior probability is rather low so that we remain unable to infer the intentions and goals of the actually observed movement and kinematics in the other person.

Neuronal hypothesis IIa: incompatibility between goal-orientations and movements

The mirror neurons—that is, the MNS—raise some important questions with regard to predictive coding in general. Kilner et al. (2007a and b) focus on the question of the temporal dimension, more specifically the temporal precedence of the other's goal orientation when compared to the observation of the other's actual movements.

They argue that the other's goal orientation cannot be inferred from the observation of the other's movements alone, and instead requires an additional prediction of a possible goal orientation as the predicted input, which must temporally precede the actual input, the observed movement. Such a predicted goal orientation can then be matched and compared with the actually observed movement, the actual input.

How is such matching and comparison between predicted goal orientation and actual movement possible? One would expect that different movements can be compared and matched with each other as, for instance, flexion and extension. Thereby it may not matter so much whether their origin is attributed to either the own or the other person since, in both cases, the movements will show the same physical features, i.e., the movement kinematics, though in different degrees. Since they refer to the same physical features, the movement kinematics of one's own and others' movements can be well compared and matched with each other and remain therefore independent of the persons who actually execute them.

The same may hold for different goal orientations; they all reflect goals and thus the same kind of contents and physical features, though in different degrees. This is, for example, manifested in the intention to throw a ball, where it does not matter for the intention itself with which person it is associated that is whether it is myself or someone else. If I observe another person throwing a ball, I can infer her intention from my own intention when throwing a ball. Intentions are thus compared with intentions in very much the same way that movements can be compared with movements, no matter which person executes them. While movements can well be compared and matched with movements and goal orientations with goal orientations, the comparison between movements and goal orientations may be rather problematic. Why? Because both involve different physical features. Unlike a movement, a goal-orientation cannot be characterized by kinematics and the respective spatial and temporal trajectories. Movements and goal-orientation are thus rather incompatible, which makes their direct comparison and matching rather difficult if not impossible.

Neurometaphorical comparison I: why we cannot compare apples and oranges

How can we better illustrate the difference between movements and intentions with regard to physical features? If one wants to compare intentions and movements with each other, one, metaphorically speaking, compares apples with oranges rather than apples with apples and oranges with oranges. And just as one cannot compare apples and oranges, one cannot compare goal orientation and movements with each other.

Let's dwell a little more on the example with apples and oranges. Why can we compare different kinds of apples (that is, "tokens" as the philosopher would say) with each other? Because they all belong to the same type of fruit subsumed under one and the same umbrella concept, that is apples; the different apples therefore show the same physical features that define the concept of apple (as "type" as the philosopher would say).

In contrast, the physical features themselves may not differ in kind, but they may nevertheless differ in their degrees, as manifest in the different kinds (or "tokens") of apples. Different kinds of apples may then be characterized as the variation in the degree of the same physical features that signify apples (as "type") *as* apples.

Oranges, in contrast, show different physical features and are therefore a different fruit and thus a different "type" of fruit. If one now directly compares apples and oranges, one simply confuses different fruits, that is, different "types" of fruits and compares therefore apples and oranges in both literal and figurative senses.

Why can one speak of confusion here? One mixes and thus confuses different types, i.e., different fruits, and thus different physical features. The take-home message is thus that any kind of direct comparison between apples and oranges, be it literal or figurative, remains impossible.

Neuronal hypothesis IIb: The need for a "common code" between predicted goal-orientations and observed movements

Such a direct comparison is, however, exactly what Kilner et al. (2007) must presuppose if they want their assumption of predictive coding in the MNS to hold. They must propose that the predicted goal-orientations are directly compared with the observed movements. That means that different physical features, the ones associated with movements and intentions, are directly compared with each other. This, however, as I claim, remains impossible in the same way that one cannot directly compare and match apples and oranges.

What can we do now? We can discard the model by Kilner and reject his assumption of predicted goal-orientations. This would abandon the need for direct matching and comparison between predicted goal-orientations and observed movements, and thus the comparison between apples and oranges. That, however, conflicts with his other, empirically supported assumptions described earlier.

Alternatively, we may need to search for some kind of neuronal mechanism that makes possible the direct interaction between predicted goal-orientations and observed movements. In other words, we have to search for some feature or property that commonly underlies both apples and oranges. This will be the focus in the next section.

Neuronal hypothesis IIc: Difference-based coding as "common code"

How is it possible for the brain to directly compare and match goal orientations and movements? I hypothesize that this is possible only by presupposing a common underlying code.

What is such a common code? In the case of apples and oranges the answer is easy. Both apples and oranges share the physical features that are associated with fruits as distinguished from, for instance, plants in general. The common code that commonly underlies apples and oranges thus consists in, metaphorically speaking, their encoding as fruits.

What, then, links goal-orientations and intentions in the same way apples and oranges are linked by their common coding as fruits? I postulate that the encoding of spatial and temporal differences and thus difference-based coding provides such a common code between goal-orientations and movements.

Both goal orientations and movements and their respective physical features are encoded in terms of their respective spatial and temporal differences, and thus, as we have seen in Chapters 1 through 3, on the basis of their respective statistical frequency distributions, their statistics. One may thus say that the statistically based encoding in terms of spatial and temporal differences supersedes the physical differences between goal-orientations and movements.

How does the statistically based encoding of both goal-orientations and movements in terms of their spatial and temporal differences make possible their direct matching and comparison? If both goal-orientations and movements are encoded in terms of spatial and temporal differences, their direct comparison and matching amounts to a comparison of different degrees of spatial and temporal differences rather than to a comparison between different physical features.

Accordingly, the encoding in terms of spatial and temporal differences provides a common code. This common code allows us to directly compare and match goal-orientations and movements with each other, independently of their different physical features and different origins.

NEURONAL HYPOTHESIS IID: STATISTICALLY BASED MATCHING BETWEEN PREDICTED GOAL-ORIENTATIONS AND OBSERVED MOVEMENTS SUPERSEDES THEIR PHYSICAL DIFFERENCES AND DIFFERENT ORIGINS

This is rather abstract so far. We need to specify the coding of differences related to both goal orientation and movement. Let's start with the observed movement as the actual input.

Relying on sparse coding (see Chapters 1–3), the actual input does not consist of a particular stimulus and its respective physical features. Instead, the actual input corresponds rather to a difference, the differences between different discrete points in physical space and time; that is, the stimuli statistical frequency distribution, their natural statistics (see Part I). This means that the actual input, like an observed movement, is encoded in terms of a difference, a statistically based spatiotemporal difference that reflects the actual input's natural statistics.

How about the predicted input? I suggest that the predicted input may be related to the resting-state activity and more specifically to its continuous changes as manifested in its spatiotemporal activity patterns, i.e., rest–rest interaction as one may want to say. As discussed in Chapters 4 through 6, the neural activity in the resting state's spatiotemporal activity pattern is also encoded in terms of statistically based spatiotemporal differences reflecting its "neuronal statistics" (see Chapters 5 and 6).

How, then, is the predicted input itself generated by the resting state's neuronal statistics? I will leave this open at this point and will discuss this in detail in Chapter 9. How can predicted and actual inputs be compared and matched with each other? The statistically based encoding of both actual input and predicted input in terms of spatial and temporal differences makes possible their direct comparison and matching, irrespective of their physical differences and different origins. If actual input and predicted input, i.e., movement and goal-orientation, are compared and matched with each other, two different degrees of spatial and temporal differences and thus two different statistics, neuronal and natural, are matched and compared with each other.

Accordingly, the common coding of goal-orientations and movements in terms of statistically based spatiotemporal differences supersedes their physical differences and different origins. Such common coding makes possible the direct comparison and matching. Based on such statistical comparisons and matching, the observing person can then directly infer the other person's goal orientation (see Fig. 7-3).

How does that stand in relation to our metaphorical comparison with apples and oranges? Both oranges and apples encode varying degrees of the physical features that link them under the concept of fruit. The same now holds in the case of goal-orientations and movements. They are encoded in terms of varying degrees of one and the same feature, spatial and temporal differences, which ties them together and ultimately makes possible their direct comparison and matching. Accordingly, what the concept of "fruit" is for oranges and apples corresponds to differences, i.e., difference-based coding, in the case of goal-orientations and movements.

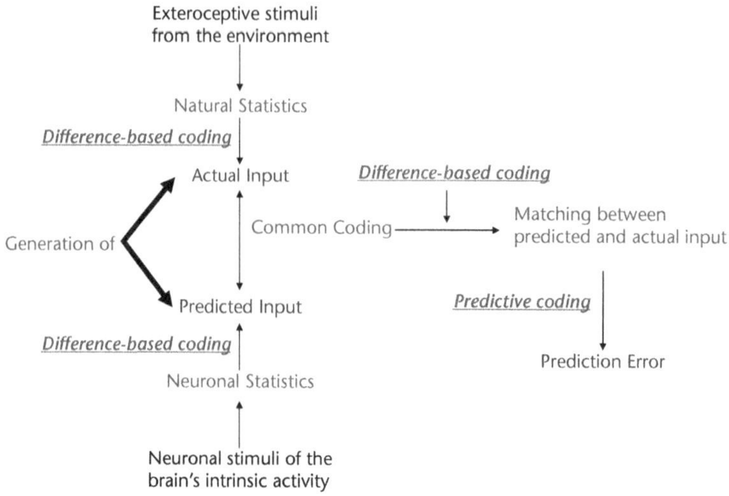

Figure 7-3 Common coding in the generation of predicted and actual input. The figure shows how the generation of both predicted input and actual input presupposes the encoding of spatial and temporal neural differences into neural activity as common code, i.e., difference-based coding. Difference-based coding as common code makes possible the direct matching and comparison between predicted and actual input and therefore the prediction error. The generation of the actual input presupposes the encoding of the stimulus' natural statistics; that is, its statistical frequency distribution across time and space (*left upper part*). That means that statistically based spatiotemporal differences are encoded into neural activity; that is, difference-based coding. In the same way, the generation of the predicted input presupposes the encoding of the resting state's activity frequency distribution across the different discrete points in physical time and space, that is, its neuronal statistics (*left lower part*); this again presupposes difference-based coding. Despite the encoding of different statistics, that is, neuronal and natural, neural activity underlying predicted and actual inputs nevertheless share a common code, statistically based spatiotemporal differences (*middle part*). This, in turn, makes possible their direct comparison and matching (*right part*) with the consecutive generation of the prediction error.

Neuronal hypothesis IIe: Difference-based coding is required in all three stages of predictive coding

What does this imply for Kilner's account of the mirror neuron and the MNS? His assumption of goal-orientation as the predicted input must be complemented by the assumption of the encoding of both predicted and actual input in terms of spatial and temporal differences, that is, difference-based coding. Otherwise their direct matching and comparison in gestalt of the prediction error remains impossible; goal orientation and observed movement can then not be linked and associated with each other.

Accordingly, Kilner must presuppose a common code for predicted and actual inputs, for example, for goal orientation and observed movements, in order for his assumption of predictive coding in MNS to hold. I suppose this common code to consist in difference-based coding as distinguished from stimulus-based coding.

What does the assumption of difference-based coding imply for the empirical characterization of predictive coding? I postulate that difference-based coding is presupposed in predictive coding in a double sense.

First, as discussed in my first hypothesis, the prediction error itself can be considered an instance of difference-based coding. More specifically, the matching and comparison between predicted and actual input are possible only if one presupposes difference-based coding of the neural activity associated with the generation of the prediction error that is, the stimulus-induced activity.

Second, difference-based coding is not only required for the matching and comparison between predicted and actual inputs but also for the generation of both inputs by themselves. The generation of both predicted input and actual input must be based on the encoding of spatial and temporal differences, i.e., difference-based coding, rather than on the encoding of their respective discrete points in physical time and space. This is necessary since otherwise there would be no common code between both inputs any more, which would make their direct matching and comparison and consequently the prediction error itself impossible.

Taken together, I hypothesize that predictive coding presupposes difference-based coding in all its different stages in all three stages: generation of the predicted input, generation of actual input, and the constitution of the prediction error as the matching between predicted and actual inputs.

Neurometaphorical Excursion IIa: Market and Money

Let me get back to the world of metaphorical comparisons. Imagine an encounter between two merchants in a market who want to make a business deal about apples and oranges. One wants to sell apples and the other wants to sell oranges. Everything is easy as long as they determine the price of their respective goods; the money is then the common currency or code that allows them to exchange, match, and compare their respective offers.

Things become more difficult, however, once one person insists on the number of apples while the other prefers to calculate in terms of money. Then there is no common currency anymore; the absence of a common code makes direct comparison and matching of their respective offers impossible.

How does that example relate to predictive coding? The different price offers, presupposing money as common currency, from our two merchants in the market correspond to the two inputs, the predicted and actual input, which can be compared and matched with each other.

This is so because both presuppose a common currency or code, difference-based coding (as the analogue to money) that makes it possible for them to overcome the principal differences in their respective goods, apples and oranges. The different price offers for their respective goods correspond to the different degrees of spatial and temporal differences that are encoded as predicted and actual input.

Neurometaphorical Excursion IIb: Brain as Market and Code as Money

Let's return from the neuronal market of the brain to the daily market of fruits and other goods. Such a common code between predicted and actual input and thus between the two merchants' offers is absent, however, if one of them prefers to trade in terms of apples rather than money. This makes direct comparison and matching between their respective offers impossible. Correspondingly, in the absence of difference-based coding as common code, actual and predicted input could no longer be compared and matched with each other so that the subsequent generation of a prediction error becomes impossible, too.

What does this example tell us about the brain in general? The whole idea of a market as an exchange of different goods is based on a common currency. If there were no common currency, any exchange between different goods would prove rather difficult, if not impossible. In that case, only the same goods could be exchanged with each other, like apples against apples and oranges against oranges. In contrast, apples could no longer be exchanged with oranges and vice versa.

The same is true in the case of the brain. If a common code like difference-based coding were lacking and were replaced by, for example, stimulus-based coding, the possible exchanges between different stimuli as well as between brain and stimuli, as in the case of the prediction error (i.e., between predicted and actual input) would be rather limited, if not impossible. Accordingly, in the same way as the market is based on money as common currency, our brain and its neural processing of different kinds of inputs like predicted and actual input may presuppose the encoding of differences as its common "currency."

Open Questions

One question concerns the problem of whether predictive coding is not only neuronally and behaviorally relevant, as discussed here, but also phenomenally relevant; that is, for consciousness (see, e.g., Seth et al. 2011). We here excluded any reference to phenomenal states and focused only on behavioral states like sensory and motor states. Since predictive coding has been associated with more cognitive functions, it may also be considered cognitively relevant. We thus investigated here the neuro-sensory, neuro-motor, neuro-behavioral, and neuro-cognitive relevance of predictive coding. This, however, left open the neuro-phenomenal relevance of predictive coding for consciousness.

Do I consider predictive coding to be phenomenally relevant? As I understand it, predictive coding is a functional hypothesis that is also applied to the neuronal level of the brain. As such, it can well account for the individual variability of behavior and its associated contents and their underlying stimulus-induced activity. However, the kind of functional and neuronal mechanisms described by predictive coding do not imply anything about consciousness and why and how it can be associated with the behavioral and neuronal states. This means that predictive coding may be neuronally and behaviorally relevant, but not phenomenally.

Another question concerns the relationship between difference-based coding and predictive coding. I postulate that predictive coding can be regarded a subset or specific instance of difference-based coding. However, it remains unclear how exactly the encoded spatial and temporal differences can signify predictions and thus the predicted input. One would suggest that, analogous to the actual input, the predicted input may be characterized by certain spatial and temporal features and thus a particular spatiotemporal structure.

How, though, can a mere spatial and temporal difference as encoded into neural activity via difference-based coding acquire a spatiotemporal structure and thus constitute a predicted input? To answer this, we must search for the neuronal mechanisms that underlie the constitution of a spatiotemporal structure in the resting state where the predicted input is generated. And we must discover how such a spatiotemporal structure is transformed into a particular input or stimulus, the predicted input, in such way that it mirrors the spatial and temporal features of the actual input from the environment. This will be specifically targeted in Chapter 9.

We are here confronted with the problem of how the predicted input is generated. Predictive coding seems to more or less take the generation of the predictive input for granted or as given. However, the question cannot be as easily discarded.

There is no specific stimulus in the case of the predicted input. The predicted input is supposed to be generated prior to the arrival of the actual stimulus or input so that it must be traced back to the preceding resting-state activity in the brain itself. How, though, can the resting-state activity acquire the information about a stimulus that may eventually occur in the environment? One may propose that there must be some special information encoded into the resting-state activity itself that makes the generation of the predicted input possible. This will be discussed in further detail in Chapter 9.

Before focusing on the predicted input and how it is generated by itself, we first need to be clearer about the nature of the actual input. This includes the investigation of the neuronal mechanisms that allows generating the actual input. As we will see in the next chapter, the answer to that question seems to be easy but will turn out to be rather complex and difficult. The following chapter, Chapter 8, will reveal that different stimuli and complex neuronal mechanisms underlie what is described as actual input in the context of predictive coding.

Notes

1. The converse may also hold. Hence, both sensory and motor consequences of ongoing motor action are predicted in the gestalt of forward and inverse models.

CHAPTER 8
Predictive Coding and Social and Vegetative Statistics

Summary

I discussed the concept of predictive coding in Chapter 7 and exemplified it by predominantly sensorimotor functions. Now I want to give a more complex example of predictive coding with reward. "Reward" describes the assignment of value to exteroceptive stimuli in the environment. Recent imaging investigations demonstrate that value assignment does not only depend on the to-be-valued stimuli themselves but also on the stimuli occurring in the respective social context, as demonstrated in recent neuroeconomy. Since the respective social context provides further exteroceptive stimuli, one may want to speak here of extero–extero interaction. Such extero–extero interaction implies that in addition to the specific to-be-valued exteroceptive stimulus' natural statistics, its "social statistics," i.e., its relation to the accompanying exteroceptive stimuli, may also be encoded into the reward system's neural activity. The term "social statistics" describes the statistically based co-occurrence of the specific exteroceptive stimulus' with other more unspecific exteroceptive stimuli in its respective social context. In addition to the exteroceptive stimuli's social statistics, the interoceptive stimuli from the own body also impact and modulate neural activity in the reward system. This again is possible by encoding the interoceptive stimuli's statistical frequency distribution across the different discrete points in physical time and space; that is, their "vegetative statistics." One may consequently suggest that the neural activity in the reward system may be determined by three different kinds of statistics: the natural statistics of the exteroceptive stimulus to which value is assigned, the social statistics of the exteroceptive stimuli in the respective social context, and the vegetative statistics of the interoceptive stimuli from the own body. I propose that the three different statistics, social, vegetative, and natural, are matched and compared with each other; this results in what the theory of predictive coding describes as actual input (and ultimately as prediction error); that is, the neural activity change in the reward system during value assignment. Such prediction error as the matching and comparison between different stimuli and their respective statistics is possible, however, only on the basis of coding the differences between the different stimuli, that is, difference-based coding, rather than coding the stimuli themselves, that is, stimulus-based coding. Hence, the example of reward demonstrates again predictive coding to presuppose difference-based coding. Furthermore, our discussion of reward shows that the concept of the prediction error and more specifically the one of the actual input needs to be specified (and expanded) by the matching and comparison between different statistics; that is, natural, social, and vegetative.

Key Concepts and Topics Covered

Reward, predictive coding, neuroeconomics, social statistics, interoception, vegetative statistics, framing effects, prediction error

Neuroempirical Background I: Predictive Coding and Reward

So far, I have discussed predictive coding mainly in the context of sensory and motor functions.

To further illustrate the concept of predictive coding and how it relates to the one of difference-based coding, I now turn to the example of reward that will further clarify especially the generation of what is described as actual input in predictive coding.

There has been much literature on reward itself and how it is related to predictive coding (see, for instance, Schultz 2006, 2007a and b; Montague and Berns 2002; Montague et al. 2006), but it would be beyond the scope of this chapter to recount all the literature and the different accounts in full detail. The main aim here is to point out the basic principles of predictive coding in reward and how those relate to different-based coding.

Neuronal findings Ia: Prediction error and behavior during reward

Investigations in the reward system describe its neural activity and behavioral effects to be determined by the "prediction error" (Schultz 2006, 2007a and b; Montague et al. 2002, 2006). Let us start with the behavioral side of things by giving the following example.

Imagine that you are confronted with a situation where you might get some benefit or reward. If deciding, for instance, to -click the right mouse button, you expect to get a food item, like orange juice. In contrast, if you -click the left mouse button, you will get an electric shock. Due to the repetition of that pattern, you already predict that you will receive an electric shock when erring and clicking the left mouse button.

Now imagine that you click the left mouse button and get no electric shock but some orange juice; there is some error in your anticipation or prediction, resulting in a mismatch between the anticipated input and the actual input; that is, the prediction error. The prediction error describes the relationship between two different inputs, the predicted input and the actual input, whether they match, and if not how much they differ from each other.

Most important, what is crucial for determining the degree of reward you assign to the stimulus is not so much the actual input itself but rather its relationship to your prediction, the predicted input: if anticipated outcome and actual input are identical—that is, if the prediction error is zero—you will assign low or non-reward value to the actual input. If, in contrast, you anticipate an electric shock and receive orange juice instead, there is a significant positive prediction error. You will consequently assign a greater reward value to the orange juice.

Now the converse situation: you anticipate orange juice and receive an electric shock instead. There again is some prediction error though a negative one leading to the assignment of a negative value so that you will experience the electric shock as aversive and punishing. If, however, you anticipate an electric shock and also receive it, your prediction error is zero (that is, signaling no difference between anticipated and predicted inputs). Despite receiving the same physical stimulus, you may then experience the electric shock as less aversive and less punishing when compared to the case where you anticipated orange juice.

Taken together, it is the relationship between the anticipated input and the actual input that accounts for the degree of value assignment, that is, reward and punishment, rather than the actual input itself.

Neuronal findings Ib: Encoding of the prediction error into neural activity during reward

What about the neuronal mechanisms underlying reward and its assignment of value to exteroceptive stimuli? Reward value has been associated with neural activity in specific brain regions like the ventral striatum and the nucleus accumbens (VS/NACC), the ventromedial prefrontal cortex (VMPFC), and the midbrain with the ventral tegmental area (VTA) (Breiter et al. 2001; Montague and Berns 2002; Knutson et al. 2001, 2003, 2005; Montague et al. 2006; O'Doherty et al. 2004; Schultz 2006; Glimcher 2011). The very same regions have also been associated with salience (Zink et al. 2003, 2004) and product preference (Erk et al. 2002; Deppe et al. 2005; Knutson et al. 2007;

McClure et al. 2004; Paulus and Frank 2003; Menon 2011).

Moreover, the prediction error is quite well established in the neuroscientific literature on reward in both animals and humans (see Schultz 2006, 2007; Montague et al. 2002, 2006; van Duuren et al. 2008). Various studies demonstrate direct parametric dependence of the reward system's neural activity on the degree of the prediction error (see, Hampton et al. 2008; O'Doherty 2011a and b; Tricomi et al. 2010).

The larger the prediction error, the stronger the neural activity changes in these regions of the reward circuitry during either a positive or negative prediction error, that is, reward or punishment. What is encoded into the reward circuitry's neural activity is thus not so much the single stimulus by itself—the actual input—but its relationship to the anticipated or predicted input: the prediction error.

Neuronal findings Ic: Encoding of the social context into neural activity during reward

Neural activity in reward circuitry, however, is not only determined by the relationship between predicted input and actual input. In addition, the relationship of the actual input to the social context may also need to be considered. The recently emerged discipline of neuroeconomics (see, for instance, Hare et al. 2008; Rilling et al. 2004; Krueger et al. 2008; Montague 2007; Fehr and Camerer 2007; Camerer and Fehr 2007; Glimcher 2011; Rustichini 2009; Schaefer 2009; Sharp et al. 2012; Engelman and Hein 2013) presents particularly striking examples of how social inputs and thus the respective social contexts modulate neural and behavioral activity changes during reward.

Let us give a paradigmatic example of an earlier functional magnetic resonance imaging (fMRI) study. Using fMRI, Fliessbach et al. (2007) demonstrated that the activity in reward circuitry (like the ventral striatum) was highest when the person in the scanner received $30 in a gambling task and knew that another fictive player got less— $10. However, neural activity in reward circuitry decreased when the fictive player got $60, even though the person in the scanner still received the same amount as before: $30 (see Fig. 8-1).

How is this possible? One would expect the neural activity in the reward system to remain the same in both cases since the person receives the same amount of money; that is, $30. But this is not the case. Neural activity increased when the person in the scanner received a higher amount than the person outside, whereas the opposite was the case in the reverse scenario.

Hence, neural activity in reward circuitry is determined not so much by the actual stimulus itself and its specifically associated value; that is, the $30. Instead, neural activity seems to be rather determined by the relationship between the actual stimulus, the $30, and the stimuli in the respective social context, the other person receiving either $10 or $60.

Things become even more complicated when considering another example from neuroeconomics, the so-called endowment effect. The endowment effect describes the tendency to associate greater value with items that one owns when compared to those that one does not own. Knutson et al. (2008) showed that the medial prefrontal cortex exhibits greater neural activity changes during buying of a low-priced good when compared to the selling of the same good for the same price.

Since buying concerns oneself and ownership, the difference between selling and buying implies a difference in the socio-personal context concerning either oneself or the other person. The results show that the medial prefrontal cortical neural activity changes are sensitive to ownership as manifest in their difference between selling and buying as related to oneself and other persons. Interestingly, the degree of neural activity in the insula even predicted the ownership, whether the item for selling was owned by oneself or another person (Knutson et al. 2008).

Taken together, these (and other not mentioned here) results demonstrate that neural and behavioral effects of reward are very much dependent on the respective social and personal context and their respective stimuli.

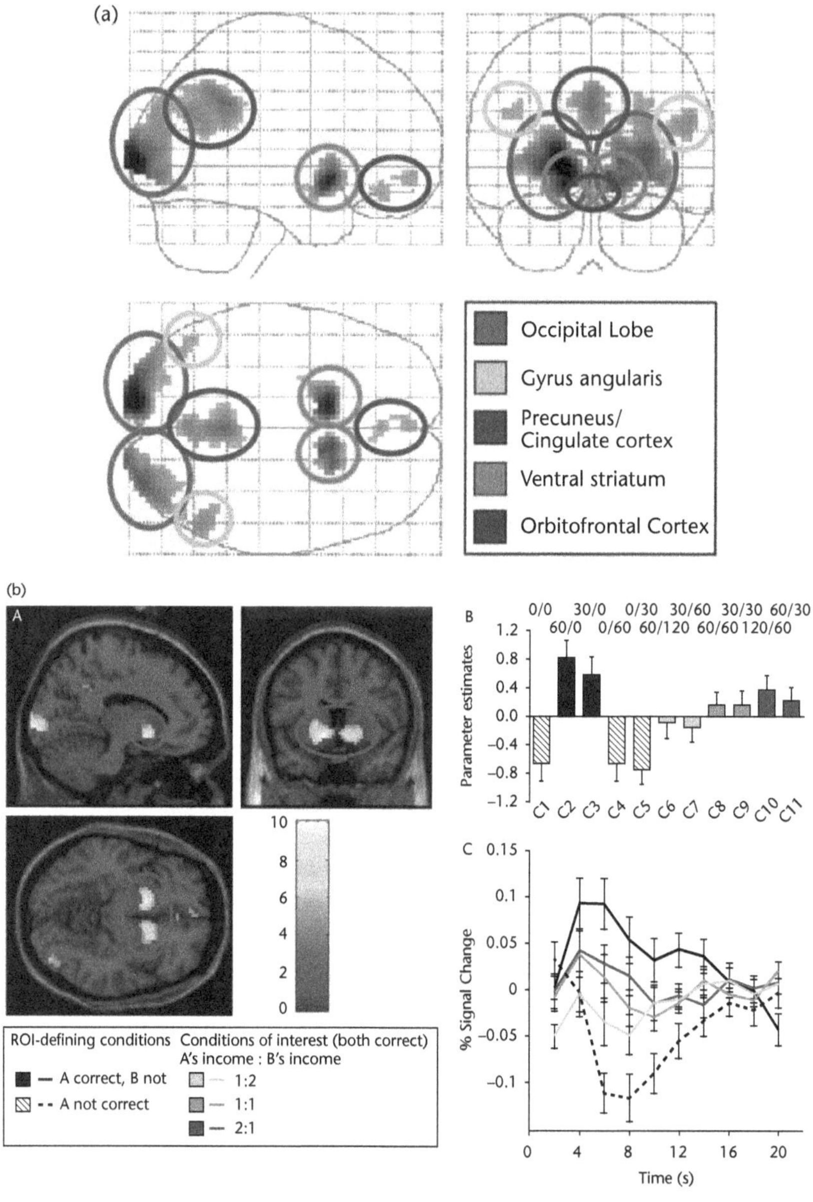

Figure 8-1a and b **Social context dependence of neural activity during reward. (*a*) Glass brain projection of brain regions showing stronger BOLD responses in conditions in which a subject received a reward while the other did not (C2 and C3), compared with conditions in which a subject did not receive a reward at all (C1, C4, and C5). (*b*) (A) T-Map projected on a single subject template for the contrast between C2, C3 > C1, C4, C5 with focus on the activation maximum in the left ventral striatum (TAL: X, –12; Y, 8; Z, 8). (B) Parameter estimates for suprathreshold voxels from this contrast show a dependency of the activation on the relative reward level. (C) Event-related signal changes after the reward feedback collapsed over trials in which a subject received a reward while the other did not (+SEM) (C2, C3), trials where a subject received no reward (C1, C4, C5, black dashed line), and different relative reward levels (1:2,; 1:1,; 2:1,). (Reprinted with permission of *Science*, from Fliessbach K, Weber B, Trautner P, Dohmen T, Sunde U, Elger CE, Falk A. Social comparison affects reward-related brain activity in the human ventral striatum. *Science*. 2007 Nov 23;318(5854):1305–8.)**

NEURONAL HYPOTHESIS IA: SOCIAL CONTEXT DEPENDENCE OF NEURAL ACTIVITY DURING REWARD

The first study demonstrated that neural activity in the reward system depended on whether the person inside the scanner receives a higher or lower amount of reward than the one outside the scanner. How is that possible? This is possible only when assuming that what is encoded into neural activity of reward is not the absolute amount of the actual stimulus itself, the $30, the person in the scanner receives by itself. Instead, the relationship or better the difference between the two stimuli, that is, the difference in the amounts of money between the two persons inside and outside the scanner, must be encoded into the reward system's neural activity.

Both stimuli, the amounts of money, are apparently compared and matched with each other, with the result of this process determining the degree of neural activity in the reward system. This means that the social relationship signified by the difference between the own and the other person's amounts of money is encoded into the neural activity change of the reward circuitry.

An analogous dependence on the respective context can be observed in the second study. Here, too, neural activity did not depend only on the stimulus itself, which was the same in both situations, that is, during buying and selling. Instead, the social and more specifically the personal context in which the person finds herself, whether she sells or buys, determines here the neural activity in, for instance, the medial prefrontal cortex and the insula.

Taken together, both examples (and many other examples from neuroeconomics) share the dependence of the behavioral and neural activities on the respective social-personal context. One may consequently speak of what I describe as "context dependence."

What do I means by the concept of context-dependence? Context dependence means that both the reward value assigned to the stimulus and the reward circuitry's neural activity do not only depend on the stimulus itself and its specific properties. Instead, both reward value and neural activity seem to depend on the stimulus' relation to other stimuli occurring at the same time in the respective social (and personal) environment, that is, another person also receiving reward or buying/selling. Since here it concerns the social environment, I speak of "social context dependence" (we will later touch upon other forms of context dependence).

NEURONAL HYPOTHESIS IB: DIFFERENCE-BASED CODING ACCOUNTS FOR THE SOCIAL CONTEXT DEPENDENCE OF NEURAL ACTIVITY DURING REWARD

How is it possible for such social context dependence to determine both behavioral and neural effects of reward? Let's discuss the exact underlying processes.

The exteroceptive stimulus that signifies the reward the person receives in the scanner must interact with the exteroceptive stimulus about the other person's reward. One may consequently postulate interaction between both exteroceptive stimuli in the brain of the person in the scanner, thus implying what I describe as extero–extero interaction in the following. This extero–extero interaction seems to determine both the reward value and the reward circuitry's neural activity the person in the scanner shows.

While extero–extero interaction may well allow for the alleged social context dependence, its exact neuronal mechanisms remain unclear. For extero–extero interaction to determine behavioral and neuronal activity, both exteroceptive stimuli must directly interact and be integrated with each other. This presupposes interactive-integrative coding rather than parallel-segregated coding (see Chapters 5 and 6 for details) of the two (or more) exteroceptive stimuli.

As detailed in Chapters 5 and 6, such interactive-integrated coding is possible, however, only if one presupposes difference-based coding rather than stimulus-based coding. This means that what is encoded into both neural and behavioral activity is the difference and thus the relationship between the two (or more) exteroceptive stimuli rather than the stimuli themselves, independent of each other.

How does that apply to our study with persons inside and outside the scanner receiving different amounts of money? This difference in the amount of money the two persons receive is different in the two situations:. the difference between $30 and $10 is different from the one between $30 and $60. I consequently postulate that the encoding of stimuli in terms of difference-based coding (rather than stimulus-based coding) accounts for the social context dependence of reward.

Neuronal hypothesis Ic: Encoding of the stimuli "natural statistics" into neural activity during reward

How it is possible for the reward system to encode the difference between different exteroceptive stimuli rather than coding the exteroceptive stimuli by themselves? This is the point where we can learn from sparse coding.

As discussed in part I, sparse coding claims that what is encoded into neural activity of the sensory cortex does not correspond to the stimulus' physical feature themselves at one particular discrete point in physical time and space. Instead, the occurrence of the stimuli and its physical features across different discrete points in physical time and space (within a certain temporal and spatial span) is encoded into the sensory cortex's neural activity.

This means that the statistical frequency distribution of the stimuli's physical features and thus what is called the stimuli's natural statistics is encoded into neural activity. What is meant by the concept of "natural statistics"?

The concept of natural statistics describes the statistical differences in the occurrence of the stimuli and their physical features across different discrete points in physical time and space (see Chapter 1 for details). The encoding of the stimuli's natural statistics into neural activity is consequently possible only when encoding their spatial and temporal differences, that is, the ones between their discrete points in physical time and space at which the stimuli occur. Since it is based on the coding of spatial and temporal difference, the encoding of the stimuli's natural statistics presupposes difference-based coding (see Chapters 1 and 2 for details). How now does the concept of natural statistics apply to the current context of reward? The behavioral and neural activity may depend on the encoding of the natural statistics of the to-be-valued exteroceptive stimulus, that is, the amount of money the person in the scanner receives. This, however, is not the case since then neural and behavioral effects should remain independent of the amount of money the person outside the scanner receives.

Instead, it is the difference between both exteroceptive stimuli that is encoded into both behavioral and neural activity. This means that, in addition to the natural statistics of the exteroceptive stimulus received by the person inside the scanner, the natural statistics of the one received by the person outside the scanner must also be encoded. One may consequently hypothesize that the natural statistics of the exteroceptive stimuli from both persons inside and outside the scanner may be encoded into neural activity.

This, however, is not fully correct either. Such encoding of the two exteroceptive stimuli's natural statistics would amount to parallel-segregated coding. In that case, one would propose that the person in the scanner encodes the absolute sum of both amounts separately, that is, the one it receives by itself and the one the person outside the scanner receives. This, however, is not in full accordance with the data that do not suggest the encoding of the absolute amount of money by itself. Instead, the data suggest, as discussed earlier, that it is the relation, that is, the difference, between the two exteroceptive stimuli, that is encoded.

More specifically, the person in the scanner encodes its exteroceptive stimulus, that is, its amount of money, in relation or difference to the sum the person outside the scanner receives. This means that the absolute sum the person outside the scanner receives is not so relevant for the encoding of the neural and behavioral activity by the person inside the scanner. Accordingly, it is not so much the natural statistics of the exteroceptive stimulus from the person outside the scanner that is encoded by the person inside the scanner. Instead, the relative difference and thus the relation to its own sum, that is, its own exteroceptive stimulus, may be encoded by the person inside the scanner. Such encoding of the relationship between two (or more) different exteroceptive stimuli that is, target and contextual stimuli may be described by the concept of "social statistics."

Neuronal hypothesis Id: Encoding of the stimuli "social statistics" into neural activity during reward

What exactly do I mean by the concept of "social statistics"? The concept of social statistics describes the co-occurrence of other exteroceptive stimuli in addition to the target exteroceptive stimulus. More specifically, it describes the statistical relationship between the target stimulus and the other stimuli, with the latter occurring in the social context of the former.

This means that the concept of social statistics describes the statistical frequency distribution in the co-occurrence between target and contextual stimuli. As such, the social statistics concerns explicitly the encoding of the social context of the target stimulus rather than the encoding of the target stimulus itself (and/or of the co-occurring stimulus as second target stimulus).

How does the concept of social statistics stand in relation to the concept of natural statistics? In the case of the natural statistics, the target stimulus' statistical frequency distribution across different discrete points in physical time and space is encoded. In social statistics, in contrast, it is not so much the co-occurring stimulus itself whose statistical frequency distribution is encoded; instead, it is only the statistical frequency distribution of its co-occurrence with the target stimulus that is supposed to be encoded.

In sum, I postulate that the concepts of "social and natural statistics" can be distinguished by distinct stimuli—that is, target and contextual stimuli—as well as by the different basis of their respective statistical frequency distributions; that is, based on either the stimuli themselves or on the co-occurrence between different stimuli.

Neuronal hypothesis Ie: The prediction error is determined by the relationship between natural and social statistics

One may now want to ask how the concept of social statistics stands in relation to the concept of the prediction error in both empirical and conceptual regard. Let us start with the empirical implications and develop some more specific experimentally amenable hypotheses. I would hypothesize that the degree of spatial and temporal differences between natural and social statistics predicts the degree of difference encoded into reward system's neural activity via difference-based coding: the larger the spatiotemporal differences between natural and social statistics, the larger the encoded differences and the higher the changes in subsequent neural activity. Conversely, lower spatiotemporal differences between both statistics may lead not only to lower differences but also to lower or even absent changes in subsequent neural activity.

This hypothesis could be well tested by operationalizing the statistical frequency distribution of both target and occurring stimuli, including the development of measures for the spatial and temporal differences in their co-occurrence. I hypothesize that these measures predict the neural effects of reward in a social context.

This implies that the behavioral effects and thus the degree of reward value assigned to the stimulus in question is directly dependent upon the degree of difference-based coding and the correspondence between social and neuronal statistics: the higher the degree of difference-based coding, the larger (that is, positive or negative) the degrees of reward value that can possibly be assigned to the stimulus. This entails that the degree of value also depends on the correspondence between social and neuronal statistics: the less both social and natural statistics match, the more positive or negative the value that can possibly be assigned to the target stimulus.

What does our assumption imply for the concept of the prediction error? By assuming the matching and comparison between natural and social statistics, I presuppose a more specific and complex picture of the prediction error and more specifically the actual input as one ingredient (besides the predicted input) entering the prediction error. This shall be briefly summarized in the following discussion.

First, I propose the prediction error to presuppose difference-based coding as already discussed in Chapter 7 and further supported in the present context of reward. Second, I postulate that the to-be-valued actual input is not encoded by itself at its discrete point in physical time and space, but rather in terms of its statistical frequency distribution across different discrete points in physical time and space; that is, its natural statistics. This needs to be demonstrated and supported in future studies on reward.

Third, and most important, I suggest that what is called "actual input" in the context of the prediction error needs to be specified. I here distinguished between target and contextual stimuli and their respective statistics; that is, natural and social statistics. What is described as actual input in the prediction error may then result already by itself from a prior matching and comparison process, the one between natural and social statistics.

Neuronal hypothesis IF: from "social statistics" to "socio-cultural statistics"

Our investigation of reward revealed that the actual input by itself, its behavioral and neural effects, is more complex than the simple processing of an isolated exteroceptive stimulus. The actual input itself can already be considered a complex amalgam of different exteroceptive stimuli like target and contextual stimuli whose relationship and more specifically co-occurrence are encoded in terms of their difference in a statistically based way that is, "social statistics."

Future investigation may want to broaden the concept of "social statistics" from the context of reward as sketched here to the brain in general and its various functions like perception, attention, and so on. This is currently being investigated in the fields of social and cultural neuroscience.

"Cultural neuroscience" focuses on the impact of culture and cultural differences on the brain and its neuronal activity (see, e.g., Han and Northoff 2008; Han, Northoff et al. 2013). One may suggest that cultural differences can ultimately be traced to differences in statistical frequency distributions of the same stimuli including both their natural and social statistics.

For instance, even if the target stimulus is the same in different cultures, their contextual stimuli may nevertheless differ from each, which then will also be encoded into neural activity. One may then be inclined to speak of "socio-cultural statistics" rather than mere "social statistics."

Neuronal findings IIA: interoceptive stimuli from the body impact reward

So far, I have considered the social context and how different exteroceptive stimuli are encoded into neural activity during reward via difference-based coding. However, there may be more to reward than only exteroceptive stimuli from the social context. The exteroceptive target stimuli are confronted in the brain not only with other exteroceptive stimuli from the respective social context but also with the stimuli that originate from the own body, the interoceptive stimuli. There may thus be not only extero–extero interaction but also what I describe as intero–extero interaction taking place in reward.

There are many studies on reward and interoception, especially in the context of food, taste, hunger, appetite, and obesity (see, for instance, Rolls 2011 for an excellent review). Hunger and appetite obviously presuppose the involvement of the own body state and thus of interoceptive stimuli. I do not go into detail, however, about this literature, which would be beyond the scope of this chapter. Instead, I only give a brief and abbreviated account of the main anatomical pathways of the intero–exteroceptive interaction during reward.

Montague argues in a series of papers that the temporal difference prediction error (TD-PD, which describes the difference between the predicted and actually occurring stimulus value; see Fiorillo et al., 2008 and Schultz 2007a and b) model of reward neglects the input from the organism itself (i.e., its internal stimuli as manifest in interoceptive stimuli; Montague, 2007a and b; Montague and King-Casas, 2007; Rangel,

2008). This is even more relevant when considering the fact that the value assigned to the external stimulus may very much depend on the organism's internal state and thus on its interoceptive stimuli (Krebs et al., 1978).

How can we further illustrate such dependence of reward on the interoceptive state of the body? For instance, a particular exteroceptive stimuli associated with cold water may be rewarding only if it is extremely hot and the organism itself is very hot, showing high temperature (see Fig. 8-2a). If, in contrast, the organism is rather cold, showing low temperature, cold water may not be regarded as a rewarding stimulus and thus be assigned a rather low value (see Montague and King-Casas, 2007 for this example).

This means that the same exteroceptive stimulus, the cold water, may be assigned a different value in the context of different bodily states and consequently different interoceptive stimuli. Hence, there must be some kind of intero–extero interaction during the assignment of value and thus reward. This is indeed empirically supported by studies showing differences of reward in the presence of different electrolyte concentration or delivery of food (see for instance Kirk et al. 2011; Northoff and Hayes 2011).

Neuronal findings IIb: Subcortical regions mediate the impact of interoceptive stimuli on reward

How is such interaction between intero- and exteroceptive stimuli mediated neuronally? Intero–extero interaction may be mediated specifically by subcortical regions. These subcortical regions include the PAG, the tectum, the colliculi, the hypothalamus, and the VTA that all show extensive convergence between intero- and exteroceptive afferences (see Part VIII in Volume II for a more detailed description of subcortical regions).

In addition to the subcortical regions, cortical regions like the insula are also central. The insula has been implicated in the processing of interoceptive stimuli from one's body and subsequent bodily awareness (see Craig 2003, 2004, 2009a and b; Wiebking et al. 2010). This goes well with the insula's connectivity pattern that is characterized by afferents from both intero- and exteroceptive sensory modalities (Augustine 1996). Interestingly, the insula has also been shown to be recruited during especially social reward tasks (see Montague 2007; Krueger et al. 2008 Kirk et al. 2011; Naqvi et al. 2007, Naqvi and Bechara 2009, 2010).

The subcortical regions and the insula, including the latter's close connection to the supragenual anterior cingulate cortex (SACC; see also Craig 2009a and b, 2010), are considered core regions of what is described as the "salience system" (see Menon 2011 for a recent summary). The salience system is supposed to be central in registering the need of the organism to dedicate and reallocate resources on the basis of its own states and the relevance, that is, salience, of the stimuli for itself given its own present bodily state (see Fig. 8-2b).

The salience system is distinguished from the default-mode network (that includes midline regions), and the central executive network and its predominantly lateral cortical regions (see Chapter 4 for details, as well as Menon 2011). Interestingly, many of the regions included in the salience system, especially insula, amygdala, SACC, and VTA, are also recruited during reward, thus suggesting strong overlap (some authors also propose identity between both) between reward and salience.

Taken together, the findings suggest involvement of interoceptive stimuli in reward. This is evidenced by the well established dependence of reward value on the body's interoceptive, that is, vegetative functions. Such assumption is further supported by the involvement of the regions of the salience system that mediates interoceptive and thus vegetative functions.

Neuronal findings IIc: "Vegetative context-dependence" and the "framing effect"

The findings described here underline the relevance of the body for reward. The body and its interoceptive stimuli may thus be regarded as yet another context that needs to be considered. More specifically, it is the vegetative state of the

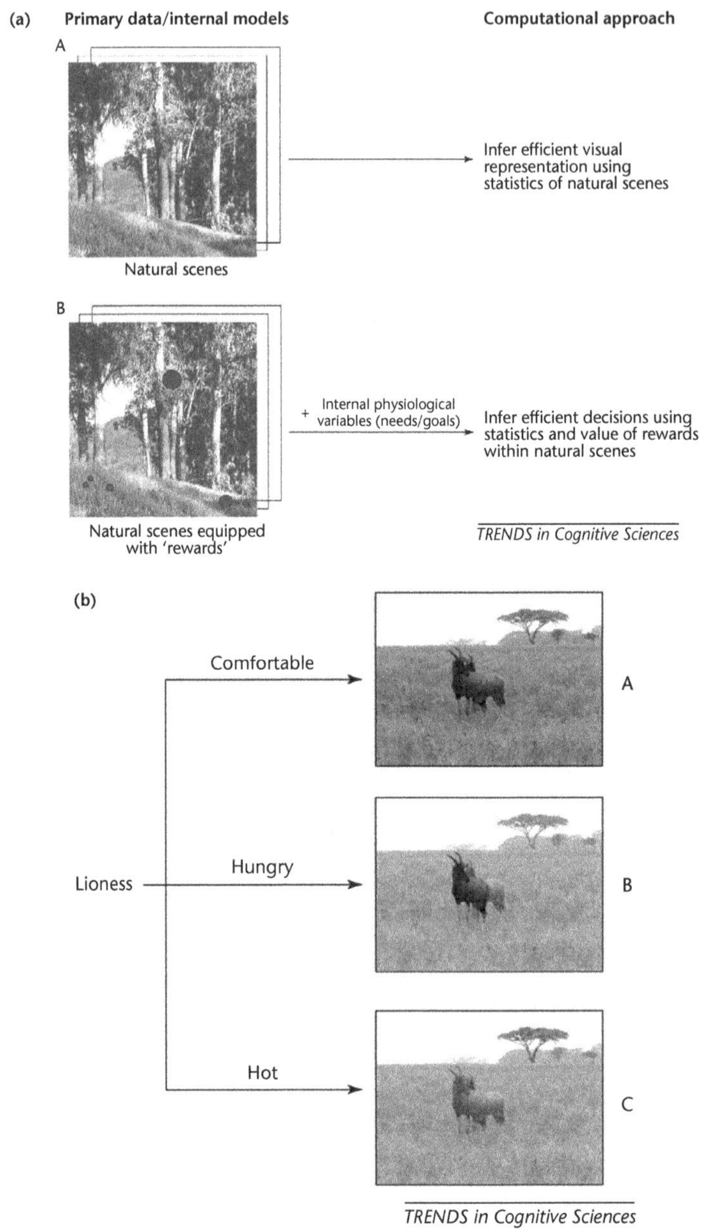

Figure 8-2a–c **Vegetative context dependence of reward. (*a*) Defining the "natural reward-harvesting statistics" problem. (A) The work of Horace Barlow crystallized an approach to vision by asking for the kinds of responses one should expect from visually sensitive neurons if they were efficient representations of "natural visual statistics." The natural visual statistics approach has expanded greatly in recent years to show that many aspects of the visual world are "matched" in an efficient way by visual neural responses. Two features are particularly pertinent: first, local spatiotemporal correlations abound—the visual statistics from one point in visual space are highly correlated with neighboring points; second, scale invariances also abound in natural visual statistics. (B) The reward-harvesting problem must have its own "natural reward-harvesting statistics." This kind of description of the reward acquisition problem would need to include at least two novel elements not naturally present in the visual problem and not usually included in optimal-foraging theory. The first is the need to consider the differential costs of exploring an environment to obtain the (possible) rewards present there. The second is the need to take account of the agent's state-of-motivation for the reward in question. Since rewards can be abstractly defined, it is now particularly important to generate good models of motivation.**

(c)

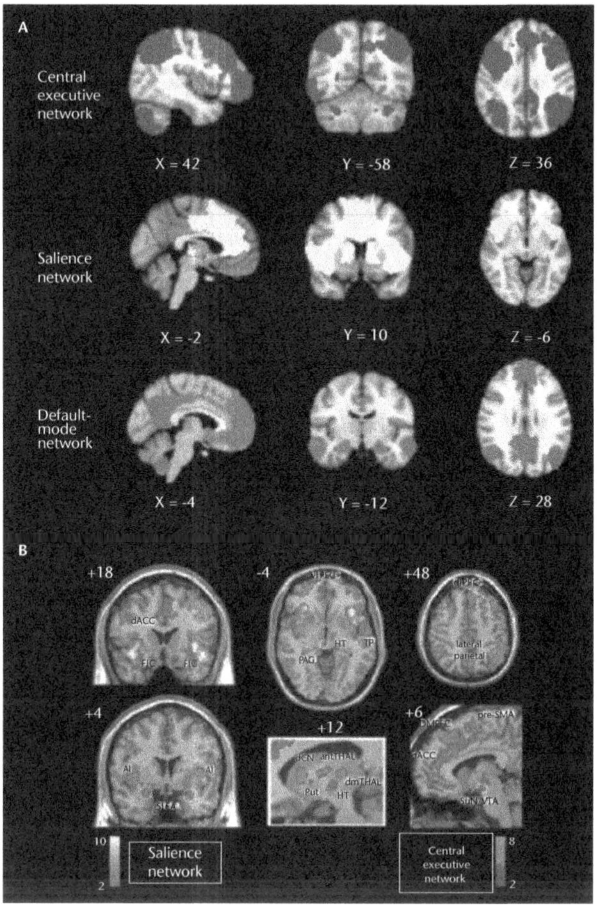

TRENDS in Cognitive Sciences

(*b*) Matching interoceptive and perceptual representations. The internal states of an animal dramatically change the value of objects in its world. A hypothetical "lioness" views a visual scene in three different states: (A) sated and comfortable; (B) hungry; and (C) sated but hot. These are not literal examples of how interoceptive states couple to visual perceptual representations, but they highlight the fact that there must be natural interoceptive statistics that have yet to be quantified, and the resulting representations should have an intimate connection to perceptual processing in the service of decision-making. Neuroeconomics, to be complete, must take on all these levels. (*c*) Three core neurocognitive networks. (A) The CEN, SN, and DMN. The frontoparietal CEN (shown in black), anchored in the dlPFC and the PPC, plays an important role in working memory and attention. The SN, shown in white, is important for detection and mapping of salient external inputs and internal brain events. The SN is anchored in the FIC and dorsal dACC and features extensive connectivity with subcortical and limbic structures involved in reward and motivation. The DMN (shown in grey), anchored in the PCC and medial PFC, is important for self-referential mental activity. (B) The CEN and SN are both coactivated during a wide range of cognitive tasks but have distinct patterns of intrinsic cortical connectivity in the dorsomedial prefrontal cortex (DMPFC) dACC, dlPFC, vlPFC and lateral parietal cortex and subcortical connectivity in the anterior thalamus (antTHAL), dorsal caudate nucleus (dCN), dorsomedial thalamus (dmTHAL), hypothalamus (HT), periaqueductal gray (PAG), putamen (Put), sublenticular extended amygdala (SLEA), SuN/VTA and the temporal pole (TP).Figures 8-2a and b: Reprinted with permission of *Trends in Cognitive Sciences,* from Montague PR, King-Casas B. Efficient statistics, common currencies and the problem of reward-harvesting. *Trends Cogn Sci.* 2007. Dec;11(12):514–519. (Reprinted with permission from Menon V. Large-scale brain networks and psychopathology: a unifying triple network model. *Trends Cogn Sci.* 2011 Oct;15(10):483–506.)

body as signified by its interoceptive stimuli that strongly impacts reward. One may consequently want to speak of a bodily or "vegetative context dependence" as distinguished from the "social context dependence" described earlier.

The concept of vegetative context dependence comes close to what Martin Paulus (2007) calls "framing effects." Martin Paulus is a German born psychiatrist who moved from the often rainy Germany to the rather sunny California in San Diego. His research focuses on the neuronal mechanisms of the body and how its healthy and abnormal states impact our decision making and reward systems. Paulus (2007) proposes that the body's interoceptive stimuli and thus its homeostasis are central in reward and decision making. The value to the stimulus is not only assigned on a purely rational, for example, cognitive, basis but also by considering its value for the interoceptive, that is, homeostatic state of the body and the organism in general.

Paulus speaks of an "interoceptive valuation" that describes the following: by providing interoceptive input to regions implicated in reward and decision making, the body and its actual vegetative state have a strong say in valuing the different options and thus to determine the degree of reward value that is assigned to the exteroceptive target stimulus.

The value of the different options depends then not only on the predictability or probability and the reward magnitude of the exteroceptive stimulus but also on the actual interoceptive state of the body. This means that the interoceptive state and thus the bodily state can impact the degree of reward value and the consecutive set of preferences in subsequent decision making.

By providing different interoceptive inputs, changes in bodily state can shift the valuing of the different options and hence set the preferences. These may, for instance, be abnormal, as Paulus (2007) argues, in addiction where the abnormal bodily vegetative state may lead subjects to assignment of abnormal reward values and ultimately to abnormal decision making.

Paulus uses the concept of "framing effects" to describe the impact of the bodily vegetative state on reward and value assignment (and subsequent decision making). This is more or less identical to what I mean by "context dependence" and more specifically "vegetative context dependence." The question, however, is what kind of neuronal mechanisms make possible such vegetative context dependence of reward and decision making; this shall be the focus in the next section.

NEURONAL HYPOTHESIS IIA: DIFFERENCE-BASED CODING AS "COMMON CURRENCY" BETWEEN INTERO- AND EXTEROCEPTIVE STIMULI

How can we further specify the dependence of reward and decision making on the interoceptive stimuli of the body and thus what Paulus describes as a "framing effect"; that is, vegetative context-dependence? Let us recapitulate briefly the earlier sections in this chapter.

I suggested that the exteroceptive stimuli's natural and social statistics are encoded into neural activity. Thereby, the encoding of their statistical frequency distribution, the natural and social statistics, provided the common currency for the two different exteroceptive stimuli, that is, target and contextual stimuli, to be directly matched and compared with each other. This, in turn, is possible only when presupposing difference-based coding (rather than stimulus-based coding) of the different stimuli's different spatial and temporal distributions.

What does this imply for intero–extero interaction? As in the case of extero–extero interaction, we are confronted with two different stimuli, interoceptive and exteroceptive stimuli. However, unlike in extero–extero interaction, the stimuli in intero–extero interaction have different origins. While in extero–extero interaction they both originate in the environment, they show different origins in inter–extero interaction; namely, body and environment. This raises the question of how stimuli from such different origins, body and environment, can directly interact with each other. For direct interaction to be possible, intero- and exteroceptive stimuli must share a common currency according to which both are processed. In short, they need to be processed in a common code as their common or shared currency (see also Chapter 7 for the question of a common code). If now extero- and interoceptive stimuli are encoded into neural activity by themselves at their different discrete positions in physical time and space, they will not share a common currency. Such stimulus-based coding would only allow for parallel-segregated coding of intero- and exteroceptive stimuli, which makes their direct interaction impossible.

In contrast, we may rather presuppose difference-based coding as encoding strategy for both intero- and exteroceptive stimuli. In this case the common currency, or better, the shared or common code, consists of differences that reflect the respective stimuli's statistical frequency distributions across their different discrete points in physical time and space. The statistical frequency distributions of both intero- and exteroceptive stimuli must consequently be encoded into neural activity.

Neuronal hypothesis IIb: Encoding of "vegetative statistics" into neural activity and its interaction with "natural and social statistics"

Analogous to the exteroceptive stimuli's natural and social statistics, one may therefore want to speak of what I describe as "vegetative statistics". The concept of "vegetative statistics" describes the statistically based occurrence of the interoceptive stimuli from their body across the different discrete points in physical time and space.

Based on these considerations I postulate that, despite their different origins in body and environment, intero- and exteroceptive stimuli nevertheless share the same code. Such common currency or code consists of the encoding of spatial and temporal differences that reflects the statistical frequency distributions of the different stimuli; i.e., natural, social, and vegetative statistics.

Such statistically based encoding makes it possible for the interoceptive stimuli from the body and their vegetative statistics to directly interact with the natural and social statistics of the exteroceptive stimuli from the environment. Hence, the suggested "framing effects," or social context dependence, of reward and decision making may be based on difference-based coding of intero- and exteroceptive stimuli in terms of their statistically based spatial and temporal differences.

Neuronal hypothesis IIc: "Actual input" as "complex amalgam" of different stimuli and their respective statistics

How does the assumption of the interoceptive stimuli's vegetative statistics and its matching and comparison with the natural and social statistics of the exteroceptive stimuli stand in relation to the concept of predictive coding and more specifically the prediction error? We remember from Chapter 4 (and see especially Chapter 32 in Volume II) that the insula is one of the key regions in mediating interoceptive stimuli.

Bossaerts (2010) proposes that the insula (see also Chapter 32 in Volume II for more details), based on its massive interoceptive input, generates predictions about the interoceptive state of the body. There may thus be "interoceptive prediction error" so that the involvement of the insula in interoceptive processing may be well compatible with the concept of predictive coding.

The assumption of a specifically "interoceptive prediction error," however, neglects that the insula not only processes interoceptive stimuli—in addition to the interoceptive input, it also receives major exteroceptive input from basically all five sensory modalities (see Craig 2002, 2003, 2009a and b; Northoff 2008). Furthermore, exteroceptive stimuli also induce major signal changes in the insula, such as, for instance, during the awareness of tones, that is, exteroceptive awareness (see Farb et al. 2012; Wiebking et al. 2010, 2011; as well as Chapter 32 for more details on the insula). Hence, we may need to consider both intero- and exteroceptive inputs in the insula with their difference determining subsequent neural and behavioral activity (see Chapter 32 for details as well as Wiebking et al. (2011) for support in this direction).

What does this imply for the alleged "interoceptive prediction error" of the insula? It means that the "interoceptive prediction error" may not be as purely interoceptive as suggested. Instead, the actual input fed into the "interoceptive prediction error" may include both intero- and exteroceptive stimuli and thus the intero-extero difference rather than the interoceptive input alone. This implies that the concept of the actual input cannot be limited exclusively to interoceptive stimuli alone but must include exteroceptive stimuli too.

One may therefore hypothesize that the actual input results from the matching and comparison between intero- and exteroceptive stimuli and their respective statistics, that is, vegetative and natural statistics. The concept of the "interoceptive prediction error" may thus need to be reformulated as "interoceptive (intero-extero) prediction error."

How can we now make more concrete empirical assumptions? One may hypothesize that the degree of value assigned to the exteroceptive stimulus may depend on its degree of statistically based matching with the interoceptive stimuli: the more intero- and exteroceptive stimuli overlap in their respective spatiotemporal statistical frequency distributions, that is, their natural and vegetative statistics, the lower the degree of value (positive or negative) that can possibly be assigned to the exteroceptive stimulus in question. Conversely, the larger the discrepancies between natural and vegetative statistics, the higher the degree of value that can possibly be assigned to the exteroceptive stimulus in question.

This means that the actual input itself is more complex and elaborated than it is often (tacitly) presupposed in predictive coding where it is considered (more or less) as given and simple. I here supposed that the actual input results from a complex process, the statistically based matching between different statistics; that is, vegetative, natural, and social statistics.

This makes it clear that the actual input itself already represents a complex amalgam of different stimuli and their respective statistics. That, however, is a tentative hypothesis at this point, which warrants more detailed empirical and conceptual characterization in the future (see Fig. 8-3).

Neurometaphorical excursion: How Godiva truffles can surprise you in the desert and in Brussels?

Let me illustrate the central relevance of the actual input by the following example. Imagine that you are extremely hungry and crave a chocolate, which reflects the vegetative statistics of your body's interoceptive stimuli. You are, however, in the middle of a desert; thus, you consequently do not expect your craving for a chocolate to be fulfilled because of the social context, that is, the desert, you are in.

Hence, if you do not get any chocolate while being in the desert, you are not really disappointed because you did not expect it anyway. This is so because social and natural statistics match well, which in turn may also affect (and hopefully down-modulate) your craving for chocolate and thus your interoceptive stimuli's vegetative statistics.

However, even the desert may not be without surprises. Suddenly, you see a person coming along who offers you your favorite chocolate, Godiva truffles, for free. This is a positive surprise since you did not expect or anticipate such a treat after having been in the desert for the last 3 weeks and having not encountered anyone. There is thus a major discrepancy between the exteroceptive target stimulus and its natural statistics, the co-occurring stimulus' social statistics, and your body's interoceptive stimuli's vegetative statistics.

This discrepancy between the three different statistics will transform into the assignment of a high value to the exteroceptive target stimulus, the Godiva chocolate, as made possible by high degrees of neural activity changes in your reward system. Hence, even though the desert is usually devoid of rewards like chocolate, this can nevertheless tell us a lot about the brain's underlying neuronal mechanisms.

Now imagine the same scenario to take place not in the desert but in the chocolate shop in Brussels, Belgium, the home of Godiva truffles. After your five-week adventure tour in the desert (without any truffle surprises), you travel to Brussels to get your beloved your beloved Godiva truffles. You expect the chocolate shop to have them.

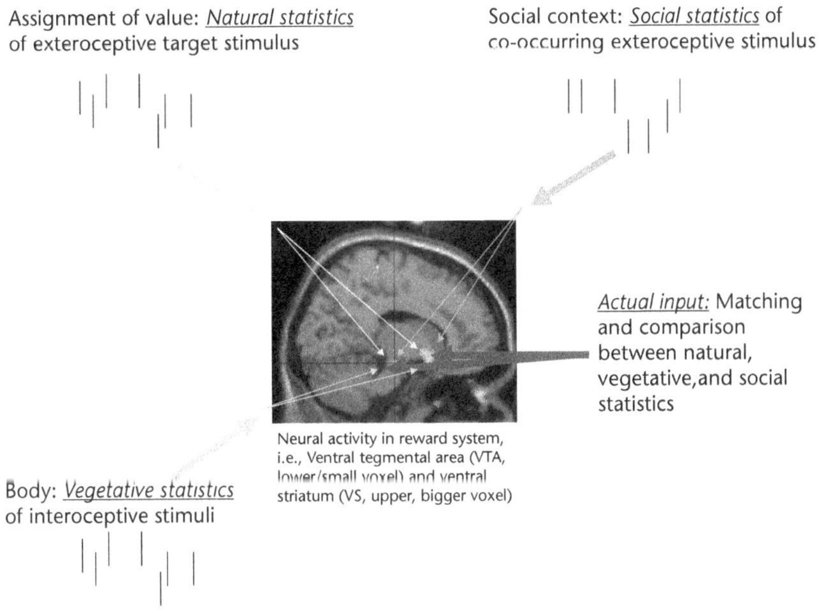

Figure 8-3 Constitution of the actual input on the basis of different stimuli. The figure demonstrates the generation of the actual input on the basis of different stimuli entering neural processing in the reward system; the latter's core regions, that is, ventral striatum (VS) and ventral tegmental area (VTA), are indicated by the brain in the middle. (*Upper left*) There is the exteroceptive stimulus, the target stimulus, to which value and thus reward shall be assigned. The exteroceptive target stimulus is encoded in the neural (and behavioral) activity on the basis of its statistical frequency distribution, its natural statistics. This is indicated by the different vertical bars at different discrete positions in physical time and space. (*Lower left*) This is complemented by the encoding of the statistical frequency distribution of the body's interoceptive stimuli and thus its vegetative statistics. (*Upper right*) In addition to the exteroceptive target stimulus, one may also need to consider the social context and thus its co-occurring exteroceptive stimuli. They are also encoded according to the statistical frequency distribution of their co-occurrence with the exteroceptive target stimulus as described by the concept of social statistics. (*Lower right*) The actual input into the reward system, as presupposed in predictive coding, is supposed to result from the interaction and thus the matching and comparison between the three statistics, natural, social, and vegetative. One may thus speak of "natural-socio-vegetative statistics" to characterize the actual input that therefore needs to be considered as complex amalgam of different stimuli and their respective statistics.

Now another surprise, yet a negative one: the chocolate shop has every kind of chocolate but Godiva truffles. You are seriously disappointed. Your body and its interoceptive stimuli were craving and thus predicting Godiva truffles. Instead, all your body gets is a high prediction error with high activity changes in the interoceptive-related brain regions.

This makes it clear that all three stimuli, exteroceptive, social, and interoceptive, and their respective statistics, natural, social, and vegetative, closely interact. And it this interaction which determines the actual input as one central ingredient of the prediction error.

Neuroconceptual Remark IA: Valuation as "Common Currency" of Behavior and Neuronal Activity

I demonstrated that exteroceptive target stimuli, exteroceptive stimuli from the social context, and interoceptive stimuli from the own body, are involved in constituting the actual input; while, as will become clear in the next chapter, neuronal stimuli and their respective neuronal statistics are implicated in generating the predicted input. Most important, all these stimuli can by themselves be assigned value and thus be experienced as rewarding by the respective subject. In other terms, extero- and interoceptive as well as neuronal stimuli can be rewarding, as it will be explicated in further detail later.

How is it possible that different stimuli of different origins can all be assigned value and thus be rewarding? Some authors associate neural activity in the NACC, the VMPFC, and the VTA with a so-called valuation system (Montague et al. 2002, 2006). Such "valuation system" does not only code the stimuli's immediate relevance, the reward value, but also their long-term value for the organism, their importance and relevance for the organism itself.

What exactly does the proclaimed "valuation system" do? Value or salience provides a common format or "common currency" for the different exteroceptive stimuli that allows them to be "converted to a common valuation scale," mirroring thereby their importance or relevance for the organism. Montague and Berns (2002, 280) suggest that value as the "common currency" is mediated by the valuation system and thus the orbitofrontal-striatal circuit:

> We strongly suspect the existence of a more generalized valuation system. We propose that the OFS circuit (i.e., orbitofrontal-striatal) computes an ongoing valuation of potential payoffs (including rewards), lo[s]ses, and their proxies (predictors) across a broad domain of stimuli. This is a different proposal from the prediction-error signal discussed above for midbrain dopamine neurons (...) and proposed for many other brain regions (...). The prediction error signal guides the system to learn the time and amount of future rewards, and may, as reviewed above, direct some forms of simple decision-making. Our specific proposal for one function of the OFS is that it computes a valuation of rewards, punishments, and their predictors. By providing a common valuation scale for diverse stimuli, this system emits a signal useful for comparing and contrasting the value of future events that have not yet happened—a signal required for decision-making algorithms that assign attention, plan actions, and compare disparate stimuli. (Montague and Berns 2002, 275–276)

Neuroconceptual remark Ib: Value-driven behavior and difference-based coding

How does such determination of value as "common currency" stand in relation to my account? The concept of value in Montague and Barns is restricted to exteroceptive stimuli. I demonstrated that other stimuli are implicated, too, social, neuronal, and interoceptive. Are they valued, too? Do interoceptive stimuli have a specific value for us? This is suggested by Paulus, who speaks of interoceptive valuation (see earlier). And even the brain's intrinsic activity and thus its neuronal stimuli may generate value, that is, neuronal value, as we will see in the next chapter; this is, for instance, well apparent in dreams and the reward value of their various contents (see Chapter 26 in Volume II for details).

If interoceptive, social, and neuronal stimuli are assigned value, for example, relevance and importance for the organism, they may undergo the same processes that take place in the value assignment of exteroceptive stimuli. And they may then be processed in the very same system, the valuation system, as Montague and Barns suggest it for the different exteroceptive stimuli. Behaviorally, this entails that not only exteroceptive stimuli may be rewarding for us but also interoceptive stimuli from the body and even neuronal stimuli from the brain itself (reflecting its intrinsic or resting-state activity).

Is there any phenomenological and behavioral evidence for that? Yes, there is. Interoceptive stimuli from the body can also be assigned a specific reward value as well, as visible in athletes or in patients with hypochondria who have an increased focus on their own bodies. Based on these observations, one would postulate that interoceptive stimuli may also be assigned value and thus undergo reward processing in the very same way, for example, in the same regions (the valuation system) and with the same processes (the interaction with the respective other stimuli) as the exteroceptive stimuli do.

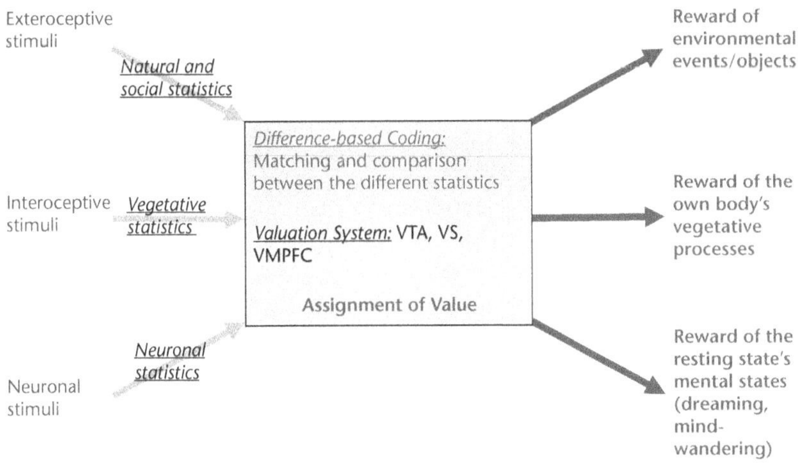

Figure 8-4 Valuation system and difference-based coding. The figure demonstrates the input (*left*) and output (*right*) of the proposed valuation system (*middle*) as mediated by regions like the ventral striatum (VS), the ventromedial prefrontal cortex (VMPFC), and the ventral tegmental area (VTA). The input into the valuation system consists of the brain's neuronal stimuli, the body's interoceptive stimuli, and the environment's exteroceptive stimuli (*left*). These, more precisely their respective natural, social, vegetative, and neuronal statistics, are processed in the valuation system. Here all the different statistics are matched and compared with each other, resulting in changes in the neural activity of the valuation system. This, in turn, leads to the assignment of value to the stimuli (*middle*). Such value assignment is then manifest (*right*) in the reward of the environment's objects/events, the reward of the own body's vegetative processes, and the reward of the mental in the resting state as, for instance, during dreaming and mind-wandering.

This is also the case with the brain's neuronal stimuli, which may also be assigned a certain value and thus reward (see Fig. 8-4). This can, for instance, be observed in dreaming (while being asleep and thus in a resting state) or in mind wandering, where certain internal thoughts and perceptions can turn out to be more rewarding than the external contents (see Chapters 25 and 25 for details on both mind wandering and dreaming).

NEUROCONCEPTUAL REMARK IC: DIFFERENCE-BASED CODING AND VALUE AS "COMMON CURRENCIES" OF NEURAL ACTIVITY AND BEHAVIOR

What does this imply for the concept of value? The concept of value may then be understood in a wider sense as concerning and being applicable not only to exteroceptive stimuli but also to interoceptive and even neuronal ones. Hence, the concept of value may be the "common currency" between these different stimuli in behavioral regard, that is, the "behavioral common currency." Such a wider concept of value may come close to the concept of value as a "candidate underlying principle" of brain function in general.

We should be careful, however. Value may indeed be a "candidate underlying principle" in the context of behavior. Why? The concept of value is a behavioral concept that describes our behavior and may therefore match well with the context of behavior. Hence, value may be a "candidate underlying principle" for our behavior that may consequently be described as "value driven and value based."

In contrast, value cannot be regarded a "candidate underlying principle" in the context of the brain and its neuronal function. Why? Because that would require a purely neuronal concept to match the neuronal context of the brain rather than a behavioral concept like value.

Based on my assumptions in this and the other chapters, I would regard the neuronal mechanisms underlying the generation of value to be a "candidate underlying principle" of our brain's neuronal function. The encoding of different stimuli in terms of their spatial and temporal differences; that is, their statistical frequency distributions across different discrete points in physical time and space, may be the common currency that makes their direct interaction with the consecutive generation of value possible.

One could consequently postulate the encoding of neural activity in terms of spatial and temporal differences and thus difference-based coding to be the "candidate underlying principle" of our brain and its neuronal function. In the same way, our behavior is value-based and -driven, our brain and its neuronal functions may be difference-based and -driven.

To put it in a nutshell, our behavior is value-driven by default. Analogously, the brain by default cannot avoid encoding intero- and exteroceptive stimuli into neural activity in terms of spatial and temporal differences. I now postulate that both the encoding of neural activity in terms of difference-based coding and the value-driven nature of behavior are intimately linked to each other by default. That, however, needs to be shown on separate grounds. This is the purpose in the next chapter.

Open Questions

What about consciousness? We said at the end of the previous chapter that predictive coding does not imply anything about phenomenal states; that is, consciousness. Given the complexity of the actual input as described, one may be inclined to revise that stance. Since consciousness is also includes contextual and bodily information, one may want to argue that the actual input and its complexity very much entail consciousness.

This, however, confuses the actual input and its functional and neuronal states with a phenomenal state, or consciousness. The functionally and neuronally defined actual input does not imply anything about a phenomenal state.

Moreover, one should not confuse cause and consequence. The actual input and its processing are often considered the causes of consciousness as it is tacitly presupposed in the neural correlates of consciousness (see Introduction I in Volume II for details). Consciousness is then considered to be the consequence of the actual input as its underlying cause.

One may also see things in a reverse way, though. Consciousness as phenomenal state may then be considered to precede the actual input and its subsequent perceptual, motor, and cognitive states, which all occur on the basis of and thus within the field of consciousness. Consciousness and its associated neuro-phenomenal mechanisms may then provide the ground for the subsequent neural processing of sensory, motor, cognitive, and affective functions, which then occur on the basis of the former. In this case the neuro-phenomenal functions underlying consciousness must be assumed to precede the neuro-sensory, neuro-motor, neuro-cognitive, and neuro-affective functions (see second Introduction in Volume II as well as Chapters 17 and 24 for more extensive discussion of this point).

The second question pertains to the interaction between social, vegetative, and natural statistics. I here demonstrated empirical support in favor of the interaction between natural and social statistics, as exemplified by examples of the social context dependence of reward. And I supported the assumption of the interaction between natural and vegetative statistics with examples from the bodily vegetative context dependence of reward. This leaves open a third interaction, namely the one between social statistics and vegetative statistics, and how that, in turn, affects the assignment of value to an exteroceptive (target) stimulus.

More specifically, the question is how the social context interacts with the vegetative state of the body and how that, in turn, impacts the assignment of value to specific exteroceptive stimuli. To test that experimentally, one would need to develop a complex 2x2x2 interaction design; that means including two variations of the social context and its co-occurring exteroceptive stimuli, two variations of the target stimuli that are to be valued, and two variations of the bodily state, that is, its interoceptive stimuli.

A third question points out a neglect. We focused mainly on the actual input in this chapter, showing that it is rather complex and not as simple as tacitly presupposed in the concept of predictive coding. This left open how the predicted input itself is generated, a question that was already briefly touched on in Chapter 7. Hence, after the detour to the actual input in this chapter, we may now want to return to this question and focus on the predicted input itself in more detail in the next chapter where we will continue to further elaborate the example of reward.

CHAPTER 9
Predictive Coding and the Brain's Neuronal Statistics

Summary

I discussed the concept of predictive coding in Chapter 7 and exemplified it by predominantly sensorimotor functions. Chapter 8 focused on how the actual input is based on the matching and comparison between different stimuli and their respective statistics; that is, natural, social, and vegetative statistics. How now is the predicted input itself generated? This is the focus in the present chapter. I first investigate the relationship between reward-related activity and resting-state activity; recent studies demonstrated considerable overlap between both in especially anterior cortical midline regions like the ventromedial prefrontal cortex (VMPFC) and the perigenual anterior cingulate cortex (PACC). Therefore I hypothesized that the predicted input can be generated on the basis of changes in the resting-state activity; that is, rest–rest interaction. How are the spatial and temporal changes in the resting-state activity encoded into neural activity? I propose that the spatial and temporal differences and thus the statistical frequency distribution of the changes in the resting-state activity are encoded by themselves into the resting-state activity. I therefore speak of what I describe as "neuronal statistics" that signifies the encoding of the spatial and temporal changes in the resting-state activity itself into neural activity. How does the resting state's neuronal statistics generate the predicted input? Usually, the generation of the predicted input is associated with the application of a cue that triggers the generation of the former. This means that the cue-triggered "as-if exteroceptive stimulus" and its "as-if natural statistics," as I describe it, interact with the resting state's neuronal statistics. Behaviorally, such interaction may be manifest in what Kent Berridge described as "wanting," the longing or craving for a particular object or event and its associated value. Such wanting must be distinguished from what Jaak Panksepp signifies as "seeking," the disposition of the organism to search (i.e., seek) for objects in the environment that could possibly be associated with value. The behavioral distinction between "seeking" and "wanting" suggests a corresponding underlying neuronal distinction during the generation of the predicted input. I suggest that corresponding neuronal stages, a completely spontaneous one and a subsequent cue-related one, need to be distinguished during the encoding of spatial and temporal changes in the resting-state activity. Taking both stages spontaneous and cue-related will allow for generating a predicted input. Taken together, this shows that the generation of the predicted input cannot be regarded simply as given and simple but rather as resulting from different and rather complex neuronal mechanisms that already operate in the resting state itself. The chapter concludes with the question for the kind of necessary neuronal conditions, that is, neural predispositions, that enable and thus make possible the transformation of neuronal into behavioral states.

Key Concepts and Topics Covered

Resting-state activity, reward-related activity, neural overlap, anterior midline regions, as-if natural statistics, neuronal statistics, predictive coding, predicted input, seeking, wanting, spatiotemporal structure

Empirical background: predicted input and the brain's resting-state activity

The theory of predictive coding claims three core elements: the actual input, the predicted input, and the prediction error (resulting from the comparison and matching between the former two). Chapter 7 focused on the prediction error, assuming that it presupposes difference-based coding. This was mainly illustrated by sensory functions and the mirror neurons. Thereby, I hypothesized that for the matching and comparison between actual input and predicted input to be possible, that is, the prediction error, both inputs need to share a common code.

I suggested that such a common code consists in the encoding of statistically based spatial and temporal differences; that is difference-based coding, into neural activity during the generation of both predicted input and actual input. By encoding their respective underlying neural activity in terms of spatial and temporal differences, both predicted and actual inputs share the same code and can therefore directly be matched and compared with each other.

The assumption of predictive coding presupposing difference-based coding was further specified in Chapter 8. There I discussed how the actual input is generated. It turned out that different kinds of stimuli and their respective statistical frequency distributions constitute what is described as actual input in predictive coding. This means that the actual input cannot be presupposed as simple and taken for granted in the theory of predictive coding as so often (rather tacitly) seems to be the case.

Let us be more specific with regard to the actual input. The actual input included the exteroceptive target stimulus' natural statistics, the co-occurring exteroceptive stimuli in the respective social context and their respective social statistics, and the vegetative statistics of the interoceptive stimuli from the body. The matching and comparison between all three statistics, natural, social, and vegetative, was supposed to constitute the actual input as described in predictive coding. Accordingly, the actual input must be considered a complex amalgam of different stimuli and their respective statistics—natural, social, and vegetative.

Where does this leave us? We showed that predictive coding presupposes differences-based coding (Chapter 7) and that the actual input is a complex amalgam of different stimuli and their respective statistics—natural, social, and vegetative (Chapter 8). This however leaves open one core ingredient of predictive coding; namely, the predicted input itself. How is the predicted input generated?

As indicated in Chapter 7, the predicted input must be generated prior to the occurrence of the actual input and the subsequent prediction error. This takes us neuronally back to the brain's resting-state activity as it characterizes the brain prior to the occurrence of stimulus-induced activity, which stems from the various stimuli associated with the actual input. We discussed the resting-state activity in full detail in Chapters 4 through 6 and characterized it by a statistically based spatiotemporal structure. How now do the resting state's statistically based spatiotemporal structure and its continuous changes lead to the generation of the predicted input? This is the focus in the present chapter.

Neuronal findings Ia: hierarchical organization and prediction errors

How do the advocates of predictive coding imagine the predicted input to be generated? Karl Friston (2010) as the main advocate of predictive coding proposes a hierarchical architecture with bottom-up processing of the actual sensory input in, for instance, sensory cortex and top-down processing of cognitive functions in, for instance, prefrontal cortex to be central for generating the predicted sensory input. In addition to the lower-most and uppermost regions like the sensory and the prefrontal cortex, there are many other regions sandwiched in between. How are now all these different levels related to each other?

Friston argues that the different levels and their respective regions serve as a higher region for the respective next lower region while, at the same time, they serve as a lower region for the next higher region. When serving as a higher region for the next lower region, their neural activity signifies predictions for the next actual input and signal of the next lower region. This prediction, that is, the predicted input for the next lower region, serves also as actual input when considering the same region as lower region for the next higher region, which then generates the predicted input for the former. Accordingly, depending on its relationship to either the next-lower or -higher region, the region's neural activity serves either as actual input (for the next-higher region) or as predicted input (for the next-lower region).

Since the same region's neural activity serves as both predicted input (for the next-lower one) and actual input (for the next-higher one), continuous matching and comparison processes going on between lower and higher regions' neural activities. Due to the fact that it provides the predicted input, the region's neural activity is matched and compared with the neural activity level of the next-lower region's activity. At the same time, that same region's neural activity and its actual input are also matched and compared with that of the one in the next higher region.

These continuous matching and comparison processes extend throughout the whole brain and enable the continuous generation of prediction errors at each level as resulting from the comparison between the respective actual and predicted inputs. Does the neural activity in the different regions of the brain indeed signify such a continuous generation of prediction errors? After all, this model is a theoretical model that, if empirically plausible, presupposes a corresponding hierarchical organization in the brain with the clear distinction between different layers according to their level in the hierarchy.(see Fig. 9-1a).

Neuronal findings Ib: Hierarchical organization and the brain

Carhart-Harris and Friston (2010) and Friston (2010) postulate a hierarchical organization in the anatomical structures of the brain. They suggest that the thalamic nuclei, the unimodal sensory regions, and the other subcortical limbic and paralimbic regions are the lowest level in the anatomical hierarchy of the brain. The next-higher levels are the salience and dorsal attention systems, while the highest level can be found in the default-mode network (DMN).

Let us briefly explain the different levels and their respective networks or systems (see also Chapter 4 for more details of the different networks). The salience system includes the dorsal anterior cingulate cortex, the fronto-insula cortices, the amygdala, and the ventral midbrain (see also Menon 2011). The dorsal attention system includes the dorsolateral prefrontal cortex, the frontal eye fields, the dorsal medial prefrontal cortex, the intraparietal sulcus, and the superior parietal lobule (see Carhart-Harris and Friston 2010, 6, for details and references). Finally, the third and top level is to be found in what is called the default-mode network (DMN) that includes cortical midline regions like the ventromedial prefrontal cortex (VMPFC), the dorsomedial prefrontal cortex (DMPFC), and the posterior cingulate cortex (PCC) as well as the lateral parietal cortex and the hippocampus (see Part II for details of the DMN).

How are now these different levels related to each other in their neural activity? These three levels, the DMN at the top, the attention systems in the intermediate level, and the sensory/limbic/paralimbic regions at the lowest, form an anatomical and functional hierarchy. Each level has its own energy, that is, free energy, with which it is trying to suppress the free energy of its respective subordinate (through minimizing the prediction error) at the next-lower level.

Spontaneous activity, such as frequency fluctuations in the DMN, suppresses and contains spontaneous activity in the regions of the attention systems via top-down modulation. The same kind of top-down modulation can then be observed between the attention system and the next lower level in the hierarchy.

This means that the spontaneous activity in the attention networks controls and inhibits neural activity changes induced by exogenous sensory input in thalamic and sensory cortical

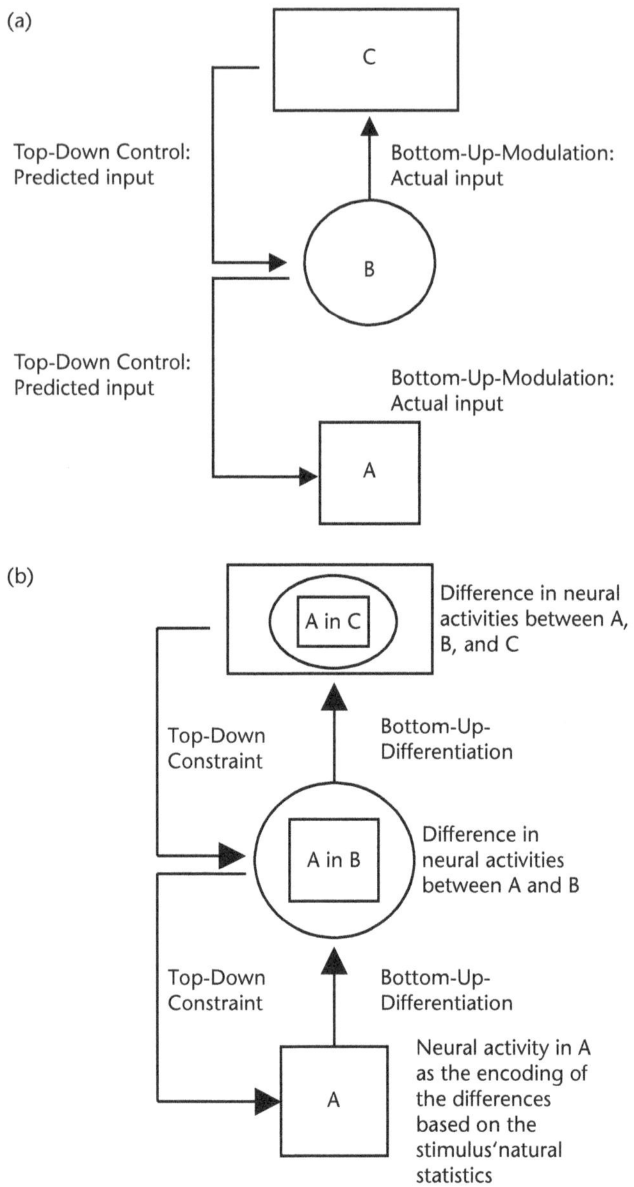

Figure 9-1a and b **Different forms of anatomical organization and neural coding. The figure describes two different forms of anatomical organization, hierarchical (*a*) and nested (*b*), and the respectively associated coding strategy. (*a*): In the hierarchical organization, the different levels are clearly separated from each other as indicated by the different shapes that do not overlap. They interact with each other from lower to upper levels signifying bottom-up modulation with the actual input, while the upper levels interact with the lower ones via top-down modulation and the predicted input. Hence, the hierarchical organization is closely tied and linked to predictive coding. (*b*): In the nested organization, in contrast, the different levels are not clearly separated from each other since they are embedded, with the lower one embedded and integrated into the next higher one, and so forth. This is indicated by the shapes from the lower levels reoccurring inside the next higher one. That necessitates the intrinsic activity of the higher level to be encoded in relation to the resting-state or stimulus-induced activity of the lower one. Such organization entails difference-based coding rather than stimulus-based coding as (tacitly) presupposed in predicted input and actual input as in predictive coding.**

regions (see Carhart-Harris and Friston 2010, 11–12, for details, as well as Wacongne et al. 2011 for a recent empirical study supporting such hierarchical processing yielding predicted inputs and prediction errors between different anatomical levels).[1]

The proponents of predictive coding propose a hierarchical structure with the generation of predicted and actual inputs at different levels of the hierarchy. This leads to the generation of prediction error as the interaction between higher and lower levels. Such hierarchical structure corresponds well to the anatomo-structural and functional organization of the brain where different levels, i.e., different neural networks and systems, interact with each other via bottom-up modulation and top-down modulation.

Neuronal findings Ic: "segregated hierarchy" versus "nested hierarchy"

One may now doubt whether such clear-cut hierarchical organization with the segregation between its different levels is empirically plausible and thus applies as such to the brain. This may be especially questionable given the multiple structural and functional connections between the different levels and systems.

Rather than such clear-cut segregation between the different levels, one may suggest that each level resurfaces and is redeployed within the next higher one, resembling the differently sized Russian dolls being nested within each other. This amounts to what Todd Feinberg describes as "nested hierarchy" (Fig. 9-1b; see Feinberg 2009, 2011,; Northoff et al. 2011).

One may thus distinguish between different forms of hierarchy. There is the "segregated hierarchy" as advanced by Friston. Here the different levels, lower and higher ones, can be clearly segregated from each other and are related to each other via bottom-up and top-down modulation.

Such a "segregated hierarchy" must be distinguished from the "nested hierarchy" where each lower level resurfaces in the next higher one, and so forth. In this case there is no longer clear-cut segregation between the different levels, because one cannot distinguish anymore in the higher level what is due to the contribution of the higher level itself and what is rather related to the lower level's resurfacing in the higher level.

How is such a "nested hierarchy" related to the brain and its anatomo-structural organization? Feinberg proposes that the brain and its anatomical structure can indeed be characterized by such a nested hierarchy rather than a segregated hierarchy. For that, though, we have to abandon the traditional distinction between lower subcortical and higher cortical regions. Instead of segregating subcortical and cortical regions, we have to consider them as integrated subcortical-cortical systems that act as functional unities. This is where the threefold anatomo-structural organization as discussed in Chapter 4 in full detail comes in.

Let us briefly recall the brain's threefold anatomo-structural organization. The Dutch anatomist Niewenhuys distinguishes between three different subcortical-cortical rings: an inner ring with subcortical and cortical regions around and adjacent to the ventricles, an outer ring at the outer surface of both subcortical and cortical territories, and a middle ring sandwiched between inner and middle rings (see Chapter 4 for details). Most important, subcortical and cortical regions within each ring act as functional unity in an integrated subcortical-cortical way.

Such integrated action makes the segregation between subcortical and cortical regions as suggested by the hierarchical organization impossible. For instance, as based on the predominant interoceptive input, the inner subcortical-cortical ring mediates the interoceptive state of the body while the outer ring, due to its predominant exteroceptive input, processes an exteroceptive state of the environment. The middle ring does not receive direct input from outside the brain, which led me to characterize it by the predominant input from the brain itself, the neuronal stimuli (see Chapter 4 for details).

How does such a "nested hierarchy" stand in relation to the "segregated hierarchy"? The main distinction in the "nested hierarchy" is no longer the vertical and thus hierarchical distinction between lower subcortical and higher cortical regions as in the "segregated hierarchy." Instead, the main distinguishing feature here is the anatomical proximity to the ventricles that allows for the distinction between inner, middle, and outer rings. In addition, the predominant stimulus input, intero- or exteroceptive or neuronal (and other neuro-anatomical features; see Chapter 4) also allows us to further distinguish the different rings from each other.

Neuronal hypothesis Ia: "nested hierarchy" and predictive coding

What does such a "nested hierarchy" imply for the generation of the predicted input? Unlike in the "segregated hierarchy", there are no clearly segregated vertically based levels of hierarchy anymore in the "nested hierarchy." This, however, makes the clear-cut association of predicted and actual inputs with lower and higher level regions impossible as implied by the model of predictive coding: the assumption that the interplay between the vertically defined lower and higher levels of neural activity accounts for the generation of the prediction error can then no longer be maintained.

This account of the "nested hierarchy" needs to be specified, though. Metaphorically speaking, one can say that "one can no longer distinguish 'what serves for what as what'" Let us briefly shed some light on the three "what's," starting with the first "what."

One cannot distinguish anymore different vertically defined regions from each other within the rings themselves. Determining and segregating lower and higher regions from each other remains impossible, so that one can no longer single out what region serves as starting point for generating predicted or actual inputs. This concerns the first "what" that undermines one central presupposition of the predictive coding model, the clear-cut vertically based hierarchical distinction into lower and higher regions as either sender or receiver of the respective other regions' neural activity.

How about the second "what"? Due to the integration of subcortical and cortical regions' neural activities during their encoding of spatial and temporal neural differences across different regions (within and across the different rings) (presupposing difference-based coding rather than stimulus-based coding), one can no longer determine the exact contribution of each region. The association of either a predicted input or an actual input with a particular region and its neural activity consequently becomes impossible. This concerns the second "what" that undermines another central presupposition of the predictive coding model, the association of a specific contribution with the neural activity of a particular region.

Finally, we need to tackle the third "what." Where are we so far? The first two "what's" showed two main points: (i) the regions are no longer anatomically segregated in a vertically based way and (ii) their neural activity is integrated and encoded in the gestalt of spatial and temporal differences. This makes it also impossible to single out where the neural activity of a particular region goes, and which subsequent region's activity it impacts.

One can then no longer distinguish between top-down modulation and bottom-up modulation (see also Northoff 2002, where I distinguish between horizontal and vertical modulation) and, most important, associate the former with the predicted input and the latter with the actual input. This concerns the third "what," which undermines the assumption in the predictive coding model that the receiver, i.e., the receiving address, of a region's neural activity can be clearly determined and associated with receiving either the predicted input or the actual input.

The model of the "nested hierarchy" undermines some of the central assumptions of the predictive coding model for the generation of the predicted input. While I am fully aware that this needs to be discussed in more detail, we nevertheless have to move on and see how we could better explain the generation of the predicted input. In order to get some idea, we may want to briefly shed some light on the kind of conditions or criteria an explanatory model would need to fulfill.

Neuronal hypothesis Ib: predicted input and resting-state activity

What kind of neuronal processes or mechanisms must occur in order to make possible the generation of the predicted input? Let me formulate some of the neural conditions or criteria an explanatory model for the generation of the predicted input must fulfill.

First, the predicted input must share the coding strategy with the actual input in order for them to interact. Since the actual input presupposes difference-based coding, the generation of the predicted input also requires difference-based coding. Hence, the predicted input must reflect and be based upon the encoding of spatial and temporal differences; i.e., difference-based coding.

Second, the difference upon which the predicted input is supposed to be based must be a statistically based difference. We saw in the case of the actual input that it is based upon the matching of different statistically based differences; that is, natural, social, and vegetative statistics. Analogously, one would propose that the predicted input is based on the matching and comparison between different statistical differences whose origin, though, remains unclear for now.

Third, the predicted input must be generated prior to and thus temporally precede the encounter with the actual input. This means that neuronally it must precede the generation of stimulus-induced activity as associated with the actual input and its matching with the predicted input. That implies, however, that the predicted input must be generated during the period when the brain is at rest being characterized by its intrinsic activity, that is, its resting-state activity. One would consequently suggest that the brain's resting-state activity is central in generating the predicted input.

If the brain's intrinsic activity is indeed relevant in generating the predicted input in, for example, the case of reward, one may hypothesize neural overlap between the regions recruited during reward and those showing high resting-state activity. More specifically, one would expect that the resting-state activity to be closely related to specifically the predicted input in reward tasks, i.e., the predicted or expected reward value, and also, at least in part, the degree of the prediction error, the actual reward, and its associated stimulus-induced activity (especially in those instances where the prediction error is low so that the impact of the predicted input is rather high).

Taken together, the criteria make it clear that we need to go back to the resting-state activity itself in order to explain the generation of the predicted input in neuronal terms. The distinction between predicted input and actual input may then correspond to the distinction between resting state and stimulus-induced activity rather than to the one between higher and lower regions as suggested in the predictive coding model.

We therefore turn now back to the brain's resting-state activity, its intrinsic activity, as was already discussed in detail in Chapters 4 through 6. However, the focus is now no longer on the resting-state activity itself and its spatiotemporal structure (see Chapters 4–6) but rather on how it can possibly generate the predicted input.

NEURONAL FINDINGS IIA: NEURAL OVERLAP BETWEEN RESTING-STATE ACTIVITY AND REWARD-RELATED ACTIVITY IN *CORTICAL* REGIONS

There has been much research in neuroscience about both reward and resting state, while investigations of their relationship in humans are less common. Given that other functions like perception and decision making have been shown to be modulated by the level of the resting-state activity (see Parts I and IV for details), it would be rather strange if this were not the case in reward.

This is especially suggested by the fact that regions like the VMPFC and the ventral striatum (VS) that are core regions of the reward circuitry do also show high levels of resting-state activity (see Chapter 7). While there has been plenty of literature in both fields of resting state and reward, their direct linkage and interaction remains to be investigated on the regional level of neural activity using, for instance, brain imaging.

Taking a first step in this direction, Niall Duncan from our group therefore conducted a meta-analysis of recent human imaging studies on reward and resting state (see Duncan et al. 2013). There was a strong overlap in the regional neural activity patterns between resting-state activity and reward-related activity. Such neural overlap was visible in the anterior midline regions, especially the VMPFC and the adjacent PACC.

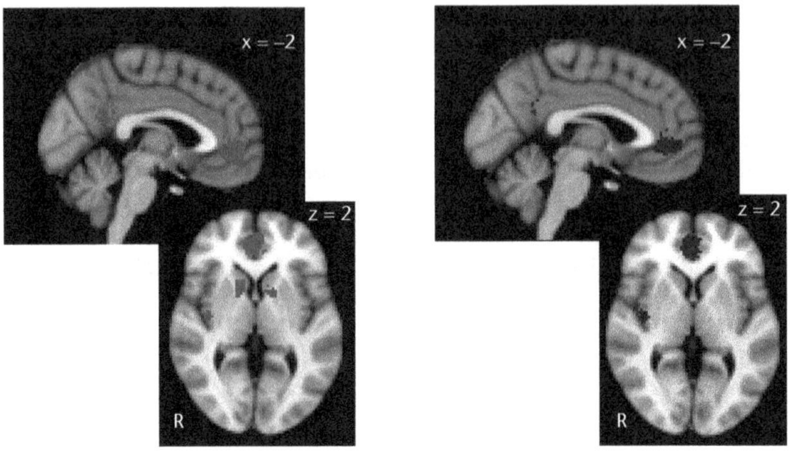

Overlap of rest and active reward tasks   Overlap of rest and passive reward tasks

Figure 9-2 **Neural overlap between resting-state activity and reward-related activity. The figure demonstrates the results from a meta-analysis of human imaging studies of reward and resting state (see Duncan et al. 2013). Thereby, reward studies are distinguished according to whether subjects passively received a reward (passive; *right side*) or had to actively engage in order to receive it (active; *left side*). The black and grey voxels in the pictures signify the neural overlap between resting-state activity and reward-related activity. In both cases (passive, active) there is considerable overlap in the anterior cortical midline structures like the ventromedial prefrontal cortex (VMPFC) and the perigenual anterior cingulate cortex (PACC). The overlap in the posterior midline region of the posterior cingulate cortex (PCC) is especially strong in the active reward tasks (*left*) while being rather weak and small in the passive conditions (*right*).**

Another neural overlap was manifest in the posterior midline regions, the PCC. This holds for both active and passive reward tasks, which were distinguished from each other according to either receiving (i.e., passive) or acquiring (i.e., active) a reward in the tasks applied by the respective studies (see Fig. 9-2).

This is even more interesting given the fact that many studies on reward and predictive coding demonstrated that the predicted input can be associated with neural activity in especially the VMPFC (see Schultz 2006, 2007a and b; Montague et al. 2002, 2006; O'Doherty et al. 2006; van Duuren et al. 2008). Taken together with our findings of an overlap between resting-state and reward-related activity, this suggests that the brain's intrinsic activity, its resting-state activity, may possibly be centrally involved in generating the predicted input (see for more details in the next section).

NEURONAL FINDINGS IIB: NEURAL OVERLAP BETWEEN RESTING-STATE ACTIVITY AND REWARD-RELATED ACTIVITY IN *SUBCORTICAL* REGIONS

How about the subcortical regions? Regions like the central tegmental area (VTA) and the ventral striatum (VS) are supposed to be central in reward. When comparing the reward-related conditions versus their respective control conditions, that is, non-reward conditions, we clearly observed the VTA and the VS. However, once we compared the reward-related conditions against the resting-state studies, this involvement of the subcortical regions was no longer visible. In contrast, when comparing the non-reward condition with the resting state, subcortical regions like the VTA and VS revealed higher signal changes in the rest condition.

The absence of subcortical regions in the comparison between rest and reward may have different reasons. One of the reasons may be that reward-related activity does not much deviate from the respectively preceding resting-state activity level. Only the non-reward conditions may induce changes in the activity level when compared to the preceding resting state. This is indeed supported by recent studies of ours in which we plotted the raw data and observed decreased signal changes only during the non-reward control condition while not much activity change was observed during the reward condition itself (see deGreck et al. 2008). If so, one would hypothesize that the intrinsic activity, the resting-state activity, in the subcortical regions may already be involved in some kind of value assignment, that is, reward-related activity, during the resting state itself (see the end of this chapter for details on that).

Alternatively, the reason for the lack of the neural overlap between rest and reward in subcortical regions may be found in methodological confounds. Subcortical regions are much more difficult to visualize in functional magnetic resonance imaging (fMRI) since they show low degrees of signal changes when compared to cortical regions. Hence, we cannot exclude a cortical bias in the data on both reward and rest at the expense of the subcortical regions. Moreover, the resting state studies in fMRI focus usually on cortical regions and their functional connectivity exclusively while often neglecting subcortical regions (except the thalamus). Hence, the lack of subcortical overlap between rest and reward may also stem from insufficient data from resting-state studies.

In sum, the empirical evidence available on humans hints at neural overlap between resting-state activity and reward-related activity in especially the anterior cortical midline structures like the VMPFC and the PACC. This is especially remarkable given the fact that studies on reward in both animals and humans associated neural activity in these regions with the generation of the predicted input.

Neuronal findings IIc: prediction of reward-related activity by resting-state activity

We so far have described the results of a meta-analysis that showed neural overlap between reward and resting-state activity, especially in anterior midline regions. How about a more direct support? For that, Niall Duncan from our group conducted a combined resting state and reward study in fMRI (Duncan et al. 2013). The resting state condition included a six-minute period of eyes closed without any stimulation or task. This allowed us to measure the spontaneous variability of the resting-state activity as accounted for by standard deviation (SD), the amplitude of the low frequency fluctuations (ALFF), and entropy (EP).

In addition to the resting-state condition, he also applied a standard reward paradigm, the Monetary Incentive Delay task (MID) where subjects have to bet for money by deciding between a right or left mouse click. They are shown a cue where they have to anticipate in a purely mental way the possible reward and their decision or, in a control condition, no reward at all. After the anticipation period that lasted 4-6s, subjects were instructed to click the mouse to indicate their decision, which is followed by the display of the reward (or the non-reward) they receive—the feedback period. The design also included control conditions where subjects had to merely anticipate without any reward and did not receive anything in the feedback period.

What were the results? As expected and as shown in other studies, the anticipation-of-reward period (when compared to anticipation of no reward) yielded significant signal changes in the typical reward regions like the ventral striatum, the caudate, the putamen, the VTA/SN, and the thalamus. In addition, signal changes were observed in cortical regions like the precuneus, the dorsal anterior cingulate cortex, and the premotor cortex. This differed from the feedback period (when compared to feedback without any reward) where subjects showed activity changes in anterior and posterior cortical midline regions like the VMPFC, the DMPFC, and the posterior cingulate cortex (PCC), and precuneus.

How now are the activity changes during the anticipation and feedback of reward related to the resting-state activity as measured during eyes closed? For that we correlated resting-state and stimulus-induced/task-related activities with each other. Let us start with the anticipation period.

The degree of SD and ALFF in the resting state in the visual cortex, the precuneus, and the thalamus negatively predicted the degree of stimulus-induced activity during the anticipation period in the same regions: the higher the degrees of SD and ALFF in the resting state in these regions, the lower the degree of stimulus-induced activity during the anticipation period. This rest-stimulus correlation pattern was specific for the anticipation period, since we did not observe the same pattern with the signal changes from the feedback period. Moreover, the rest-stimulus correlation was specific for those anticipation periods where subjects had to anticipate reward whereas it was not observed where they had anticipate no reward. How about the feedback period? We here observed that the resting state measures of SD, ALFF, and EP in VMPFC, PCC, and precuneus predicted the feedback-related signal changes in the same regions in a positive way. The stronger the SD, the ALFF, and EP in the resting state, the stronger signal changes during the feedback period were induced in these regions. And again, as in the case of the anticipation period, these rest-stimulus correlations were specific for the feedback period; the correlation of the resting state measures with the anticipation-related signal changes did not yield any significant relation in these regions.

Our findings clearly support direct relationship between the variability of resting-state activity and the degree of stimulus-induced or task-related activity during reward. More specifically, our results show that the variability (as measured with SD and EP) of the resting-state activity's fluctuations in the low frequency range (as measured with the ALFF) predicts the degree of subsequent stimulus-induced activity specifically during reward conditions (as distinguished from non-reward as it was controlled in our experimental design).

In sum, our findings highlight the importance of the variability of the resting-state activity (as measured with SD, ALFF, and EP), which reflects its continuous changes and thus rest–rest interaction (see below for further explanation). The degree of the resting-state activity's spontaneous changes is apparently central in determining the degree to which a reward-related stimulus or task can induce stimulus-induced or task-related activity. Most interesting, the resting state variability in different regions seems to be related to different aspects of reward like anticipation or feedback. This strongly suggests that the resting-state activity in different regions seems to contain different information about the distinct aspects of reward.

Neuronal hypothesis IIa: Resting-state activity as rest–rest interaction

The data indicate neural overlap and prediction between resting-state activity and reward-related activity especially in the anterior midline regions like the VMPFC and the PACC. What does this mean for the generation for the predicted input, which may be generated during the brain's resting state and thus by its intrinsic activity?

As detailed in Part II of this volume, there is already plenty of interaction going on in the resting state. There is interaction between the different regions of the brain as manifest in functional connectivity (see Chapter 4). In addition, there is plenty of interaction in the resting state across different discrete points in physical time as manifest in the fluctuations of the resting state's activity in different frequency ranges (see Chapter 5). This is well manifested in the measures of the variability of the resting state as applied in the study on rest-reward by Duncan et al. (2013), the standard deviation (SD), the amplitude of low frequency fluctuations (ALFF), and the entropy (EP).

Taken together, various interactions with continuous changes in the spatial and temporal activity patterns occur already in the resting state itself. This is what can be subsumed under the concept of rest–rest interaction that describes the continuous changes in the resting state's spatiotemporal activity patterns, which operationally are manifested in measures of the resting-state activity's variability.

How can we describe such rest–rest interaction in further detail? Let us learn from the interaction between different stimuli, as discussed in Chapter 8 (see also Chapter 10). There we described interaction between different exteroceptive stimuli, that is, extero–extero interaction, and the interaction between intero- and exteroceptive stimuli, that is, intero–extero interaction. Despite the different origins of the different stimuli, both intero–extero and extero–extero interactions were made possible by a common coding strategy in the encoding of the different stimuli into neural activity. This common coding strategy consisted of coding the statistical frequency distribution of the different stimuli; that is, their natural, social, and vegetative statistics. This in turn allowed for their direct matching and comparison and thus for their interaction.

How does that now apply to the resting state and its rest–rest interaction? Here (taken ideally) too we are dealing with different stimuli, different neuronal stimuli that are generated and originate in the brain itself (see Chapter 4 for details). These neuronal stimuli are generated in different regions and thus at different discrete points in physical space and time. Rest–rest interaction can consecutively be regarded as an interaction between different neuronal stimuli and their respectively associated different discrete points in physical time and space.

Neuronal hypothesis IIb: Encoding of the "neuronal statistics" of rest–rest interaction into the resting state's neural activity

I postulate the actual resting-state activity level, i.e., its level at one particular discrete point in time and space, to result from rest–rest interaction and more precisely from the interaction between different neuronal stimuli. How must the different neuronal stimuli be encoded in order to generate the resting-state activity level? As in the case of intero- and exteroceptive stimuli, I hypothesize that the different neuronal stimuli and their subsequent rest–rest interaction are encoded in a statistically based way and thus on the basis of their statistical frequency distribution. The encoding of different statistical frequency distribution should then lead to different and continuously changing resting-state activity levels; this is indeed the case as manifest in the various measures of resting state variability (SD, EP, ALFF) as described earlier.

What exactly does the encoding of statistical frequency distribution mean? This means that the spatial and temporal differences between the different discrete points in physical time and space at which the various neuronal stimuli occur are encoded into neural activity, that is, the resting-state activity. The resulting level of neural activity in the resting state is thus difference based rather than stimulus based. Rather than on single neuronal stimuli at their different discrete point in physical time and space, the resting-state activity is based on the encoding of the neuronal stimuli's statistical frequency distribution across their different discrete points in time and space.

Analogous to natural, vegetative, and social statistics, one may therefore speak of the encoding of the neuronal stimuli's "neuronal statistics" into the resting state's neuronal activity (see also Chapter 6 for the introduction of the concept of "neuronal statistics"). The concept of neuronal statistics describes the resting state's encoding of neural activity changes; it describes the encoding of the spatial and temporal differences of its neuronal stimuli across their different discrete points in time and space. In short, I characterize the resting-state activity by the encoding of its own "neuronal statistics."

Neuronal hypothesis IIc: The resting-state activity's neuronal statistics contain information about the predicted input

How is the resting state's encoding of its own neuronal statistics related to the generation of the predicted input?

I postulated that the predicted input was generated during the resting state and thus by rest–rest interaction. If now rest–rest interaction can be traced back to the encoding of the neuronal stimuli's neuronal statistics, one may suggest that the resting state's neuronal statistics is central in generating the predicted input. In a nutshell, I suggest that the generation of the predicted input is directly related to the encoding of the resting state's neuronal statistics into its own neural activity.

Let's be more concrete. The resting state was characterized by functional connectivity and fluctuations in different frequency ranges (see Part II). One may now suggest that the predicted input is generated by specific (though yet unclear) changes in the resting-state activity triggered during rest–rest interaction. This means that the predicted input and its underlying neuronal activity in the resting state should be directly related to and thus predicted by the resting-state activity's neuronal statistics. This is strongly supported by our rest-reward findings as described earlier.

What we measured as resting state variability with SD, EP, and ALFF reflects nothing but the resting-state activity's neuronal statistics, the distribution of its activity across different discrete points in physical time (and space). We now observed that the resting-state activity's variability (that is, SD and ALFF) predicted the degree of neural activity change during the anticipation period. This means that the resting-state activity's neuronal statistics predict the reward-related activity.

What does this tell us about the generation of the predicted input? The anticipation period reflects the generation of a predicted input (that is, the anticipation of reward as input). Since the neural activity during the anticipation was predicted by the resting state's variability, the neuronal statistics of the resting state's activity must already contain some information about the predicted input which was modeled as anticipation period in our paradigm.

Neuronal hypothesis IId: The cue triggers (rather than causes) spatiotemporal activity patterns as the predicted input in the resting-state activity

How does that stand in relation to the assumptions in the predictive model? Advocates of predictive coding propose that the presence of a cue triggers the generation of the predicted input (see later for details with regard to cue- and non-cued-related activity).

Let us apply that to the present context of the resting state: the cue must somehow interact with the resting-state activity and its neuronal statistics. More precisely, the cue must modulate the resting-state activity's functional connectivity and its frequency fluctuations in the same way as the predicted stimulus did the last time that the brain's resting-state activity encountered it as actual input (see, for instance, the experimental settings by Schultz 2006, 2007a and b; Montague et al. 2002, 2006; van Duuren et al. 2008).

What now happens, exactly, during the exposure of the cue that is supposed to trigger the generation of the predicted input? Being exposed to a cue that indicates a specific input will eventually occur changes the resting state and its neuronal statistics: the resting-state activity's spatial and temporal pattern take on the same constellation as was elicited when the stimulus that is supposed to be predicted actually occurred and was processed as actual input.

I postulate that the cue only triggers, but does not cause, the occurrence of specific spatiotemporal activity patterns in the resting-state activity itself. These spatiotemporal activity patterns are supposed to be more or less similar to those that occurred during the last encounter with the actual input that is now predicted. The resting state itself and its actual spatial and temporal activity pattern may then make it more or less likely that the respective spatiotemporal activity patterns as related to the predicted input can be triggered again by the cue.

This implies that the resting-state activity itself, prior to the cue, should already contain some information about the predicted input. If so one, would expect the resting-state activity itself, prior to and independently of any cue, to predict the degree of neural activity during the subsequent presence of the cue and its predicted input. This is exactly what our findings demonstrate: they show that the resting-state activity variability (as measured completely independently of the reward paradigm) predicted the degree of neural activity during the cue-related anticipation period (see earlier).

Neuronal hypothesis IIe: Predicted input results from the matching between "neuronal statistics" and "as-if natural statistics"

How can we describe the situation in further conceptual and empirical detail? We are de facto still in the resting state and thus within the realm of its neuronal statistics. However, due to the cue as trigger, the resting-state activity takes on a spatiotemporal activity pattern that signifies specific exteroceptive (or interoceptive) stimuli, the actual input. One may thus want to say that brain's processes exteroceptive stimuli in "as-if way": the concept of "as if" refers to a neural activity pattern in the brain that, despite the absence of the exteroceptive stimuli is more or less similar to the activity pattern that is elicited during the presence of the respective stimulus.

The resting-state activity may then be characterized by the neural processing of "as-if exteroceptive stimuli." The concept of an "as-if exteroceptive stimulus" describes a state wherein the exteroceptive stimulus has not yet occurred but is already processed (in a virtual or fictive and thus as-if way) by the brain's resting-state activity and its spatiotemporal activity patterns (see also Northoff 2011 for the "as-if" concept).

What is then encoded into the resting state's activity? It is no longer exclusively the neuronal statistics of the resting-state activity itself that are encoded. Instead, it is the presumed statistics of the exteroceptive stimulus whose prediction is triggered by the cue. Analogous to the concept of the "as-if-exteroceptive stimulus", one may therefore want to characterize its statistical frequency distribution as "as-if natural statistics."

The concept of "as-if natural statistics" describes the statistical frequency distribution of the possible occurrence of an exteroceptive stimulus that has not yet occurred. The term "as-if natural statistics" thus refers to the probability estimate of that stimulus' occurrence in the future as based on its statistically based occurrence in the past.

What does this imply for the generation of the predicted input? I suggest that the predicted input results from the interaction between the resting-state activity's neuronal statistics and the "as-if exteroceptive statistics" of the cue and its triggering of "as-if exteroceptive stimuli." The predicted input results then from the matching and comparison between two different statistically frequency distributions, the neuronal statistics of the resting-state activity itself and the "as-if natural statistics" of the "as-if exteroceptive stimulus" (see Fig. 9-3a).

The assumption of such "as-if" natural statistic's in the generation of the predicted input is well in line with the simulation model of Rao and Ballard 1999 (see Chapter 7 for details). They demonstrated that the predicted input by itself must reflect the previous statistical frequency distribution of the input that is to be predicted. Our own results also support the matching hypothesis, though only in an indirect way via the correlation between resting-state and stimulus-induced activity.

More direct empirical support comes from recent animal studies (see, for instance, Fukushima et al. 2012; Berkes et al. 2011). A study by Berkes et al. (2011) investigated visual cortex (V1) activity in developing animals (awake ferrets), and recorded stimulus-induced and spontaneous activities. They observed similarity between spontaneous and stimulus-induced activity pattern that were specific to responses evoked by natural scenes and increased with age.

Another study, in monkeys, using chronic microelectrocorticography (Fukushima et al. 2012) observed the spontaneous activity in auditory cortex to exhibit the same spatial co-variation as during the auditory stimulation and its tonotopic maps in auditory cortex. This, as I will claim in Chapter 11, is only possible when one presupposes a specific interaction of the stimulus with the resting-state activity entailing what I will call "stimulus–rest interaction."

Taken together, these data strongly suggest that the resting-state activity encodes the natural statistics of the stimuli into its own neuronal activity, its own neuronal statistics. Any spontaneous changes in the resting state's neuronal statistics may then evoke the original stimulus and its natural statistics and thus what I describe as "as-if natural statistics."

NEURONAL HYPOTHESIS IIF: DIFFERENCE-BASED CODING ALLOWS FOR THE GENERATION OF THE "AS-IF NATURAL STATISTICS" AND THE PREDICTED INPUT

How does the resting-state activity's generation of such "as-if natural statistics" stand in relation to difference-based coding? As discussed in detail in Parts I and II, such a matching and

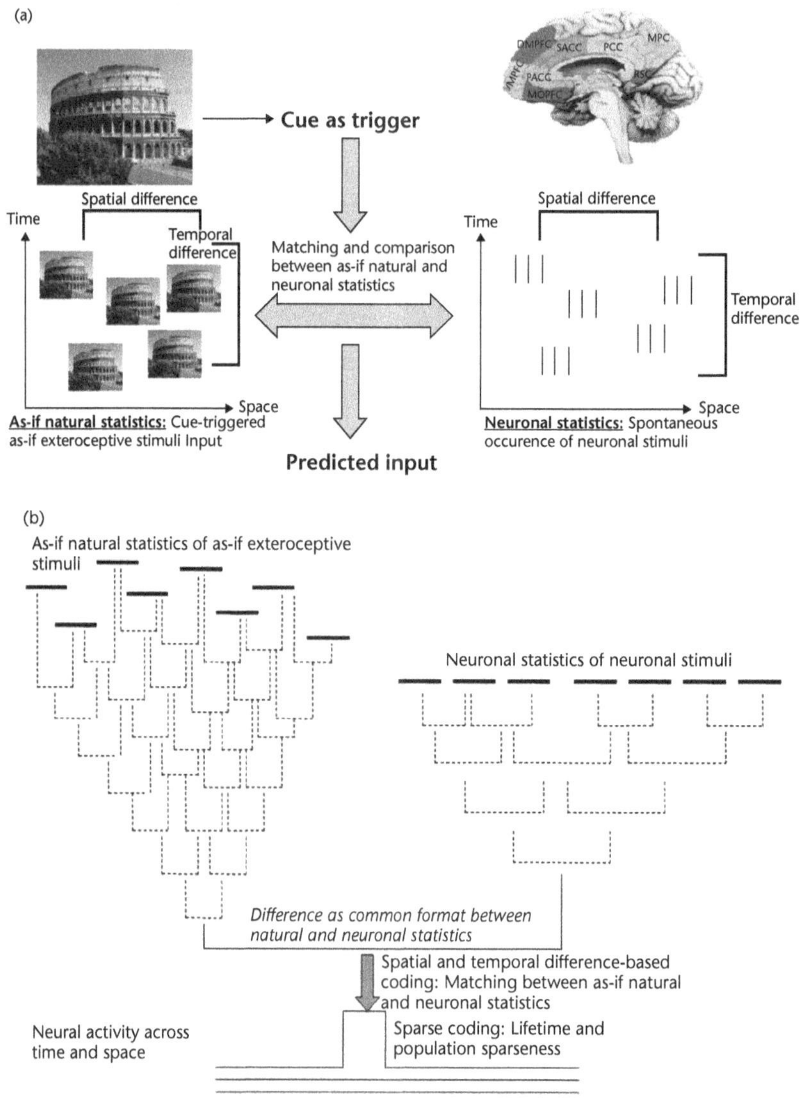

Figure 9.3 Generation of the predicted input. (*a*) Matching and comparison between as if natural statistics and neuronal statistics. (*b*) Difference-based coding and sparse coding of neural activity underlying the generation of the predicted input. The figure shows the neuronal mechanisms underlying the generation of the predicted input. How as-if natural statistics of the as-if exteroceptive stimuli is matched with the brain's intrinsic activity's neuronal statistics (*a*), and how that is mediated by difference-based coding and sparse coding (*b*). (*a*): The figure shows on the left the spatiotemporal frequency distribution of the as-if exteroceptive stimuli (as triggered by the cue) across time and space; this is described as "as-if natural statistics." The as-if exteroceptive stimuli's as-if natural statistics are matched and compared with the statistical frequency distribution of the brain's intrinsic activity across time and space; i.e., its neuronal statistics, as indicated in the right part of the figure. Hence, there is matching and comparison between two different statistics, as-if natural and neuronal statistics. (*b*): The figure shows that the comparison and matching between the as-if exteroceptive stimuli's as-if natural statistics and the brain's neuronal statistics (upper part) is possible because they presuppose the same coding strategy. The common code consists in coding statistically based spatial and temporal differences reflecting both kinds of stimuli's statistical frequency distributions across time and space (middle part). The difference as common code makes possible their mutual matching and the consequent sparsening of neural activity; this leads to the activation and recruitment of a lower number of neurons (when compared to the number of stimuli and the number of total number of available neurons) (lower part) across time (lifetime sparseness) and space (population sparseness).

comparison process between different statistics is possible only on the basis of difference-based coding as common underlying code. Different statistical differences are thus matched and compared during the encounter between the resting state's neuronal statistics and the "as-if exteroceptive stimulus" and its "as-if natural statistics."

As explicated in Chapters 1 through 3 and 6, such matching and comparison between different statistically based differences goes along with the temporal and spatial sparsening resulting in sparse coding. The generation of the predicted input may thus be related to the temporal and spatial sparsening of the neural activity in the resting-state activity as triggered by the cue; that is, the "as-if exteroceptive stimulus" and its "as-if natural statistics" (see Fig. 9-3b).

Based on the results described earlier, one may now postulate that such matching and comparison between the neuronal statistics and the as-if natural statistics may occur especially in anterior midline structures like the VMPFC and PACC. This is well in accordance with our results (Duncan et al. 2013) where the resting-state activity's variability in midline regions like the VMPFC (and PCC and precuneus) predicted the degree of stimulus-induced activity during the feedback period of reward (see earlier).

Why are the midline regions especially relevant for the matching between the different statistics? One may assume the following: (1) these regions have been shown to strongly overlap between resting-state activity and reward-related activity (see earlier); (2) their neural activity during reward has specifically been associated with the predicted input; and (3) neural activity in these regions has also been associated with the predicted input in functions other than reward, such as, sensory (visual) functions (see Chapter 7).

Neuronal Findings IIIa: Seeking as the Behavioral Manifestation of Unconditioned Resting-State Activity

So far, I have considered only the neuronal activity during the resting state and the anticipation or prediction of reward, while leaving open its corresponding behavioral manifestation. Thereby we may need to distinguish two distinct behavioral manifestations, the one during the resting state itself and the one during its interaction with the cue.

We need to first search for the behavioral correlate of the continuous changes in the resting state itself and its neuronal statistics. This may consist of what is described by Jaak Panksepp as "seeking."[2] Second, the behavioral correlate of the matching between the resting state's neuronal statistics on the one hand, and the as-if natural statistics" of the 'as if exteroceptive stimulus" on the other oeeds to be discussed. This may be associated with what Kent Berridge subsumes under the concept of "wanting." In this section, I want to discuss the concept of seeking in further detail, and in the next section I will shed some light on "wanting."

Let us start with seeking. We considered the social and bodily context of reward as discussed in Chapter 8. There is, however, more to reward than social environment and body. What does this "more to reward" consist of on a behavioral level? There seems to be a particular disposition to go out and search for rewards and assign value to stimuli. This is a purely spontaneous tendency of the organism that remains independent of any particular stimuli or cues. However, that tendency or disposition may strongly impact whether we can get a cue or a possibly rewarding stimuli into our focus at all. The value assigned to a particular stimulus may thus not only depend on social and bodily contexts but also on a disposition to search for possible rewards. This is what neuroscientist Jaak Panksepp (1998, 2011a and b) calls the "seeking disposition" (see later for detailed explanation).

Before seeking the neuronal mechanisms underlying seeking, let us first seek the person of Jaak Panksepp a little. He was originally born in the Baltic states, but, due to political turmoil, came to the United States as a young child. There he dedicated his life and his research to subcortical regions and their central role in processing affect and emotions, which, by founding and pioneering affective neuroscience, has had most profound implications for our understanding of the brain in general (see Chapter 31 in Volume II for the discussion of emotions and affect in the context of consciousness).

Now we are ready to seek the neuronal mechanisms underlying "seeking" itself. Coarsely and preliminarily defined, the concept of seeking refers to the spontaneous behavior of animals (and humans) in the absence of any specific stimulus or cue. Being exposed to at best only unspecific stimuli, Panksepp argues that animals (and humans, too) display a tendency in their behavior to search for (or seek) potentially rewarding stimuli in the environment.

Following Panksepp, seeking is a spontaneous unconditioned (and thus unlearned) and therefore intrinsically ingrained behavior. There is no conditioning at all involved in seeking, which distinguishes it from other related concepts like anticipation and wanting (see later in the next section). Since it is not triggered by any kind of acquisition or learning processes, seeking must be considered an intrinsic feature that as such comes as part of the organism's biological equipment.

Neuronal findings IIIb: Seeking and predictive coding

How can we put the concept of seeking into the context of predictive coding? Let us briefly rewind. Empirical investigations in both animals and humans associate neural activity in reward circuitry, and specifically dopamine, with the prediction error and hence with reward (see Montague et al. 2002, 2006; Schultz 2006). The prediction error is supposed to be determined exclusively by the actual input and its relation to the predicted input.

Panksepp (1998; Alcaro et al. 2007; Alcaro and Panksepp 2011), however, argues that this is only half of the story. The other half consists of the motivation and the organism's internal drives as part of its intrinsic biological equipment. These intrinsic drives are supposed to first and foremost make it possible for the organism to get excited by, become engaged in, and to consequently approach stimuli that could be potentially rewarding.

How can we describe the seeking disposition in more concrete empirical terms? Consider, for instance, subjects with a rather low seeking disposition and subsequent low degrees of searching for novelty in their environment; that is, novelty-seeking. This is the case in subjects with depression who often suffer from abnormally low seeking disposition, as is well manifested in low novelty-seeking scores (see Panksepp 1998; Alcaro et al. 2010; and see Chapter 27 for more details on depression).

The low seeking disposition makes it rather difficult for the depressed patients to assign value to stimuli and to consecutively experience them as rewarding and pleasurable. Due to their low seeking disposition with low novelty-seeking scores, depressed patients remain unable to even approach and engage in potentially rewarding stimuli, let alone to experience them as rewarding and pleasurable.

The decrease in seeking results in their inability to experience pleasure, which is described by the term "anhedonia" as one of the hallmark symptoms of depression (see Northoff et al. 2011 for details). The example of depression thus tells us that seeking, though occurring in the absence of any particular stimuli or tasks, has major effects and reverberations on the subsequent behavior, including especially the affective functions. Seeking thus seems to concern the behavioral predispositions of possible reward; this distinguishes it from predictive coding, which is about actual rather than merely possible rewards.

Unlike in conditioned and thus learned behavior (like wanting or anticipation) that is triggered by some kind of extrinsic stimulus, the purely unconditioned seeking reflects a contribution or input that the organism itself and its brain provide prior to the exposure to any particular stimulus or cue. Hence, Panksepp searched for the necessary but not sufficient neural and behavioral conditions; that is, the neural predispositions (as distinguished from the neural correlate; see Introduction I in Volume II for details on that difference) of reward.

This differs from predictive coding that concerns the actual rather than possible reward; namely, its necessary (predicted) input, and sufficient (prediction error) conditions of reward. Accordingly, the main difference between seeking and predictive coding consists in the difference between possible and actual reward and consecutively between behavioral/neural predisposition and behavioral/neural correlates of reward.

I have focused so far on describing seeking only in behavioral terms. How about its underlying neuronal mechanisms? Based on numerous empirical data in animals, Panksepp (1998) proposed a so-called seeking system in subcortical brain regions, more specifically in mesolimbic dopaminergic brain regions, including the VTA, the VS/NACC, and others like the lateral hypothalamus.

Following Panksepp, dopamine is responsible for the organism's internal drive to seek curiosities and novelties, to engage in pleasurable activities, and to get excited by them, and hence to approach, engage, and ultimately receive reward. According to him, the mesolimbic dopamine system makes possible the seeking disposition and thus the organism's intrinsic tendency to search and seek possible rewards in the environment.

Neuronal findings IIIc: "wanting" and cues

What Panksepp calls "seeking" must be compared with concepts described by other researchers. I therefore want to (only briefly) venture into this rather complex discussion. Jeffrey Gray (1995), for instance, speaks of a "behavioral activation system" that is associated also with more or less similar subcortical (and cortical) regions as the seeking system. There seems to be a strong similarity between Panksepp's seeking system and Gray's behavioral activation system in both behavioral and neuronal terms.

Another related concept is the one of "wanting" as introduced by Kent Berridge (2000, 2003, 2004, 2007, 2012). "Wanting" with quotation marks refers to subconscious implicit motivation, while wanting without quotation marks describes conscious desire. In the following discussion, I focus on the former meaning of "wanting"; that is, the implicit, unconscious meaning. "Wanting" in this sense describes the (unconscious) longing or urging for a particular object, more specifically for its motivational value, the "object-associated motivational value." Based on such a definition, "wanting" describes the organism's behavioral and psychological state as related to the object's motivational value before receiving the actual reward itself as associated with the object. Following Berridge, the subsequent presentation of the actual object itself, including its associated value, induces what he describes as "liking." Let us dwell more on the "wanting" in the following discussion.

"Wanting" a particular object and more specifically its associated motivational value presupposes that some value must already be present, though only mentally; that is, in mental representation. However, the object that is associated with that value is not yet physically present. How is such mental representation of the object and its value generated? Usually this is made possible by some kind of cue indicating that the object, including its associated value, is most likely to physically appear soon. The cue is supposed to trigger the mental representation of that object, more specifically its associated motivational value. The need for the presence of a cue in "wanting" implies some kind of prior conditioning and learning; this is so because without such a cue, the organism would not be able to generate the mental representation of a specific possible object and its associated value. This is different from seeking. In contrast to "wanting," seeking does not presuppose prior conditioning at all. Instead, as pointed out earlier, seeking remains completely unconditioned, requiring neither a stimulus nor any kind of cue.

Neuronal findings IIId: "seeking" and "wanting"

How can we further specify the difference between "wanting" and seeking? Seeking describes the organisms' intrinsic disposition for possible conditioning rather than the actual conditioning itself, as "wanting" does. Hence, the crucial difference seems to lie here between actual and possible conditioning and consecutively between intrinsic and extrinsic generation: "wanting" presupposes prior actual conditioning by an extrinsic cue and is therefore ultimately extrinsically generated. In contrast, seeking describes an intrinsic predisposition that makes possible subsequent actual conditioning by an extrinsic cue, while by itself remaining independent of both extrinsic cue and prior learning/conditioning. This implies that seeking must occur prior to "wanting," with the latter therefore presupposing the former.

Let me formulate the difference between seeking and "wanting" again, specifically with regard to value and the cue. "Wanting" goes along with the mental representation of a particular object-associated motivational value; this is triggered by a cue that indicates the high probability of the subsequent occurrence of the object and its respective motivational value. In contrast to "wanting," seeking is not triggered by a particular cue indicating the potential presence of a particular object and its associated value. Instead, seeking occurs prior to the occurrence of any specific cue and any kind of value. As such, seeking only reflects the organisms' disposition or tendency to search (and thus seek) for cues and values and thus for objects in general in the environment that could possibly be associated with value (see Fig. 9-4). Hence, unlike "wanting," seeking is neither associated with a particular cue nor a specific value (as associated with an object).

Since "wanting" describes the psychological and behavioral state associated with a specific cue and its associated value, the question for it being conscious or unconscious arises. Berridge (2004) argues that "wanting" as the longing or craving for a specific possible reward remains unconscious and thus implicit. As such, the implicit "wanting" may be distinguished from what is described as anticipation, where the implicit longing is rendered explicit (and thus represented) on the cognitive level. How does seeking stand in relation to unconsciousness and consciousness? Since it is prior to even "wanting", one may be inclined to say that it remains unconscious as well. However, one may object

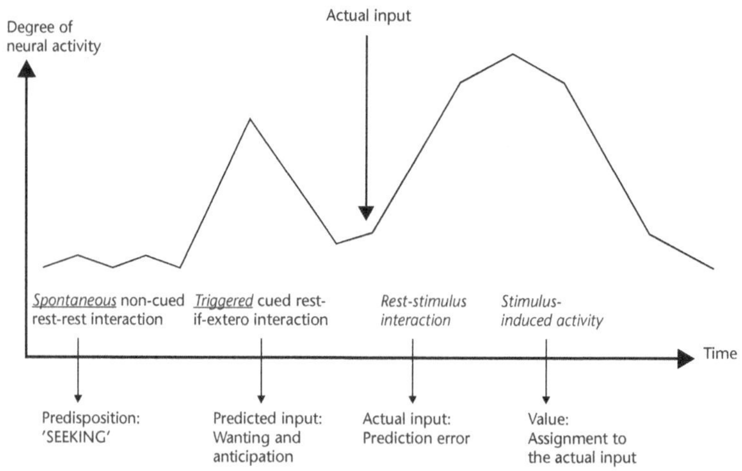

Figure 9-4 Neuronal mechanisms underlying seeking, "wanting," and value. The figure illustrates the different processes across time (x-axis) underlying seeking, wanting/anticipation, and value (x-axis) and their underlying degree of neural activity (y-axis). There is intrinsic activity or resting-state activity that behaviorally corresponds to seeking as non-cued behavioral manifestation of spontaneous activity fluctuations in the resting state (most left on x-axis). The resting state itself may then be modulated by a cue that triggers interaction with the resting state, which results in the generation of a predicted input and associated "wanting" (second from left on x-axis). This may go along with a considerable increase in neural activity during the resting state (as seen in relation to the y-axis). Now the brain encounters a specific stimulus, an actual input, that is compared and matched with the predicted input, thereby yielding the prediction error; this presupposes rest–stimulus interaction (see third from left on x-axis). That, in turn, yields activity changes in the resting-state activity level, which result in what is described as stimulus-induced activity (most right on x-axis). Behaviorally, such stimulus-induced activity may then be associated with the assignment of value to the stimulus.

that even the unconscious, at least in the sense of the cognitive unconscious (see Volume II, introduction II) is still tied to the (implicit) mental representation of specific objects. This, however, is not the case in seeking that, as described earlier, neither presupposes any specific value (as associated with an object) nor any kind of cue.

If so, seeking, being value- and cue-free, cannot be considered unconscious and implicit in the same sense as Berridge characterizes his concept of "wanting" as unconscious: seeking does not presuppose yet any objects or a particular value in either a physical or mental way. This is different in 'wanting' where an object and its related value are presupposed in an implicit and purely mental way. Accordingly, seeking seems to consequently presuppose a more basic form of the unconscious, one that may reach more deeply into the kind of unconscious Sigmund Freud and other psychoanalysts described when they use the concept of the "dynamic unconscious (see Northoff 2011; Panksepp 1998).

Neuronal hypothesis IIIa: Neuronal mechanisms of "seeking" and "wanting"

So far, I have discussed only behavioral ingredients of reward, seeking and "wanting," while leaving out the underlying neuronal processes. Both seeking and "wanting" are supposed to be generated by neural activity in the reward system, including the VTA, the VS, and the VMPFC. Such a regional characterization leaves open, however, the exact mechanisms of where such neural activity comes from. As is clear in both cases, the neural activity cannot come from the actual input, the actual stimulus, since that would be to neglect their occurrence prior to the onset of the rewarding stimulus.

Where does the neural activity associated with seeking and "wanting" come from? The advocate of "wanting" may want to argue that it is induced by the cue that triggers the activation of the object-associated motivational value and thus the associated "wanting." Such triggering does depend, of course, on both the cue itself, the strength of the associated value, and the internal state of the organism whether it is, for instance, hungry or not.

However, as the seeking proponent argues, even the cue and its effects presuppose some prior neural activity; otherwise the cue could not modulate anything and produce the kind of neural activity changes that are associated with "wanting." In short, "wanting" may presuppose seeking not only behaviorally, but also neuronally.

The search for the neural mechanisms underlying seeking and "wanting" converges with my quest for the neuronal mechanisms underlying the generation of the predicted input. Based on the first hypothesis in this chapter, I propose the following. I hypothesize that what Panksepp describes as seeking may be mediated by the continuous changes in the resting-state activity and its neuronal statistics; while "wanting" may be related to the interaction between the resting state's neuronal statistics and the cue-related "as-if exteroceptive stimulus" and its "as-if natural statistics" (see earlier for details).

Neuronal hypothesis IIIb: Resting state and behavior

We so far discussed the neuronal mechanisms that underlie seeking and wanting. This however left open one central question. How is it possible that the cue-triggered matching and comparison between the resting state's neuronal statistics and the as-if exteroceptive stimulus and its as-if natural statistics, can yield some kind of behavioral manifestation; that is, "wanting"? And how it is possible that the mere resting-state activity and its neuronal statistics generate a behavioral manifestation; namely, "seeking"?

These questions touch upon a deeper and more basic issue. The question here is why and how neuronal states are associated with behavioral states at all. Considered in a purely logical world (that is, as detached from the natural and thus actual world), one could imagine plenty of ongoing neural activity that is not associated with any kind of behavior. Neuronal activity and behavioral manifestation would then be decoupled or dissociated from each other. There seems to be indeed some empirical support for such dissociation between neuronal activity and behavioral manifestation: patients in vegetative state show stimulus- and task-related activity which however, unlike in healthy subjects, does not translate into behavioral activity (see Chapter 28 and 29 in Volume II for details).

What predisposes our brain to associate its own neuronal states with behavioral states? I postulate that the encoding of both neuronal statistics and the "as-if natural statistics" in terms of spatial and temporal differences may be central here. Only by encoding spatial and temporal differences into neural activity can the latter be associated with behavioral activity like seeking and wanting. I thus argue that difference-based coding is not only neuronally but also behaviorally relevant. Let us explicate this point further.

How is it possible for the neuronal activity to become associated with behavioral states like seeking and wanting? Behavior is spatiotemporally structured, meaning that it occurs across different discrete points in physical time and space. Let us now recall the characterization of the brain's intrinsic activity as discussed in Part II. There I suggested that the brain's intrinsic activity constitutes a spatiotemporal structure that is statistically based and spans across different discrete points in physical time and space.

One may now hypothesize that the spatiotemporal structure of the behavior is very much predisposed and thus made possible, that is, as a necessary (though not sufficient) condition, by the spatiotemporal structure of the brain's intrinsic activity. Let us be more specific: Any changes in the brain's resting-state activity may go along with changes in its statistically based spatiotemporal structure.

These changes in the resting state's spatiotemporal structure may signify changes in its spatiotemporal constellation or configuration. And if large enough, the changes in the resting state's spatiotemporal structures may lead to changes in the spatiotemporal configuration and position of the organism as a whole, and thus to its behavior.

NEURONAL HYPOTHESIS IIIC: SPATIOTEMPORAL CONFIGURATION OF BEHAVIOR DEPENDENCE AND THE SPATIOTEMPORAL STRUCTURE OF THE RESTING STATE

Such a change in the resting state's spatiotemporal structure may, for instance, be triggered by stimuli like exteroceptive stimuli presupposing rest–stimulus interaction (see Part IV for details). However, even a cue triggering the interaction between the resting state's neuronal statistics and the as-if exteroceptive stimulus and its as-if natural statistics may yield large enough changes in the resting state itself and its spatiotemporal structure to yield "wanting" as its behavioral manifestation. I consequently postulate that the presence of the cue is by itself not sufficient to induce the generation of the predicted input and the associated "wanting." Instead, the degree of change in the activity level of the resting state as triggered by the cue must be regarded the sufficient neural condition of "wanting."

The stronger the as-if natural statistics of the as-if exteroceptive stimulus is able the change and impact the resting state's neuronal statistics, the more likely the presentation of the cue will be associated with the generation of a behavioral state; namely, "wanting." Future studies may therefore want to probe different cues and more specifically investigate the impact of their associated "as-if natural statistics" on the neuronal statistics of the resting state.

One may also need to consider the level of the resting state itself. More specifically, different levels of resting-state activity by themselves may predispose the resting state and its associated neuronal statistics to different degrees of possible change by the cue: the more volatile and labile the resting state's neuronal statistics, the more it is prone to possible changes by the "as-if natural statistics" associated with the cue, and the more likely a behavioral state, such as "wanting", will be associated. If, in contrast, the resting state's neuronal statistics is more stable and less flexible, the less likely the as-if natural statistics will have a possible impact. And the less likely a behavioral state like "wanting" will be generated.

How about seeking? The stronger the changes in the resting state's spatiotemporal structure and its neuronal statistics, the stronger the spatiotemporal changes, and the more likely the spatiotemporal changes on the neural level will transform into changes in the spatiotemporal configuration of the organism as manifest in its behavior (like seeking).

In short, larger changes in the resting-state activity's spatiotemporal structure should go along with larger degrees of seeking.

NEUROCONCEPTUAL REMARK IA: NEURO-BEHAVIORAL ISOMORPHISM

We should, however, be fully aware that these are rather tentative neuro-behavioral hypotheses that need to be specified empirically and experimentally in the future. These tentative hypotheses imply some degree of correspondence between the changes in the resting state's spatiotemporal structure and the spatiotemporal structure of the associated behavior. Whether such a correspondence between both the resting state's change in neural activity and the behavior's spatiotemporal structures amounts to one-to-one correspondence must remain open at this point.

What do I means by "the spatiotemporal structure of behavior"? Operationally, one would suggest that the spatial and temporal coordinates and their changes across the different discrete points in physical space and time can account for the spatiotemporal structure of the behavior. This means that the spatiotemporal structure of the behavior concerns ultimately the statistical frequency distribution of the organisms' spatial and temporal coordinates in relation to the environment.

That amounts conceptually to what one may want to describe as "behavioral statistics" that refers to the statistical frequency distribution of the organisms' spatial and temporal positions and its changes in relation to the environment. In short, the spatiotemporal structure of behavior can be determined by the "behavioral statistics."

How, now, is such behavioral statistic related to the resting state's neuronal statistics? I propose that there is a certain correspondence in a yet unclear way between the neuronal statistics of the brain's resting-state activity and the organism's behavioral statistics. The better both neuronal and behavioral statistics match, the more likely it is that the neuronal state will be associated with a behavioral state. Due to such correspondence, one may conceptually be inclined to call this "neuro-behavioral isomorphism."

We have to be careful, though, concerning both, what is isomorphic and about the isomorphism itself. In general, the concept of Isomorphism implies that two distinct phenomena more or less correspond to each other in a one-to-one basis. What exactly are those two phenomena in our case of neuro-behavioral isomorphism? The isomorphism here is neither between cue/stimulus and behavior, nor between resting state and behavior. Instead, the neuro-behavioral isomorphism is assumed to consist in the correspondence between the resting state's statistically based spatiotemporal structure and the spatiotemporal structure of the behavior; i.e., its spatiotemporal coordinates. Accordingly, I postulate an isomorphism between neuronal and behavioral statistics and their respectively associated spatiotemporal structures (rather than between the resting state itself and the behavior itself).

NEUROCONCEPTUAL REMARK IB: NARROW VERSUS WIDE NEURO-BEHAVIORAL ISOMORPHISM

We also have to be careful in defining the concept of isomorphism itself. Roughly, one can understand it in a strict or narrow way, with one-to-one correspondence between both neuronal and behavioral statistics. That would basically mean that the resting-state activity itself is both a necessary and a sufficient condition of behavior, while the stimulus itself, the cue, has essentially no major impact.

Such a strict definition of isomorphism, however, is empirically implausible given that the cue does have a significant impact on behavior. The resting-state activity seems to be only a necessary but not a sufficient condition of behavior, with the stimulus, the cue, providing the sufficient condition. Instead of one-to-one correspondence, neuronal and behavioral statistics would then correspond in a one-to-many or many-to-one way. Conceptually, this implies a loose or wide rather than strict or narrow form of neuro-behavioral isomorphism.

How can we tackle the assumption of such wider or loose neuro-behavioral isomorphism in more experimental terms? One could, for instance, construct a quantifiable spatiotemporal matrix or grid from the spatiotemporal coordinates and configuration of both the changes in the resting-state activity and the associated behavior.

If the assumption of a wider or low form of neuro-behavioral isomorphism holds, one would hypothesize that the resting state's spatiotemporal structure and its neuronal statistics predict the spatiotemporal coordinates of the associated behavior and thus its "behavioral statistics." One could construct statistically based spatiotemporal trajectory maps for both behavior and the resting-state activity and see how both are related to each other.

In addition to its behavioral relevance, the resting state's neuronal statistics may also be phenomenally relevant; that is, for consciousness. As we will see in Volume II, the resting-state activity's spatiotemporal organization may predispose the association of the purely neuronal stimulus-induced activity with consciousness and its phenomenal features.

Most important, I will claim that the spatiotemporal structure of the resting-state activity resurfaces in the spatiotemporal structure of the phenomenal features that signify consciousness. There may therefore be a certain wide or loose isomorphism between the resting state's neuronal statistics and the "phenomenal statistics" of consciousness (if one wants to say so), a wide or loose neuro-phenomenal isomorphism.

Open Questions

The first question concerns the mechanisms and processes underlying the generation of the predicted input. I indicated neural overlap between high resting-state activity and predicted input generation in VMPFC and PACC, anterior midline regions. This left open the question of whether subcortical regions are also associated with generating predicted inputs.

As mentioned in Chapter 7, even a region as early involved as the primary visual cortex (and possibly subcortical regions) seems to generate some kind of predicted input during visual perception. If so, one would suggest the same to apply in the case of reward, where early resting-state processing in the subcortical regions may generate some kind of predicted input. As said earlier, the exclusive association of the predicted input with cortical regions in human imaging studies does not rule out the involvement of the subcortical regions that are rather difficult to visualize in fMRI.

In addition to subcortical regions, one may also want to investigate the neuronal mechanisms underlying the interaction between resting state and predicted input as well as the subsequent interaction between predicted and actual inputs. One may propose nonlinear mechanisms here as they are suggested by studies on rest–stimulus interaction in other functional domains such as perception (see Chapters 9–12, and 28–29 in Part IV for details). The neuronal mechanisms underlying rest–stimulus interaction will be discussed in more detail in Part IV.

Finally, one may ask what our assumption about the generation of the predicted input tells us about the brain in general. Based on the continuous changes in its resting-state activity and its spatiotemporal structure, the brain seems to continuously, almost by default in an almost unavoidable and necessary way, generate predictions or anticipations of what could possibly happen next (see Llinas and Roy 2009; Llinas et al. 1998; Linas and Ribary 2001; Deco et al. 2009, 2010, 2011). One may consequently say that the brain generates a "hypothesis" about its environment: "In more general terms, one might ask if such intrinsic cortical states represent the brain's 'current hypothesis' about the state of the external world" (Ringach 2003, 913).

Therefore, Gustavo Deco et al. (2009), a Spanish neural network expert and his colleagues, compare the brain's resting state to a tennis player awaiting his opponent's serve: the tennis player makes small moves and steps along the lines in order to bring himself into the best possible position to return the serve he expects. Analogously, the brain continuously changes its resting-state activity and its associated spatiotemporal structure in small increments in order to prepare itself for possible changes in the spatiotemporal configuration of the environment. Behaviorally, such continuous changes result in seeking, while even stronger changes in the resting state and its associated spatiotemporal structure can be triggered by specific cues that then may lead to "wanting."

Notes

1. Interestingly, Carhart-Harris and Friston (2010) associate this hierarchical model with Freud's psychodynamic concepts of id and ego as well

as with primary and secondary processes. They argue that the top-down control of the highest level, the DMN, over the subsequent lower levels corresponds to the ego, binds energy, and is associated with secondary processes, while the lowest level of the hierarchy is related to the id, free energy, and primary processes. Both interact with each other in that DMN suppresses the limbic regions in very much the same way the ego and its secondary processes contain the id and its primary processes by binding their free energy (Carhart-Harris and Friston 2010, 3, 7, 11, 11–12). This, however, is not the topic of this book; it is dealt with in my recent book *Neuropsychoanalysis in Practice* (Northoff 2011).

2. Although Panksepp used all capital letters in his terminology ("SEEKING"), we will use lowercase letters herein.

PART IV
Encoding Extrinsic Activity

General background

The starting point of this volume was how the brain encodes extrinsic stimuli from the environment, discussed in Part I. This revealed that the stimuli's statistical frequency distribution across different discrete points in physical time and space—that is, their natural statistics—is encoded into the neural activity of the neurons and the regions, rather than the stimuli themselves at their particular points in physical time and space. Since this allows for coding many stimuli into one particular neural activity, such a coding strategy is referred to as *sparse coding*.

Sparse coding describes the spatial and temporal sparsening of neural activity and, I claim, is only possible on the basis of encoding spatial and temporal differences between different stimuli at their different discrete points in physical time and space. Such difference-based coding is to be distinguished from stimulus-based coding that describes the encoding of the extrinsic stimuli themselves at their different discrete points in physical time and space a. In short, sparse coding presupposes difference-based coding rather than stimulus-based coding.

We then moved on from the environment and its extrinsic stimuli to the brain itself and its intrinsic activity. The brain's intrinsic activity and its spatial and temporal structure were the subjects of Part II. The constitution of such statistically based spatiotemporal structure is possible only when the brain's encodes its own intrinsic activity in terms of spatial and temporal differences and in a sparse way thus presupposing difference-based coding and sparse coding. Accordingly, the brain applies the same coding principles to its own intrinsic activity as to the extrinsic stimuli.

How are such difference-based coding and sparse coding realized? Based on single-cell and population data as well as on regional evidence, I postulate that neural inhibition and GABA play a major role in the encoding of the intrinsic activity's spatial and temporal differences that reflect the statistical frequency distribution of its own activity across different discrete points in physical time and space. This, in turn, makes it possible for the intrinsic activity to constitute a spatiotemporal structure that is statistically based rather than reflecting the biophysical-computational features of the neurons/regions themselves.

What does brain's intrinsic activity and its spatiotemporal structure imply in functional terms? The continuous changes in the neural activity and the spatiotemporal structure of the brain's intrinsic activity may be manifested in what we describe as predictions or anticipations of possible actual inputs, the predicted input. This is the assumption of predictive coding as discussed in Part III.

Predictive coding claims the neural activity results from the matching and comparison between predicted and actual inputs, thereby yielding what is described as prediction error.

The prediction error is based on the difference between predicted and actual input, whose degree is supposed to determine the degree of stimulus-induced activity associated with the actual input. This means that the prediction error and its associated stimulus-induced activity are difference-based signals, which, as such, presuppose difference-based coding.

We have so far described various mechanisms the brain itself applies to the neural processing of both extrinsic stimuli and its intrinsic activity. This concerns especially the coding strategy and the intrinsic activity: the brain encodes changes into its neural activity in terms of spatial and temporal differences, amounting to difference-based coding (and sparse coding) as distinguished from stimulus-based coding (and local/dense coding) (Part I). And the brain generates and organizes its own intrinsic activity in terms of a virtual statistically based spatiotemporal structure (Part II) that continuously changes and generates predictive coding (Part III).

Since both encoding strategy and intrinsic activity have their origins in the brain itself and, most importantly, define its particular way of neural processing, they may be described as intrinsic features of the brain that define the brain (see Introduction in Volume II for further details on the distinction between intrinsic and extrinsic features of the brain). These intrinsic features of the brain were the main focus in Parts I through III.

The brain's intrinsic features must be distinguished from its extrinsic features, which have their origin outside the brain and do therefore not define the brain's particular way of encoding its neural activity and its neural processing. Such extrinsic features of the brain concern (for example) its stimulus-induced activity (or task-related activity) as related to extrinsic stimuli (and tasks) from outside the brain that originate in either body or environment. These extrinsic features of the brain and thus its extrinsic stimulus-induced activity will be the focus in the final part of this volume, Part IV.

General overview

How do the brain's intrinsic features, the encoding of the stimuli's natural statistics and the brain's intrinsic activity (including its predictive coding), impact the extrinsic features of the brain, its stimulus-induced activity as associated with particular stimuli or tasks? This is the focus of Part IV.

The central question here is the following: How does the brain itself provide the transition from its own intrinsic activity, the resting-state activity, to its extrinsic activity, the stimulus-induced activity as elicited by extrinsic stimuli from outside the brain? To address this question, I will investigate how different extrinsic stimuli interact with each other in the brain and what we can learn from that for the interaction between the extrinsic stimuli and the brain's intrinsic activity.

Chapter 10's focus is on the interaction of different extrinsic stimuli in the neural activity of the brain, i.e., stimulus–stimulus interaction. For that purpose, I take cross-modal interaction as the paradigm. This reveals functional principles like spatial and temporal coincidence, inverse effectiveness, and nonlinearity that guide stimulus–stimulus interaction and its subsequent stimulus-induced activity in cross-modal interaction. These functional principles presuppose difference-based coding of cross-modal interaction, which otherwise, in the case of stimulus-based coding, would remain impossible. Finally, various objections to difference-based coding during stimulus–stimulus interaction and stimulus-induced activity as well as different possible coding strategies are discussed here.

Chapter 11 focuses on the application of these functional principles to the interaction of the extrinsic stimulus with the brain's intrinsic activity; that is, rest–stimulus interaction. Based on recent findings, I show how the preceding resting state impacts subsequent stimulus-induced activity so that there is direct interaction between resting-state and stimulus-induced activity. Such direct interaction between intrinsic and extrinsic activity is supposed to be possible only on the basis of encoding of spatial and temporal differences into the resulting stimulus-induced activity.

This presupposes difference-based coding rather than stimulus-based coding of the brain's extrinsic activity, its stimulus-induced activity, in the same way as it applies to the brain's intrinsic activity. Due to the application of the same coding strategy (difference-based coding), there is a neuronal continuum between the brain's intrinsic and extrinsic activity and thus between resting state and stimulus-induced activity (see Appendix 1 for further details of this "continuity hypothesis").

Chapter 12 focuses on the coding of stimulus-induced activity and more specifically on neural inhibition and sparse coding of rest–stimulus interaction. How is difference-based coding implemented during the rest–stimulus interaction? This leads us back to neural inhibition as mediated by GABA as discussed in previous parts (see Chapters 3 and 6).

Recent findings demonstrate that GABA seems to mediate the transition from resting-state to stimulus-induced activity with the latter's degree being directly dependent upon the degree of former, that is, GABAergic-mediated neural inhibition. This, in turn, makes the encoding of spatial and temporal differences, i.e., difference-based coding, into the resulting stimulus-induced activity unavoidable and thus necessary. That results consequently in the spatial and temporal sparsening of the spatiotemporal activity pattern as observed during stimulus-induced activity, thus reflecting sparse coding on a regional level of neural activity.

CHAPTER 10
Stimulus–Stimulus Interaction and Neural Coding

Summary

The brain receives continuous exteroceptive input from the environment. Thereby various stimuli with different features occur at the same time. This raises the question for the kind of neuronal mechanisms that underlie the interaction between the different exteroceptive stimuli, that is, stimulus–stimulus interaction, in the brain's neural activity during stimulus-induced activity. I here take cross-modal interaction to be a paradigmatic example of such stimulus–stimulus interaction. Based on recent empirical data, this reveals four principles: spatial and temporal coincidence, inverse effectiveness, and nonlinearity. The implementation of these four principles in guiding neural activity during cross-modal interaction is presumed to be possible only by the encoding of spatial and temporal differences into neural activity. This presupposes difference-based coding, because such cross-modal interaction would remain impossible in the case of stimulus-based coding. Such difference-based coding can be exemplified, for example, in the temporal dimension where it allows for the alignment of the ongoing oscillatory phase to the temporal onsets of the stimuli across time; this is described as "phase resetting." Finally, based on recent data, I discuss possible objections to difference-based coding in both the spatial and temporal dimensions of stimulus-induced activity. This reveals not only the high degree of empirical plausibility of difference-based coding, but also its encoding of both spatial and temporal dimensions in an integrated way. Difference-based coding can consequently be characterized as a statistically based spatiotemporal encoding strategy that codes and determines the brain's extrinsic activity, its stimulus-induced activity.

Key Concepts and Topics Covered

Cross-modal interaction, spatial and temporal coincidence, nonlinearity, inverse effectiveness, phase resetting, higher order cognitive top-down modulation, parallel coding strategies, unifying coding strategy, difference-based coding, spatiotemporal coding strategy

Neuroempirical background: Encoding and resting-state activity precede stimulus-induced activity

In Part I, we investigated how the brain encodes extrinsic stimuli from the environment by focusing on sparse coding as a variant of difference-based coding. The same principles of neural coding— sparse coding and difference-based coding—were then shown to also hold in the case of the brain's intrinsic activity, its resting state (see Part II). That, in turn, made it possible for the brain to predict inputs and thus to anticipate signals as it has been discussed in the context of predictive coding (see Part III).

What happens if such a brain, which is equipped with different-based coding of its resting-state activity and prediction of inputs, actually encounters a real-life stimulus from the outside the brain, the environment (or the body, which is completely neglected in our account here; see Chapter 32 in Volume II)? In other words, we are now ready to "finally" turn our attention to stimulus-induced activity (or task-related activity, which conceptually will be subsumed in the following discussion under the term "stimulus-induced activity").

Why "finally"? I say here deliberately "finally" because usually stimulus-induced activity is considered the starting point for any neuroscientific investigation and its exploration of the neural basis of sensory, motor, cognitive, affective, and social functions. As already discussed in the introduction in this volume (see also Appendix 1 in Volume II), I consider the sensory, motor, affective, cognitive, and social functions of the brain and their respective extrinsic activity, stimulus-induced (or task-related) activity, to be dependent on the brain's intrinsic activity and its particular coding strategy.

This made it necessary to first discuss the brain's intrinsic activity in detail; namely, its encoding strategy and its intrinsic activity. These intrinsic features may then set the stage for the brain's processing of the subsequent extrinsic stimuli from the environment (and body), including the associated sensory, motor, affective, cognitive, and social functions. Since I discussed the brain's intrinsic features in detail in Parts I through III, I can now "finally" revert to the brain's extrinsic functions, its stimulus-induced activity as related to sensory, motor, affective, cognitive, and social functions.

Neurometaphorical excursion I: prelude and fugue

Let us compare the situation to a prelude and fugue. In a musical piece, the prelude sets the stage for the subsequent fugue. The same now holds in the case of the brain's intrinsic and extrinsic features. The brain's intrinsic features, its encoding strategy and its intrinsic activity, set the stage for any subsequent neural processing of extrinsic stimuli from outside the brain.

What do I mean by "setting the stage"? I mean that the brain's encoding strategy and intrinsic activity determine the kind and degree of stimulus-induced activity that extrinsic stimuli (or tasks) can possibly trigger in the brain. In the same way as a particular prelude excludes (or better) predisposes particular keys and harmonies in the subsequent fugue, the brain's encoding strategy and intrinsic activity prevent or facilitate certain ways in the subsequent neural processing of extrinsic stimuli and their associated stimulus-induced activity.

Accordingly, the brain's intrinsic features, its coding strategy and intrinsic activity, can be considered the prelude for the subsequent fugue, the brain's extrinsic features as related to stimulus-induced activity. After having extensively worked on the prelude itself, I am now "finally" ready for the fugue and thus to discuss the brain's extrinsic features; namely, stimulus-induced activity. This will be the focus in this chapter.

Neuronal findings IA: cross-modal interaction

After my prelude, I come back to empirical matters: more specifically, to stimulus-induced activity. Even stimulus-induced activity is not as simple as we often think. What we as neuroscientists observe as stimulus-induced activity does not usually reflect simply the neural activity elicited by a single stimulus in a one-to-one way. Instead, what we describe as stimulus-induced activity results usually from the interaction between different stimuli and their respective features. This means that stimulus-induced activity implies the interaction between different stimuli and features, that is, stimulus–stimulus interaction.

In the following I want to investigate the mechanisms and processes underlying stimulus–stimulus interaction in both spatial and temporal detail. For that, I take cross-modal interaction, the interaction between stimuli from different sensory modalities as the paradigmatic example of stimulus–stimulus interaction.

What is cross-modal interaction? Interaction between exteroceptive stimuli from different sensory modality (auditory, visual, olfactory, somatosensory, gustatory) are subsumed under the umbrella term "cross-modal interaction." The traditional view is that the different sensory cortex themselves are unimodal, meaning they only process stimuli from one particular modality. For instance, the auditory modality only processes auditory stimuli, the visual modality visual stimuli, and the same applies to the remaining sensory modalities.

Interaction and integration between stimuli from different sensory modalities are traditionally associated with higher-order regions in either subcortical (like the superior colliculi) or mainly cortical (intraparietal cortex, the premotor cortex, the lateral prefrontal cortex, and the superior temporal sulcus) regions. Since these higher-order regions allow for the integration between the stimuli from the different sensory modalities, one may describe the traditional view as "higher-order view."

The traditional higher-order view of cross-modal interaction is challenged, however, by recent results that show cross-modal interaction already in auditory and visual cortex itself. For instance, using electroencephalography (EEG), Murray et al. (2005) observed that electrophysiological potentials, auditory-evoked potentials, in auditory cortex evoked by an auditory tone were enhanced by a simultaneous somatosensory stimulus.

Moreover, this enhancement occurred rather early, 50ms after stimulus onset, which makes it rather likely that it is related to neural activity in the auditory cortex rather than elsewhere like in prefrontal cortex, in which case it would occur later, like after 100–200ms. These findings suggest that auditory-somatosensory interaction must have taken place in the auditory cortex itself. However, while EEG studies provide excellent temporal resolution, their spatial resolution remains weak, meaning that exact localization of cross-modal interactions in the auditory cortex cannot be inferred from the EEG data alone. This means that we need to consider both spatial and temporal dimensions in cross-modal interaction and thus results from both EEG and fMRI.

I will focus in this section mainly on the work by C. Kayser and N. Logothetis, who describe different principles of cross-modal interaction (see Kayser and Logothetis 2007; see also subsequent studies confirming and refining those principles: Kayser et al. 2010; Lurilli et al. 2012 with a commentary by Kayser and Remedios 2012; Kayser 2010 commenting on Lemus et al. 2010; Panzeri et al. 2010). Later sections will discuss the cross-modal interaction studies by Schroeder and Lakatos (2009). I am well aware that this leaves out many others' work, but given our focus on the main principles, we need to concentrate on a few paradigms.

In addition to the many other authors' findings on cross-modal interaction, we also leave out the observations in the context of synaesthesia, where two (or more) sensory modalities are experienced in conjunction. As said earlier, the main idea here is to elucidate general functional principles of stimulus–stimulus interaction, which then later, in Chapter 11, shall be applied to rest–stimulus interaction.

Neuronal findings Ib: "Principle of nonlinearity"

In his earlier work, Kayser et al. (2005) conducted functional magnetic imaging (fMRI) studies in measuring auditory cortical activity in monkeys while applying both tactile and auditory stimuli. The auditory cortex showed activity during auditory stimuli alone and a weaker response when tactile stimuli were applied in isolation.

Most important, responses in auditory cortex (primary and predominantly secondary auditory cortex, the so-called "auditory belt") were enhanced when both stimuli, auditory and tactile, were presented simultaneously. Such enhancement concerned both spatial extension, that is, the activated cortical volume, as well as the strength (i.e., signal percent change) of the activation in auditory cortex.

How can we describe such cross-modal enhancement in more detail? First, the enhancement of auditory cortical activity, that is, strength and extension, was stronger than the mere addition or sum of both auditory and tactile activities alone as measured independent of each other. The enhanced activity can consequently not result from mere superposition, that is, linear addition or summation, of both activities but rather from their specific interaction.

Such interaction must consequently be characterized as nonadditive and nonlinear. This is what Kayser et al. (2005) (as well as Kayser and Logothetis 2007) describe as "the principle of nonlinearity." The principle of nonlinearity describes that the resulting stimulus-induced activity during two (or more) stimuli cannot be traced back to the merely linear addition or summation of each stimulus' stimulus-induced activity by itself. Instead, there must be some interaction between the different stimuli that makes it possible for the resulting stimulus-induced activity to be either higher or lower than the mere linear summation or addition of the different stimuli's stimulus-induced activities (see Fig. 10-1a).

How is such nonlinearity in cross-modal interaction realized and implemented? This leads me to the second principle, the "principle of spatial co incidence."

Neuronal findings Ic: "Principle of spatial coincidence"

One important measure is the spatial dimension, meaning the spatial extension of the activated cortical volumes. The cortical volumes recruited during combined auditory-tactile stimulation were far greater than the mere sum or addition of the cortical volumes obtained during auditory and tactile stimulation alone. The extension of cortical volumes during cross-modal interaction was particularly strong in the regions of the auditory belt, the secondary or association auditory cortex, whereas it was rather weak in primary auditory cortex.

The observation of such cross-modal enhancement is in accordance with observations that the secondary auditory cortex does indeed receive afferents from somatosensory cortex as related to the processing of tactile stimuli. The somatosensory afferents in auditory cortex make then possible the larger spatial extension of the neural activity during simultaneous presentation of tactile and auditory stimuli, thus accounting for what Kayser et al. (2005; see also Kayser and Logothetis 2007) refer to as the "principle of spatial coincidence" (see also Kayser et al. 2010; Lurilli et al. 2012 with a commentary by Kayser and Remedios 2012; Kayser 2010 commenting on Lemus et al. 2010).How can we define the "principle of spatial coincidence"? The "principle of spatial coincidence" describes that the interaction between the interacting stimuli nonlinearly enhances the degree of spatial extension in the resulting stimulus-induced activity beyond their mere linear spatial addition or summation. This leads me to the following assumption: the more two stimuli overlap, or coincide, in their spatial extension, the more the stimulus-induced activity resulting from their interaction will be spatially extended in a nonlinear way (see Fig. 10-1b).

Neuronal findings Id: "Principle of temporal coincidence"

The same study also tested how the temporal relationship between auditory and tactile stimuli affects the cross-modal enhancement in auditory cortex. They applied both auditory and tactile stimuli in either a synchronous or asynchronous way. Both forms of application led to enhancement of activity in the auditory cortex when compared to auditory and tactile stimuli alone.

However, the cross-modal enhancement in auditory cortex was significantly stronger during the synchronous application when compared to the asynchronous one. This means that temporally coincident auditory and tactile stimuli show stronger cross-modal interaction when compared to temporally noncoincident ones.

Most generally, these results show that the temporal relationship between different stimuli is crucial for their interaction and thus for their mutual enhancement. The authors here speak of the "principle of temporal coincidence." The "principle of temporal coincidence" describes that the temporal overlap between the interacting stimuli nonlinearly enhances the strength of the resulting stimulus-induced activity beyond their mere linear addition or summation (see Fig. 10-1c).

This leads to the following assumption: the more two stimuli overlap, that is, coincide, temporally, the stronger the stimulus-induced activity resulting from their interaction (see also Kayser et al. 2010; Lurilli et al. 2012 with a commentary by Kayser and Remedios 2012; Kayser 2010 commenting on Lemus et al. 2010).

Neuronal Findings Ie: "Principle of Inverse Effectiveness"

Finally, the authors also tested how the strength of auditory stimuli may affect their degree of

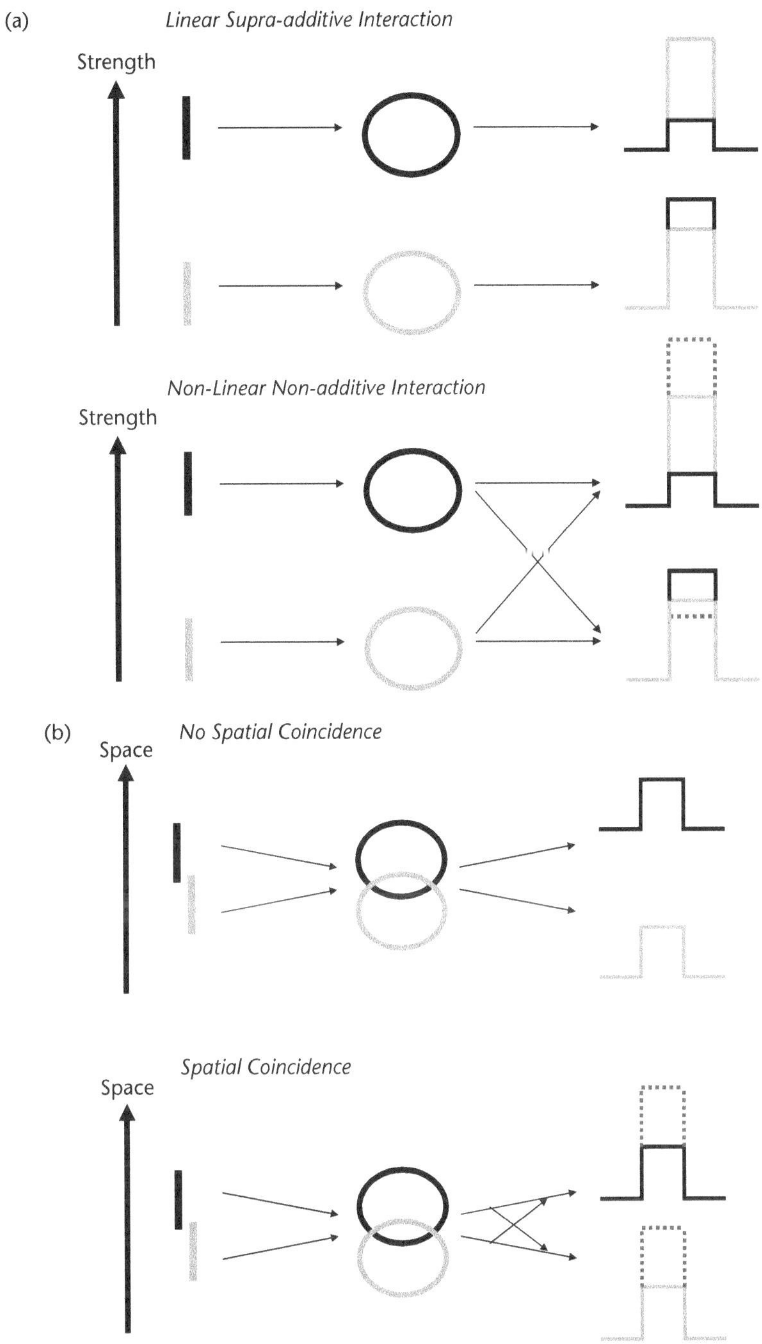

Figure 10-1a, b, c, and d **Neuronal principles of stimulus–stimulus interaction. The figure shows a graphic illustration of the different principles (*a*–*d*) of how different stimuli interact with each other. The stimuli are shown on the very left in forms of bars; the circles in the middle stand for the regions in the brain. Finally, the bars on the very right indicate the degree of neural activity elicited by the stimulus after it interacted with the region's activity related to the respective other stimulus. Grey and black lines indicate the contributions of the respective stimulus to the degree of neural activity. The remaining part (dotted lines) indicates the part of neural activity that cannot be traced back directly to either stimulus by itself; instead it can result only from the interaction between the stimuli as indicated by the crossing arrows (second from the right). (*a*): This figure describes the principle of nonlinearity. The interaction consists of merely adding (or subtracting) the other' stimulus' contribution to the other region's neural**

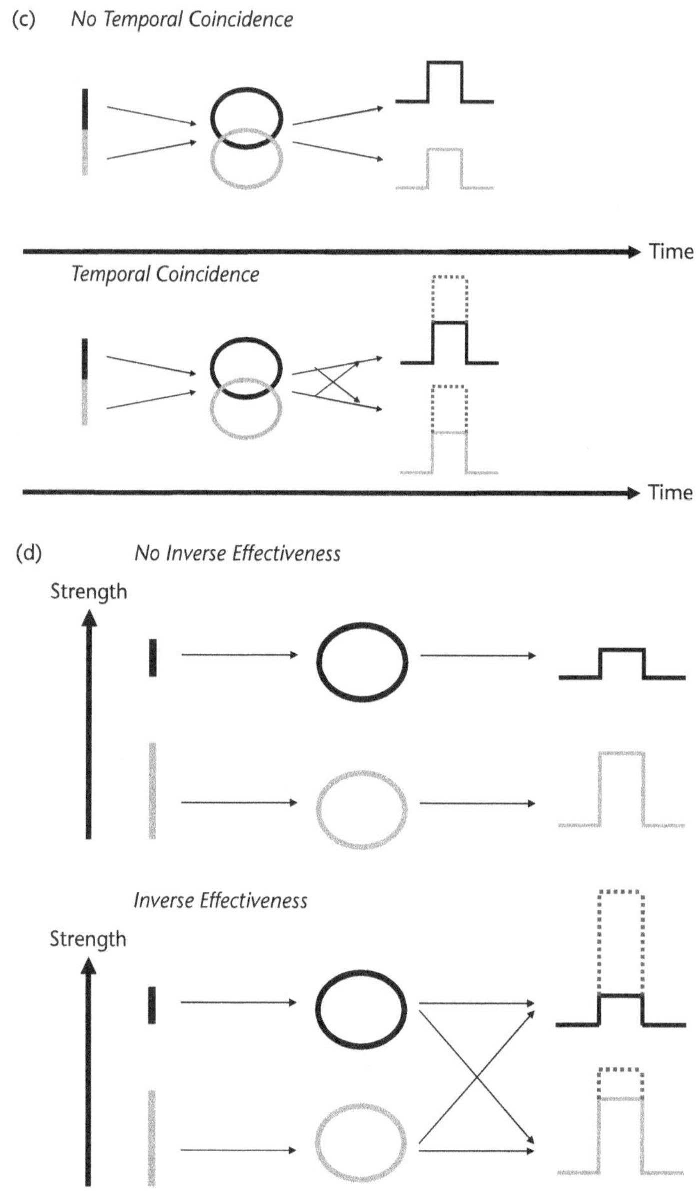

activity, resulting in nonlinear interaction (*upper part*). Or the region's activity is either higher or lower than the mere addition (or subtraction) of the neural activity related to both stimuli, implying nonlinear interaction (*lower part*).(*b*): The figure describes the principle of spatial coincidence. If the two stimuli overlap in space, their respective region's neural activity may also overlap, leading to an increase in their neural activity as indicated by the red part (*lower part*). However, such an increase cannot be observed in the absence of spatial coincidence between the two spatial stimuli (*upper part*).(*c*): The figure describes the principle of temporal coincidence. If the two stimuli overlap in time, their respective region's neural activity may also overlap temporally, leading to an increase in their neural activity as indicated by the red part (*lower part*). However, such an increase cannot be observed in the absence of temporal coincidence between the two spatial stimuli (*upper part*).(*d*): The figure describes the principle of inverse effectiveness. If one of the stimuli is strong and the other is weak (inverse strength), both regions' neural activity may be stronger than being related to the stimulus alone as indicated by the red part (*lower part*). However, such an increase in neural activity remains absent if there is no inverse effectiveness (*upper part*).

cross-modal interaction with tactile stimuli. They presented weaker and stronger auditory stimuli with the one being 10 db louder than the other one. As expected, the weaker stimuli induced less activity in the auditory cortex than the stronger ones when presented alone.

This pattern, however, reversed during cross-modal interaction. In conjunction with the tactile stimulus, the weaker auditory stimulus elicited stronger cross-modal interaction effects, that is, a larger cortical volume and a higher strength, than the stronger one. This means that a weaker stimulus elicits stronger cross-modal interaction than a stronger one, thus obeying the "principle of inverse effectiveness," as Kayser et al. (2005) call it.

The "principle of inverse effectiveness" describes that the interaction between different stimuli depends on the integrated constellation of their strength rather than on the mere summation or addition of their respective strengths alone. The degree of interaction between different stimuli is strongest when one stimulus' strength is weak, while the other stimulus is rather strong. If, in contrast, both interacting stimuli are strong, their interaction may become rather weak. Hence, the constellation between the two stimuli has to be inverse, that is, weak and strong, for the interaction to be strong (see Fig. 10-1d).

One may postulate four principles guiding and underlying the interaction between different stimuli, or stimulus–stimulus interaction, during cross-modal interaction (see Kayser and Logothetis 2007, 122–123). The four principles are nonlinearity, spatial coincidence, temporal coincidence, and inverse effectiveness. We now want to know how compatible they are with difference-based coding; this is the focus in the next sections.

Neuronal hypothesis Ia: Nonlinear cross-modal interaction and difference-based coding

How are these principles of cross-modal interaction related to difference-based coding? I hypothesize that all four principles are possible only on the basis of encoding spatial and temporal differences into the resulting stimulus-induced activity during cross-modal interaction. Accordingly, I propose cross-modal interaction to presuppose difference-based coding rather than stimulus-based coding.

Let me be more specific. Cross-modal interaction does not refer to merely additive and thus linear effects in the interaction between different sensory stimuli. Instead, the effects are supra-additive and nonlinear and can therefore not be explained by the mere addition of the activations elicited by each stimulus alone. This means that what is encoded into the neural activity underlying cross-modal interaction cannot result from the mere addition of the neural activities associated with each of the stimuli alone.

Such addition or summation would, for instance, be possible if the stimuli were encoded into neural activity separately and independent of each other as it is implied by stimulus-based coding. Stimulus-based coding in this sense seems to be presupposed in the traditional view of cross-modal interaction. Here the sensory regions are suggested to encode the respective unimodal stimuli themselves in isolation and independence of the other sensory stimuli, thus presupposing stimulus-based coding in sensory cortex. That, however, is not compatible with the data that suggest nonlinear interaction rather than mere addition or summation.

What, however, must be encoded into the neural activity of the sensory cortex to make possible the nonlinear interaction as it is observed during cross-modal interaction? I hypothesize that such supra-additive nonlinear effects are possible only if the spatial and temporal differences, rather than the mere addition between the two stimuli, are encoded into neural activity.

Rather than the sum of the activities of each stimulus alone, the spatial and temporal difference between both determines and predicts the subsequent degree of stimulus-induced activity. The stimulus-induced activity thus presupposes difference-based coding rather than stimulus-based coding.

Neuronal hypothesis Ib: Encoding of temporal differences during cross-modal interaction

Let us specify such difference-based coding in spatial and temporal regard: the less the two stimuli overlap in their respective temporal position (i.e., at their respective discrete point in physical time), the weaker their possible interaction effects. This means that the temporal difference between the two stimuli must be encoded; otherwise the degree of their interaction could not be dependent on the stimuli's degree of temporal difference (see Brasselet et al. 2012; Kayser et al. 2010 for first empirical support).

How would two temporally differing stimuli be encoded in the case of stimulus-based coding? In the contrasting case of stimulus-based coding, such dependence of the interaction effects on the degree of the stimulus' degree of temporal difference would be impossible. This is so because the temporal position of each stimulus would then be encoded independently and isolated of each other. Whether the two stimuli overlap temporally or not, would not matter at all anymore. The degree of their temporal difference would no longer impact the degree of the subsequent stimulus-induced activity (see later discussion of objections to my hypothesis of difference-based coding).

This is clearly different in the case of difference-based coding. Unlike in stimulus-based coding, the degree of the stimuli's temporal difference matters very much for their possible degree of interaction: the smaller their temporal difference, the more likely their interaction will proceed in a nonlinear way, and the higher the degree of the subsequent stimulus-induced activity.

If, in contrast, their temporal difference is rather large, the more both stimuli will interact in a linear rather than nonlinear way and the lower the subsequent stimulus-induced activity. Accordingly, the degree of temporal difference is central in determining the degree of nonlinearity during cross-modal interaction, including the respectively associated stimulus-induced activity.

Neuronal hypothesis Ic: Encoding of spatial differences during cross-modal interaction

How about difference-based coding in the spatial domain? I propose that, as in the temporal domain, differences are also encoded in the spatial domain. The above-described results showed the "principal of spatial coincidence." Very much like in the temporal domain, the degree of spatial difference between different stimuli may determine the degree of possible nonlinearity during their interaction and consequently the degree of their stimulus-induced activity.

This again contrasts with the case of stimulus-based coding. In the contrasting case of stimulus-based coding the degree of spatial differences between the respective stimuli and their respectively underlying neurons would not matter at all: either they overlap spatially and allow for cross-modal interaction, or they do not overlap spatially at all, implying the complete absence of any cross-modal interaction effects.

This, however, is not compatible with the empirical data. I consequently hypothesize that neural activity must be encoded in terms of spatial differences, that is, difference-based coding, in order for the principle of spatial coincidence to be possible and thus to hold true.

Neuronal hypothesis Id: Inverse effectiveness presupposes difference-based coding

We so far have shown that three principles of nonlinearity and spatial and temporal coincidence are not only quite compatible with difference-based coding but that, in the opposite case of stimulus-based coding, they would remain impossible. How about the fourth principle, the principle of inverse effectiveness?

I suppose that, like the other three principles, the principle of inverse effectiveness also presupposes difference- rather than stimulus-based coding. If stimulus-based coding holds, one would expect the mere summation of the two stimuli's strength to elicit stronger stimulus-induced activity during stimulus–stimulus interaction. In that case, two strong stimuli should induce the strongest neural activity. This, however, was not the case, as the data show.

Instead, the constellation of a strong with a weak stimulus showed the strongest interaction effects. This is possible only if the difference in strength between the two stimuli is encoded into neural activity rather than the strength of each stimulus alone independent of the respective other (as in stimulus-based coding). In short, the principle of inverse effectiveness is possible only if presupposing difference-based coding rather than stimulus-based coding.

Taken together, I hypothesize that the four principles of cross-modal interaction are not only compatible with difference-based coding but, even stronger, that they must presuppose it in order to be possible. This holds for the principles of spatial and temporal coincidence that presuppose difference-based coding in spatial and temporal domains and the associated principle of nonlinearity. And it holds for the principle of inverse effectiveness that must presuppose nonlinear interaction as it is possible only on the basis of difference-based coding as distinguished from stimulus-based coding (see later for objections to my hypothesis of difference-based coding).

Neuronal hypothesis IE: nonlinearity and consciousness

Why do I emphasize so much the linkage of both spatial and temporal coincidence and inverse effectiveness with nonlinear changes in neural activity? I showed that increases in spatial and/or temporal coincidence are relevant in that they go along with higher degrees of both nonlinearity and subsequent stimulus-induced activity. This pertains to the neuronal relevance of nonlinearity.

In addition to its mere neuronal relevance, the nonlinearity may also be relevant for consciousness and thus phenomenally relevant. I suppose that the degree of nonlinearity predicts not only the degree of the purely neuronal stimulus-induced activity but also the degree to which the latter can be associated with consciousness and its phenomenal features.

In order to fully understand this, we need to go back to the brain's intrinsic activity and its interaction with extrinsic stimuli. The more the extrinsic stimuli coincide temporally and spatially with the spatiotemporal structure of the brain's intrinsic activity, the more likely it is that both extrinsic stimuli and intrinsic activity will interact in a nonlinear way. And the higher the degree of their interaction, the more likely it is that the resulting purely neuronal stimulus-induced activity will be associated with consciousness. The neuronal details of such nonlinear rest–stimulus interaction will be discussed in the next chapter, Chapter 11, while the exact neuro-phenomenal mechanisms will be explored in Chapters 28 and 29 in Volume II.

Neurometaphorical excursion IIA: sidewalk and stimuli

After having discussed stimulus-induced activity by the example of cross-modal interaction and its coding strategy, I am now ready to investigate the impact of the resting state on subsequent stimulus-induced activity. This will be the focus in Chapter 11. First, though, let me briefly illustrate the four principles of cross-model interaction in particular and stimulus–stimulus interaction in general by the following metaphorical comparison.

Imagine that two persons are walking down a street. If the street is large, containing four lanes, there may be sidewalks on both sides. If the two persons walk on the different sides and their respective sidewalks, there is almost no chance for them to meet and interact.

Now imagine they walk on the same side on the same sidewalk; however, the sidewalks are big and the number of people walking is large. The two persons walking on the opposing ends of the same sidewalk have almost no chance to meet and interact with each other within the crowds pushing through the sidewalk.

Let's now imagine that the very same sidewalk is almost empty and thus devoid of people, while both persons are still walking on the sidewalk's opposite ends. Even though neither person has changed her spatiotemporal coordinates, the chance of them meeting is now much higher than before.

Why? Because now their respective spatiotemporal position can more easily be directly related to the one of the respective other than before, where their relationship could at best be indirect that is through the other people. This means that the actual spatiotemporal position of one person is encoded into the relationship and thus relative spatial and temporal difference from the ones of the respective other(s).

I do not need to say that this is exactly what happens in the brain during cross-modal interaction. The more directly both persons can be connected and linked to each other in spatial and temporal regard, the more likely they will meet, thus presupposing the "principles of spatial and temporal coincidence."

NEUROMETAPHORICAL EXCURSION IIB: STAGE AND BRAIN

Now stretch your imagination one more time. The two persons finally recognize each other and start interacting. One is in a rather gloomy mood, whereas the other one's mood is somehow indifferent. The one in the indifferent mood state remembers a funny occurrence during her last encounter, which she now tells to the other person. Suddenly, the gloomy mood of the other person changes drastically, a smile lighting up his face.

This, in turn, makes the person who told the episode happy, too. Hence, both persons' moods are changed suddenly and more or less drastically (from gloomy or indifferent to joyful); this corresponds to what in the case of the brain is described as the "principle of inverse effectiveness" and "principle of nonlinearity."

Is our brain like a sidewalk? Probably not. The brain can be better compared with a theater stage than with a sidewalk. The actors and dancers interact on the stage of the theater; this corresponds to the way the stimuli interact with the brain and its intrinsic activity. The spatiotemporal configuration of the theater's stage determines the kind of moves that can possibly be made by the actors and the dancers. If the stage is not completely horizontal but tilted slightly vertically, certain moves by the dancers will be impossible.

The same is true in the case of the brain. If the brain's intrinsic activity and its spatiotemporal structure are configured in a certain way, this may allow the stimuli to exert its action along the lines of, for instance, the aforementioned four principles. In order to understand why and how the brain applies the four principles to its stimulus-induced activity, we must therefore go back to the brain itself and its intrinsic activity, the resting-state activity, and how that impacts its neural processing of extrinsic stimuli. This shall be the focus in the next chapter. First, though, we need go into more detail about the exact neuronal mechanisms underlying stimulus–stimulus interaction.

NEURONAL FINDINGS IIA: CROSS-MODAL INTERACTION AND PHASE RESETTING

Let me now go into more detail about the neuronal mechanisms underlying stimulus–stimulus interaction in cross-modal interaction by going back to the cellular and population level of neural activity. Besides the excellent studies by C. Kaysers as described earlier, C. Schroeder and P. Lakatos are other authors investigating cross-modal interaction on a cellular level (see also Chapters 20 and 21 in Volume II for more details of their work and studies).

C.Schroeder and P. Lakatos (2009) (see also Schroeder et al. 2008 as well as Kayser 2009) investigated cell recordings during cross-modal sensory interaction in auditory cortex of monkeys. An auditory stimulus induces a feedforward response that starts in layer 4 of the auditory cortex and subsequently elicits strong action potentials, increases in oscillatory power, and stronger phase coherence across various frequencies (gamma, beta, alpha, delta, theta). The auditory stimulus may thus be regarded as a "driving input" for auditory cortical activity (see also Schroeder and Lakatos 2009; Lakatos et al. 2009).

In contrast, a somatosensory stimulus has little impact on both local action potentials and oscillatory power and thus the lower cortical layers (layers 3 and 5) in auditory cortex. In contrast, the somatosensory stimulus does induce changes in auditory cortical supragranular layers (layer 1 and 2). More specifically, unlike the auditory stimulus, the somatosensory stimulus exerts a strong impact on the phase coherence between the different frequency bands (gamma, alpha, delta, theta); such resetting of their phases results in what is described as "phase synchronization." (see later for details).

Based on these observations, Schroeder and Lakatos propose that the somatosensory stimulus corresponds to what they describe as "modulatory input" for the auditory cortex (see also Schroeder and Lakatos 2009; Lakatos et al. 2009). Unlike the driving input, the modulatory input does not modulate the strength of the resulting neural activity but only its timing by resetting its phases, that is, phase synchronization. Phase resetting means that the stimuli and their onsets (that is, stimulus onset) are temporally always located in the same relation to the ongoing oscillatory phase, that is, at their same time points, across the different trials (see Fig. 10-2a-c) (see also Chapters 14, 15, and 20 for more details).

Schroeder and Lakatos suggest that such phase resetting characterizes cross-modal interaction. By resetting the phase of the ongoing neural activity in the uni-modal sensory cortex, the cross-modal stimulus may pave the way (or alternatively, open the door) for the uni-modal stimulus to elicit stronger neural activity changes; that is, in power or amplitude. Hence, rather than driving the neural activity in the uni-modal sensory cortex as the uni-modal stimulus itself, the cross-modal stimulus modulates the neural activity.

Neuronal findings IIb: Phase resetting and oscillatory activity

In a subsequent study, Schroeder and Lakatos could show that the modulation of phase coherence, that is, phase resetting, is not only related to cross-modal stimulation but also to attentional mechanisms (see Lakatos et al. 2009; see also Kayser 2009 for a commentary). They now recorded in monkey primary visual cortex during attention/nonattention to either visual or auditory stimuli and investigated power/amplitude and phases in the respectively resulting stimulus-induced activity. Let's start with the visual stimuli and their effects on visual cortex. Attended visual stimuli induced an increase in both the power, that is, amplitude, of the excitation/activation and the phase resetting of oscillations (mainly in the theta and gamma frequency)., This pattern differed in nonattended visual stimuli. Nonattended visual stimuli (attention is on the auditory stimuli) also induced an evoked response, but, unlike the attended stimuli, they did not affect the phase of ongoing oscillations.

How about the auditory stimuli and their effects on the visual cortex? Auditory stimuli that were attended did induce phase resetting in visual cortex (mainly in the theta and gamma frequency), while the amplitude (power) was not affected. This distinguished them from non-attended auditory stimuli that neither affected the power nor the phase of ongoing oscillatory activity. The attended auditory stimuli thus also exerted an impact in visual cortex by resetting its phases, thus reflecting cross-modal interaction.

Such phase resetting occurs though only if the auditory stimulus is attended, while nothing happens in the case of nonattended stimuli. Phase resetting may consequently be regarded a mechanisms of cross-modal attentional selection. This implies that the auditory stimulus functions as a modulatory input for the visual cortex, while the visual stimuli themselves are the "driving inputs."

Taken together, these results show that cross-modal interaction and the attentional selection of stimuli operate temporally via phase resetting. This means that the phases of the ongoing unimodal oscillatory activity are aligned to the cross-modal stimulus, the modulatory input, which thereby sets the stage for the unimodal stimuli, the driving input, to exert stronger amplitude, or power, changes.

Neuronal hypothesis IIa: Phase resetting and encoding of temporal differences

How do the results by Schroeder and Lakatos relate to difference-based coding? Schroeder and Lakatos show that cross-modal integration is achieved by resetting the phases in the ongoing oscillatory activity. This results in neural synchronization of the phases in the different frequency bands, which can be independent of and occur without accompanying changes in the power of the oscillations (see also Sauseng and Klimesch 2008; Fell and Axmacher 2011; and Canolty and Knight 2010 for recent review papers in this regard).

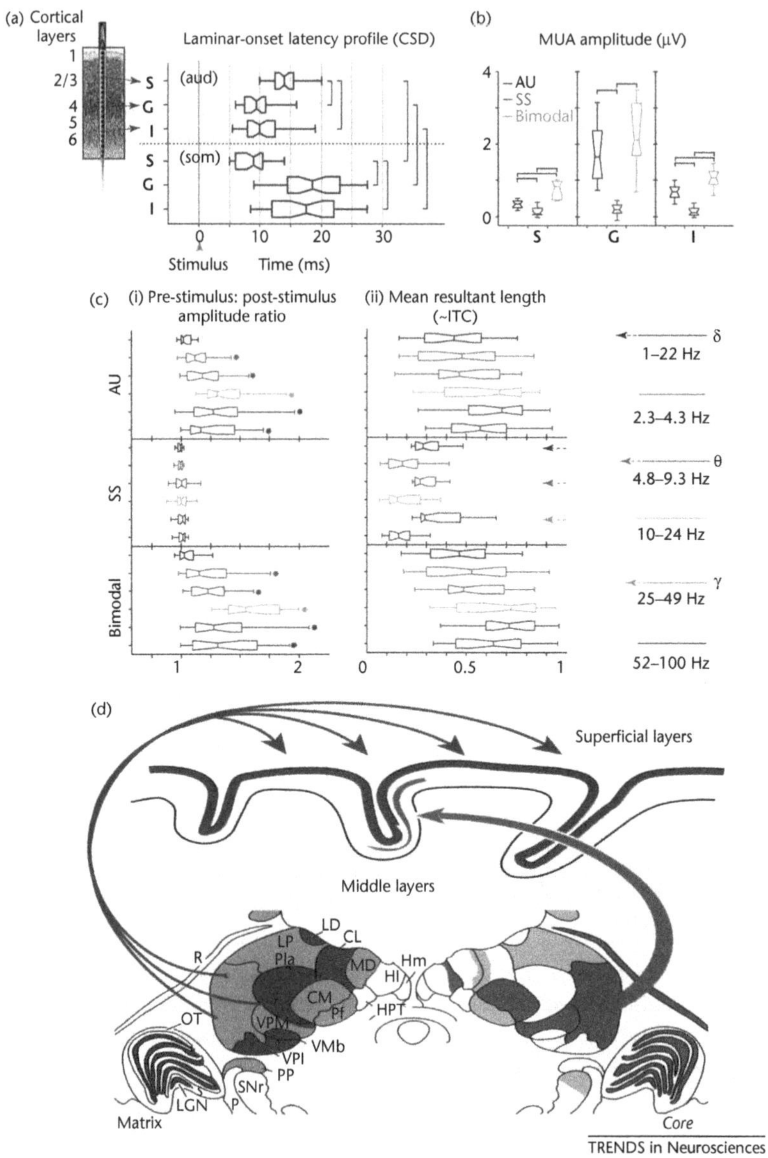

Figure 10-2a, b, c, and d **Neuronal mechanisms of "driving and modulatory inputs." (*a*) Box plots show pooled onset latencies of the characteristic frequency-tone- (aud) and somatosensory stimulus (som)-related CSD response in supragranular (S), granular (G), and infragranular (I) layers across experiments. The boxes have lines at the lower quartile, median, and upper quartile values, and the notches in boxes graphically show the 95% confidence interval about the median of each distribution. Brackets indicate the significant *post hoc* comparisons calculated using Games-Howell tests ($P < 0.01$). (*b*) Box plots show pooled ($n = 38$) CSD and MUA amplitudes on the selected channels (S, G, and I) averaged for the 15–60 ms time interval for the same conditions as (*a*), plus the bimodal condition. Brackets indicate the significant *post hoc* comparisons calculated using Games-Howell tests ($P < 0.01$). (*c*) (i) Pooled ($n = 38$) post-stimulus:pre-stimulus single-trial oscillatory amplitude ratio (0 to 250 ms: −500 to −250 ms) for different frequency intervals (different colors) of the auditory (AU), somatosensory (SS), and bimodal supragranular responses. Stars denote where the amplitude ratio is significantly different across the pre- and post-stimulus periods (one-sample t tests, $P < 0.01$).**

How is such phase synchronization independent of power changes possible? I hypothesize that it is possible on the basis of difference-based coding (see later for objections to my hypothesis of difference-based coding), whereas such independent phase synchronization would remain impossible in the case of stimulus-based coding. Let me be more specific. Schroeder and Lakatos demonstrate phase synchronization during cross-modal interaction. Such phase resetting is possible only by encoding the temporal position of the actual stimulus in relation, for example, in difference, to the temporal position of the phase in the ongoing oscillatory activity.

If this temporal difference is small tending toward zero, phase resetting is not necessary. If, in contrast, the temporal difference between actual stimulus and oscillatory phase is large, the latter's temporal course, its phase onset, is reset and aligned with the temporal position of the former, the actual stimulus. One would consequently postulate the following relationship: the larger the temporal difference between stimulus and phase, the larger the degree of (possible and necessary) phase resetting.

This relationship holds, however, only within a certain spectrum of temporal differences. If the degrees of the temporal difference are either too large or too small, they may exceed the minimally or maximally necessary values that can still possibly be processed within the framework provided by the brain's (species-specific) biophysical-computational range, as reflected for instance in the phase durations of its different frequency bands (see Chapters 1, 2, 11, and 21 for details). Hence, one may hypothesize that the postulated relationship between the degree of temporal difference and the degree of phase resetting holds within the range of the brain's biophysical-computational spectrum.

Neuronal hypothesis IIb: Stimulus- versus difference-based coding of phase resetting

How about stimulus-based coding? In such a case, the temporal position of the actual stimulus would be encoded by itself, independently of its relationship to the ongoing phase. This, though, would make it impossible to reset the phase in orientation on the stimulus' temporal position because the former would have no orientation on how and to which degree to reset its phase.

How about the converse scenario, encoding of the phase of the ongoing oscillatory activity independent of the stimulus' temporal position? In this case, phase resetting would remain equally impossible, since only the stimuli from the oscillatory activity would then be encoded into neural activity, thus presupposing again stimulus-based coding rather than difference-based coding.

Pointing to yet another scenario, one could also imagine that phase resetting could be operated via changes in oscillatory power. The

---

(ii) Pooled intertrial coherence (ITC) expressed as a vector quantity (mean resultant length) measured at 15 ms post-stimulus (the time of the initial peak response). Note that, in the case of somatosensory events, an increase in phase concentration only occurs in the low-delta (1–2.2 Hz), theta (4.8–9.3 Hz), and gamma (25–49 Hz) bands, indicated by colored arrows on the right. (*d*) Relative distributions and concentrations of calbindin-positive matrix cells (bottom left) and parvalbumin-positive core cells (bottom right) in a frontal section through the middle of a macaque monkey thalamus. The projections of the matrix to superficial layers of cortex over a wide extent and unconstrained by areal borders is shown at the top. Core cells restricted to individual nuclei (e.g., the ventral posterior nucleus) project in a topographically ordered manner to the middle layers of single functional cortical fields. *Abbreviations:* CL, central lateral nucleus; CM, center median nucleus; Hl, lateral habenular nuclei; Hm, medial habenular nuclei; LD, lateral dorsal nucleus; LGN, lateral geniculate nucleus; LP, lateral posterior nucleus; MD, mediodorsal nucleus; OT, optic tract; P, color-coded retinal ganglion cells; Pla, anterior pulvinar; PP, peripeduncular nucleus; R, reticular nucleus; s, s laminae; SNr, substantia nigra pars reticularis; VMb, basal ventral medial nucleus; VPi, ventral posterior inferior nucleus; VPM, ventral posterior medial nucleus.Reprinted with permission of Elsevier from Schroeder CE, Lakatos P. Low-frequency neuronal oscillations as instruments of sensory selection. *Trends Neurosci.* 2009 Jan;32(1):9–18.

observed phase resetting would then result as secondary consequence of the more primary stimulus-based activity; that is, encoding of power or strength (see also Sauseng and Klimesch 2008; Fell and Axmacher 2011; and Canolty and Knight 2010 for recent review papers in this regard).

This would again presuppose stimulus-based coding where the oscillatory power is encoded independently of the stimulus and its subsequent phase resetting. However, such a scenario would presuppose that phase resetting and phase synchronization always go hand in hand with power changes and would thus no longer remain at least partially independent. This is not the case, as the data from Schroeder and Lakatos clearly show.

Neuronal hypothesis IIc: Encoding of content versus encoding of temporal and spatial features

Finally, one may put forward yet another objection. The data from Schroeder and Lakatos show that phase resetting presupposes the encoding of the stimulus' temporal position in relation to the ongoing oscillatory activity. What they do not show, however, is that the encoding is exclusively based on the stimulus' temporal features independent of its respective auditory content.

For that to show, one would need to conduct an interaction design where different auditory stimuli (with equal spatial and temporal features) are presented in the same temporal relation to the ongoing oscillatory activity in visual cortex. If now both induce phase resetting (in more or less the same degree), the underlying neural activity must indeed be entirely based on the encoding of statistically based temporal features of the stimuli; that is, their temporal positions indicating the statistical frequency distribution across time. This is exactly what I postulate. I posit that difference-based coding is allows for the encoding of the statistically based spatial and temporal features of the stimuli (across their different discrete points in physical time and space), independently of the content associated with the respective stimulus at its particular discrete point in physical time and space. This is to be distinguished from the encoding and processing of the respective content itself, which would amount to stimulus-based coding (see Chapters 18–20 for the constitution of content on the basis of difference-based coding).

In sum, I propose that difference-based coding operates in both spatial and temporal domains during cross-modal interaction in particular and stimulus–stimulus interaction in general. This presupposes that any neural activity on any level of the brain, from primary sensory cortex to higher-order regions as well as from subcortical to cortical regions, is encoded in terms of spatial and temporal differences across the different discrete points in physical time and space associated with the different stimuli.

Such difference-based coding must be distinguished from stimulus-based coding. The stimuli would then be encoded on the basis of their discrete spatial and temporal points in physical time and space independent of their spatial and temporal difference relative to each other and the brain's ongoing resting-state activity (see Chapter 11 for details on the latter).

Neuronal hypothesis IId: Phase resetting and consciousness

Why is the supposed difference-based coding of phase resetting relevant? We so far have discussed the neuronal relevance of phase resetting in that it determines the degree of neural activity a particular stimulus can induce. This concerned stimulus–stimulus interaction and stimulus-induced activity.

We already saw in Chapter 5 that analogous mechanisms of phase resetting also occur during the resting-state activity itself, by means of which a temporal (or better, spatiotemporal) structure is constituted. This means that phase resetting is relevant not only for stimulus-induced activity but also for the resting state and how it constitutes the statistically based spatiotemporal structure of its neural activity.

Most important, we will argue in Volume II that phase resetting is highly relevant for consciousness and thus phenomenally relevant. I suppose the following: the better the ongoing intrinsic resting-state activity can shift and align the phase onsets of its low frequency fluctuations to the onsets of the extrinsic stimuli, the more likely it is that the resulting stimulus-induced activity will be associated with consciousness. This means that phase resetting may be not only neuronally relevant but also phenomenally relevant (see Chapters 18–20 and 28–29).

Neuronal findings III: Binding between different features of the stimulus

My assumption of difference-based coding holding during stimulus-induced activity and s naturally evokes some objections, which shall be discussed briefly in the following. The first objection argues that what I associate with the encoding of spatial and temporal differences in lower-order sensory regions must rather be associated with cognitive mechanisms in higher-order regions like the prefrontal cortex that from the top-down modulate lower-order sensory cortical activity. To demonstrate this objection and how it can be countered, I want to discuss an example of an imaging study that investigated the binding between different features of a stimulus.

Seymour et al. (2009, 2010) conducted fMRI studies in human subjects by exposing them to visual stimuli. There were three distinct types of visual stimuli. The visual stimuli were determined by their color alone independent of form and motion, or they were determined according to their form and motion independent of the color. Or, finally, the stimuli were determined by the conjunction of both color and form/motion.

To test whether voxels in the different areas of the visual cortex (V1, V2, V3, V4, MT/V5) are associated with either color, form/motion, or the conjunction of both, Seymour et al. (2009, 2010) applied a multivariate classifier analysis to their fMRI data.

What are their results? The multivariate classifier analysis allowed them to distinguish the voxels specifically related to the conjunction from the voxels that were either related to form/motion or color. They observed that particular voxels in almost every visual region, including V1, were specifically related to the conjunction of both color and form/motion. This pattern was prevalent in all visual regions except in V4 where only color-specific voxels were observed and in MT/V5 with only motion-specific voxels (as expected from what is known about these regions).

In sum, these results demonstrate that the linkage between color and form/motion and thus their binding by synchronization (see later for details) occurs already in V1. Otherwise there would not be voxels in V1 specifically related to the conjunction of color and form/motion.

Such binding by synchronization seems to occur at every level of visual processing as suggested by the observation of conjunction-specific voxels in all visual areas (see later for further results from that study as well as Chapters 11 and 12 as well as Chapters 18 and 19 for further details on such binding by synchronization).

Neuroempirical objection Ia: "Higher-order objection" and higher-order cognitive regions

How do these results stand in relation to difference-based coding? The results by Seymour et al. (2009, 2010) provide direct support for the assumption that there is binding by synchronization already on the level of V1 and also on all subsequent stages of visual processing and its respective visual regions. This is suggested by the observation of voxels specifically related to the conjunction of color and form/motion.

Such conjunction between color and form/motion is possible only on the basis of encoding differences between form/motion and color as manifest in the conjunction voxels. These voxels reflect neuronal activity that can be yielded only on the basis of encoding the relative difference between color and form/motion thus being difference-based rather than stimulus based as based on either form/motion or color alone.

One may now want to argue that such difference-based coding does not occur in primary visual cortex, that is, V1, itself but is due to the top-down modulation of V1 by higher-order regions like the prefrontal cortex. This means that there is no difference-based coding in V1 itself and that it only looks as if there is. Instead, the top-down modulation from, for instance, the prefrontal cortex links form/motion and color that are encoded by themselves and thus isolated and independently of each other in V1. Hence, what I diagnose as difference-based coding in V1 turns out to be stimulus-based coding.

However, this higher-order objection, as I call it, backfires and feedbacks to its proponent in very much the same way it describes the relationship between higher-order cognitive and lower-order sensory regions. Let's start with the higher-order cognitive regions. How can they compute the conjunction between form/motion and color?

The only way to do that is to directly match and compare them and thus to encode their relative (spatial and temporal) difference. This means that the higher-order cognitive regions' neural activity must be based on the encoding of spatial and temporal differences between different stimuli rather than on the stimuli themselves (and their discrete points in physical time and space).

Accordingly, the conjunction between form/motion and color in higher-order regions themselves presuppose difference- rather than stimulus-based coding in these regions (see also Chapter 3). This provides one half of our argument that difference-based coding is necessary for making possible conjunction between form/motion and color.

Neuroempirical Objection Ib: "Higher-Order Objection" and Lower-Order Sensory Regions

How about the other half of our argument, the primary visual cortex, V1? In the higher-order scenario, V1 is supposed to encode its neural activity in terms of stimulus-based coding; this means that its neural activity is determined by form/motion and color alone and independent of each other and their relative difference. How now is it possible that conjunction voxels between form/motion and color can be observed in V1? This is realized by top-down modulation as relayed from prefrontal to primary visual cortex.

Now two scenarios are possible. First, some of the voxels encoding form/motion and color alone are modulated by the prefrontal input. In that case, neural activity in V1 and thus the observed voxels must encode the difference between its own neural activity related to form/motion or color alone and the prefrontal input, that is, the conjunction. What is encoded in V1, then, is the relative difference between its own stimulus-based activity and the activity relayed from the higher-order cognitive regions. This amounts to difference-based coding rather than stimulus-based coding already holding in V1.

Second, another scenario for the prefrontal input to affect V1 would be that it modulates those cells/cell assemblies in V1 that did not encode either form/motion or color alone. There would thus be three different cells/cell assemblies in V1 with each encoding a different feature, form/motion, color, or the conjunction of both. This would be compatible with the observation of three different types of voxels as described earlier.

However, even this scenario would still presuppose difference-based coding namely of the difference between the prefrontal input and the primary visual cortical activity. Otherwise the former could not target only those voxels that did not encode either form/motion or color alone. Hence, even in this scenario, one would have no way other than to propose difference-based coding in V1, which, however, operates side by side with stimulus-based coding in a parallel way.

The "higher-order objection" against difference-based coding does not hold. Even the assumption of higher-order processing accounting for the conjunction voxel cannot help but presuppose difference-based coding in both higher- and lower-order regions. The only point the "higher-order objection" can made is to plead for stimulus-based coding to occur in parallel to difference-based coding in V1. This, however, is not an argument against the necessity of difference-based coding, but rather one for some kind of parallelism between difference- and stimulus-based coding.

Neuroempirical Objection IIa: "Segregation Objection"

The opponents of difference-based coding may want to bring forth yet another argument. In addition to the voxel specifically related to the conjunction, voxels only related to either form/motion or color were also observed in all visual regions. These voxels seem to be based on the exclusive coding of one particular feature while explicitly excluding any conjunction between the two features.

This means that the neural activity underlying these voxels can only be based on the features themselves rather than on their differences, thus entailing feature- or stimulus-based coding rather than difference-based coding. Since all three stimuli are encoded in isolation and independently in terms of stimulus-based coding, they would be processed in a segregated way. One may consequently suggest segregated processing of color, form/motion, and their conjunction in the different subregions of the visual cortex. This is what I describe as the "segregation objection." which may be considered an argument against difference-based coding.

Is such segregated processing compatible with difference-based coding? Yes and no. It is compatible with difference-based coding since it may hold at least for the conjunction-specific voxels. In contrast, segregated processing is not compatible with the assumption of difference-based coding as the main and only coding strategy, since the other voxels, the ones specifically related to either form/motion or color alone, seem to presuppose stimulus- rather than difference-based coding.

Neuroempirical objection IIb: functional independence versus functional dependence

Do the form/motion- and color-specific voxels really presuppose stimulus-based coding? If so, one would expect not only functional segregation but also functional independence between all three types of voxels (form/motion, color, and conjunction).

Why is there functional independence? Stimulus-based coding presupposes the encoding of different stimuli in isolation and independently of each other so that the one stimulus does not interfere with the respective other, and vice versa (see Fig. 10-3a).

Functional independence implies that the three voxels do not correlate at all and thus do not stand in any relation to each other. This was not the case, however, in the results by Seymour et al. (2009, 2010). Instead, form/motion-, color-, and conjunction-specific voxels, were negatively related to each other: for instance, the better a voxel coded for color, the worse it coded for motion/form. Importantly, this also holds for the conjunction-specific voxels: the better a voxel in V1, V2, and V3 coded the conjunction, the worse it coded color. Hence, there was a negative correlation, or even stronger, an anti-correlation between the three different voxels.

As Seymour et al. (2010, pp. 1951) themselves remark, this suggests that even those voxels that code best for one particular feature still contain some information about the respective other features. How is it possible that one voxel coding for one particular feature contains some information about the respective other features?

Despite being functionally segregated, the three types of voxels are not functionally independent of each other since otherwise there would be no correlation at all, whether positive or negative. The negative correlation thus indicates that there must be some degree of functional dependence among the three types of voxels. While the voxels are spatially segregated, they still seem to be functionally dependent on each other since otherwise they would not anti-correlate.

How is such functional dependence possible? One could, of course, argue again with feedback connections and top-down modulation from higher regions, as I claimed earlier. That, however, turned out to be empirically implausible since in either case it presupposed some kind of difference-based coding in both lower- and higher-order regions (see earlier). Alternatively, one could propose that they are coded within V1 itself in terms of difference-based coding and thus in dependence on each other.

The resulting voxels are then based on the difference between the three different features rather than on the features themselves. In short, one would opt for difference-based coding rather than (feature- or) stimulus-based coding.

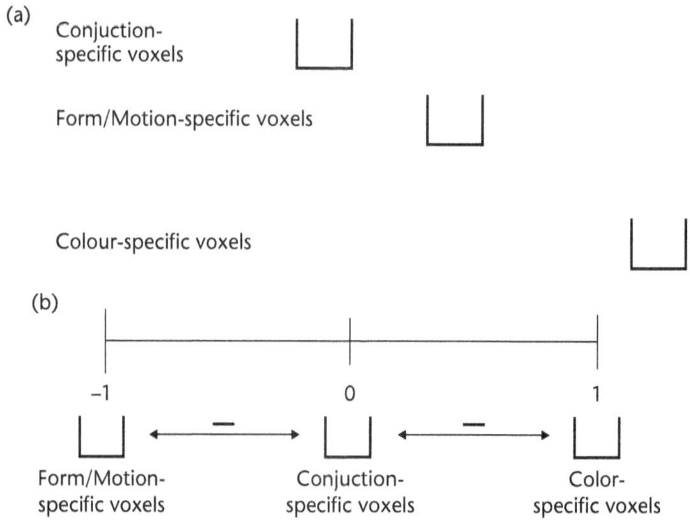

Figure 10-3a and b **Coding of form and motion. The figure illustrates two different ways, stimulus-based (a) and difference-based coding (b), of the voxels related to form, motion, and their conjunction. (*a*) In the case of stimulus-based coding, all three voxels are coded in neural activity in a segregated and independent way, entailing different voxels for all three features, motion, form, and conjunction. (*b*) In the case of difference-based coding, all three—form, motion, and conjunction—are encoded in a segregated but dependent way. They are encoded in different voxels, but the degree of activity in each of the voxels depends on the degree of activity in the respective other voxels; this is indicated by the arrows. The degree of activity or intensity in each other the voxels is consecutively encoded on a continuum between −1 and +1 (artificially assumed as minimal and maximal degrees of possible activity) as indicated by the upper line.**

The "segregation objection" is not compatible with the empirical data that show negative functional dependence, i.e., anti-correlation, rather than functional independence with no correlation at all among the three voxels. Such functional dependence whether positive or negative implies that the one voxel contains some kind of information about the respective other voxels.

This, however, is possible only by encoding relative differences between different voxels rather than the voxels by themselves in an isolated and independent way. Accordingly, the data themselves, the anti-correlation, refute the "segregation objection" and make necessary or unavoidable the assumption of difference-based coding rather than stimulus-based coding.

Neuroempirical objection IIc: segregation as a necessary or unavoidable outcome

The assumption of difference-based coding requires more detailed explanation. In the case of conjunction-specific voxels, difference-based coding makes perfect sense because here functional dependence is not accompanied by functional segregation but rather functional overlap.

The case is more difficult for the form/motion- and color-specific voxels where functional dependence goes along with functional segregation. Their functional segregation suggests stimulus-based coding while their apparent functional dependence is better compatible with difference-based coding. How is it possible for one and the same voxel to be associated with two contradictory coding strategies, stimulus- and difference-based coding?

I hypothesize that what looks as stimulus-based coding to us in the form/motion and color voxel can be traced back to the encoding of differences, or difference-based coding. More specifically, I suppose that the color- and form/motion-specific voxels represent extremes on the continuum between minimally (−1) and maximally (+1) possible differences between form/motion and color. In these voxels, one particular feature predominates over the respective other and this predomination corresponds to a negative relationship as observed in the empirical data: the larger difference at the one end (−1), as, for instance, the form/motion end, is negatively correlated with the larger difference at the other end (+1), the color end.

Both form/motion and color voxels may then represent extremes of a continuum of different differences. In contrast, the conjunction-specific voxels may rather be "located" in the middle of the continuum between both extreme differences, the color and form/motion voxels. If so, the "conjunction voxels" should negatively correlate with the larger differences at both extreme poles of the continuum. This is exactly what the data show.

How is that related to the observed functional segregation between the three voxels? The degree of difference may correspond to the degree of spatial segregation between the three voxels: the larger their difference, the more spatially they may be separated from each other. Smaller differences, in contrast, may go along with lower degrees of spatial segregation, which ultimately may result in functional overlap, as observed in the conjunction voxels.

I hence propose that the degree of spatial (and thus functional) segregation of the three voxels is dependent upon their respective degree of (spatial and temporal) difference between the three features. And to extend this hypothesis even further: the more spatially and functionally segregated the three voxels are from each other, the more negatively they are related to each other, which is well compatible with the observed data, that is, the anti-correlation (see Fig. 10-3b).

Taken together, the "segregation objection" cannot be used as an argument against difference-based coding. Instead, spatial and functional segregation of the three different types of voxels are well compatible with their functional dependence and ultimately difference-based coding. One may put it even more strongly. Due to the presumed link between the degree of encoded differences and the degree of spatial segregation, one may suggest that difference-based coding is necessarily or unavoidably accompanied with functional segregation between spatially distinct voxels as the necessary or unavoidable outcome..

Neuronal findings IVa: "Binding by convergence" versus "Binding by synchronization"

Let us move away from the findings by Seymour to German neuroscientist Wolf Singer. Singer is famous for his detection of the neuronal synchronization in the gamma-frequency range in visual cortex; he thereby made major contributions to the binding and synchronization of cell assemblies and stimuli's features. This also strongly touches upon consciousness, as it will be discussed in volume II (see especially Chapter 19). Here let us consider what he has to say about the neural code.

Singer (1999, 49–50, 55) proposes binding of neural activity on the basis of spatial convergence when axonal projections from different neurons converge onto one and the same neuron. He calls such strategy "binding by convergence" or "binding by conjunction cells." In such case, the given neuron always signals the same conjunction of input signals as being based on the (anatomo-structural) spatial convergence of the neuron's underlying axonal projections.

This entails fixed labeling ("labeled line coding"), which is realized by enhancing the discharge rate of the given neuron via the conjunction of the respective input signals; that amounts to neural coding based on the discharge rate, that is, "rate coding" as reflected in (for instance) the firing rates of neurons (see Introduction for a brief explanation of rate coding).Such "binding by convergence" on the basis of rate coding must be distinguished from another binding strategy, binding by synchronization. In this case, as described earlier, two (or more) neuronal inputs are tied together not by their spatial and thus axonal convergence but rather temporally via their respective temporal position and coherence. In his review paper from 1999, Singer calls such binding by synchronization "dynamic binding" and distinguishes it from "binding by convergence."

Since it is based on temporal rather than spatial convergence, "dynamic binding" presupposes a different coding strategy, "relational coding" or "assembly coding," as Singer calls it; this is so because here different neurons are tied together into a (transitory rather than permanent) relationship or cell assembly. Such "relational coding" and its temporal dimension, i.e., temporal convergence, must be distinguished from the earlier mentioned rate coding that is rather dominated by the spatial dimension, or spatial convergence.

Neuronal findings IVb: "Parallel coding strategies"

Can such double binding, that is, binding by convergence and binding by synchronization, and their associated coding strategies, that is, rate coding and relational coding, be supported by empirical data? The difference between binding by convergence and binding by synchronization seems to somehow mirror the distinction between "driving inputs" and "modulatory inputs" as described earlier in the findings by Lakatos and Schroeder. Driving inputs may rely on spatial and thus axonal convergence and, following Singer's assumptions, impact the discharge rate, thus presupposing rate coding.

In contrast, modulatory inputs seem to rely rather on temporal convergence and "relational coding" or "assembly coding." Hence, though not entirely accordant, the distinction between driving and modulatory inputs may more or less be compatible with the assumption of parallel and complementary binding and coding strategies like "binding by convergence"/rate coding and "binding-by-synchronization"/relational coding. Such parallelism of binding and coding strategies can ultimately be traced back to a parallelism between the processing of spatial and temporal dimensions in neural activity.

Can we support the assumption of such parallel coding strategies by empirical data? Further empirical support for parallel coding strategies comes from a recent study on stimulus–stimulus interaction by the group around Singer (Biederlack et al. 2006). They investigated single-cell activity in cat visual cortex (V1) multisite recording during visual perception of a center grating; the latter's perceived brightness was changed by varying the orientation or relative spatial phase of a surrounding grating.

Discharge rates in response to the center were significantly enhanced by increasing the orientation contrast between the center and the surround: the more different center and surrounding, the more the discharge rates in response to the visual fixation on the center increased. In contrast, high similarity between center and surrounding decreased the discharge rates in response to the visual fixation on the center.

Most important, the degree of synchronization between different neurons decreased once the orientation contrast between center and surrounding was introduced; however, unlike the rate discharge (the firing rate), the degree of synchronization did not decrease further with increasing degrees in the orientation contrast.

This was different when the phase relations between the gratings of the center and the surrounding were changed. Changes in phase relations did not induce changes in discharge rates (firing rates), while they did induce changes in the degree of synchronization. The more offset phase relations (while orientations were kept the same), the higher degrees of synchronization were observed between the different neurons' neural activities.

These data provide support in favor of different parallel and complementary coding strategies. The degrees of both discharge rates, or firing rates, and synchronization are modulated by different features of the stimulus, that is, orientation and phase relations. This indeed suggests different encoding strategies—that is, rate coding and relational coding—for the different features of the stimuli in terms of discharge rates, or firing rates, and synchronization between neurons.

Singer suggests two parallel coding strategies to operate during the encoding into neural activity. There is rate coding, as manifested in binding-by-convergence that concerns mainly the spatial dimension. That must be distinguished from relational coding with its binding-by-synchronization that takes place mainly in the temporal dimension.

Neuronal findings IVc: neural coding and psychological contents

How is this predominantly neuronal distinction related to the psychological level of stimuli and their content? The psychological level is more explicitly addressed in a later review paper by Singer (2009). Here, the two binding strategies of binding by convergence and binding by synchronization resurface in the coding strategies of "chunking" and "relating."

Briefly "chunking" describes how different features (or stimuli) are grouped into a chunk, which may concern particular and fixed features in a fast, rigid, and more or less *a priori* defined way. This presupposes "binding by convergence" and rate coding. "Relating," on the other hand, concerns the binding and linkage among different features (or different stimuli) in dependence on their respective context, which is rather slow and flexible and not *a priori* defined. This presupposes binding-by-synchronization and relational coding.

Especially the latter ("relating") has been closely associated with what is described as "binding," which concerns the contents of our psychological states, such as during perception. Since "binding" is closely related to consciousness and its phenomenal states, for which it has been suggested as a possible neural correlate, I will discuss it in further detail in Volume II (see Introduction I as well as Chapters 18 and 19).

NEURONAL HYPOTHESIS IIIA: ENCODING OF SPATIOTEMPORAL DIFFERENCES INTO NEURAL ACTIVITY

Do these different binding strategies, chunking/binding by convergence and relating/binding by synchronization, really presuppose different coding strategies? Put into our framework, one may want to argue that relating/binding by synchronization is compatible with difference-based coding as mirrored in Singer's characterization of "relational coding." While chunking/binding by convergence may rather presuppose stimulus-based coding that is based on stimulus-specific modulation of discharge rates, that is, rate coding.

Are the different coding strategies really parallel and complementary? Singer's distinct codes basically reflect spatial and temporal codes. Binding by convergence and rate coding presuppose basically a spatial code that relies on spatial convergence (see earlier), whereas binding by synchronization is a temporal code that accounts for temporal convergence. I now hypothesize that difference-based coding is well suited to underlie both spatial and temporal encoding strategies of binding.

More specifically, I hypothesize that the spatial code is not as purely spatial as implicitly presupposed in rate coding. The resulting discharge rate is also very much dependent on the temporal positioning of the different inputs and thus their relative temporal position to each other.

Most important, the spatial position of the stimulus is not encoded in isolation of its own and other stimuli's temporal position in space. Instead, the spatial position of the stimulus is encoded in relation and thus relative difference to other stimuli's temporal position in space. Hence, what appears to be exclusively spatial turns out to be intrinsically spatiotemporal (see Fig. 10-4a,b).

NEURONAL HYPOTHESIS IIIB: DIFFERENCE-BASED CODING IS AN INTRINSICALLY SPATIOTEMPORAL CODING STRATEGY

This means that binding by convergence/chunking may also presuppose difference-based coding rather than stimulus-based coding. If so, both binding by convergence and binding by synchronization presuppose one and the same coding strategy, difference-based coding.

Both rate and relational coding must be regarded as two variants of the same underlying coding strategy; that is, different-based coding, rather than as two different and parallel operating coding strategies. Difference-based coding allows for the encoding of stimuli in both domains, spatial and temporal, at the same time, without segregating them from each other into parallel coding strategies.

This means that difference-based coding must be characterized as a unifying and intrinsically spatiotemporal coding strategy that applies the same code to both spatial and temporal dimensions of stimulus-processing and subsequent neural activity. More radically put, difference-based coding makes superfluous the assumption of segregated, parallel coding

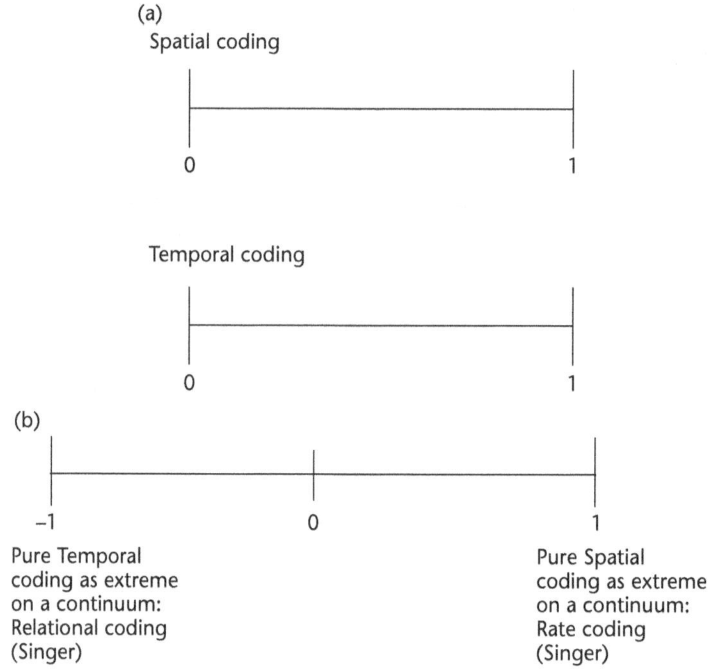

Figure 10-4a and b **Functional segregation and continuum. The figure illustrates two different forms, stimulus- and difference-based coding, of the relationship between spatial and temporal coding of neural activity. (*a*) Stimulus-based coding implies segregated and independent coding of spatial and temporal dimensions into neural activity, with each dimension showing its own distinct continuum. (*b*) Difference-based coding codes spatial and temporal dimensions on a continuum common to both. Here spatial and temporal dimensions are no longer considered as segregated and independent but rather as extremes on a common continuum. What W. Singer calls "relational coding" and "rate coding," indicating the coding of temporal and spatial dimensions respectively, are then just extreme instances on a continuum common on to both dimensions.**

strategies for spatial and temporal dimensions of neural activity.

The characterization of difference-based coding as unifying spatiotemporal encoding strategy changes the view on spatial and temporal coding of neural activity. While Singer seems to suppose that temporal and spatial coding are different and extrinsic, both coding strategies may turn out to be distinct and intrinsic aspects of the same underlying coding strategy; namely, difference-based coding.

More specifically, the seemingly purely spatial and temporal forms of coding must then be regarded as extremes on the continuum of different possible spatiotemporal differences encoded into neural activity. What Singer describes as purely spatial coding turns out to be a spatiotemporal difference whose balance is tilted strongly toward the spatial pole, whereas the converse holds for the seemingly purely temporal forms of coding.

Neuroconceptual remark: brain versus observer

Why does Singer nevertheless propose two different coding strategies for spatial and temporal dimensions? I suggest that this can be traced back to his need as an observer to experimentally distinguish between spatial and temporal dimensions in his operational variables—for instance, the one he measures in fMRI or EEG. From his acquisition of both spatial and temporal variables in segregated ways, he then seems to infer that they must also be *encoded* by different encoding strategies, spatial and temporal.

While the data acquisition and the parsing between spatial and temporal measures can be taken as given (for the sake of simplicity), the inference from the data about the brain to the brain itself and its coding strategy may nevertheless be put in doubt. The way we as observers can (and cannot) measure and thus observe the brain does not need to correspond one-to-one to the way the brain itself, independently of us and our observation, encodes its neural activity.

In other words, we need to distinguish between the observer's experimental measures and the brain's neuronal measures. The distinction between observer-based experimental measures and brain-based neuronal measures implies that we as observers need to refrain from projecting our own role as observers and its experimental requirements onto the neuronal function of the brain itself, such as its encoding strategies.

Therefore, pending more experimental support for difference-based coding in the future, I postulate the following: the distinction between parallel and segregated spatial and temporal coding strategies may turn out to be more related to us and our roles as observers of the brain (observer-based) than to the brain itself, as it is independent of us and our observation, i.e., brain-based (see also appendix 3 in this Volume I for more details on brain- vs. observer-based concepts).

Open Questions

The first main question is whether phase resetting described here is also behaviorally relevant. I have only focused on the neuronal mechanisms to describe stimulus–stimulus interaction in order to set a template for rest–stimulus interaction. Phase resetting and especially gamma synchronization have been observed to be relevant in a variety of different functions, including sensorimotor, visual, and cognitive. Since gamma synchronization especially may also be phenomenally relevant (i.e., for consciousness), I will delegate their discussion to Volume II (see Chapters 14, 15, and 18–20).

Another issue pertains to the question of whether the discussion of parallel versus unifying coding strategies is only theoretically relevant or also empirically, that is, neuronally, important. Empirical importance would, for instance, be given if a particular psychological function is possible only on the basis of one or the other coding strategy, the unifying approach of difference-based coding or the parallel coding strategies of rate and relational coding.

As demonstrated in this chapter, this also pertains to the question of how spatial and temporal dimensions are encoded into neural activity. I will argue that consciousness is possible only on the basis of a unifying coding strategy like difference-based coding. In contrast, the association of a neuronal state with a phenomenal state, or consciousness, would remain impossible if spatial and temporal dimensions were encoded separately and independently into neural activity as in stimulus-based coding. This is the subject of volume II.

Why do we need a common coding strategy for the encoding of spatial and temporal dimensions into neural activity in order to associate a phenomenal state, consciousness, with the neuronal states? Because only an encoding strategy common to both spatial and temporal dimensions allows for their intrinsic integration in neural activity. This will allow us to understand how the brain can predispose consciousness where spatial and temporal dimensions remain inseparable in our subjective experience, that is, phenomenal states. This will be explained in detail in Volume II.

CHAPTER 11
Rest–Stimulus Interaction and Difference-Based Coding

Summary

The brain receives continuous exteroceptive input from the environment. However, the exteroceptive stimuli do not encounter a passive empty brain but rather a highly active brain that constitutes a statistically based spatiotemporal structure (see Part II) and generates predictions (see Part III). This means that the exteroceptive stimuli have no chance other than to interact with the brain's resting-state activity if, metaphorically speaking, "they want to be processed and leave their trace in the brain." This amounts to what I call rest–stimulus interaction. What are the neuronal principles and mechanisms underlying rest–stimulus interaction? My assumption is that the very same principles underlying stimulus–stimulus interaction (see Chapter 10) do also apply to rest–stimulus interaction (and also to the converse direction in stimulus–rest interaction). Recent data from both animals and humans show that the degree of stimulus-induced activity, including the associated behavioral measures, can be predicted by the degree of the preceding resting-state activity level. How is this possible? For this to be possible, the stimulus-induced activity must be linked and connected to the resting-state activity. This is, as I assume, possible by encoding the extrinsic stimulus in spatial and temporal relationship, that is, relative difference, from the brain's intrinsic activity, thus presupposing difference-based coding. Why and how can the preceding resting-state activity be relevant for and even predict the stimulus as processed in subsequent stimulus-induced activity? Based on previous empirical data, one may hypothesize that previous stimuli left their traces in the resting-state activity via stimulus–rest interaction. The preceding stimulus–rest interaction thus predisposes the resting state for the prediction of stimulus and consequently for rest–stimulus interaction. Based on their actual state, the resting state's spatial and functional features, for example, functional connectivity and low-frequency fluctuations, may then provide a "spatiotemporal window of opportunity" for subsequent rest–stimulus interaction. The degree of the resting state's "spatiotemporal window of opportunity" may then also determine the degree of difference-based coding (and its balance to the degree of stimulus-based coding) the resting state can possibly apply to its own processing of the extrinsic stimulus during rest–stimulus interaction. This means that the resting state's activity level predisposes, not only the degree of difference-based coding, but also the degree of stimulus-induced activity and its associated behavioral and phenomenal effects.

Key Concepts and Topics Covered

Spatial and temporal coincidence, nonlinearity, rest–stimulus interaction, difference-based coding, stimulus–rest interaction, biophysical-computational limits, spatiotemporal window of opportunity

Neuroempirical background I: stimulus-induced activity and resting state activity

I discussed the neuronal mechanisms and principles guiding stimulus–stimulus interaction in the last chapter. Earlier, in parts II and III, I demonstrated the neuronal mechanisms underlying the brain's intrinsic activity and its continuous changes with the constitution of a statistically based spatiotemporal structure. The question is now whether and how the brain's resting-state activity impacts stimulus-induced activity. I here hypothesize that thereby the same neuronal principles and mechanisms are at work as during stimulus–stimulus interaction.

There have been several studies in both animals and humans that demonstrate indeed that the resting-state activity strongly shapes and modulates stimulus-induced activity (see Northoff et al. 2010 for a recent review). For heuristic purposes, I distinguish between intra- and transregional rest–stimulus interaction. Intraregional rest–stimulus interaction is given when the resting state of one particular region impacts the stimulus-induced activity in the very same region. In contrast, I speak of transregional rest–stimulus interaction when the resting-state activity in one region/network impacts the stimulus-induced activity in another region/network.

One of the pioneers of investigating rest–stimulus interaction in human functional imaging is Andreas Kleinschmidt. Andreas Kleinschmidt is a German neuroscientist who works in both Frankfurt, Germany, and Paris, France. He may thereby be able to combine the fin, light French cuisine with the sometimes rather heavy German food. While I do not know whether and how he combines French and German food, he clearly combines the investigation of resting-state activity and stimulus-induced activity in extraordinary ways. Henceforth, I will focus on his studies to reveal some of the neuronal mechanisms underlying rest–stimulus interaction. But I remain unable to describe all studies by other authors in full detail, which would be beyond the scope of this chapter (see the following, however, for a tentative overview).

Neuronal findings Ia: intra-regional rest–stimulus interaction

One functional magnetic resonance imaging (fMRI) study from Kleinschmidt's group focused on the auditory cortex (Sadaghiani et al. 2009). They let subjects perform an auditory detection task and presented broadband noise stimuli in unpredictable intervals of 20–40 ms. The subjects had to press a button when, and only when, they thought they heard the target sound; otherwise, they did not hit the button. This allowed the researchers to compare the neural activity preceding hits with the one preceding instances where subjects did not hear the target sound.

Interestingly, successful detection was preceded by significantly higher prestimulus activity, for example, resting-state activity, in auditory cortex, when compared to misses. That means that the level of resting-state activity in auditory cortex impacted the degree of perception, that is, whether subjects could hear the auditory stimuli.

How about rest–stimulus interaction in a sensory modality other than the auditory? Kleinschmidt's group also investigated rest–stimulus interaction in the visual modality (see Hesselmann et al. 2008). Higher prestimulus resting-state activity levels in the fusiform face area were related to subsequent perception of a face rather than a vase in the Rubin's ambiguous vase-face figure. This means that the higher resting-state activity in the fusiform face biases the subsequent perceptual content toward seeing the face, rather than the vase (see Fig. 11-1a).

Analogous findings were observed with another visual stimulus like visual motion: the resting-state activity in the visual motion area in the middle temporal cortex (V5/MT) predicted the degree of the subsequent perception of coherent motion (Hesselmann et al. 2008). They also related prestimulus resting-state activity and peak stimulus-induced activity with behavioral performance: the less prestimulus resting-state activity and peak stimulus-induced activity correlated each other, the better the subjects' subsequent behavioral performance, for example, the motion perception. Hence, better behavioral performance went along with increased distinction of stimulus-induced activity from the preceding resting-state activity.

The authors postulate in another paper (Hesselmann et al. 2008) and a subsequent review paper (Sadaghiani et al. 2010) nonlinear interaction between the resting state and the stimulus

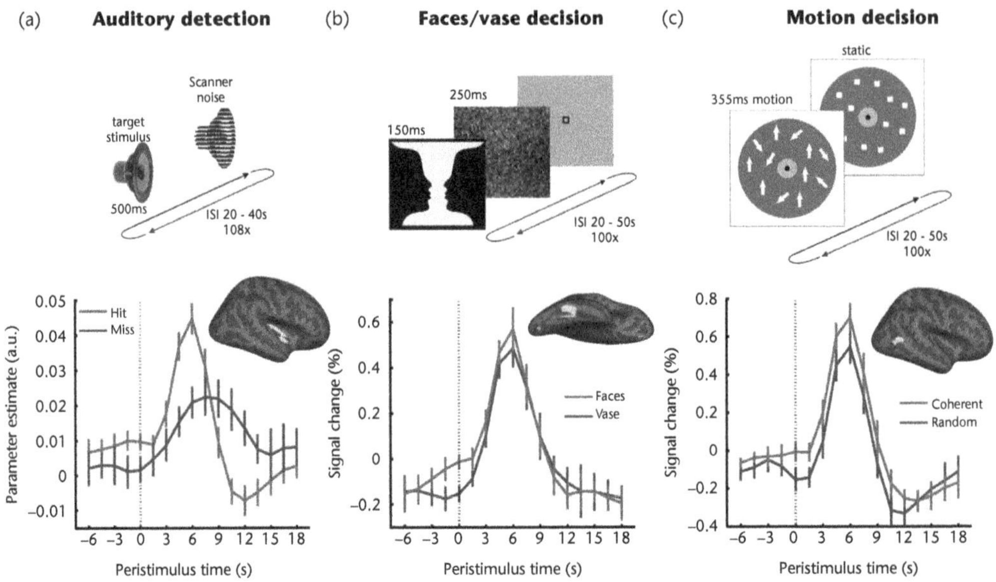

Figure 11-1a **Local spontaneous variations in ongoing activity of specialized sensory regions impact perception. The upper part illustrates the paradigm: (*a*) auditory detection experiment: in a free-response setting subjects detected an auditory target stimulus presented at perceptual threshold. (*b*) Perceptual decision on an ambiguous figure: subjects reported either faces or vase perception in response to flashes of the faces-vase ambiguous figure. (*c*) Motion decision experiment: random dot motion was presented at motion coherence threshold and subjects decided trial by trial whether motion was coherent or random. In all experiments, trials followed at long and unpredictable intervals. In each experiment, the pre-stimulus BOLD signal (dotted vertical line marking stimulus onset) was examined as a function of perceptual outcome and sampled from accordingly specialized sensory areas. The corresponding regions of interest (early auditory cortex, FFA and hMT+, respectively) are presented on a canonical inflated cortical surface of the right hemisphere. In all experiments, higher pre-stimulus time course in the respective sensory region biased towards perceiving stimulus properties for which these regions are particularly sensitive. Error bars represent standard error across subjects. (Figure 3 reprinted from Sadaghiani S, Hesselmann G, Friston KJ, and Kleinschmidt A (2010). The relation of ongoing brain activity, evoked neural responses, and cognition. *Front Syst Neuroscie* 2010, June 23, 4:20.)**

during the generation of stimulus-induced activity. They argue that rest–stimulus interaction does not result from mere addition or summation of the levels of both resting-state activity and stimulus-induced activity.

Instead, the resting-state activity seems to exert a specific mechanism by itself, by means of which it is able to impact subsequent stimulus-induced activity. Thereby the level of the resting-state activity itself may set the threshold for the degree to which the nonlinear mechanism can be exerted and imposed upon stimulus-induced activity (see Chapter 12 for more details on non-linearity during rest-stimulus interaction)

Does intraregional rest–stimulus interaction also hold in regions other than the sensory cortex? Kleinschmidt's group (Coste et al. 2011) conducted a Stroop task wherein the names of colors interfered with the color in which the respective color names were presented (the word "green" was, for instance, presented inside the color "red"). Subjects had to push a button to determine the color and whether it was congruent or incongruent.

They again showed that the pre-stimulus activity in relevant regions like the anterior cingulate cortex (ACC) and the dorsolateral prefrontal cortex (DLPFC) predicted subsequent behavioral performance, that is, reaction times: the higher the pre-stimulus resting-state activity in the ACC and the DLPFC, the faster the subsequent reaction times in response to the stimuli.

While this concerns cognitive regions like the ACC and the DLPLFC, the reverse relationship was observed in sensory regions involved in color and word processing: the higher the pre-stimulus resting-state activity in the right color-sensitive area and the visual word form area, the slower the subsequent reaction times. These data clearly show that rest–stimulus interaction is mediated by both higher order cognitive and lower order sensory regions but in different ways.

Neuronal findings Ib: transregional rest–stimulus interaction

So far we have discussed only intra-regional rest–stimulus interaction. How about the impact of the resting-state activity in one region on the stimulus-induced activity in another region? This may be subsumed under the concept of "trans-regional rest–stimulus interaction."

A more or less analogous observation of transregional effects in humans was first shown in a study by Greicius and Menon (2004). They investigated how the default-mode network (DMN), the task-negative network, impacts subsequent stimulus-induced activity in visual and auditory tasks during passive sensory tasks within each subject.

The level of activity in the DMN during stimulation predicted the degree of neuronal activity in both visual and auditory cortex during the auditory and visual tasks: the lower the activity in the task-negative regions of the DMN during auditory/visual stimulation, the higher the stimulus-induced neuronal activity in task-positive regions like the auditory and visual cortex. Hence, the level of resting state activity in the task-negative regions of the DMN impacts the stimulus-induced neuronal activity in task-positive regions.

Support for the impact of the DMN on sensory cortex also comes from the aforementioned auditory detection study by Sadaghiani et al. (2009; see also Boly et al. 2007; Mennes et al. 2011; Liu et al. 2011, for analogous results that demonstrate the impact of the DMN's resting state on subsequent stimulus-induced activity in other regions). In addition to the auditory cortex (see earlier), other regions like the precuneus, the anterior insula, the thalamus, the medial prefrontal cortex, and the anterior cingulate cortex also showed higher pre-stimulus activity that preceded hits but not the misses: the higher the pre-stimulus activity in these regions, the better the subsequent behavioral performance; that is, successful detection of the target sound.

Interestingly, pre-stimulus activity in the regions of the dorsal attention system, including the parietal and lateral frontal cortices, was biased toward misses. The higher the pre-stimulus resting-state activity in these regions, the more likely subjects were to miss and not hear the target sound. This again underscores that transregional rest–stimulus interaction may occur throughout the whole brain, though in different ways in different regions and networks.

What about functional connectivity during stimulus-induced activity? Smith et al. (2009) collected data from various fMRI activation studies that focused on stimulus-induced activity during different kinds of stimuli and tasks. In addition (and independently), they also investigated resting-state connectivity in a separate sample of subjects.

In both cases (meta-analysis of their subject groups), they used independent component analysis (ICA) to delineate the regions whose time series correlated with each other to investigate the neural overlap of the resting state networks with those during stimulus-induced activity. Interestingly, the networks that yielded functional activity (FC) during the stimulus-induced activity resembled very much the FC during resting state activity. Going one step further, they also demonstrated that the resting state networks persisted more or less during the stimulus-induced activity. This means that the neural networks are continuously connected and are thus 'active' during both resting state and stimulus-induced activity with the latter only modulating the FC of the former.

In sum, the neural networks and their FC during stimulus-induced activity do seem to be very much predisposed by the ones during the resting state. The networks and their functional connectivity in the resting state may be regarded as necessary though non-sufficient condition of the kind of neural networks and their degrees of functional connectivity that can possibly be elicited by the stimulus. Hence, there is transregional rest–stimulus interaction, which also predicts the behavioral (and also mental; see Volume II for details) states associated with the respective stimulus-induced activity.

Neuronal findings IIA: Causal interaction between resting-state and stimulus-induced activity in animals

These data clearly demonstrate that the resting-state activity level has an impact on subsequent stimulus-induced activity and its behavioral effects. What one needs to show, however, is that the resting-state activity causally impacts the stimulus-induced activity. One strategy here may be to vary the overall global level of resting-state activity and then to see how that impacts stimulus-induced activity during particular tasks. This was done in animals in a study by the group around Robert Shulman.

You may remember from part II, Robert Shulman is the physicist at Yale University who investigated the baseline metabolism of the brain and how it impacts the latter's intrinsic activity level. Now he went one step further and tested how the baseline metabolism impacts subsequent stimulus-induced activity in an animal study by Maandag et al. (2007).

Maandag et al. (2007) induced pharmacologically (using anesthetic drugs halothane and chloralose that are supposed to act, at least in part, via GABA) high and low levels of resting-state activity (RSA) in rats and measured their neural activity in fMRI during forepaw stimulation. The high level of resting activity was associated with widespread activity across the cortex and rather weak evoked activity in sensorimotor cortex during the forepaw movement. This pattern was reversed in the low RSA where neural activity was stronger in the sensorimotor cortex but more or less absent in other cortical regions.

These results demonstrate that the level of RSA may modulate the distribution and intensity of stimulus-induced activity in different ways in different cortical regions (see also Shulman et al. 2009a and b; and van Eijsden et al. 2009, for discussion of the results by Maandag on a conceptual level). Most important, they provide evidence in favor of a causal impact of the resting-state activity on both intra- and transregional stimulus-induced activity.

Neuronal findings IIB: Causal interaction between resting-state activity and stimulus-induced activity in humans

How about such causal rest–stimulus interaction in humans? For that, Pengmin Qin (Qin et al. 2013) from our group devised a clever experimental design by taking advantage of the distinction between different baselines.

Recall that we distinguished in Chapter 4 between different baselines in the brain. The "exteroceptive baseline" signifies the brain's resting state during unspecific exteroceptive stimuli during eyes open, while the "interoceptive baseline" describes the resting state when the eyes are closed and the unspecific interoceptive stimulus predominates. What did Pengmin Qin do in order to test for rest–stimulus interaction? He delivered the same auditory stimuli once during eyes open and once during eyes closed. This allowed him to test for the causal impact of two different resting states, that is, intero- and exteroceptive baselines, on the stimulus-induced activity related to the same stimulus.

First, based on a special acquisition technique in fMRI, for example, sparse sampling, Pengmin Qin determined the impact of the scanner noise on the auditory cortex and compared that condition to the complete absence of any scanner noise. As expected, this yielded strong activity changes in the bilateral auditory cortex in the comparison of noise versus no noise. This served to determine and locate the auditory cortex's resting-state activity, albeit indirectly, via the comparison of noise versus no noise. He then used the exact location in auditory cortex as the region of interest for the subsequent analyses.

In a second step, he conducted data acquisition in fMRI during eyes open and closed to investigate the resting-state activity in visual cortex and its modulation by a very basic stimulus, eyes open. Analogous to the auditory cortex, this served to determine the visual cortex's resting-state activity albeit indirectly via eyes open; this region was then used as a region of interest in subsequent analyses. Data in both eyes open and closed conditions were acquired in two different modes, in 20-s periods ("block design"), which allowed for the generation of BOLD changes, that is, neural activity, and 6 min periods to determine functional connectivity of the visual cortex to other regions, for instance, the auditory cortex.

Finally, in a third step, Qin et al. (2012) investigated auditory name perception in two conditions, eyes open and closed, by letting subjects listen to the same names during both conditions: closed and open eyes. This served

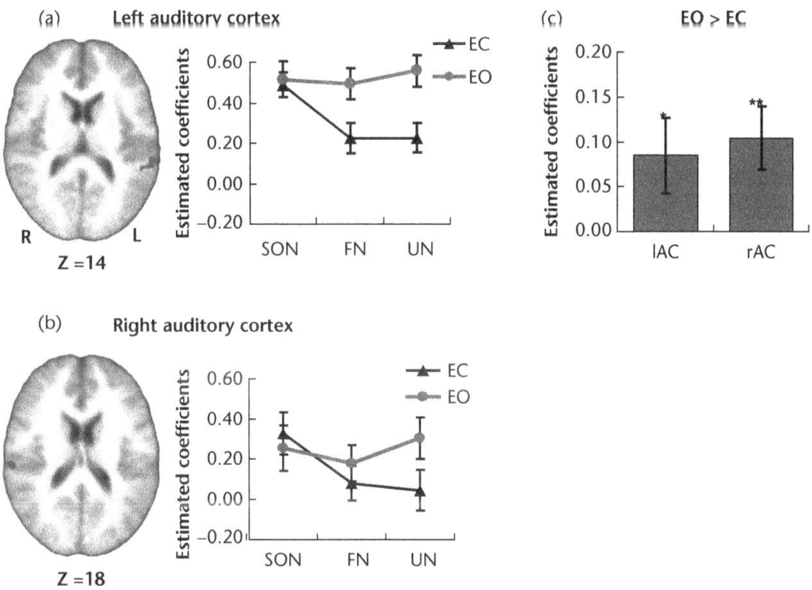

Figure 11-1b **Nonlinear rest–stimulus interaction in auditory cortex. The figure describes the outcome/signal changes in left and right auditory cortex (lAC, rAC) of a functional magnetic resonance imaging (fMRI) study by Qin et al. (2013), where the same auditory stimuli (subject's own name/SON as indicated by red bars; unknown name/UN as indicated by black bars) were presented during two different resting-state conditions, eyes closed (EC) and eyes open (EO). (*a*) The figure shows the signal changes (bar diagrams) for the two conditions (own and unknown name) in both right and left auditory cortex. While the subject's own name elicited the same degree of signal change during both EC and EO, this was not the case in the unknown name; here the signal change was much stronger during EO than EC. Since the stimuli were the same in both EC and EO, this can only be due to the difference in the resting-state activity itself, that is, the change from EC to EO. This difference with regard to the unknown name during EC and EO is further illustrated by figures (*b*) (based on real data) and (*c*) (schematically) showing that it can only be related to the difference in the resting-state activity caused by the difference between EC and EO. The differential reactivity of the resting state during EC and EO to the same stimulus, that is, the unknown name, while showing similar reactivity to another stimulus, the subject's own name, is strongly indicative of nonlinear (rather than linear) rest–stimulus interaction.**

to investigate the impact of eyes open and closed, mirroring different baselines (i.e., extero- and interoceptive baseline; see Chapter 4) on stimulus-induced activity associated with the same stimulus (see Fig. 11-1b).

How about the impact of the different resting states on stimulus-induced activity? During eyes closed, the subject's own name induced significantly stronger activity in auditory cortex than the other person's name. This difference disappeared, however, when the same names, his own and others, were presented during eyes open. Since the stimuli were the same in both cases, i.e., his own and other names, the absence of any difference in signal change between one's own and other names during eyes open can only be due to the resting state itself and thus to the difference between eyes closed and open.

This means that the resting-state activity in auditory cortex must have undergone some changes when opening the eyes, thereby apparently changing its sensitivity to especially the other names' stimuli. While we currently do not know what exactly changed in the resting state itself, this demonstrates the causal impact of the resting-state activity level on subsequent stimulus-induced activity in auditory cortex.

Taken together, these findings show that different levels of resting-state activity in auditory cortex (during eyes open and closed) impact subsequent stimulus-induced activity, that is, name perception, in the very same region. This indicates that there must be some interaction between the resting-state activity and the stimulus-induced activity in auditory cortex. Hence, the amount or degree of stimulus-induced activity is not only determined by the stimulus itself but also by the level of the resting-state activity. The exact neuronal mechanisms underlying the resting state's impact on stimulus-induced activity remain unclear (see later for further discussion).

Neuronal hypothesis Ia: difference-based coding of rest–stimulus interaction

What kind of neural coding and which neuronal mechanisms mediate the reported intra- and transregional rest–stimulus interaction? The observed dependence of the possible degree of stimulus-induced activity on the preceding resting-state activity level is possible only if the activity the stimulus elicits, that is, stimulus-induced activity is encoded in its relative (spatial and temporal) difference from the resting-state activity level.

The degree of stimulus-induced activity is consequently determined by the degree of the "virtual" difference between resting-state activity and stimulus-induced activity (if it were induced independent of the brain's resting-state activity). In short, I presume difference-based coding during rest–stimulus interaction.

If, in contrast, there were stimulus-induced activity, the resulting stimulus-induced activity should be completely and exclusively traced back to the stimulus itself, while the preceding resting-state activity should have no impact at all. That contradicts, however, the findings by the group around Kleinschmidt and others (see earlier discussion, as well as Northoff et al. 2010, for a recent review).

The assumption of stimulus-based coding also contradicts the findings by Qin et al. (2013): if stimulus-based coding holds, hearing the same name should lead to the same degree of stimulus-induced during both eyes open and closed. This, however, is not the case, as described earlier. Instead, the resting-state activity level impacts and predicts subsequent stimulus-induced activity, including its associated behavioral (and mental) states.

Based on these observations, I hypothesize that what is encoded into stimulus-induced activity is the (virtual spatiotemporal) difference between the actual resting-state activity level and the degree of stimulus-induced activity if it were induced isolated and independent of any resting-state activity. In short, I postulate that rest–stimulus interaction presupposes difference-based coding rather than stimulus-based coding.

Neuronal hypothesis Ib: difference-based coding of rest–stimulus interaction and consciousness

Why is the characterization of rest–stimulus interaction by difference-based coding so important? I hypothesize that difference-based coding of rest–stimulus interaction is relevant not only neuronally but also phenomenally; that is, for consciousness. If the stimulus is encoded in terms of stimulus-based coding, it is processed more or less independently and isolated from the resting-state activity. This means that there is no real interaction between rest and stimulus in the case of stimulus-induced activity.

Based on recent empirical data (see Chapters 28 and 29 in Volume II for details) I propose that this is exactly what happens in patients with vegetative state (VS) who have lost their consciousness. Due to (presumably) their lack of metabolic energy, these patients are apparently no longer able to encode extrinsic stimuli relative to the resting state activity in terms of spatial and temporal differences. Their degree of difference-based coding during rest–stimulus interaction is consequently rather low, while the degree of stimulus-based coding is rather high.

What does such reduced difference-based coding imply for the processing of the stimulus? The stimulus can no longer properly interact with the resting-state activity. For reasons that will become clear in Volume II, I deem proper rest–stimulus interaction necessary in order to associate the resulting purely neuronal stimulus-induced activity with consciousness and its phenomenal features. The loss of proper rest–stimulus interaction, due to the extremely low degree of difference-based coding, may then go along with loss of consciousness as is observed in VS patients (see Chapters 28 and 29 for details). Accordingly, I suggest that difference-based coding of rest–stimulus interaction is relevant not only neuronally, but also phenomenally.

Neuronal hypothesis IIa: Rest–rest interaction precedes rest–rest interaction

How can we specify the neuronal mechanisms underlying difference-based coding of rest–stimulus interaction? Let us remember what I stated earlier, in the context of stimulus–stimulus interaction. There I described four functional principles, spatial and temporal coincidence, inverse effectiveness, and nonlinearity, which presuppose difference-based coding rather than stimulus-based coding (see Chapter 10 for details).

If we can now show that the same principles also hold for and determine rest–stimulus interaction, one must postulate that the latter also presupposes difference- rather than stimulus-based coding. Accordingly, since the same functional principles apply, I postulate that difference-based coding applies to rest–stimulus interaction in very much the same way as it seems to operate during stimulus–stimulus interaction.

Let us be more concrete and discuss each principle separately, starting with the principle of spatial coincidence. The principle of spatial coincidence states that the degree of stimulus-induced activity is dependent on the degree to which different stimuli and their underlying neuronal activity converge spatially. How is transregional rest–stimulus interaction, such as that between the DMN's resting-state activity level and the sensory cortical stimulus-induced activity, possible?

I propose that there must be some prior transregional interaction within the resting state itself, that is, rest–rest interaction in that the DMN's resting-state activity must modulate the resting-state activity level of the sensory cortex (see Qin et al. 2013 for empirical support). Hence, transregional rest–stimulus interaction seems to presuppose transregional rest–rest interaction, which in turn predisposes the possible range of subsequent stimulus-induced activity.

Neuronal hypothesis IIb: "Spatial coincidence" during rest–stimulus interaction

What does this tell us about the spatial nature of rest–stimulus interaction? I hypothesize that there must be spatial coincidence between resting-state activity changes and the neural activity changes as they can potentially be induced by the stimulus. More specifically, the spatial pattern of the preceding rest–rest interaction must coincide with the spatial and temporal pattern related to the stimulus. What do I mean, however, when I speak of coincidence between rest and stimulus?

The reference to spatial (and temporal) pattern refers to what we described in parts I and II as the stimuli's statistical frequency distribution across different discrete points in physical time and space; that is, the stimuli's natural statistics. As discussed in the preceding chapters (see Chapters 6 and 9), the same holds on the side of the brain and its resting-state activity: analogously, the brain's intrinsic activity shows a statistical frequency distribution in its neural activity, its neuronal statistics (see Chapters 6 and 9) as they are manifested in what I described as the resting state's "spatial structure" (see Chapter 4).

What does this imply for rest–stimulus interaction? This means that the degree of spatial coincidence between the resting state's and the stimuli's statistically based spatial (and temporal) pattern ultimately comes down to the degree to which natural and neuronal statistics match and compare with each other. I henceforth hypothesize the principle of spatial coincidence to also apply to rest–stimulus interaction: This principle is determined by statistically based spatial coincidence between the resting state's spatial structure, its neuronal statistics, and the stimuli's different discrete points in physical space, their natural statistics.

NEURONAL HYPOTHESIS IIC: "TEMPORAL COINCIDENCE" DURING REST–STIMULUS INTERACTION

What about the principle of temporal coincidence? The principle of temporal coincidence states that the degree of stimulus-induced activity is dependent on the degree to which, and how, different stimuli and their underlying neuronal activity converge temporally.

Electroencephalography (EEG) studies (see Northoff et al. 2010 for an overview as well as Chapters 5 and 10 for more details) clearly show that the temporal occurrence of the stimulus in relation to the resting-state activity is important to elicit and modulate stimulus-induced activity. This means that the temporal difference between, for instance, the slow wave oscillations of the resting-state activity and the temporal occurrence of the stimulus may determine and thus code subsequent stimulus-induced activity. This will be further discussed and supported by empirical examples in Chapter 12 as well as in Chapters 14, 15, 19, and 20).

Analogous to the spatial domain, the temporal features of the resting-state activity, for example, the timing of the phase onsets and durations of its frequency fluctuations and its functional connectivity, need to coincide with the temporal coordinates of the stimuli. Thereby it is the statistical frequency distribution across the different discrete points in physical time of both the resting-state activity and the stimulus that is central. In other words, as in the spatial domain, the resting state's neuronal statistics and the stimuli's natural statistics may be compared and matched with each other in their temporal features.

More specifically, I hypothesize that the degree of temporal coincidence corresponds to the degree of matching or difference between the natural statistics of the stimulus' occurrence across time and the neuronal statistics of the resting state's frequency fluctuations. That is possible only if the statistically based temporal differences between resting state and stimuli are encoded into neural activity (rather than encoding both separately and parallel; that is, independently).

This means that such statistically based temporal coincidence presupposes difference-based coding rather than stimulus-based coding. Accordingly, as in the spatial domain, difference-based coding makes possible the principle of coincidence during rest–stimulus interaction, while it would not be compatible with stimulus-based coding.

NEURONAL HYPOTHESIS IIIA: "INVERSE EFFECTIVENESS" DURING REST–STIMULUS INTERACTION

We also need to discuss the principle of inverse effectiveness. We recall from Chapter 10 that the principle of inverse effectiveness states that the degree of weakness of a particular stimulus enhances its possible interaction effects with another, rather strong, stimulus when compared to the state of both stimuli's being strong (see Chapter 10).

How does that apply to rest–stimulus interaction? One may want to argue that the level of resting-state activity may predispose the possible range of the subsequent stimulus-induced activity. But we need to be more specific: the stronger the degree of the resting state's functional connectivity and the more power its frequency fluctuations show, the less the stimulus will be able to elicit strong stimulus-induced activity. One would consequently hypothesize an inverse relationship between the strength or power of the resting-state activity and the possible degree of stimulus-induced activity. The weaker the one, the stronger the other, while the converse is also true.

How can we empirically support this assumption of inverse effectiveness during rest–stimulus interaction? Some initial, more indirect support for that assumption comes from the animal study by Maandag et al. (2007). They did indeed observe higher resting-state activity to go along with decreased activity in motor cortex, while low resting-state activity led to increased motor cortical activity (see earlier for details).

Neuronal Hypothesis IIIb: "Trait" versus "State" Resting-State Activity and "Inverse Effectiveness"

We need to be careful, however. The current data, especially from the group around Kleinschmidt, do not lend direct support to the assumption that a lower resting state makes possible higher stimulus-induced activity. They rather observed the opposite: namely, that a higher pre-stimulus interval leads to higher subsequent stimulus-induced activity and stronger behavioral effects.

How can we explain that? We need to distinguish among different kinds of rest–stimulus interaction in orientation on the temporal scale. The group around Kleinschmidt tested for the effects of the actual resting-state activity level in each trial, i.e., trial-based, which thus concerns a state-dependent resting-state activity.

This differs from a more long-term resting-state activity across several trials, as investigated in the studies by Qin and Shulman; they therefore target trait rather than state features in the resting-state activity. In short, based on the different time scales and the use of either one or several trials, one may want to speak of "state resting-state activity" and "trait resting-state activity."

How does that relate to the principle of inverse effectiveness? The principle of inverse effectiveness may apply to the "trait resting-state activity" and may thus be regarded a trait feature of the resting-state activity. In contrast, it may not apply to the "state resting-state activity" and is therefore not a state-dependent feature of the resting-state activity that, for instance, may be more manifest during particular events or single trials (as put in operational terms). Since the group around Kleinschmidt focused on the "state resting-state activity," their findings could not conform to the principle of inverse effectiveness.

Neuronal Hypothesis IIIc: Range of the Resting-State Activity and "Inverse Effectiveness"

Another issue may be the range of the resting-state activity level. One may, for instance, want to distinguish between optimal and non-optimal ranges of resting-state activity for subsequent stimulus-induced activity. Increases in resting-state activity within its optimal range may make possible higher stimulus-induced activity.

This may imply that recruitment in the resting-state activity's optimal ranges may go along with increased degrees of the principle inverse effectiveness, which may indicate increased degrees of reactivity or sensitivity of the resting state to extrinsic stimuli.

In contrast, increases in the resting-state activity outside its optimal ranges may go along with a decrease in the possible degree of subsequent stimulus-induced activity. That may signify decreased degrees of the principle of inverse effectiveness which indicates that the resting-state activity is simply no longer as reactive to stimuli anymore. This may be the case in psychiatric disorders like depression, where the resting-state activity shows abnormally high levels of activity in certain regions that seem to be closely related to decreased stimulus-induced activity in the same regions (see Chapter 27 for details).

However, we currently do not know much, if anything, about the optimal and nonoptimal ranges of the resting-state activity for subsequent stimulus-induced activity. This may also be related to the biophysical-computational features of the neurons and the resting-state activity itself, which will be discussed later (see Fig. 11-2a).

Neuronal Hypothesis IVa: "Nonlinearity" During Rest–Stimulus Interaction

What about the principle of nonlinearity? The principle of nonlinearity states that the stimulus-induced activity results, not from the mere addition or summation of two stimuli or resting state and stimulus-induced activity—instead, the resulting stimulus-induced activity is either higher or lower than their mere addition or summation, which can only be due to nonlinear effects in their interaction.

The earlier described data by Pengmin Qin from our group provide tentative empirical support in favor of nonlinearity in rest–stimulus interaction. The same stimuli,.i.e., the subject's own name, elicit different degrees of stimulus-induced activity during different resting-state conditions. And, most important, this was different for different stimuli, i.e., one's own and another's name, that interacted in different ways with the different resting-state activity levels during the conditions of eyes open and closed. Such differential interaction of the different stimuli with the different resting-state activity lets one suppose nonlinear rather than linear interaction.

The same may be inferred from the results by the group around A. Kleinschmidt (see earlier discussion as well as Hesselmann et al. 2008). However, future studies may want to apply measures of nonlinearity and see whether they predict neural activity changes during rest–stimulus interaction.

I tentatively hypothesize that nonlinearity requires a specific constellation between the resting state's neuronal statistics and the stimuli's natural statistics (see Fig. 11-2b). There must be a specific statistically based spatiotemporal difference in order for the stimulus to elicit nonlinear deviation from the actual resting-state activity level. If, in contrast, the "right" statistically based spatiotemporal difference is not met, the stimulus will be able to only elicit linear rather than nonlinear changes in the brain's resting-state activity.

However, what the "right" and "wrong" statistically based spatiotemporal differences are remains unclear at this point. Moreover, the neuronal mechanisms underlying such nonlinearity during rest–stimulus interaction remain unclear, too (see Fig. 11-2b); these will be discussed in further detail in Chapter 12 herein, as well as in Chapters 28 and 29 in Volume II.

Neuronal Hypothesis IVb: "Nonlinearity" During Rest–Stimulus Interaction and Consciousness

The assumption of nonlinearity in rest–stimulus interaction is not only neuronally relevant, but may also be of central relevance for consciousness; that is, phenomenally relevant. I assume, for instance, that patients in a vegetative state (VS), as defined by the loss of consciousness, may suffer from a lack of nonlinearity during rest–stimulus interaction (see Chapters 28 and 29 for details).

If so, the degree of nonlinearity during rest–stimulus interaction may be related to the degree of consciousness: The higher the degree of nonlinearity during rest–stimulus interaction, the more likely the resulting purely neuronal stimulus-induced activity will be associated with consciousness and its phenomenal features. If, in contrast, there is a high degree of linearity (rather than nonlinearity) during rest–stimulus interaction, the lower the likelihood that consciousness will be associated with the resulting stimulus-induced activity.

Since this reaches deeply into the realm of consciousness, I will discuss the exact underlying neuronal mechanisms in Volume II, especially in Chapters 28 and 29. What is clear at this point is that nonlinearity during rest–stimulus

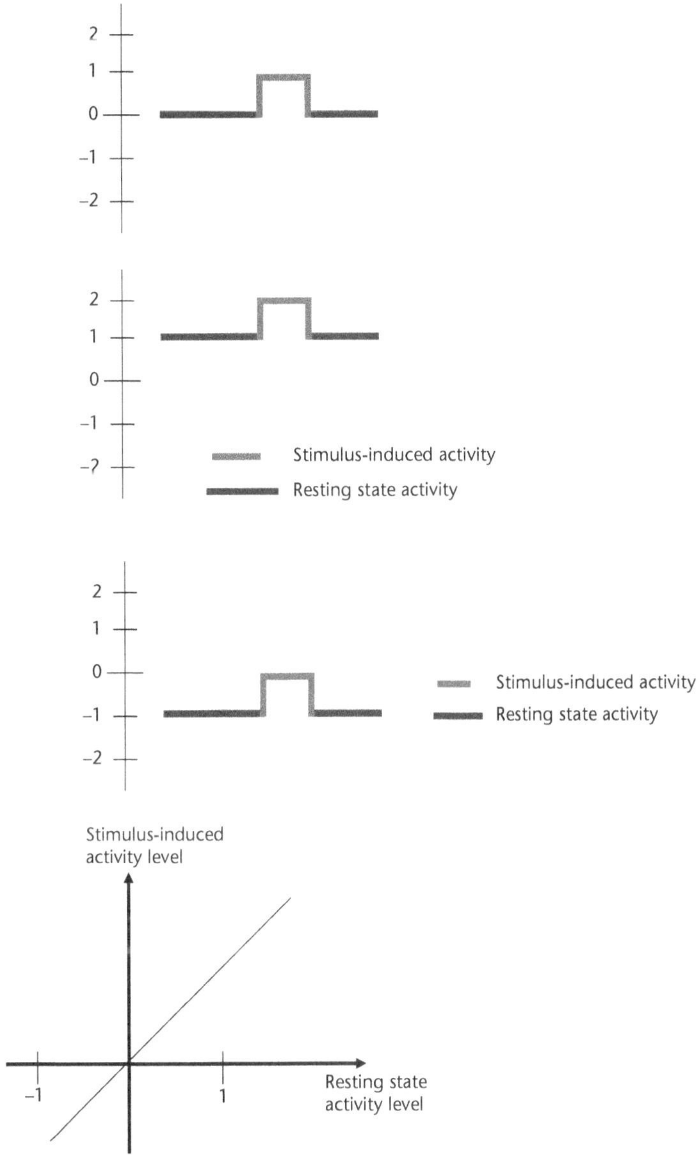

Figure 11-2a and b **Inverse effectiveness and nonlinear interaction during rest–stimulus interaction. The figure illustrates the relationship between inverse effectiveness and nonlinearity in neural activity. Different levels of resting-state activity (black, -1, 0, 1) are shown and how they impact subsequent stimulus-induced activity(grey). This is illustrated in the upper three graphs in each figure, that is, *a* and *b*. While the fourth graph in each figure (*a*, *b*) summarizes this by plotting the degree of stimulus-induced activity (y-axis) in dependence on the different degrees of resting-state activity (x-axis). In the case of no inverse effectiveness, the different degrees or levels of resting-state activity (-1, 0, 1) elicit the same degree of stimulus-induced activity (first three graphs), resulting in linear relationship between both (fourth graph). In the case of inverse effectiveness, the different degrees or levels of resting-state activity (-1, 0, 1) elicit different degrees of stimulus-induced activity (first three graphs), resulting in nonlinear relationship between both (fourth graph).**

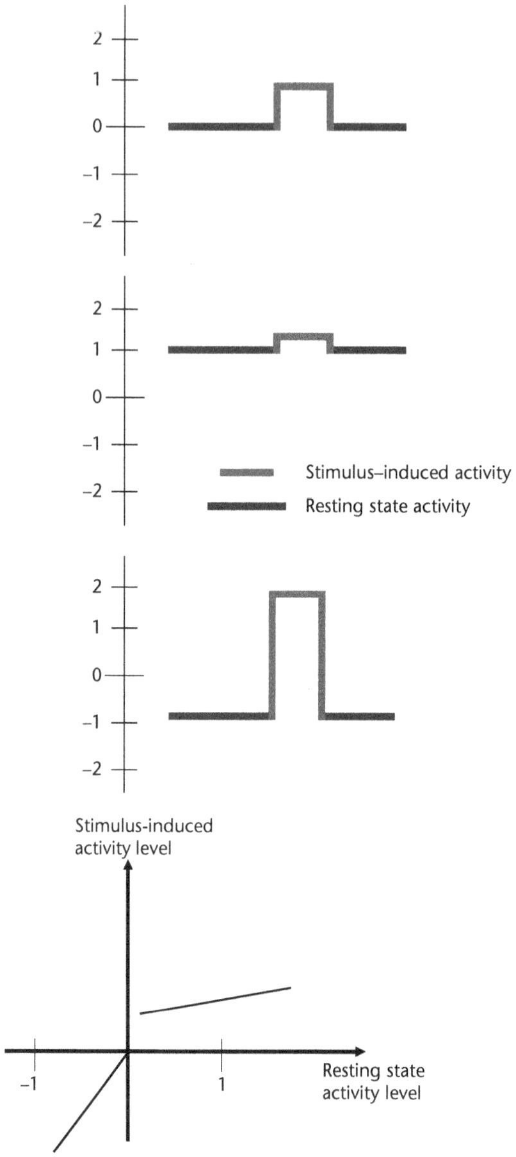

Figure 11-2a and b (*continued*)

interaction is not only neuronally but also phenomenally relevant.

Neuronal Findings IIIa: Stimulus–Rest Interaction During Sensory and Motor Stimuli

So far I have demonstrated that the brain's resting-state activity exerts an impact on subsequent exteroceptive stimuli and their associated stimulus-induced activity in either the same or other regions. This is what I subsumed under the concept of rest–stimulus interaction.

There may be the reverse kind of interaction going on with the stimulus-induced activity modulating the resting-state activity level in either the same or other regions. This is what I subsume under the general concept of "stimulus–rest interaction" (see also Northoff et al. 2010). Unlike in the case of rest–stimulus interaction, there are not yet many studies showing the impact of stimuli on subsequent resting-state activity. In the following I want to describe some of the earlier studies while not covering the whole territory. One study in humans investigated the effects of motor learning on resting-state activity in humans (Albert et al. 2009). Resting-state activity was investigated in fMRI before and after an 11-minute visuomotor training session. Neural activity in lateral frontal and parietal regions and the cerebellum was significantly increased after the visuomotor training session when compared to before the session.

Interestingly, the same network was not recruited during mere motor performance; changes in the resting-state activity in this network may thus be more closely related to visuomotor learning rather than mere visuomotor performance. Accordingly, the neural effects of both motor learning and motor performance could be distinguished from each other with regard to their networks and their time period (i.e., stimulus- versus resting-state period).

Another study by Lewis et al. (2009) investigated the effects of visual perceptual learning on resting-state connectivity. The subjects trained in a shape-identification task constrained to one visual quadrant. After several days of training, subjects underwent fMRI, which was done during the visual training task. This revealed an effect of the training of the respective side; that is, the respective visual quadrant, in the visual cortical activation when compared to the untrained side.

How about the impact of the training on the functional connectivity in the resting state? Subjects also underwent two sets of fMRI resting-state scans with visual fixation before and after behavioral training. The training led to a difference in the resting-state connectivity between the visual cortex and other regions, including task-positive (i.e., frontoparietal regions involved in spatial attention) and task-negative (i.e., DMN) regions. These findings clearly demonstrate the impact of visual perceptual learning on the resting-state functional connectivity inside and outside the DMN.

Analogous effects were observed in rat visual cortex (Han et al. 2008). The repetitive presentation of a visual stimulus induced not only stimulus-induced activity in the visual cortex but also impacted subsequent spontaneous ongoing activity in the same region. The subsequent spontaneous activity pattern in the visual cortex resembled very much the spatiotemporal pattern of the preceding stimulus-induced activity. The authors called this "wave-mediated reverberation," and postulated that it may contribute to the consolidation of the transient effects of sensory experience onto long-lasting cortical modifications.

Such stimulus–rest interaction is also suggested by other recent animal studies (Berkes et al. 2011; Fukushima et al. 2012). Based on recording cellular and multicellular activity, they demonstrate that spontaneous activity patterns in either visual (Berkes et al. 2011) or auditory (Fukushima et al. 2012) cortex resemble very much the stimulus-induced activity pattern in their spatial and temporal pattern. Fukushima et al. (2012) showed that the spontaneous activity in monkey auditory cortex exhibits the same spatial covariation as the stimulus-induced tonotopic maps in the same region. The same could be observed in visual cortex (V1) in ferrets, whose spontaneous activity resembled more and more the activity during stimulus-induced activity and the stimuli's natural statistics (see Berkes et al. 2011; see also Chapter 9 for such stimulus–rest interaction).

In sum, these initial studies demonstrate that stimuli can exert their effects on the subsequent resting state amounting to stimulus–rest interaction. It should be noted that the neural effects concerned mainly long-term effects as averaged across different trials of stimulus-induced activity. This suggests that the stimulus–rest interaction effects reported here concern mainly trait rather than state features of the resting-state activity and thus the "trait resting state" as distinguished from the "state resting state" (see earlier for this distinction). Moreover, the animal studies suggest that the encoding of the stimuli's natural statistics into the resting-state activity and its neuronal statistics (see Chapter 9) may be the central encoding mechanism that provides the bridge from the stimulus-induced to the resting-state activity.

Neuronal findings IIIb: stimulus–rest interaction during cognitive and emotional stimuli

These studies show effects of the stimulus on the subsequent resting-state activity in sensory cortex; this concerns mainly what we described as the "exteroceptive baseline" of the resting-state activity, since it is maintained by continuous unspecific sensory input (see Chapter 4 for details). How about the resting-state activity in other networks and regions of the brain, such as the "neural baseline," the midline regions as part of the default-mode network where the input from the brain itself, the neural stimuli, predominates? Some studies also investigated the effects of sensorimotor stimuli and their stimulus-induced activity on the resting-state activity in the DMN.

A study by Pyka et al. (2009) investigated the activation of the DMN following different loads (1- and 2-back) in working-memory tasks compared to the activation in the DMN after the same task without any load (0-load). As expected, the different task difficulties— the 0-, 1-, and 2-back loads—yielded different degrees of deactivation; that is, negative BOLD response, in the regions of the DMN (perigenual anterior cingulate cortex, posterior parietal, and posterior cingulate cortex) during the working-memory task.

Interestingly, the resting-state periods following the working-memory task also differed in their degree of activation; that is, positive BOLD response. The resting-state periods following the 1- and 2-back tasks showed significantly higher signal changes in the aforementioned regions when compared to the ones following the 0-back task. This suggests that the subsequent resting-state period was differentially modulated by the different loads of the preceding working-memory task, indicating stimulus–rest interaction.

An analogous modulation of the resting-state activity level in the DMN by the preceding stimuli could be observed for the stimuli's degree of self-specificity in a study by Felix Schneider from our group (Schneider et al. 2008). Higher degrees of self-specificity in the preceding stimuli led to higher degrees of activity in the subsequent resting-state period in ventro- and dorsomedial prefrontal cortex and the posterior cingulate cortex (when compared to stimuli with lower degrees of self-specificity; see Schneider et al. 2008, as well as Chapter 23 for more details).

Focusing on emotions, Eryilmaz et al. (2011) investigated the impact of fearful, joyful, and neutral movie clips (50-sec presentation) on subsequent resting-state activity (90-sec eyes closed). They asked the participants after the resting-state period about their thoughts while lying in the scanner during fMRI. This revealed behaviorally that the subjects' personally relevant issues in their thoughts were increased after neutral movies, less increased after joyful movies, and significantly decreased after fearful movies. These results show a clear behavioral or better psychological effect of emotions on the thought contents in subsequent resting-state periods; fearful movies seem to leave apparently the strongest traces in the subsequent resting state's thought contents.

Neuronally, as measured with fMRI, the same subjects showed higher neuronal activity in subcortical regions (pallidum, anterior thalamus, hypothalamus) during the resting-state periods after seeing the fearful faces when compared to the ones following neutral movies (rest after fearful larger than rest after neutral). Most interestingly, the reverse comparison (rest after neutral larger rest after fearful) revealed higher signal changes in various regions of the DMN (VMPFC, PACC, DMPFC, STG) (see also Sreenivas et al. 2012 as well as Wiebking et al. 2011 for analogous overlap between emotion processing and the DMN).

This means that the inclusion of fearful emotions in the preceding movie had a clear effect on the level of the subsequent resting-state activity. The stronger resting-state effects of the preceding frightening movies are further confirmed by the more delayed recovery of the signal changes during the resting-state period (90s) after emotional movies.

Taken together, these studies demonstrate that stimulus-induced activity impacts the level of resting-state activity in both subcortical and cortical regions. However, due to the low number of studies, this conclusion must be considered preliminary, hence awaiting further empirical support.

Moreover, we need to be careful in distinguishing between state-related and trait-related effects: if studies show resting-state effects in single trials, the latter may concern state-related features, as in the studies on working memory and emotions. If, in contrast, the effects occur over several trials on a more long-term basis, the stimuli may rather affect trait features of the resting-state activity. We have to be clear, however, that neither the exact neuronal mechanisms underlying both state and trait features of the resting-state activity, nor their differential manipulation by stimuli, are currently known.

Neuronal hypothesis VA: spatial and temporal coincidence during stimulus–rest interaction

These examples clearly demonstrate that there is bilateral traffic between the resting state and stimuli. The resting state impacts the stimulus-induced activity, which in turn leaves its traces in the resting-state activity on either its state or trait features. This means that rest–stimulus and stimulus–rest interaction go hand in hand and may, metaphorically speaking, be considered two sides of one and the same coin.

I assumed that rest–stimulus interaction presupposes difference-based coding, which in turn makes possible the application of the four principles discussed earlier, spatial and temporal coincidence, inverse effectiveness, and nonlinearity. Without going into details, I now suggest the same to hold for stimulus–rest interaction.

Let me specify this for the principles of spatial and temporal coincidence. The stimulus-induced activity must spatially and temporally coincide with the subsequent resting-state activity in order to modulate the latter. The resting-state activity may thus show (or be constrained or imposed by the stimulus) the same spatial and temporal activity pattern as during the preceding stimulus-induced activity.

One would then postulate similarity or resemblance in spatiotemporal activity patterns between stimulus-induced activity and resting-state activity, which is indeed empirically supported, as demonstrated in the study on rat visual cortex by Han et al. (2008) and the other above mentioned studies by Berkes et al. (2011) and Fukushima et al. (2012). There may thus be spatial and temporal coincidence between stimulus-induced activity and resting-state activity, which suggests that the principles of spatial and temporal coincidence also hold for stimulus–rest interaction.

We have to be careful, however, since there is one difference. In the case of rest–stimulus interaction, the resting state and the stimulus had to spatially and temporally coincide. As detailed earlier, spatial and temporal coincidence describes a statistically based spatiotemporal coincidence of the resting state's neuronal statistics with the stimuli's natural statistics when the resting state impacts the stimulus. Such statistically based spatial and temporal coincidence is accompanied by nonlinear interaction and inverse effectiveness during rest–stimulus interaction. .

However, the situation is different in the case of stimulus–rest interaction. Here, the stimulus-induced activity and its spatial and temporal statistical frequency distribution, i.e.,, the stimuli's natural statistics, must spatially and temporally coincide with the resting state activity itself, i.e., the neuronal statistics. This means that the direction of spatial and temporal coincidence is no longer directed from the brain's resting-state activity to the stimuli from the environment, but rather in reverse, from environmental stimuli to the brain's resting state. While there may be spatial and temporal coincidence between stimulus-induced activity and resting-state activity, the question is whether such stimulus-rest interaction still is related to nonlinearity and inverse effectiveness. This will the discussed in the next section.

Neuronal hypothesis VB: nonlinearity during stimulus–rest interaction

How about nonlinear changes in the level of the resting-state activity itself after the exposure to the stimuli when compared to before stimuli?

The degree of the resulting resting-state activity changes may not be accounted for by the mere addition or summation between the degree of stimulus-induced activity and the degree of the resting-state activity level prior to the stimulus. Instead, the resulting resting-state activity level after the stimulus may be either higher or lower than their mere addition or summation would account for.

How would such nonlinearity impact the neuronal and behavioral effects of the stimulus–rest interaction? One would suggest the following: the higher the degree of nonlinearity during stimulus–rest interaction, the stronger the neuronal and behavioral effects that the stimulus can exert on the subsequent resting-state activity. This means that the resting-state activity and its spatiotemporal activity pattern would be highly sensitive and reactive to changes and modulations by the stimuli including its behavioral effects.

In contrast, lower degrees of nonlinearity in stimulus–rest interaction may lead to lower behavioral and neuronal effects of the stimulus on the subsequent resting state. Here the resting-state activity may be less sensitive and reactive to changes and modulations in its spatiotemporal activity pattern by the stimuli.

This may be the case in patients with vegetative state (VS) who have lost their consciousness. Here the stimulus may still elicit stimulus-induced activity, as has been demonstrated in various imaging studies applying cognitive tasks in VS patients (see Chapters 28 and 29). However, the stimulus may no longer affect the resting-state activity anymore because the latter, probably due to lacking energy, is no longer sensitive and reactive to the modulation of its spatiotemporal activity pattern by stimuli (see Chapters 28 and 29 for details). This means that the occurrence of nonlinearity may not only be neuronally relevant, that is, for stimulus–rest interaction, but also phenomenally, that is, for consciousness.

Neuronal hypothesis VIa: resting-state activity predisposes rest–stimulus interaction

Why are the resting state and its spatiotemporal activity pattern sensitive and reactive to stimuli as suggested by stimulus–rest interaction? As described earlier, the data show statistically based resemblance and similarity in the spatiotemporal activity pattern between stimulus-induced activity and resting-state activity.

What does such a similarity in their statistically based spatiotemporal activity pattern imply for the relationship between resting-state activity and stimulus-induced activity? By encoding the extrinsic stimuli's natural statistics into its own spatiotemporal activity pattern and its neuronal statistics, the brain's intrinsic activity may "prepare itself" optimally for the subsequent processing of the same extrinsic stimuli. In other words, by letting its own spatiotemporal activity pattern be modulated and changed by the stimuli during stimulus–rest interaction, the brain and its resting state provide the "optimal ground" for subsequent rest–stimulus interaction.

I hypothesize that rest–stimulus interaction may be predisposed by prior stimulus–rest interaction. There is consequently bilateral relationship between resting-state activity and stimulus-induced activity, with both mutually impacting, changing, and modulating each other's statistically based spatiotemporal activity pattern as manifested in rest–stimulus and stimulus–rest interaction. Such bilateral relationship makes possible that the effects of the one, stimulus–rest interaction, are conveyed and transferred to the respective other, rest–stimulus interaction.

How now can we describe such a transferal of the effects of stimulus–rest interaction onto subsequent rest–stimulus interaction in further detail? This leads us back to the resting-state activity itself, which commonly mediates both.

I propose that the resting-state activity provides a spatiotemporal predisposition for the possible ranges of subsequent rest–stimulus and stimulus–rest interaction. The resting state's configuration of its spatiotemporal structure, that is, its neuronal statistics, may open up the possibility for various stimuli and their respective natural statistics to interact strongly with the resting state. Or, alternatively, the resting state's neuronal statistics may be spatiotemporally configured in such way that it rather narrows and limits the possible degrees of subsequent rest–stimulus and stimulus–rest interaction.

Neuronal hypothesis VIb: Resting-state activity provides a "spatiotemporal window of opportunity"

How can we better illustrate the resting state and the kind of predisposition for subsequent rest–stimulus and stimulus–rest interaction? The resting state's predisposition may be compared to a spatiotemporal window of opportunity the resting state itself provides for its subsequent processing of the stimuli. I therefore speak of a "spatiotemporal window of opportunity." The concept of "spatiotemporal window of opportunity" describes the resting state's predisposition for its subsequent interaction with stimuli.

How is the resting state's "spatiotemporal window of opportunity" mediated? I postulate that the resting state's "spatiotemporal window of opportunity" consists in the particular configuration or constellation of its statistically based spatiotemporal activity pattern.

Neuronally, that may for instance be manifested in the resting state's functional connectivity pattern and its low and high frequency fluctuations, including the coupling of their phase onsets and amplitudes (see Chapters 4 and 5 for details). This is suggested by the observations of spatial and temporal coincidence between resting-state activity and stimulus-induced activity, as reported in the findings on rest–stimulus and stimulus–rest interaction.

By providing such a "spatiotemporal window of opportunity," the resting-state activity can impact the subsequent processing of the stimulus and thus stimulus-induced activity. The resting-state activity may restrict or enlarge the range in the degree of changes in functional connectivity or low frequency fluctuations the stimulus can possibly elicit in the brain and its resting-state activity.

If the resting-state activity is spatially and temporally configured in an optimal way, the resting-state activity may show high degrees of sensitivity and reactivity to stimuli, so that the latter may then be able to exert strong effects with possibly high degrees of nonlinearity and inverse effectiveness. In this case the resting state's "spatiotemporal window of opportunity" is wide open to possible change and modulation by stimuli.

What we here refer to as the resting state's "spatiotemporal window of opportunity" has also been described as "state dependency," the dependence of perception and cognition on the initial psychological and neuronal state of the respective subject (see Silvanto et al. 2008; Silvanto and Pascual-Leone 2008). The concept of "state dependency" has been used especially in the context of transcranial magnetic stimulation (TMS): the effects of the magnetic pulses on the visual cortex have been shown to be dependent not only upon the degree of stimulation itself, but also on the initial state of the brain and the psychological state of the person (see Najib et al. 2010; Silvanto et al. 2008).

Neuronal hypothesis VIc: Consciousness and the resting state's "spatiotemporal window of opportunity"

We can observe major changes in the resting state in psychiatric patients with depression. Here, the resting-state activity is abnormally high in for instance the anterior midline regions that show abnormal functional connectivity and low and high frequency fluctuations (see Chapter 27 for details). The resting-state activity is therefore in a less optimal range, which decreases its sensitivity and reactivity to stimuli; the range in the degrees of changes the stimuli can possibly elicit is here very much restricted and therefore limited by the resting state itself.

The resting-state activity's "spatiotemporal window of opportunity" is here no longer as wide open in depression as in healthy subjects. Since such partial closing of the resting state's spatiotemporal window of opportunity goes along with major changes in the contents of consciousness, I discuss the case of depression in full detail in Volume II (see Chapter 27).

There we will also encounter the most extreme case of when the resting-state activity closes its "spatiotemporal window of opportunity." In the case of the minimally conscious state (MCS) and vegetative state (VS), the resting-state activity's "spatiotemporal window of opportunity" seems to be partially closed, with the resting state being less sensitive and reactive to its modulation and change by stimuli. As suggested in Chapters 28 and 29, such partial closure of the resting state's "spatiotemporal window of opportunity" may be closely related to the lack of consciousness in these patients.

In the most extreme case, the resting-state activity is no longer sensitive and reactive to any kind of change or modulation in its spatiotemporal activity pattern by stimuli. This means that the resting-state activity does not provide any reactivity and sensitivity and thus an opportunity at all anymore for any kind of stimulus. Nothing happens anymore in the brain and its resting-state activity. The resting state's "spatiotemporal window of opportunity" is then not only closed, but locked. That is when we slip from coma into brain death (see Chapters 28 and 29).

On a whole, stimulus–rest interaction is assumed to be relevant in constituting the spatial and temporal structure of the resting-state activity in such way that it can optimally process stimuli during subsequent rest–stimulus interaction and stimulus–rest interaction. This leads to what I describe as the resting state's "spatiotemporal window of opportunity," which concerns the resting state's predisposition for possible changes and modulations elicited by stimuli during both rest–stimulus and stimulus–rest interaction.

In addition to its neuronal relevance, the resting state's spatiotemporal window of opportunity may also be central for consciousness and thus phenomenally relevant: the resting state's "spatiotemporal window of opportunity" seems to be partially closed in minimally conscious state (MCS) and vegetative state (VS) and then completely in coma and brain death (see Chapters 28 and 29).

Neuronal hypothesis VID: difference-based coding, nonlinearity, and the resting state's "spatiotemporal window of opportunity"

How can we further characterize and specify the resting state's "spatiotemporal window of opportunity" in neuronal terms? So far, I have characterized it by a particular constellation and configuration in the statistically based spatiotemporal activity pattern of the resting-state activity. We may, however, want to detail it further in neuronal terms; this is the focus in the next sections.

Let me start with the neuronal characterization of the resting state's "spatiotemporal window of opportunity." I demonstrated in Chapters 4 through 6 that the resting-state activity itself encodes the continuous dynamic changes in its own activity levels in terms of spatial and temporal differences, which is possible only on the basis of difference-based coding (as distinguished from stimulus-based coding). However, difference-based coding is not a matter of all-or-nothing, presence or absence. Instead, difference-based coding comes and operates in different degrees, showing a reciprocal balance with the degree of stimulus-based coding (see Chapters 1, 2, 4, and 6).

Who and what determines the degree of difference-based coding in the resting state? This is where the resting state itself and its "spatiotemporal window of opportunity" come in. By setting its level at a certain degree and showing a particular spatiotemporal configuration and constellation, the resting-state activity itself may modulate the degree of difference-based coding of neural activity. This means that certain levels of resting-state activity and particular spatiotemporal constellations and configurations may allow for a higher degree of difference-based coding (and a lower degree of stimulus-based coding) than others.

In other words, the resting state may provide an optimal "spatiotemporal window of opportunity" for high degrees of difference-based coding of its own neural activity during both the resting state and subsequent rest–stimulus interaction. The resting state's "spatiotemporal window of opportunity" may then be wide open to difference-based coding and rather closed to stimulus-based coding during rest–rest, rest–stimulus, and stimulus–rest interactions.

However, the resting state can also close its "spatiotemporal window of opportunity" for difference-based coding by changing its level and/or modulating its spatiotemporal activity pattern. In that case, the degree of difference-based coding will decrease while the one of stimulus-based coding will increase. The resting state's "spatiotemporal window of opportunity" is then partially closed for difference-based coding, while it is more open for stimulus-based coding of neural activity during the resting state itself and rest–stimulus and stimulus–rest interaction (see Figs. 11-3a).

Neuronal hypothesis VIe: Different degrees of difference-based coding modulate the "spatiotemporal window of opportunity"

Why is all that relevant? As described earlier, the degree of the various functional principles of rest–stimulus and stimulus–rest interaction is strongly dependent upon the degree of difference-based coding. More specifically, the degree to which spatial and temporal coincidence, inverse effectiveness, and nonlinearity operate during rest–stimulus and stimulus–rest interaction is dependent upon the degree of difference-based coding. Higher degrees of difference-based coding make more likely higher degrees of spatial and temporal coincidence, inverse effectiveness, and nonlinearity during rest–stimulus and stimulus–rest interaction.

What does mean for the resting state's "spatiotemporal window of opportunity"? By modulating the degree of difference-based coding via its level or spatiotemporal activity pattern, the resting state itself can impact the possible degree to which spatial and temporal coincidence, inverse effectiveness, and nonlinearity apply and operate during rest–stimulus and stimulus–rest interaction.

Higher degrees of difference-based coding will make possible higher degrees of nonlinearity, whereas higher degrees of stimulus-based coding will decrease the degree of nonlinearity and increase the degree of linearity during rest–stimulus and stimulus–rest interaction. This means that there are optimal and less optimal "spatiotemporal windows of opportunity" (or thresholds) set by the resting-state activity itself for the employment of high degrees of nonlinearity during subsequent rest–stimulus and stimulus–rest interaction (see Fig. 11-3b).

Neuronal hypothesis VIf: The resting state's "spatiotemporal window of opportunity" modulates the degree of sparse coding

As discussed earlier, the degree of nonlinearity strongly impacts the degree of stimulus-induced activity a stimulus can possibly elicit in the brain and its resting-state activity. High degrees of nonlinearity during rest–stimulus interaction may lead to high degrees of stimulus-induced activity. In contrast, low degrees of nonlinearity will only allow for a rather limited range in the degree of stimulus-induced activity. This means that the resting state's "spatiotemporal window of opportunity" is neuronally relevant in that it strongly impacts the degree of subsequent stimulus-induced activity.

The neuronal relevance of the resting state's "spatiotemporal window of opportunity" is further supported by its impact on the degree of sparse coding. We recall from Chapters 1 through 3 and Chapter 6 that the neural activity during both resting-state activity and stimulus-induced activity may be encoded into neural activity in a spatially and temporally sparse way.

This means that the relationship between the number of stimuli and the number of active cells/regions does not correspond in a one-to-one (local coding) or one-to-many (dense coding) but rather in terms of many-to-one. The stimuli and their spatial and temporal features are thus encoded into neural activity in a temporally and spatially sparse way during both resting state and stimulus-induced activity.

As in the case of difference-based coding, sparse coding is not an all-or-nothing matter, but comes rather in different degrees standing in reciprocal balance to dense/local coding (see Chapters 1 and 2). Higher degrees of sparse coding, then, are accompanied by lower degrees of local/dense coding, while increases in the degree of the latter entail decreases in the degree of the former.

Most important, I demonstrated in Chapters 1, 3, and 6 that sparse coding presupposes difference-based coding: the encoding of spatial and temporal differences into neural activity via difference-based coding leads to and entails the sparsening of the spatial and temporal activity

(a)

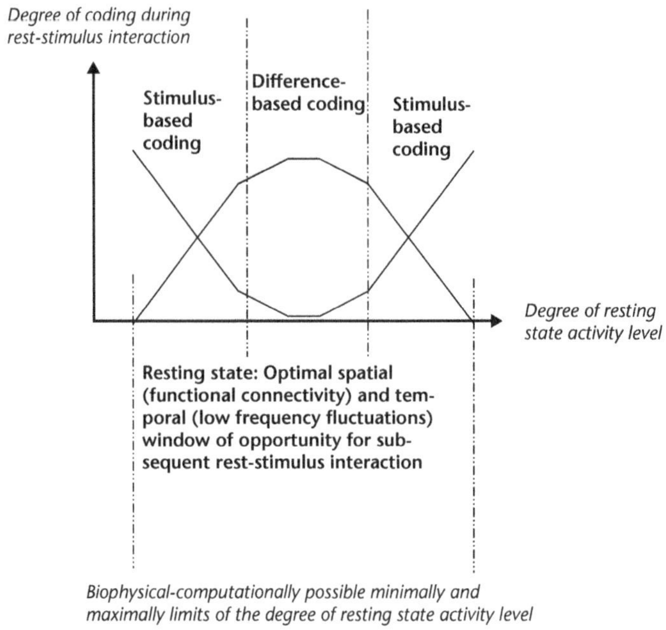

(b)

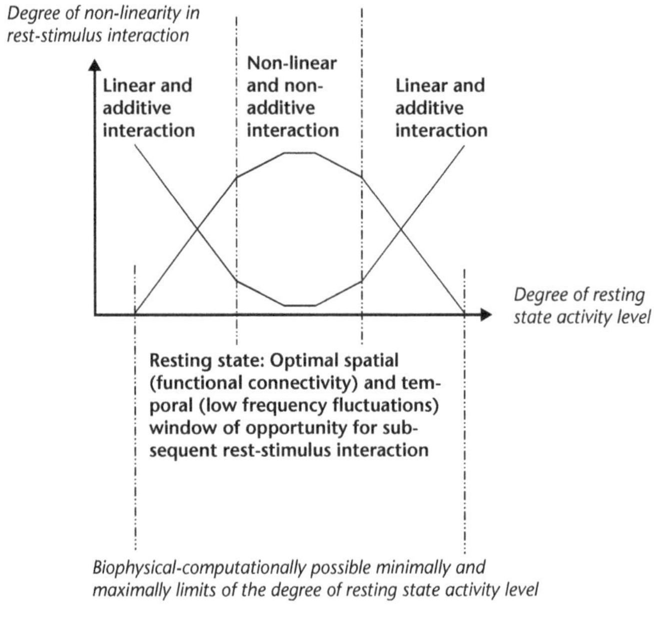

Figure 11-3a, b, c, and d Resting state as "spatiotemporal window of opportunity" for rest–stimulus interaction. The figure illustrates the dependence of the degree of coding (*a*), nonlinearity (*b*), sparse coding (*c*), and the stimuli's phenomenal (mental) and behavioral effects (*d*) during rest–stimulus (and possibly applicable also to stimulus–rest interaction) interaction (y-axis) on the degree of the resting-state activity level (x-axis) in relation to its maximally minimally possible biophysical-computational spectrum. Thereby the resting state is characterized by temporal, that is, frequency fluctuations, and spatial, that is, functional connectivity, features. These spatial and temporal features predispose the resting-state activity to interact with the stimuli in a particular way, which affects their degree of difference-based coding in stimulus-induced activity (*a*), the latter's degree of nonlinearity (*b*), the degree of sparse coding

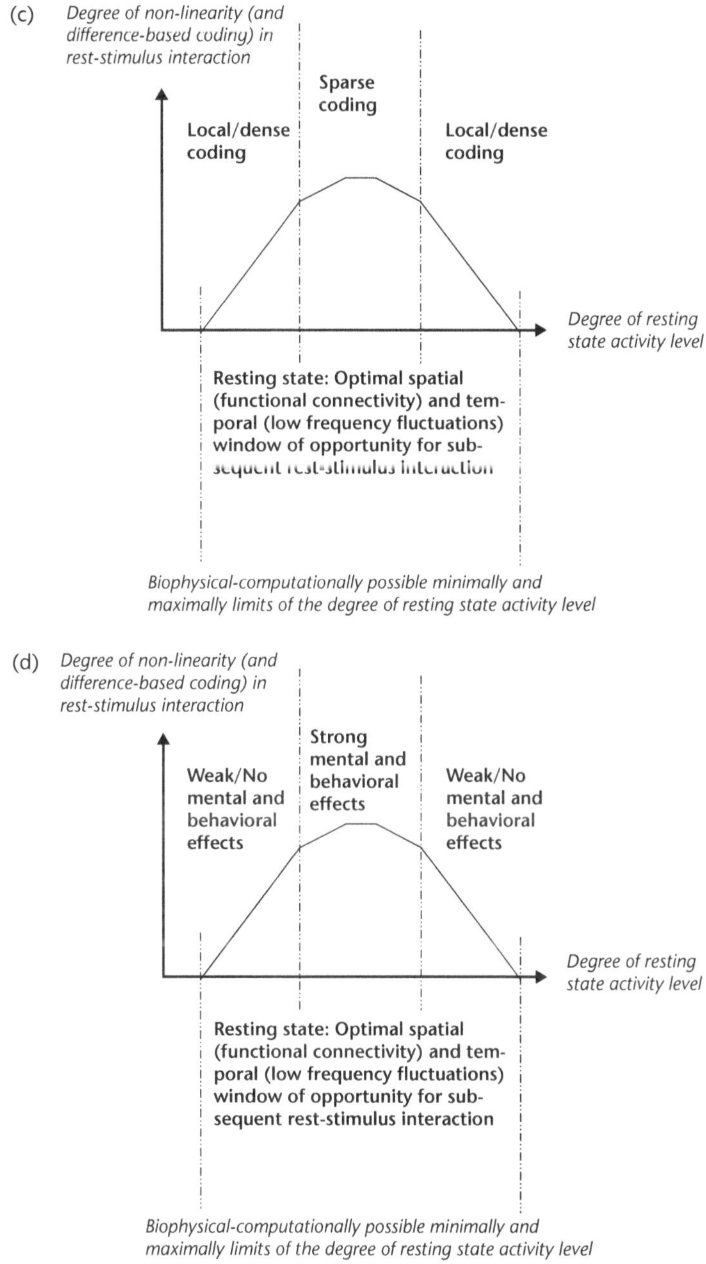

(*c*), and the stimuli's phenomenal (mental) and behavioral effects (*d*). Depending on its degree and how it relates to the brain's biophysical-computational spectrum and its maxima and minima, the resting-state activity level may provide a smaller or larger window of spatiotemporal opportunity for the stimuli to elicit the aforementioned coding, nonlinear, and phenomenal (mental)-behavioral effects. The two inner dotted lines indicate the optimal biophysical-computational range of the resting-state activity level for subsequent stimulus-induced activity, while the two outer dotted lines indicate the biophysical-computational maximum and minimum of the resting-state activity level (and its spatial and temporal measures).

patterns. The degree of sparse coding is consequently strongly dependent upon the degree of difference-based coding.

What does this dependence of sparse coding on difference-based coding imply for its relationship to the resting state's "spatiotemporal window of opportunity"? Since the resting state's "spatiotemporal window of opportunity" can modulate the degree of difference-based coding during subsequent rest–stimulus (and stimulus–rest) interaction, it also impacts the degree of sparse coding.

Optimal ranges in the resting state's "spatiotemporal window of opportunity" may then allow for high degrees of sparse coding during rest–stimulus interaction. In contrast, less optimal ranges may lead to higher degrees of local/dense coding (see Fig. 11-3c).

Neuronal hypothesis VIg: The resting state's "spatiotemporal window of opportunity" mediates behavioral and phenomenal functions

In addition to this neuronal relevance, the resting state's "spatiotemporal window of opportunity" may also be behaviorally and phenomenally (or mentally) relevant. Stronger behavioral effects may be associated with high degrees of difference-based coding and nonlinearity during rest–stimulus (or stimulus–rest) interaction. While this remains to be demonstrated explicitly in the future, the data reported here make this assumption rather likely.

Finally, the resting state's "spatiotemporal window of opportunity" may also be relevant for consciousness; that is, phenomenally (or mentally) relevant. By allowing for (or preventing), for instance, high degrees of difference-based coding and nonlinearity during rest–stimulus interaction, the resting-state activity itself may predispose the likelihood to which the purely neuronal stimulus-induced activity will be associated with a phenomenal state, or consciousness.

As will be discussed in full detail in Chapters 28 and 29, higher degrees of difference-based coding and nonlinearity during rest–stimulus interaction increase the likelihood that consciousness will be associated with the resulting stimulus-induced activity. More technically put, this means that the resting-state activity itself and its level and spatiotemporal activity pattern predispose the degree of possible consciousness during rest–stimulus interaction.

In sum, the resting state's "spatiotemporal window of opportunity" is relevant not only neuronally and behaviorally but also phenomenally. We will see later in Chapters 28 and 29 that this is highly relevant in, for instance, explaining the loss of consciousness in patients with vegetative state (VS) (see Figs. 11-3d).

Neurometaphorical excursion: Windows, apartments, and brains

I characterized the resting state as a "spatiotemporal window of opportunity" whose degree of openness strongly depends on its actual position relative to its underlying biophysical-computational continuum. How can we further illustrate this? Let's compare the situation to a real window in your house.

If the window is barely open, you as a person on the street have almost no chance of seeing anything inside the other person's house. No matter how hard you try, you have no chance of seeing anything. Why? Because the window of opportunity (in both literal and figurative senses) is nearly shut down. If, in contrast, the window is wide open, you have a good chance of seeing something inside the house.

Most important, where the window itself is open, everything else—namely, how and where the window of opportunity is given—depends on your glasses and your level on the street where you stand, and so on. The real window thus provides an opportunity or "predisposition" for you to see something inside the house, a "look inside the house." However, whether you can see inside depends now on you whether you grasp and seize that opportunity—your own position, your glasses, etc.

Analogous to the real window, the brain's resting state can be said to provide a predisposition, or a spatiotemporal window of opportunity, for possible interaction with stimuli in subsequent rest–stimulus and stimulus–rest interaction. In the same way as the real window can be more or less open, the resting state's spatiotemporal window of opportunity may also be more or less open for the stimulus to have "look inside the house," which is called the brain in our case, thus amounting to a "look inside the brain."

The stimulus goes further, though. The stimulus "looks" around in the house or apartment called "brain" and "sees" whether it can change the spatiotemporal configuration of its neuronal furniture; that is, functional connectivity and low-frequency fluctuations. The better the stimulus links itself to the resting state's spatiotemporal structure, the more it will be able to move its hosts' neuronal furniture around. Hence, the stimulus can be regarded as a rather impolite guest who intrudes and tries to impose itself upon the neuronal furniture of its host, the brain and its resting-state activity.

Of course, it is not only the stimuli themselves that determine what will happen during the stimuli's "look inside the brain." It is also the brain and specifically the resting-state activity itself that has an active role in determining what the stimuli can and cannot do inside the "house of the brain."

If, for instance, the neuronal furniture of the resting state itself is abnormally configured, with abnormal resting-state functional connectivity and low frequency fluctuations, the stimuli may elicit rather strange and abnormal changes in the resting state and thus in the "house of the brain." This can lead to rather bizarre behavioral and phenomenal states, such as in psychiatric disorders like depression and schizophrenia, as will be discussed in full detail in Volume II (see Chapters 17, 22, and 27).

NEURONAL HYPOTHESIS VIIA: "PARTIAL DEPENDENCE" OF THE RESTING STATE'S "SPATIOTEMPORAL WINDOW OF OPPORTUNITY" ON THE BRAIN'S BIOPHYSICAL-COMPUTATIONAL SPECTRUM

One may finally want to raise the question of how we can determine the possible range of the resting state's "spatiotemporal window of opportunity." This is a question for the neuronal features of the resting-state activity itself, which ultimately are determined and constrained by the biophysical-computational features of the neurons and the regions and ultimately of the brain as a whole.

We already encountered the brain's biophysical-computational features in the context of sparse coding (see Chapters 2 and 3) as well as in the resting state (see Chapter 6). We now aim to briefly discuss how the brain's biophysical-computational features determine its resting state's "spatiotemporal window of opportunity." This is not only of purely theoretical interest, but also highly relevant for consciousness, as we will see in Chapters 28 and 29.

How are the brain's biophysical-computational features related to the resting state's "spatiotemporal window of opportunity"? The biophysical-computational features provide the brain with a certain biophysical-computational spectrum upon which its resting-state activity can operate. This means that the brain's resting-state activity can vary its degree, its level, and its spatiotemporal activity pattern within the range determined by its brain's biophysical-computational spectrum.

Since different species show different biophysical-computational spectrums in their brains, the range in which their resting-state activity can possibly operate is different between for instance dogs, bats, and humans. One would consequently postulate that the resting state's "spatiotemporal windows of opportunity" are defined in different ways in different species, which in turn determines their respective stance (or point of view) within the environment (see Chapter 21 for details).

How is all this related to the resting state's "spatiotemporal window of opportunity"? The brain's biophysical-computational spectrum determines and limits the possible minima and maxima of the resting state's "spatiotemporal window of opportunity." In other words, the resting state's "spatiotemporal window of opportunity" can only operate within the range and limits determined by its brain's biophysical-computational spectrum. Figuratively put, the brain's biophysical-computational spectrum determines the degree to which the resting state can open and close its "spatiotemporal window of opportunity."

Is the resting state's "spatiotemporal window of opportunity" thus enslaved by the brain's biophysical-computational spectrum? Yes and no! Yes, there is partial dependence. The brain's biophysical-computational spectrum determines the minima and maxima and thus the possible range within which the resting state's "spatiotemporal window of opportunity" can operate. The range of the resting state's "spatiotemporal window of opportunity" is consequently predetermined and thus predisposed by the brain's biophysical-computational spectrum. This is what I mean by "partial dependence."

Neuronal hypothesis VIIb: "partial independence" of the resting state's "spatiotemporal window of opportunity" on the brain's biophysical-computational spectrum

Such dependence and predetermination, however, covers only one-half of their relationship. The other half consists of partial independence of the resting state's "spatiotemporal window of opportunity" from the brain's biophysical-computational spectrum.

We discussed earlier that there are optimal and less-optimal ranges in the resting state's "spatiotemporal window of opportunity" itself for subsequent difference-based coding, nonlinearity, sparse coding, and even behavioral and phenomenal effects. This means that the resting-state activity itself can vary, change, and modulate the degree of (for instance) difference-based coding and sparse coding.

How does that relate to the brain's biophysical-computational spectrum? Due to its ability to vary and modulate neuronal measures, the resting-state activity applies and operates different degrees of difference-based coding and sparse coding across the range of its brain's underlying biophysical-computational spectrum. The resting-state activity and its various neuronal measures, like difference-based coding, sparse coding, and nonlinearity, are thus not completely enslaved by the brain's biophysical-computational spectrum. Instead, the resting-state activity can modulate and impact the degrees of difference-based coding, sparse coding, and nonlinearity by "using" different positions within the brain's biophysical-computational spectrum.

In other words, the resting state's "spatiotemporal window of opportunity" operates across and supersedes the brain's biophysical-computational spectrum rather than being tied and corresponding to it in a one-to-one way. This means that the resting state's "spatiotemporal window of opportunity" has indeed some partial independence from and is thus not completely enslaved by the biophysical-computational spectrum of its underlying brain.

As illustrated in the preceding figures, the degree of enslavement of the resting state's "spatiotemporal window of opportunity" is strongest in the maximal and minimal ranges of the brain's biophysical-computational spectrum. This is manifested in the high degrees of stimulus-based coding, linearity, and local/dense coding and the low behavioral and phenomenal effects. In contrast, the degree of enslavement is the lowest in the middle ranges of the brain's biophysical-computational ranges where the highest degrees of difference-based coding, sparse coding, and nonlinearity, as well as strong behavioral and phenomenal effects, can occur.

Neuronal hypothesis VIIc: resting-state activity as an "active player" in the brain's field of neural activity

Why is all that relevant? We will see later in Volume II that the degree of enslavement of the resting state's "spatiotemporal window of opportunity" by the brain's biophysical-computational spectrum is relevant for the degree to which consciousness, a phenomenal state, can be associated with the brain's neuronal states.

If the brain and its resting-state activity operate at the lower or minimum end of the brain's biophysical-computational spectrum, the resting state's "spatiotemporal window of opportunity" is strongly enslaved by the latter. That, I hypothesize, decreases the likelihood that a phenomenal state— consciousness, —is associated with the purely neuronal activity during either resting state or stimulus-induced activity.

I consequently hypothesize that the resting state's "spatiotemporal window of opportunity" in patients in vegetative state operates close to the minimum end of their brain's biophysical-computational spectrum (see Chapters 28 and 29 for details). And the closer the resting state's spatiotemporal window of opportunity operates to the minimum of the brain's biophysical-computational spectrum, the less likely its neural activity will be associated with consciousness and its phenomenal features.

Taken together, the characterization of the resting state by a "spatiotemporal window of opportunity" provides the resting state with a neuronal tool of enormous impact. By varying and modulating the level and spatiotemporal activity pattern of its resting-state activity, the brain can make itself at least partially independent of its enslavement by its own biophysical-computational spectrum. That in turn makes it possible for the resting-state activity to impact and modulate its own neural activity during both resting-state activity and stimulus-induced activity, via difference-based coding of rest–stimulus and stimulus–rest interaction.

In other words, the brain and more specifically its resting-state activity must be considered an active player in modulating and determining its own neural activity. Due to this active role, the resting-state activity is able to constitute a statistically based spatiotemporal structure that supersedes and operates across the brain's biophysical-computationally based features, the biophysical-computational spectrum.

On the whole, we have to consider the difference between the biophysical-computationally based features of the brain and the statistically based spatiotemporal structure of the resting-state activity. This difference will prove central not only neuronally but also behaviorally and phenomenally, as we will see in Volume II (see Chapters 21, 28, 29). In a nutshell, the difference between the merely biophysical features of the brain and its neuronal resting state activity makes the difference between a passive recipient and an active player within the field of the brain's neural activity. This, as I will demonstrate later in volume I will prove central for making possible the difference between non-consciousness and consciousness.

Open Questions

One may first wonder why I restricted rest–stimulus and stimulus–rest interaction to exclusively exteroceptive stimuli while completely neglecting interoceptive stimuli from the subject's own body. This is even more puzzling given the fact that in the brain's intrinsic activity I distinguished the "interoceptive baseline" from the "exteroceptive baseline" (see Chapter 4). One may consequently suggest that we need to investigate both baselines, intero- and exteroceptive, separately with regard to their respective rest–stimulus interactions.

This means that one may want to distinguish between rest–extero and rest–intero interaction as well as between intero–rest and extero–rest interaction. Unfortunately, though, there are not many data currently available for the interaction between resting-state activity and interoceptive stimuli, hence my focus here on exteroceptive stimuli. This does not mean, however, that I disregard the role of the body and thus rest–intero and intero–rest interactions. I will provide more details on interoceptive processing and awareness in Volume II (see Chapter 32).

Another question here is how such rest–stimulus interaction is related to sparse coding. I assumed sparse coding to also hold on the regional level of both stimulus-induced activity (see Chapter 3) and resting-state activity (see Chapter 6). This raises the question whether rest–stimulus (and stimulus–rest) interaction can also be characterized by spatial and temporal sparsening. I will address this question in Chapter 12.

CHAPTER 12
Rest–Stimulus Interaction and GABA-ergic Neural Inhibition

Summary

Chapter 11 demonstrated the neuronal mechanisms underlying rest–stimulus and stimulus–rest interaction. However, this left open the neurophysiological mechanisms. Based on both stimulus-induced activity on the cellular level (see Chapter 2) and resting-state activity (see Chapter 6), one would hypothesize that GABA and neural inhibition may play an essential role in mediating rest–stimulus and stimulus–rest interaction. Therefore, this chapter focuses on GABA and neural inhibition and how they mediate neural activity, especially during rest–stimulus interaction. One hallmark feature of stimulus-induced activity is gamma frequency fluctuations. Recent data show that the resting state can be characterized by an ongoing gamma cycle that is dependent upon the balance between neural excitation and inhibition. That, in turn, strongly impacts stimulus-induced activity, which is possible, as I hypothesize, only if one presupposes difference-based rather than stimulus-based coding. Moreover, recent findings in humans demonstrate that the resting-state concentration of GABA predicts the degree of stimulus-induced activity in the same local region, while the resting-state concentration of glutamate seems to exert its effects in more distal and thus remote regions during both resting state and stimulus-induced activity. Taken together, the findings suggest a central role for GABA and neural inhibition in mediating the transition from resting-state to stimulus-induced activity. That is possible, as I propose, by the disproportionate increase of GABA-ergic-mediated neural inhibition relative to glutamatergic-mediated neural excitation during the resting state's encounter with the stimulus. The disproportionate increase of GABA-ergic-mediated neural inhibition may account for the nonlinear changes in stimulus-induced activity when compared to the preceding resting state as discussed in Chapter 11. Finally, as based on the findings discussed in Parts I and II, one also would suggest GABA-ergic-mediated neural inhibition to induce temporal and spatial sparsening of neural activity during rest–stimulus interaction. In short, I postulate GABA-ergic-mediated neural inhibition to be central in making possible both difference-based coding and sparse coding during rest–stimulus interaction.

Key Concepts and Topics Covered

Gamma frequencies, stimulus-induced activity, rest–stimulus interaction, neural inhibition, gamma cycle, GABA, glutamate, rest–stimulus interaction, fMRI and MRS, difference-based coding, gamma frequencies, sparse coding, resting-state activity

NEUROEMPIRICAL BACKGROUND IA: "NEURONAL CONTINUITY" BETWEEN RESTING-STATE AND STIMULUS-INDUCED ACTIVITY

So far, I have considered the coding strategy and the principles that determine stimulus–stimulus interaction (Chapter 10) and rest–stimulus (and stimulus–rest) interaction (Chapter 11). Empirical evidence in both instances speaks in favor of difference-based coding rather than stimulus-based coding as the main coding strategy. This was manifest in the principles of spatial and temporal coincidence, inverse effectiveness, and nonlinearity that were shown to apply to and operate during both stimulus–stimulus and rest–stimulus (and stimulus–rest) interaction.

What I left open, however, are the exact neurophysiological mechanisms that allow for the encoding of spatial and temporal differences into the neural activity during rest–stimulus interaction.

Let us briefly recall from the preceding parts: We discussed the central role of GABA and glutamate in the neural coding of sparse inhibition during stimulus-induced activity on a cellular and population level (see Chapter 2). And I showed how GABA and glutamate mediate difference-based coding and ultimately sparse coding of the brain's resting-state activity, that is, rest–rest interaction, on a regional level (see Chapter 6). Do GABA and glutamate also mediate the constitution of neural differences, that is, difference-based coding, on a regional level during the resting state's encounter with the stimulus, that is, rest–stimulus interaction? This is the focus in the present chapter.

The question for the constitution of neural differences by GABA and glutamate during rest–stimulus interaction is not only of importance for our understanding of how stimulus-induced activity is constituted. Reaching deeper, it also pertains to a more basic issue, namely the question of whether there is neuronal continuity between resting-state and stimulus-induced activity (see also appendix 1 for a more extensive discussion where I suggest what I describe as the "continuity hypothesis").

Neuroempirical background Ib: "More-or-less continuum" between resting-state and stimulus-induced activity

Do GABA and glutamate mediate rest-rest and rest-stimulus interaction? One would expect GABA and glutamate to mediate the neuronal continuity between rest–rest and rest–stimulus (and also stimulus–stimulus and stimulus–rest) interactions. This raises the question how the resulting stimulus-induced activity can be sufficiently distinguished from the preceding resting-state activity.

Such a distinction seems to be necessary, since otherwise we may not be able to distinguish the stimulus in our perceptions and cognitions from the brain's resting-state activity itself and its associated psychological functions like thoughts and mind-wandering (see Chapter 26 for more details on the latter). Therefore, as an alternative to the assumption of neuronal continuity, one may propose a principal distinction between resting-state activity and stimulus-induced activity.

The constitution of neural differences during stimulus-induced activity should then be mediated by neurophysiological mechanisms other than GABA and glutamate and neural inhibition and excitation. That, however, raises the question how stimulus-induced and resting-state activity are linked and connected to each other as it is suggested by the empirical evidence for rest–stimulus and stimulus–rest interaction (see Chapter 11).

As usual, the brain itself defies our all-or-nothing dichotomies and might "opt" (if it could) for a more-or-less continuum between resting state and stimulus-induced activity. Instead of mutually exclusive alternatives, the alternatives of complete neuronal continuity and principal difference between resting-state activity and stimulus-induced activity may be considered extreme cases on the maximal and minimal ends of a neuronal continuum.

How does such neuronal continuum look like? Both resting state and stimulus-induced activity may reflect different variations of the same neural activity: What we call resting-state and stimulus-induced activity may then simply refer to different degrees of change in the same neural activity that may be elicited either spontaneously during the resting-state activity itself or by the extrinsic stimuli. From the perspective of such a more-or-less continuum between resting state and stimulus-induced activity, the assumption of their principal difference seems to be more related to the observer than to the brain itself; that is, observer- rather than brain-based (see Appendix 3 for details on the latter distinction).

What does such "more-or-less continuum" between resting state and stimulus-induced activity imply for the roles of GABA and glutamate? GABA and glutamate may mediate both rest–rest and rest–stimulus (and stimulus–stimulus and stimulus–rest) interaction, thus allowing for some degree of neuronal continuity. At the same time, GABA and glutamate seem to allow for sufficient distinction of the stimulus-induced activity from the preceding resting-state activity by modulating the degree of the excitation-inhibition balance (EIB).

How is such co-occurrence between neuronal continuity and distinction between resting state and stimulus-induced activity possible? This will be the focus of the present chapter.

I will proceed in this chapter in two steps. In a first step, I will discuss the relationship between neuronal excitation and inhibition during rest–stimulus interaction. For that I will turn to recent results on gamma oscillations and how they are mediated by the balance between neural excitation and inhibition. This prepares the ground for the second step, the involvement of GABA and glutamate in modulating rest–stimulus interaction on a regional level of stimulus-induced activity that complements my accounts of the cellular level (see Chapter 2) and the regional level of the resting state activity (see Chapter 6).

NEURONAL FINDINGS IA: STIMULUS-INDUCED ACTIVITY AND GAMMA

Before going into the neurophysiological details of rest–stimulus interaction, let us recall from Chapter 10 the neuronal mechanism underlying stimulus–stimulus interaction. I showed that resetting and alignment of the phases of gamma frequency fluctuations may be central in binding different stimuli and their respective temporal positions together during stimulus-induced activity.

Such binding between the stimuli's distinct temporal positions was supposed to be possible only on the basis of encoding the stimuli's different temporal positions relative to the timing of the ongoing gamma phase. The gamma phase provides then the temporal reference frame (or temporal template) against which the different stimuli's temporal positions can be compared and matched. This, in turn, makes possible their binding (or nonbinding).

Gamma frequency fluctuations seem to be particularly central in mediating stimulus-induced activity. Gamma-band synchronization (30–80 Hz) was early observed in the cat's olfactory cortex and was related to the encoding of olfactory information (see Uhlhass et al. 2009, 2011 for reviews). This was complemented by observation of gamma-band synchronization in the 40 Hz range in cat primary visual cortex during the perception of global stimulus properties (see Singer 1999, 2009 for reviews).

These findings led to the hypothesis that synchronized gamma-band oscillations across different cells and columns of cells serve as mechanisms to coordinate and integrate distributed neuronal responses and hence to bind together different features of stimuli. This is the binding-by-synchronization hypothesis as discussed in Chapter 10, which is closely tied to the occurrence of gamma-band synchronization.

Characterizing stimulus-induced activity in general, gamma-band synchronizations have been shown to be crucially involved in various functions like object recognition, feature binding, polysensory integration, sensory-motor coordination, working memory, long-term memory, and selective attention (Fries et al. 2007; Fries 2009). Moreover gamma oscillation has also been associated with consciousness (see Koch 2004), which will be discussed in further detail in Volume II (see Chapters 18 and especially 19).

Taken together, these and other findings (see Chapters 10 and 19) suggest that gamma frequency fluctuations seem to be a hallmark feature of stimulus-induced activity in general irrespective of the type of stimulus, the region of the brain, and the kind of function. Hence, if we want to understand the neurophysiological mechanisms underlying rest–stimulus interaction, gamma frequency fluctuations may be a good candidate to start with on the side of stimulus-induced activity.

Neuronal findings Ib: gamma cycles and the timing of stimuli

Let me now go into more neurophysiological details about gamma and how it mediates rest–stimulus interaction on a cellular and population level. There is a specific temporal constellation between the discharges of GABA-ergic interneurons and glutamate-ergic pyramidal cells during gamma-band synchronization. The pyramidal cell's discharge occurs a few milliseconds earlier than the one of the interneuron (see also Chapter 2) as it has been shown for the hippocampus and the prefrontal cortex (see Buzsáki 2006, and Fries 2009, for reviews; as well as Canolty and Knight 2010, Fell and Axmacher 2011; Sauseng and Klimesch 2008; and Mazzoni et al. 2010).

Such a temporal delay may be due to the fact that the glutamate-ergic pyramidal cell excites the GABA-ergic interneurons that yield inhibition, which then in turn terminates the excitation of both pyramidal cells and interneurons (see also Chapter 2 for details). There is thus only a short time window, the time between the onset of pyramidal excitation and the onset of the interneurons' inhibition, for the pyramidal cell to exert its excitatory impact (see Chapter 2). This short time window is the time window for the gamma oscillation to start anew before the whole network is inhibited (see Fig. 12-1). Hence, these are what Fries et al. (2007) call "gamma cycles."

These gamma cycles are supposed to be continuously generated during the brain's resting state irrespective of whether stimuli are encountered. However, the stimuli can modify and thus modulate the ongoing gamma cycle by (for instance) shifting its phase onsets.

Following Fries et al. (2007; see also Fries 2009), such modulation of the gamma cycle is possible on the basis of different mechanisms. First, the timing of the gamma cycle itself and thus the temporal course of its phase(s) and phase onsets may be modified by the stimulus. Second, I suggest that the strength of the stimulus and its associated degree of neural excitation may exert an impact on subsequent neural inhibition which in turn may modulate the strength (i.e., power) and timing (i.e., phases) of the gamma cycle. Third, I propose the ongoing gamma cycle itself and more specifically its strength (i.e., power) may impact the degree to which the stimulus can (or cannot) exert its modulating effects.

Let us go into more detail and start with the first mechanism, the timing. Recording both multiunit activity (MUA) and local field potentials (LFPs) in the primary visual cortex of cats showed a clear relationship between spike timing and gamma cycle. During depolarization in the LFPs, spiking as recorded in MUA occurred earlier when compared to hyperpolarization in the LFPs where it occurred later. This means that the exact timing of the spiking activity as measured with MUA is very much dependent on its temporal relationship, its relative temporal difference, to the ongoing gamma cycle. Let me detail and explain these results, which show that the exact timing of the pyramidal excitation and the associated stimulus eliciting the spiking is extremely important. The occurrence of pyramidal excitation during moments of decreased inhibition—that is increased depolarization within the gamma cycle—leads to short temporal latencies and thus earlier onsets of the spikes. The earlier the spiking occurs, the more likely that it can impact other pyramidal cells before the GABA-ergic neural inhibition starts (and "kicks in").

If, in contrast, stimulation and subsequent pyramidal excitation occur during phases of strong inhibition, that is, hyperpolarization, within the ongoing gamma cycle, the spikes occur later with longer latencies and later onsets. Such longer latencies of the spikes makes their impact on other pyramidal cells less likely because their timing may coincide with the phases of strong inhibition in the ongoing gamma cycle (see Fries et al. 2007; Fries 2009; Buzsáki 2006; Vinck et al. 2010). Taken together, this suggests that the timing of the stimulus relative to the ongoing gamma cycle is central.

Neuronal findings Ic: gamma cycles and the strength of stimuli

How about the strength of the stimulus and the degree of neural excitation it induces? This

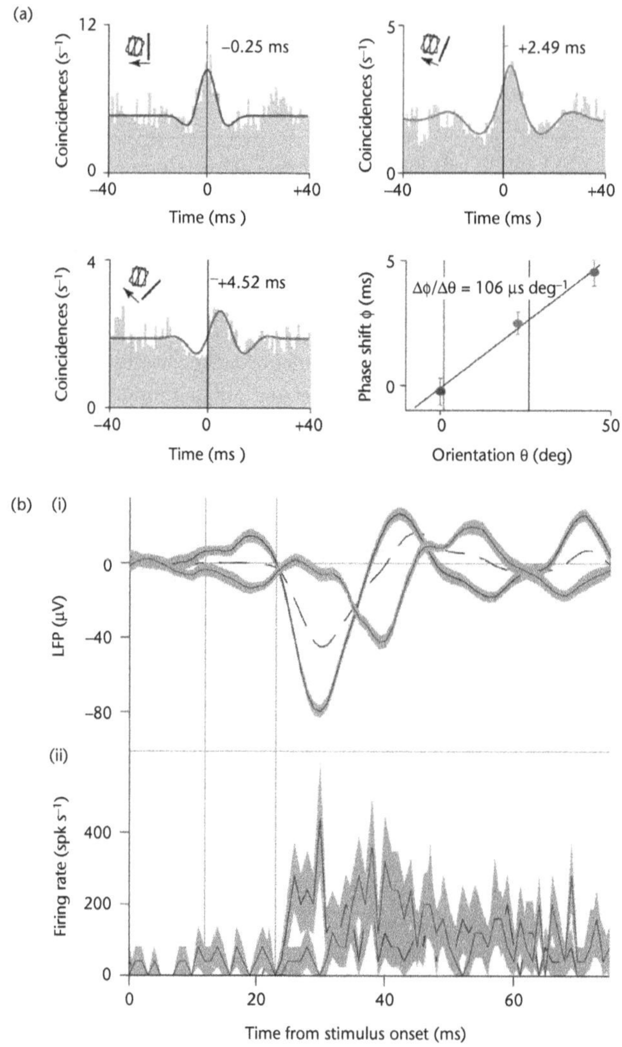

Figure 12-1a and b Neurophysiological mechanisms of the gamma cycle. Evidence for an interaction between excitation and rhythmic inhibition in the visual cortex. (*a*) Gamma-band synchronization among visual cortical spike train recordings entails phase leads and lags that depend on relative excitation levels. A pair of multi-unit activity (MUA1 and MUA2) was recorded under three different visual stimulation conditions. For each condition, the cross-correlation histogram (CCH) between the two MUAs was calculated and fitted with a Gabor function (different lines for the three stimulation conditions). A CCH peak with negative (positive) time offset indicates that MUA1 was leading (lagging) MUA2. In condition 1 (Gabor fit), MUA1 received more optimal visual stimulation than did MUA2. In condition 2 (fit), MUA2 received more optimal stimulation than did MUA1. In condition 3 (fit), the relative activation advantage of MUA2 was further increased. The results demonstrate that relative activation (and thereby excitation) strengths are translated into relative spiking phases within the gamma cycle. (*b*) Ongoing gamma-band oscillations co-determine the timing of first spiking in primary visual cortex after stimulus onset. LFPs and MUA were recorded from corresponding positions in primary visual cortex of the two hemispheres of an anesthetized cat. The average stimulus-related LFP is shown as a dashed line, defining response onset at 23 ms. Two subsets of trials were then chosen in which the LFP just before response onset was falling (rising), corresponding to spontaneous neuronal depolarization (hyperpolarization). The corresponding average LFPs are shown as different curves in (i). (ii) shows the MUA responses averaged separately for these two groups of trials. When the LFPs indicated spontaneous depolarization (hyperpolarization), the MUA response was particularly early (late). (Reprinted with permission of Elsevier, from Fries P, Nikolić D, Singer W. The gamma cycle. *Trends Neurosci.* 2007 Jul;30(7):309–16.)

touches upon the question of what the exact interaction between the excitation strength of the pyramidal cell and the gamma cycle looks like.

One would, for instance, expect that pyramidal cells with stronger excitation may interact with the gamma-band synchronization in a different way than those with weaker excitation. To put it into more technical terms, the strength of the pyramidal cell's excitation may be translated into a phase value that corresponds to the exact timing of the spikes within the ongoing gamma cycle.

This was addressed in a study by Vinck et al. (2010) (see also Womelsdorf et al. 2012). Vinck et al. (2010) investigated LFP and MUA in the primary visual cortex of rhesus monkey (n = 3) during visual stimulation of grating drift directions with 800–1000 ms pre-stimulus baseline and 800–1500 ms passive stimulus viewing (with preferred and nonpreferred orientation of stimuli). All spikes recorded during MUA were related to the average LFP recorded simultaneously from separate electrodes (at 1–3 cm distance).

This demonstrated clear phase-locking with a high number of spikes occurring particularly in the gamma-frequency band (spike-LFP pairs: peaking at around 67 Hz in monkey one and at around 40 Hz in monkeys two and three). When neurons were more strongly excited, they spiked significantly earlier in the cycle of the LFP, thus showing gamma-phase shifting (see also Fries et al. 2007). If, in contrast, the neurons less strongly excited are showing low strength in their spiking, their spikes occurred later within the ongoing gamma cycle in the LFP.

What do these results tell us about the relationship between spiking and the gamma phase? They suggest that stronger stimuli induce higher excitation levels, which in turn shift the gamma phase (including its phase onsets) when compared to the lower excitation levels of weaker stimuli. Accordingly, the strength of stimuli may have an impact on the degree of gamma-phase shifting and its temporal course.

Neuronal findings Id: Gamma cycles and the power of resting state activity

In addition to the timing and strength of the stimulus, the strength or power of the ongoing gamma cycle itself in the resting state preceding the onset of the stimulus may also exert an impact.

For instance, stronger rhythmic modulation of the gamma cycle may make it less likely for spikes, triggered by stimuli, to induce gamma-phase shifting in the ongoing gamma cycle. The stronger the power of the ongoing gamma cycle in the preceding state, the less likely the stimulus and the respectively induced spikes are able to induce a shift in the gamma phase (see also Womelsdorf et al. 2012). Accordingly, if the resting state's gamma power is strong, the stimulus-induced gamma shift should be weak. And, of course, the converse also applies with weaker resting-state gamma power leading to stronger stimulus-induced gamma shifts.

This hypothesis was tested by Vinck et al. (2010), who compared trials with high gamma-band power with those showing low gamma-band power in the resting state. Strong excitation/activation and thus strong spikes induced less phase shifting during high gamma band-band power when compared to trials with low gamma-band power. The same was observed during the baseline condition, the pre-stimulus interval. Weak gamma-band power in the pre-stimulus interval and thus in the resting state was here associated with stronger phase shifting by the subsequent spikes.

Most interestingly, Vinck et al. (2010) also tested the reverse scenario by distinguishing neurons that were strongly phase-locked to gamma rhythms from those that were only weakly phase-locked. As expected, the activation-dependent gamma-phase shifts were much stronger in those neurons that were only weakly phase-locked. This indicates a clear impact of the strength, that is, power, of the resting state's gamma rhythm on the subsequent stimulus-induced gamma-phase shift.

Taken together, these data show that the degree of the resting-state activity level, that is, gamma power, exerts a strong impact on the degree of to which a subsequent stimulus can shift the gamma cycle, the gamma phase shift. This clearly demonstrates the mutual interplay and reciprocal dependence between resting-state activity and stimulus on a cellular and population level of neural activity.

Neuronal hypothesis Ia: Temporal linkage between intrinsic activity and extrinsic stimulus

Remember that we encountered an almost analogous scenario of timing during stimulus–stimulus interaction in Chapter 10. More specifically, cross-modal interaction between visual/auditory and tactile stimuli was also made possible by linking and aligning the stimulus-induced phases of the one stimulus, the unimodal stimulus, to the temporal position of the respective other, the cross-modal stimulus. That, I proposed, is possible only by encoding the temporal position of the cross-modal stimulus relative to the timing of the phases associated with the unimodal stimulus.

This concerned stimulus–stimulus interaction. We now encounter an almost analogous scenario in the current context of rest–stimulus interaction. The incoming stimulus exerts its effects via glutamate-ergic pyramidal cells, thus inducing neural excitation. The stronger the incoming stimulus is, the more pyramidal cells spike and the stronger the degree of subsequent neural excitation.

The degree of neural excitation, however, does not act alone and independent of the level of the resting-state activity, the ongoing oscillatory power and its respective phases as manifest in (for instance) the gamma cycle. The neural excitation, as induced by the stimulus, must thus be linked temporally to the phases of the ongoing oscillatory resting-state activity in order to be processed further and exert maximally possible impact in the resulting stimulus-induced activity.

This is well reflected in the results showing that the exact timing of the neural excitation in relation to the ongoing gamma cycle is central for its subsequent effects on gamma. As in the case of stimulus–stimulus interaction, this presupposes that the actual temporal position of the stimulus-induced neural excitation must be encoded relative to the timing of the phase of the resting state's ongoing oscillatory power in the gamma cycle.

Neuronal hypothesis Ib: Gamma cycle and difference-based coding

How can we account for the observed temporal linkage between the ongoing gamma cycle in the resting state and the degree of spiking during stimulus-induced activity? The observed temporal linkage between intrinsic activity and extrinsic stimulus is possible only when presupposing the encoding of temporal differences between the actual temporal position of the stimulus-induced excitation, the spiking, and the timing of the resting state's gamma phase, the ongoing gamma cycle.

This leads me to the following hypothesis. I hypothesize that the kind of temporal alignment of the gamma cycle to the onset of the stimulus and its spiking as observed in the gamma shift is possible only when presupposing difference-based coding in temporal regard. In short, the observed gamma shift requires the encoding of relative temporal differences.

Since they are based on both the stimulus and the resting state, the encoded temporal differences should be modulated and impacted by the strength and temporal position of the stimulus and its degree of spiking, as well as by the power of the ongoing gamma cycle in the resting state. This is exactly what the data show, as described earlier, that therefore support the assumption of difference-based coding albeit indirectly.

This gamma shift would, in contrast, remain impossible if there were stimulus-based coding. In that case, the temporal position of both the stimulus-induced excitation, the spiking, and the resting state's gamma phase, the gamma cycle, would be encoded independently and isolated from each other. In this case, the single discrete points in physical time as associated with both gamma phase ad spiking would be encoded by themselves and thus isolated and independent from each other.

How would such scenario of stimulus-based coding look like in empirical regard? The power of the gamma cycle in the resting state should have no impact on the temporal position and gamma power related to the stimulus and its spiking. Nor should the latter, the stimulus and its spiking, be able to induce a shift in the resting state's ongoing gamma cycle. In other words, the gamma phase shift should remain impossible in the case of stimulus-based coding. This, however, contradicts the earlier described data, which therefore lend strong empirical support to difference-based coding as distinguished from stimulus-based coding.

Neuronal hypothesis Ic: Difference-based coding as common code between intrinsic activity and extrinsic stimulus

How can we further characterize such difference-based coding? The resulting temporal difference value may be considered the "final functional common pathway" into which both stimulus/spiking and resting state/gamma power converge. Hence, the temporal difference value may reflect the code that is shared and common to both resting-state activity, or gamma cycle, and stimulus, or neural excitation/spiking.

Such common coding is possible, however, only on the basis of difference-based coding that allows for the constitution of temporal (and spatial) neural differences between resting-state activity/gamma power and stimulus-induced activity/spiking. Stimulus-based coding, in contrast, would make such common coding impossible, since both stimulus/spiking and resting state/gamma power would then be coded independently and isolated from each other. There would thus be a binary code rather than a common code.

Why is all that important? The earlier described results and hypotheses illustrate the kind of neuronal mechanisms that underlie rest–stimulus interaction and determine the degree of stimulus-induced activity on a regional level. Such neuronal mechanisms concern the impact of the power and the timing of the ongoing gamma cycle in the resting state and how it impacts the subsequent stimulus-induced activity.

At the same time, the timing and strength of the stimulus itself exert considerable impact on the resulting stimulus-induced activity. The stimulus-induced activity can therefore be regarded a true "hybrid" between the spatial and temporal features of the stimulus itself and those of the ongoing resting-state activity (see later for a more detailed characterization of the hybrid nature of stimulus-induced activity).

In addition to such neuronal relevance, these neuronal mechanisms are also relevant for consciousness; that is, phenomenally relevant. As I will demonstrate in Volume II in detail, the degree of alignment of the stimulus and its temporal position to the ongoing phase onsets and durations of the resting state's low frequency fluctuations are central in associating consciousness to the stimulus and its stimulus-induced activity (see especially Chapter 20).

The better the brain's intrinsic resting-state activity and its spatial and temporal features can align and couple its low frequency fluctuations' phase onsets to the onset of the extrinsic stimuli and their spatial and temporal features, the more likely the resulting purely neuronal stimulus-induced activity can be associated with consciousness. The exact neuronal mechanisms of such mutual alignment between resting state and stimulus via their respective spatial and temporal features will be discussed in Volume II (see Chapters 14, 15, 20, 21, 28, and 29).

Neurometaphorical excursion Ia: Soccer and relative positions

How can we illustrate such a mutual and reciprocal adjustment between resting-state activity and stimulus-induced activity in a more easy and accessible way? Let us compare the relationship between resting state and stimulus to that of soccer with two teams playing against each other.

The action on the soccer field is neither determined by the absolute position of the one team's players in either defense or attack. Nor is it determined by the absolute position of the other team's players. What instead determines the positions and movements of all players from the one team is their respective spatial and temporal position to the ball and how that relates in turn to the positions of the other team's players. The players from the one team must thus think in terms of relative time and space by encoding their respective positions relative to the ball and the other team's players.

Thereby it does not matter whether the specific player is in the attack or the defense (or the midfield). Only his actual position relative to the ball and the other players, and thus his relative position in space and time, matters, which, most importantly, determines his role: that is, whether he will attack or defend.

This is further supported by considering the players from the other team. The players from the opposing team will not care whether the player they confront in their attacking half is originally a defense or an attack player. All they will care about is the other player's spatiotemporal position relative to the ball and themselves and how that, in turn, increases the likelihood that the other player will be able to shoot a goal.

An analogous scenario surfaces in the case of the brain. The brain and its resting-state activity, to put it metaphorically, may not so much care about whether the stimulus it processes comes from the brain itself, the body, or the environment. This corresponds to the fact that ultimately it does not matter whether the player appearing in front of the other team's goal is originally a defense or attack player.

Moreover, the brain's resting-state activity may not care so much about the absolute temporal and spatial position of the stimulus itself independently and isolated from the resting state's own spatial and temporal positions. Rather, the resting-state activity may very much care about how the stimulus' temporal and spatial position is related to the actual position of its own resting-state activity, that is, its gamma phases (and the phases of its frequency fluctuations in other ranges), and thus, more generally, the resting state's spatiotemporal structure (see Chapters 4 and 5).

What is encoded into the brain's neural activity are the relative rather than absolute temporal and spatial positions of the stimulus, its spatial and temporal position relative to the one of the resting-state activity. This corresponds to the situation that a player of the one team does not much care about whether he is at spatial position x of the soccer field at time point a. More important for him is how his position x and time point a are related to the positions and time points of the ball and the other players (from both his own and the other team).

Neurometaphorical excursion Ib: defense and resting state activity

Let us for now shift our perspective of the outside observer to a perspective from the inside of the field itself, the perspective the players themselves take while playing. This would correspond to, metaphorically, taking the perspective of the stimulus itself that approaches the brain and its resting-state activity. One may then be inclined to compare the brain's resting-state activity to the ball's and the other players' positions in space and time. Let us be more specific.

The ball and the other players serve as reference, standard, and measure for determining the spatial and temporal position of the player and his subsequent moves; namely, where and how fast he will run in the next seconds. Analogously, the brain's resting-state activity, for example, the power and phases of its ongoing gamma cycles (and its other measures), serve as reference, standard, and measure to determine the spatial and temporal position of the stimulus. Very much like the ball and the other players serve as spatiotemporal template or grid on which our player orients himself and determines his subsequent moves, the resting state's spatiotemporal structure provides a template or grid for the stimulus to align itself to the brain and its resting-state activity. Good soccer coaches tell you that nothing should happen independently of the ball, its spatial position and its temporal features (whether it moves fast or slow). The brain seems to have taken that lesson to heart (metaphorically speaking): nothing happens without the involvement of the brain's resting-state activity since a stimulus that does not involve and modulate the resting-state activity will not exert any neuronal, behavioral, and phenomenal effects. Such stimulus could then be compared to a soccer player running 90 minutes up and down the soccer field independent of the ball and the other players.

One may consequently be inclined to compare the resting state to the ball in soccer: The actual position of the ball serves as the point of orientation and reference for any player no matter from what team he is on and what position he is supposed to play. Analogously, the brain's resting state provides the spatiotemporal template, standard and measure, the point of orientation, against which any stimulus and its spatial and temporal features are processed.

This applies to all players from both teams also the referee. The same holds in the case of the brain, where it also applies to all stimuli, whether they originate in the brain itself, the body, or the environment. Like the ball itself, which does not "care" about whether the player is from this or that team (and whether he is a defense or attack player), the resting state itself does not "care" about the origin of the stimuli and the role they are supposed to play.

Accordingly, all the resting-state activity cares about is measuring and referencing all stimuli, regardless of their origin, against itself and its own spatiotemporal structure (see Chapter 25 for an extensive discussion of possible "origin-based coding" of neural activity).

Neurometaphorical excursion Ic: Resting-state activity as an active player

Is our brain nothing but a ball? There is one important difference. The ball itself is passive since it does not move and change its positions by itself; it requires the players to do that. The brain, in contrast, is active since it can change the level of its resting-state activity by itself as signified by rest–rest interaction. Accordingly, the brain may be compared to an active ball.

How is such an active ball driven? By the metabolic-energy supply it receives from the body. Hence, the body seems to take over the role of the soccer players in the case of the brain. In the same way as the players provide the energy and power that lets the ball move and fly across the space and time of the soccer field, the body supplies the metabolism and energy to the brain that let its resting-state activity constitute its spatiotemporal structure.

Now let us take the perspective of the players of the team that currently finds itself in a defensive position. If the defending players learn the soccer coach's lesson well and position themselves in space and time relative to the ball and the attacking players, they will be able to resist the attack from the other team and to consequently prevent goals.

This is also the case with the brain. If the brain and its resting state activity position themselves well and thus relative to the stimulus, this may prevent the latter from intruding and shooting the resting state's neural activity to new levels, that is, stimulus-induced activity.

Like the defending players, the brain and its resting-state activity may have the neuronal means to minimize and contain the degree of their colonization by the stimulus. In other words, like the defensive players with regard to the attacking players from the opposing team, the brain and its resting-state activity can take an active role in containing the impact of the stimuli from body and environment.

This leads us to what we defined in the last chapter as the resting state's "spatiotemporal window of opportunity." In the same way as the defending players in their own team can actively create a "spatiotemporal window of opportunity" for their own attack players to shoot a goal, the brain's resting-state activity can actively constitute and modulate its own "spatiotemporal window of opportunity" that either opens, i.e., maximizes, or closes, i.e., minimizes, the possible effects the stimuli can exert in the brain.

In sum, like the soccer players, the resting-state activity itself must be considered an active player in the neuronal field of the brain and its various "neuronal games" (which we like to call resting state and stimulus-induced activity).

Neuroempirical background II: Modulation of rest–stimulus interaction by glutamate and GABA

The previous sections in this chapter and the preceding two chapters in this part discussed the neuronal mechanisms underlying stimulus–stimulus and rest–stimulus interaction. Both stimulus–stimulus and rest–stimulus interaction were shown to be possible only on the basis of difference-based coding.

How do glutamate and GABA mediate such rest–stimulus interaction and make possible its encoding in terms of difference-based coding? This is an important question, since GABA and glutamate are the key players in constituting stimulus-induced activity.

Based on our considerations at the beginning of this chapter, there are two requirements for the glutamate- and GABA-ergic modulation of stimulus-induced activity: On one hand, GABA and glutamate must allow for some degree of neuronal continuity between resting state and stimulus-induced activity. On the other hand, they must create some degree of neuronal distinction between resting state and stimulus-induced activity to allow the stimulus (and its behavioral, cognitive, and phenomenal features) to be sufficiently different from the resting-state activity.

I suggest that glutamate and GABA, and especially their interplay in constituting the excitation-inhibition balance, are central in allowing for both neuronal continuity and distinction between resting state and stimulus-induced activity (see later for details). How can I lend support to that hypothesis? The first step consisted in showing the central role of neural excitation and inhibition and thus the excitation-inhibition balance, the EIB, in rest–stimulus interaction, as was demonstrated by the example of the gamma cycle. This is now complemented by the second step, which aims to demonstrate how the EIB is modulated by glutamate and GABA.

Let us remind the reader that we already discussed glutamate and GABA in previous chapters in this volume. I so far have demonstrated the involvement of glutamate and GABA in stimulus-induced activity on a cellular level (see Chapter 2) and in resting-state activity on a regional level (see Chapter 6). I left open, however, how glutamate and GABA mediate stimulus-induced activity and especially rest–stimulus interaction on a regional level of neural activity. This will be the focus in the remainder of this chapter.

Neuronal findings IIa: *Glutamate* modulates *intra-regional* rest–stimulus interaction

Several studies combined fMRI with magnetic resonance spectroscopy (MRS) to measure the intra- and extracellular concentration of GABA and glutamate. Combining MRS with fMRI allows us to link the investigation of neural activity (fMRI) with the measurement of its biochemical modulation by GABA and glutamate (MRS). Such combination of fMRI and MRS makes it possible to investigate the modulation of rest-stimulus interaction and stimulus-induced activity by GABA and glutamate.

Recent studies combining fMRI and MRS demonstrated that the intra-regional concentration of glutamate predicted the degree of stimulus-induced signal changes in the same region during particular tasks. For instance, Jocham et al. (2012) showed that the resting state concentration of glutamate in PACC predicted the degree of stimulus-induced activity in the same region during a reward task. Interestingly, both GABA and glutamate concentrations in PACC predicted the value-related behavioral effects as well as the associated stimulus-induced activity in the same region, though in opposing, positive and negative, ways: the higher the PACC glutamate concentration and the lower the one of GABA, the higher the PACC signal changes and the higher the behavioral value associated with the respective stimulus.

Interestingly, the same study also showed a particular temporal constellation in the effects of glutamate and GABA. Individuals with higher glutamate and lower GABA concentrations showed faster signal changes during the early phases of the trials, This was different in the later phases of the trials, where the same subjects (lower GABA, higher glutamate) showed faster termination of the signal changes. Such timing effects were observed only in difference-based signal changes that directly compared high and low values whereas they were not observed in the raw BOLD signal itself. That makes it rather likely that the effects of GABA and glutamate are related to the encoding of the stimulus' value into neuronal activity as measured with the BOLD signal in fMRI rather than to the BOLD signal itself.

Another study, by Falkenberg et al. (2012), investigated the resting state concentration of glutamate in dorsal anterior cingulate (DACC) in MRS. In fMRI subjects performed a cognitive control task with attention focused on either the main (salient) stimulus or the control (less salient) stimulus. The concentration of glutamate in DACC predicted the degree of task-related activity in the same region (and other regions like the retrosplenial cortex, the orbitofrontal cortex, and the basal ganglia): the higher the concentration of glutamate in DACC, the higher (or lower) the signal changes in the above mentioned regions during the cognitive attention task.

Moreover, they could observe that glutamate effects differed depending on the degree of task difficulty: Low levels of glutamate predicted BOLD increases when the task was difficult; that is, when the subject's attention was distracted by a less salient stimulus. In contrast, high levels of glutamate predicted increased BOLD signals during the easy part of the task when the attention was not distracted and aligned to the stimulus.

Finally, a study by Schmaal et al. (2012) demonstrated that the concentration of glutamate in the same region, the dorsal anterior cingulate cortex (DACC), predicted the behavioral measures during a reward task (delay discounting). The behavioral measures of delay discounting were in turn correlated with the degree of resting-state functional connectivity of the DACC with a subcortical spot including the ventral tegmental area/subthalamic nucleus (VTA/STN), a region that is central for reward. These results suggest that the effects of DACC glutamate on delay discounting are mediated by resting-state functional connectivity from DACC to the subcortical regions (which was supported by mediation analysis).

Taken together, these studies demonstrate that the resting state concentration of glutamate impacts intra-regional stimulus-induced activity. Most important, the study by Jocham et al. (2012) demonstrates differential—opposing—effects of glutamate and GABA on both the signal changes and their time course. This suggests that glutamate makes a differential contribution during rest–stimulus interaction on a regional level of activity when compared to the one of GABA (see later).

Neuronal findings IIb: *Glutamate* modulates *trans-regional* rest–stimulus interaction

These studies show mainly intra-regional effects of resting state glutamate on the stimulus-induced activity in the same region. How about trans-regional effects with resting state glutamate in one region modulating stimulus-induced activity in another region? This was tested for by Niall Duncan from our group in an earlier study (Duncan et al. 2011).

Using MRS, Niall Duncan from our group (Duncan et al. 2011) investigated the resting-state concentration of glutamate in the PACC and the supragenual anterior cingulate cortex (SACC). He then applied an empathy paradigm (perceiving and showing empathy with faces from the Ekman Series) in fMRI to elicit stimulus-induced activity in the very same regions in order to investigate their modulation by glutamate.

As expected, the PACC as typical DMN region showed negative BOLD response during the empathy task. In contrast, the SACC, a region not typically associated with the DMN, exhibited rather positive BOLD responses. How are the more resting state–associated negative BOLD responses in PACC related to the stimulus-induced positive BOLD responses in SACC?

It is well known that PACC and SACC as distinct parts of the anterior cingulate cortex are closely related to each other in terms of structural connectivity. Based on this structural connectivity pattern, one would expect strong functional connectivity between PACC and SACC. This was indeed the case. Duncan et al. (2011) showed strong functional connectivity between the signal changes in both regions, more specifically between negative BOLD responses in PACC and positive BOLD responses in SACC. One can thus speak here of functional connectivity across the division of resting state and stimulus-induced activity since it links the resting-state activity in PACC to the stimulus-induced activity in SACC.

However, this relationship was unidirectional: signal changes in the PACC (as seed region) covaried with the ones in SACC across time, thus indicating functional connectivity. In contrast, the reverse scenario, signal changes in SACC (as seed region) covarying with the ones in PACC, did not hold. This suggests that the PACC modulates the SACC, but the latter does not impact the former. There is thus unilateral functional connectivity (i.e., effective connectivity) from PACC and their resting state–related negative BOLD response to the stimulus-induced positive BOLD response in SACC. This further supports the assumption of trans-regional rest–stimulus functional connectivity (while the reverse direction of trans-regional stimulus–rest functional connectivity does not hold).

How is such unilateral rest–stimulus functional connectivity from PACC to SACC now related to glutamate? First, Duncan et al. (2011) observed that the resting-state concentration of glutamate in PACC predicted the signal changes in the SACC: the higher the resting-state concentration of glutamate in PACC, the stronger the stimulus-induced positive BOLD response in SACC.

Secondly, as expected, he observed that the degree of functional connectivity from PACC to SACC was also predicted by the resting-state concentration of glutamate in the PACC: the higher the resting state concentration of glutamate in PACC, the higher the degree of functional connectivity from resting state–related negative signal changes in PACC to stimulus-related positive signal changes in SACC. (see Fig. 12-2a).

Does the resting state glutamate in the PACC mediate the stimulus-induced activity in SACC directly, or rather indirectly via the resting-state activity in SACC? Duncan et al. (2011) also measured the resting state concentration of glutamate in the SACC which however did not correlate with the degree of stimulus-induced activity in the same region. Moreover, he did not observe any correlation of the concentration of glutamate in SACC with the one in PACC. Taken together with the earlier described findings, this suggests that the observed correlation of PACC resting state glutamate with SACC stimulus-induced signal changes is a direct rather than indirect trans-regional rest-stimulus interaction effect.

Accordingly, glutamate seems to exert direct transregional modulation during rest–stimulus interaction, such as, for instance, from resting-state activity in PACC to stimulus-induced activity in SACC. Unfortunately, the study by Duncan et al. (2011) did not include the measurement of GABA, so a direct comparison between GABA and glutamate with regard to trans-regional effects remains impossible.

These findings of glutamate mediating trans-regional functional connectivity during rest-stimulus interaction converge with the observation that glutamate also mediates trans-regional functional connectivity in the resting state that is rest-rest interaction. This was described in Chapter 6. One may thus postulate that glutamate mediates trans-regional effects in general irrespective of whether they are related to the resting state itself, that is rest-rest interaction, or to stimulus-induced activity and its rest-stimulus interaction.

Neuronal findings IIIa: *GABA* modulates *intra-regional* rest–stimulus interaction in *sensory and motor* regions

Using fMRI and MRS, Muthukumaraswamy et al. (2009, 2012) investigated the resting-state concentration of GABA in the visual cortex and its effects on subsequent stimulus-induced activity in the visual cortex itself and gamma frequency bands. They measured resting-state levels of GABA in the visual cortex with MRS and applied fMRI and magnetic encephalography (MEG) to measure stimulus-induced activity changes in the visual cortex.

What did they observe? The resting-state concentration of GABA in the visual cortex predicted the degree of stimulus-induced activation (positive BOLD response) and elevated gamma frequency power in the same brain region: the higher the resting-state concentration of GABA in visual cortex, the lower the positive signal changes in the same region elicited by a visual stimulus, and the lower the stimulus-induced gamma power. In contrast, such relationship could not be observed for glutamate that did not correlate with either the signal changes or the gamma power (see also Gaetz et al. 2011 for more or less analogous findings in the motor cortex).

Further confirmation of the role of GABA in mediating neural activity changes in visual cortex comes from Qin et al. (2012a). He correlated neural activity changes in visual and auditory cortex during the transition from eyes closed to eyes open with the resting state density of GABA-A receptors in the same regions.

Qin et al. (2012) observed that the degree of resting-state GABA-A receptor density in both visual and auditory cortex predicts the neural activity changes in the same regions (and other regions like the precuneus and the prefrontal cortex) during the transition from eyes closed to eyes open (see Chapter 6 for a more detailed description of this study, since it concerns mainly the resting state itself rather than stimulus-induced activity and rest–stimulus interaction).

Neuronal Findings IIIb: *GABA* Modulates Neural Inhibition During *Intra-Regional* Rest–Stimulus Interaction in *Sensory and Motor* Regions

How is GABA related to neural inhibition on a regional level of neural activity? Tentative support for the association of GABA with neural inhibition comes from studies by Stagg et al. (2011a and b). They combined the measurement of GABA and glutamate with transcranial

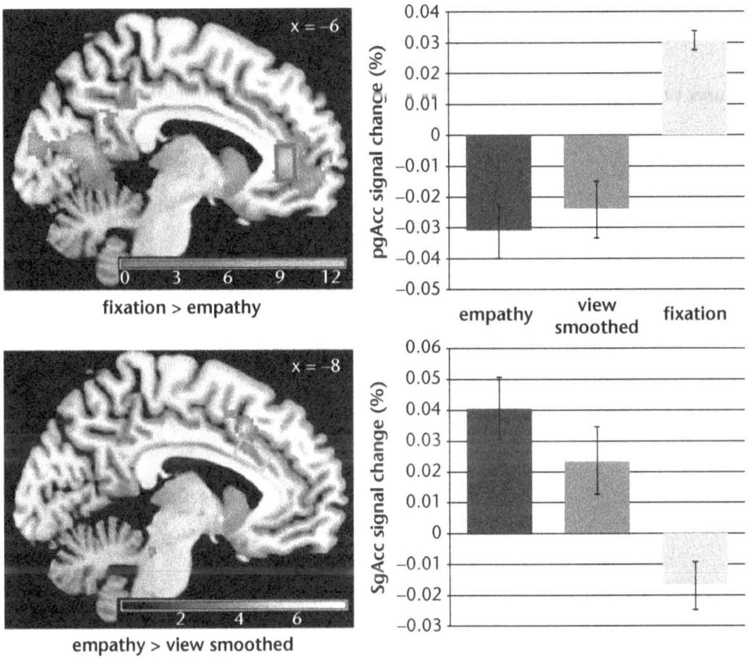

Figure 12-2a **GABA ergic and glutamatergic modulation of rest–stimulus interaction. (*a*) Areas of deactivation from rest in response to the empathy task are shown (contrast [fixation > empathy]), along with activations in response to the empathy task (contrast [empathy > smoothed]). Mean percent signal changes are shown for the viewing of emotional pictures, the viewing of smoothed pictures, and the fixation period in the pgACC (box in upper image) and sgACC (box in lower image) MRS voxels. Mean percentage signal changes were calculated using the Marsbar toolbox (available at: http://marsbar.sourceforge.net/). Error bars represent SEM. Images are shown with a threshold of P = 0.005 (unc.) for the purpose of illustration. (*b*) Unidirectional connectivity between negative signal changes in the pgACC MRS region (red box) and positive signal changes in the sgACC MRS region during the empathy task was demonstrated using PPI analyses. A relationship between the BOLD response during the same task in the sgACC and the level of glutamate in the pgACC was demonstrated using regression analyses. A plot of the regression between the mean sgACC BOLD response and pgACC glutamate at the peak regression voxel within the sgACC is shown. A combined plot of the PPI regression results for each individual subject obtained from their first level PPI analysis at the peak voxel within the sgACC (from the group level analysis) is also shown. Regression plots were produced by obtaining the fitted response at the peak voxel via the "fitted response" option of the "plot" function in SPM, and plotting these against the relevant explanatory variable in MATLAB (The Mathwork Inc., Natick, MA). Activation images are shown with a threshold *P* ¼ 0.005 (unc.) for the purpose of illustration.**

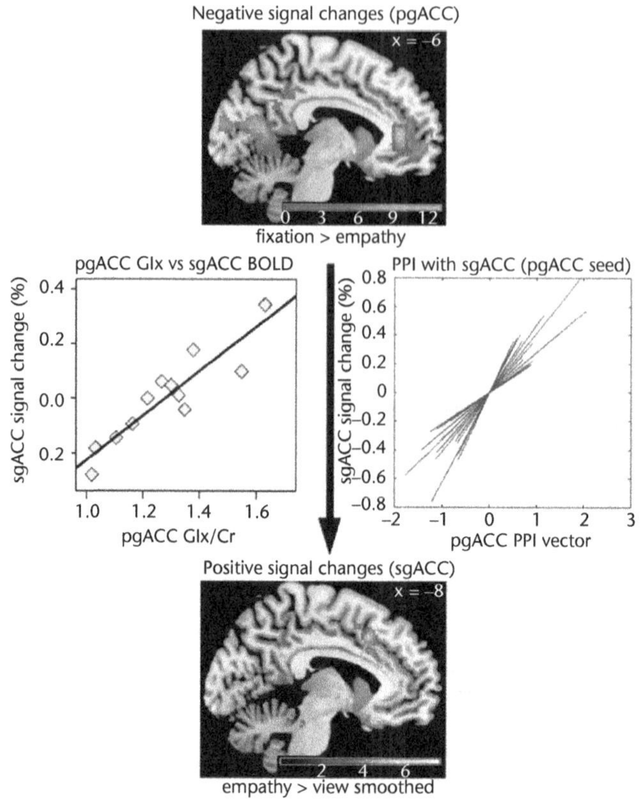

Figure 12-2a (*continued*)

magnetic stimulation (TMS) in motor cortex and measured the degrees of neural inhibition and excitation applying special TMS protocols over the motor cortex.

What do they show in their results? The degree of neural inhibition was directly related to the concentration of GABA measured in the motor cortex: the higher the concentration of GABA in motor cortex, the higher the degree of neural inhibition in the same region (see, though, Tremblay et al. 2012, who did not find a correlation of GABA concentration in left motor cortex with the silent period duration in inhibitory TMS). Furthermore, cortical excitability in motor cortex was related to glutamate: the higher the concentration of glutamate in motor cortex, the stronger the degree of cortical excitability in the same region.

There is, of course, abundant support from the animal side that links changes in GABA to changes in neural inhibition (see, for instance, Buzsáki 2006). One measure in fMRI that may be indicative of GABA-ergic-mediated neural inhibition may be negative signal changes (as distinguished from positive ones), the so-called deactivation or negative BOLD response (see Lauritzen et al. 2012 for an overview). Based on this observation, one would now expect that negative BOLD response correspond to an increase in neural inhibition as mediated by GABA (see also Lauritzen et al. 2012).

This was indeed demonstrated by Shmuel et al. (2002, 2006) in both monkey and human visual cortex. They measured both LFPs and fMRI: increase in negative BOLD response in fMRI was accompanied by a decrease in LFPs, which is indicative of increased neural inhibition (see also Goense et al. 2012 for further neurophysiological differentiation of positive and negative BOLD responses, with regard to especially their effects on cerebral blood flow and volume in different cortical layers). Unfortunately they did not include measures of GABA, which would have been necessary to close the suggested triangular relationship between negative BOLD response, GABA, and neural inhibition (see also Logothetis et al. 2010; Lauritzen et al. 2012, Northoff et al. 2007).

Taken together, these data show that the resting-state concentration of GABA in sensory and motor cortex predicts the degree of subsequent stimulus-induced activity in the same (and other) regions (see also Chapter 32 for findings on GABA in the insula). Thereby such intraregional rest–stimulus prediction seems to be specific for GABA since it was either not observed in or differed from the effects of glutamate.

Neuronal findings IIIc: *GABA* modulates *intra-regional* rest–stimulus interaction in *midline* regions

One may now question whether this applies also to other regions like the midline regions as a core part of the default-mode network (DMN). As discussed in Part II, the regions of the DMN show special neuronal features, especially in fMRI, which may also touch upon their underlying biochemical modulation. One would consequently like to see analogous GABA-ergic modulation of rest–stimulus interaction in the DMN before assuming GABA-ergic mediation of rest–stimulus interaction in general.

Using combined MRS and fMRI, a recent study from our group (Northoff et al., 2007) investigated the level of gamma-aminobutyric acid (GABA) in a typical DMN, the perigenual anterior cingulate cortex (PACC). The PACC is part of the DMN and shows predominant negative blood oxygen level dependent (BOLD) response during stimulus-induced activity in fMRI. The question was whether such stimulus-induced negative BOLD response is modulated by the resting-state concentration of GABA and must consequently be related to neural inhibition.

How now is the resting-state concentration of GABA related to the stimulus-induced negative BOLD response in PACC? The resting-state level of GABA in the PACC correlated with the degree of negative BOLD response as induced by an emotional judgment task in the very same region: the higher the resting-state concentration of GABA in the PACC, the higher was the degree of negative BOLD response in the same region during stimulus-induced activity.

Moreover, this relationship holds specifically for GABA because it was not found for glutamate; the latter was not related to the negative BOLD response. These findings thus demonstrate that the resting state concentration of GABA may be central in mediating the transition from resting-state activity to stimulus-induced activity in the PACC by mediating its degree of stimulus-induced negative BOLD responses (see Fig. 12-2b).

Neuronal findings IIId: *GABA-A receptors* modulate *intra-regional* rest–stimulus interaction in *midline* regions

The fMRI-MRS study demonstrated that the resting-state concentration of GABA in the PACC may indeed impact rest–stimulus interaction and consequently stimulus-induced activity changes in the PACC. Does this also hold true for GABA A receptors? Christine Wiebking from our group (Wiebking et al. 2012) combined measurement of stimulus-induced activity in fMRI with whole-brain measurement of GABA-A receptors using 18-F-Flumazenil positron emission tomography (PET) that allows to measure the density of GABA-A receptors in the resting state. She combined the PET with the investigation of fMRI where she tested a task for intero- and exteroceptive awareness (perception with counting of either the own heart beat or an externally presented tone).

As in the fMRI-MRS study, the resting-state GABA-A receptor density in the PACC predicted the degree of stimulus-induced activity (i.e., exteroceptive awareness during tone counting) in the same region, that is, the PACC: the higher the GABA-A receptor density in PACC, the lower the degree of stimulus-induced activity, namely negative BOLD responses, in the same region.

Since unlike MRS, 18-F-Flumazenil PET allows for whole-brain measurement of GABA-A receptor density, we could also test other regions besides the PACC. This revealed one other region; namely, the posterior cingulate cortex (PCC), where the GABA-A receptor density also predicted the degree of stimulus-induced activity in the same way. This suggests that GABA and more specifically GABA-A receptors seem to operate in similar ways in different regions of the

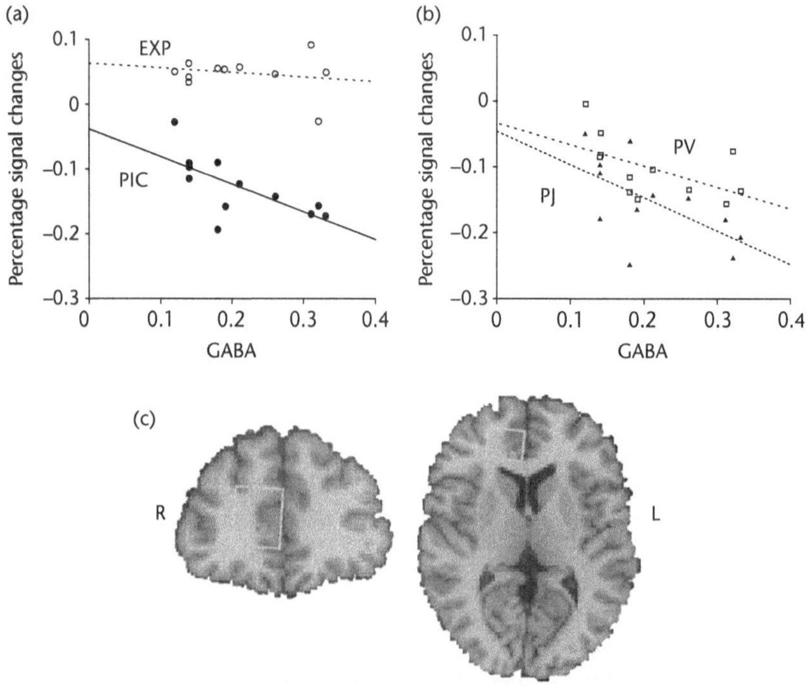

Figure 12-2b **GABA-ergic and glutamatergic modulation of rest–stimulus interaction. Correlation between GABA concentration and negative BOLD responses in the ACC.**
(*a*) Correlation between GABA concentrations (relative to creatine levels) and negative BOLD responses in the ACC for all pictures (PIC, $r = -0.713$, $P < 0.01$, filled circles and black line) and the EX (not significant, $P > 0.9$, open circles and dotted line). (*b*) Separate correlations for PV ($r = -0.554$, $P < 0.1$, open squares and open dashed line) and PJ ($r = -0.635$, $P < 0.05$, solid triangles and dense dashed line). (*c*) Local maxima of the voxel-wise simple regression analysis of the contrast [Rest > all pictures] with GABA levels in the ACC region of interest. Shown are the coronal (left) and transversal (right) sections. Orange boundaries indicating region of interest size and location correspond to the MRS voxel. Negative BOLD responses correlating with GABA concentrations are clearly restricted to the medial prefrontal gray matter in the ACC even on an uncorrected level of significance ($P < 0.005$). (Reprinted with permission of *Nature Neuroscience,* from Northoff G, Walter M, Schulte RF, Beck J, Dydak U,... Boesiger P. GABA concentrations in the human anterior cingulate cortex predict negative BOLD responses in fMRI. *Nat Neurosci.* 2007 Dec;10(12):1515–7.)

DMN (like PACC and PCC) and also in regions outside the DMN as in sensory and motor cortex as described earlier.

Interestingly, this relationship between GABA-A receptor density and stimulus-induced activity holds for only one condition: exteroceptive awareness, as tested for by tone-counting. In contrast, no such modulation by GABA-A receptor density was observed in another condition, interoceptive awareness that was measured by letting subjects counts their own heartbeat. Most important, the difference between intero- and exteroceptive awareness persisted even though there was no difference in the degree of signal change between intero- and exteroceptive awareness in PACC. That makes a psychologically specific effect of GABA-A receptors in both PACC and PCC rather likely: the GABA-A receptors in PACC and PCC mediate specifically extero- rather than interoceptive awareness (see Fig. 12-2c and d).

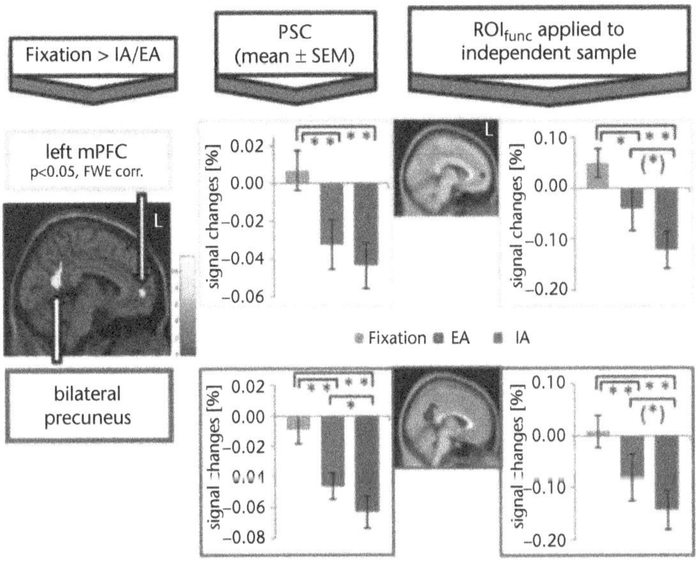

Figure 12-2c **Intero-and exteroceptive awareness and neural activity in the cortical midline regions. Cortical midline regions of interest (ROI functional) were defined by the contrast [Fixation > Internal (IA)/External Awareness (EA)] (P ≤ 0.05, FWE-corrected, k ≥ 5, n = 24 subjects; see SPM images on the left side). Bar diagrams, next to the SPM images, show percent signal changes (PSC, mean SEM) and accordingly negative BOLD responses (NBRs) during fixation, EA, and IA. Paired t-tests between the PSC were calculated (**$P \leq 0.005$, *$P \leq 0.05$, (*) $P \leq 0.1$). ROI functional were also applied to an independent data sample ($n = 30$ subjects), and paired t-tests between PSC were calculated. Note that there was no major significant difference in the degree of signal changes between intero- and exteroceptive awareness in both anterior and posterior cortical midline regions.**

NEURONAL FINDINGS IIIE: *GABA-A RECEPTORS* MODULATE *TRANS-REGIONAL* REST–STIMULUS INTERACTION IN *MIDLINE* REGIONS

How are the midline regions related to sensorimotor cortex? This question was addressed in a study by Hayes et al. (2013) from our group. He applied an aversion task (targeted to measure the contextual aversion effects) that activated the sensorimotor cortex as demonstrated in fMRI. The same subjects also underwent 18-F-Flumazenil PET to measure the density of GABA-A receptors (during the resting state) in a midline region, the ventromedial prefrontal cortex (VMPFC) (closely located to the PACC), and other regions including the sensorimotor cortex (unlike MRS, 18-F-Fluamzenil PET allows us to scan the whole brain).

He observed that the density of GABA-A receptors in the VMPFC (and also in the sensorimotor cortex) positively correlated with and thus predicted the degree of signal change during aversion in sensorimotor cortex: the higher the GABA-A receptor density in VMPFC (and sensorimotor cortex), the higher the aversion-induced signal changes in the sensorimotor cortex. This clearly suggests that the midline GABA-A receptors exert transregional effects on (for instance) the sensorimotor cortical activity.

Finally, the attentive reader may have noticed that the correlation of the stimulus-induced activity in PACC with the GABA-A receptors (PET) is positive rather than negative as in the case of the GABA concentration (MRS) (see earlier). The reasons for that are unclear. GABA-A receptors as measured with PET are obviously closely related to the intra- and extracellular concentration of GABA as measured with MRS. Their exact relationship remains unclear at this point, however. Whether the GABA-A receptor

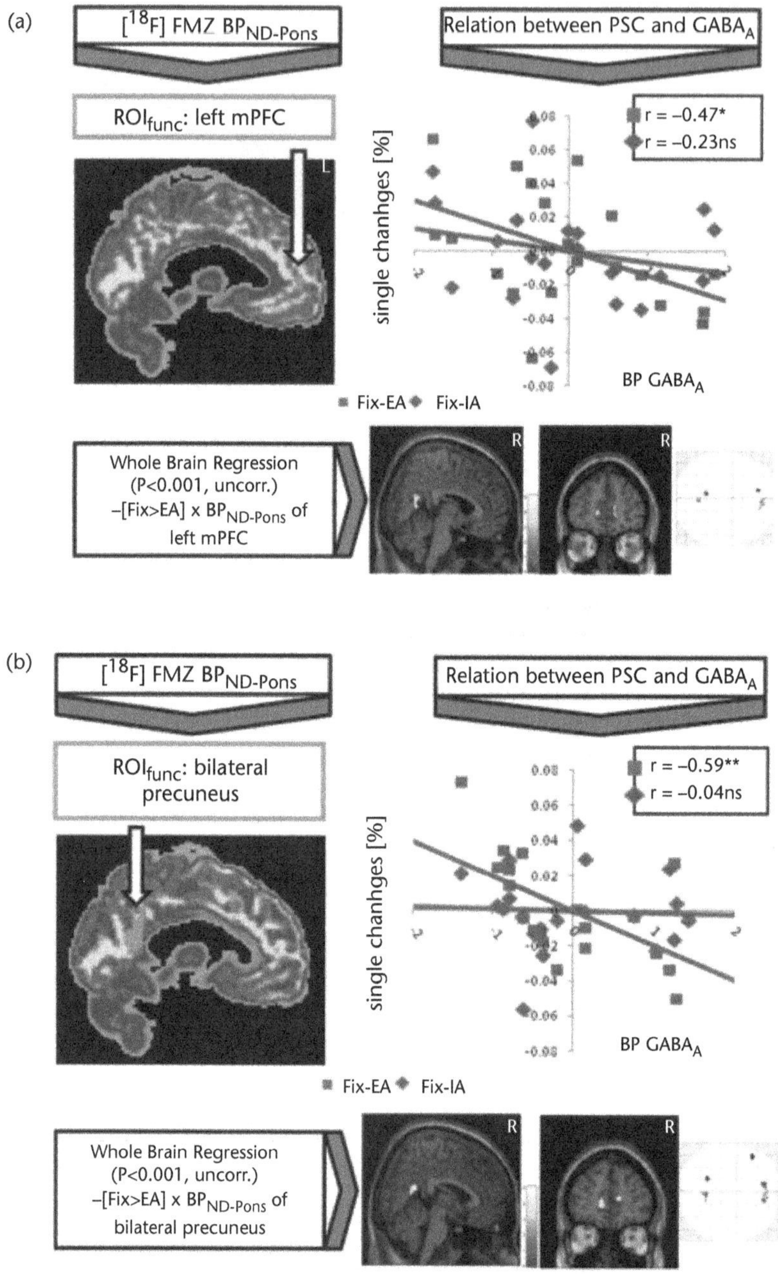

Figure 12-2d Modulation of exteroceptive awareness by GABA-A receptors. [18F]FMZ-PET imaging was used to calculate binding potentials (BPND-Pons) for GABAA receptors, applying functional regions of deactivation (ROIfunc, green color) derived from the contrast [Fixation > Internal/External Awareness] ($P \leq 0.05$, FWE-corrected, $k \geq 5$; see also Fig. 1). These values were correlated (controlled for gray matter) with percent signal changes (PSC) of the ROIs (see partial correlation graph showing the residuals of BPND-Pons and PSC, $*P \leq 0.05$, $**P \leq 0.01$). Moreover, BPNDPons values were entered into a whole brain regression analysis in SPM (controlled for the proportion of gray matter). The lower part shows a negative correlation for the contrast [Fixation > External Awareness] with BPND-Pons ($P \leq 0.001$, uncorrected, $k \geq 20$).(*a*) Shows results for the left mPFC and (*b*) for the bilateral precuneus.

density (and affinity) decreases or increases with lower or higher concentration of GABA has not been explored yet. Therefore, we remain unable to interpret the opposite correlations of GABA-A receptor density (PET) and GABA concentration (MRS) with the BOLD signal in fMRI.

Taken together, these studies (and others, see Jocham et al. 2012 as earlier) demonstrate that resting state GABA in midline regions like the PACC and PCC mediates stimulus-induced activity in the very same regions. Whether GABA mediates stimulus-specific effects as related to the respective region (as suggested in the study by Wiebking et al. 2012; see also Jocham et al. 2012 for GABA predicting stimulus-induced activity during especially rewarding stimuli) remains unclear. Accordingly, the question for psychological and regional specificity of GABA-ergic effects during rest-stimulus interaction cannot be addressed at this point in time.

Neuroempirical Background III: Neuronal Continuity and Distinction Between Resting State and Stimulus-Induced Activity

How do these various findings on glutamate and GABA account for difference-based coding that is supposed to underlie rest–stimulus interaction? Most important, we need to address this question by considering the neuronal mechanisms that allow for both neuronal continuity and neuronal distinction between resting state and stimulus-induced activity.

The resting state activity can exert some impact on the stimulus-induced activity only of the latter is continuous with the former. Such continuity is, as I will explicate in Volume II, of utmost importance to associate consciousness with the resulting stimulus-induced activity. At the same time, though, the stimulus-induced activity has to sufficiently differ from the resting-state activity in order to allow for the stimulus to induce its distinct behavioral and phenomenal effects. That is also important for our perception of the stimulus in our consciousness as sufficiently distinct from the continuously ongoing inner thoughts as related to the resting state activity.

Accordingly, the neuronal mechanisms underlying rest–stimulus interaction are "confronted" with the challenge of providing both neuronal continuity and distinction of stimulus-induced activity from resting-state activity. How is such combination of both neuronal continuity and distinction possible? For that, I suggest that the interplay between glutamate and GABA is central.

Neuronal Hypothesis IIa: Glutamate Mediates Stimulus-Induced Neural Excitation

Let us start with the glutamate and its role in rest–stimulus interaction. The findings demonstrate that the resting state concentration of glutamate increases the neural activity (as measured with the positive BOLD signal in fMRI) in different regions like the PACC and the DACC during different tasks like reward and cognitive control. In addition to such intra-regional effects, the resting state concentration of glutamate also modulates trans-regional effects on stimulus-induced activity in other regions, as shown in the study by Duncan et al. (2012; see also Falkenberg et al. 2012 for transregional effects).

What do these results imply for the neurophysiological mechanisms of glutamate in rest–stimulus interaction? Glutamate apparently increases neural activity on a regional level as is manifested in the observed stimulus-related positive BOLD responses. These positive BOLD responses have been shown to be neurophysiologically related to the power of local field potentials as measured with multi-unit activity (see Logothetis et al. 2001; Logothetis 2008; Lauritzen et al. 2012).

Since local field potentials are closely related to neural excitation, one would now suggest glutamate to exert its effects on a regional level to the modulation in the degree of neural excitation. Therefore, taking both cellular and regional levels together, I postulate that, on a regional level of neural activity, glutamate mediates the degree of neural excitation that is elicited by particular stimuli or tasks.

Most important, the level of neural excitation seems to remain independent of the degree of neural inhibition elicited by the same stimulus or task; that may be so because of the temporal delay between neural excitation and inhibition as we will discuss later (see also Chapters 2 and 6). Accordingly, the degree of stimulus-induced glutamate-ergic-mediated neural excitation may be characterized in an absolute way, as it remains independent of the degree of stimulus-induced neural inhibition.

We have to be careful, however. Glutamate-ergic-mediated neural excitation may only be independent of stimulus-related changes in neural inhibition. This may concern predominantly phasic inhibition that is modulated by the stimulus. In contrast, the glutamate-ergic-mediated neural excitation is still very much dependent on the degree of ongoing tonic inhibition.

For instance, higher degrees of tonic inhibition in the resting state may make it more difficult for glutamate to induce neural excitation during stimulus-induced or task-related activity. This leads us to explore the exact mechanisms of how glutamate mediates the transition from resting state to stimulus-induced activity.

Neuronal hypothesis IIb: stimulus-induced glutamate-ergic-mediated neural excitation is dependent on resting-state activity

The stimulus-induced glutamate-ergic-mediated neural excitation is still very much dependent on the degree of resting-state activity and its actual excitation-inhibition balance. This is suggested by the earlier described results, which show that the degree of stimulus-induced activity and its associated behavioral effects are dependent on the concentration of glutamate in the resting state. Accordingly, the degree of stimulus-induced glutamate-ergic-mediated neural excitation seems to be based and thus dependent on the resting-state activity and its level of glutamate.

What are the exact neuronal mechanisms by means of which glutamate induces neural excitation on the basis of the resting-state activity level? Some of the neuronal mechanisms may concern (for instance) the modulation of the power and/or timing of the resting state's gamma cycle, described earlier. To show that, we would need to conduct EEG studies and combine them with measurements of glutamate and GABA; this, however, remains to be reported. One would hypothesize that the gamma cycle is not only mediated by GABA, as suggested by Fries, but also by glutamate, which, however, may modulate distinct neuronal measures (like the gamma cycle's phase shift rather than its power).

In order to further reveal the neuronal mechanisms of glutamate and how it modulates the resting-state activity during the encounter with stimuli, we also need to be clearer about the resting-state activity itself. When we talk of resting-state activity here, we refer to its trait features (across time) rather than its state features (at one particular point in time) (see Chapter 11 for more details on the distinction between trait and state features of the resting-state activity).

How does the distinction between trait and state features apply to glutamate? The MRS does not allow us to measure spontaneous changes in glutamate in relation to single trials or stimuli (though some functional MRS studies have recently been carried out; see for instance Schaller et al. (2013)). The spectra obtained in MRS result from an integral of about 5-10 minutes of measurement (which for GABA is even longer). This makes it likely that what is measured in MRS concerns the trait glutamate of the resting-state activity rather than the state glutamate as related to spontaneous changes in the resting-state activity (or to stimulus-induced activity as related to single trials).

How does that relate to the earlier described findings? The findings suggests that the resting state concentration of glutamate as trait feature of the resting-state impacts the more state-related changes during stimulus-induced or task-related activity. This, however, leaves open the role of the state features of the resting-state activity itself, its spontaneous changes and dynamic fluctuations in the glutamate concentration. To measure the state changes of glutamate and its impact on subsequent stimulus-induced activity, we however need to develop better technical devices that may allow measuring the spontaneous changes in glutamate concentration in the resting state itself.

How would such spontaneous changes of glutamate in the resting state impact subsequent stimulus-induced activity? Depending on (for instance) the timing or power of the stimulus relative to the resting state's glutamate fluctuations, the stimulus may induce stronger or weaker neural excitation. In the same way that we showed how the dynamic changes in the gamma cycle impact subsequent stimulus-induced activity, we may then assume a "glutamate cycle." The assumption of such "glutamate cycle" and its specific features, however, remains speculative at this time.

Neuronal hypothesis IIc: Glutamate modulates trans-regional effects and neuronal continuity during rest–stimulus interaction

Another feature of glutamate seems that it can exert effects in distant regions, thus showing trans-regional effects. This has been nicely demonstrated in the study by Duncan et al. (2011), who demonstrated that the resting state concentration of glutamate in PACC predicts the degree of stimulus-induced activity in the SACC, including their trans-regional rest–stimulus functional connectivity. Analogous trans-regional effects were also observed in the study by Falkenberg et al. (2012) where the DACC resting state glutamate exerted effects on stimulus-induced activity in other cortical regions.

How can glutamate mediate such trans-regional rest–stimulus interaction? This, I argue, may be mainly due to the specific anatomo-structural organization (see also Buzsaki 2006 for details): glutamate and its various types of receptors (metabotropic, NMDA, AMPA) are located predominantly at pyramidal cells (mainly in layer 4 of the cortex). These show abundant afferent and efferent connections to neurons in more distant and remote regions.

Such anatomo-structural considerations predisposes the glutamate in one region to exert its effects in other regions. This may account for the observed trans-regional effects of glutamate during rest–stimulus interaction. Since this concerns anatomo-structural features, one would expect the same kind of trans-regional effects of glutamate to be manifested already during the resting state itself. This is indeed the case with glutamate modulating the degree of trans-regional functional connectivity in the resting state itself, as we described it in Chapter 6 (see especially Duncan et al. 2013).

Combining this with the apparent effects of glutamate on neural excitation, one would propose the trans-regional effects of glutamate to be mediated by the induction or spread of neural excitation across different regions. Whether such glutamatergic-mediated spread of neural activity across different regions may underlie what has been described as "travelling waves" must remain open though at this point in time. In sum, glutamate seems to be central in inducing neural excitation as related to the stimulus. This may allow the stimulus-induced activity to be sufficiently distinct from the preceding resting-state activity. At the same time, the stimulus-induced glutamate-ergic-mediated neural excitation is very much dependent on the level of the resting-state activity as (for instance) its glutamate concentration (while remaining independent of the stimulus-related phasic GABA changes; see below). This means that glutamate is central in providing the transition from resting state to stimulus-induced activity, thus allowing for their neuronal continuity.

Neuronal hypothesis IIIa: GABA and glutamate exert differential effects on the regional level of neural activity

I have so far shown that glutamate seems to provide some neuronal continuity from the resting-state activity to the stimulus-induced activity. At the same time, it induces neural excitation by means of which the stimulus-induced activity can distinguish itself from the resting-state activity.

How now can the stimulus-induced activity be even further distinguished from the resting-state activity in order to "bring out" the distinct neuronal, behavioral, and phenomenal effects of the stimulus itself? I hypothesize that GABA and its interplay with glutamate are central here.

Let us start with the results on GABA described earlier. The findings show that the resting state concentration of GABA (and/or the resting state density of GABA-A receptors) in various regions, including sensory and motor cortex and midline regions, impacts stimulus-induced activity in the same regions. This again suggests that the resting-state activity—more specifically, its concentration of GABA—exerts an impact on the degree of the subsequent stimulus-induced activity. The stimulus-induced activity is thus very much dependent upon the resting-state activity and its (trait) concentration of GABA.

We are thus confronted with the same scenario as in the case of glutamate, where an analogous dependence of stimulus-induced activity on the resting-state concentration of glutamate can be observed. This, however, is the point where the similarities between GABA and glutamate end and their differences start.

The differences between GABA and glutamate are suggested by the findings described earlier (which, however, due to the low number of studies, must be taken tentatively). GABA and glutamate differed in their temporal (i.e., early versus late; see Jocham et al. 2012), neurophysiological (i.e., neural inhibition and excitation; Stagg et al. 2011a and b), and stimulus-specific (i.e., extero- versus interoceptive awareness; Wiebking et al. 2012, 2013) effects.

Neuronal hypothesis IIIb: GABA modulates neural inhibition on the regional level of neural activity

How are such differences between GABA and glutamate possible? Their differences already start on the cellular level. As discussed in Chapter 2, GABA is associated with inhibitory interneurons that receive strong connections from glutamate-ergic-mediated pyramidal cells. These direct connections allow for the glutamate-ergic pyramidal cells to excite and activate the GABA-ergic inhibitory interneurons, which can in turn exert their inhibitory effects by introducing and increasing neural inhibition (see later for more details on that). Most important, as the results on the cellar level show, there is a temporal delay of around 10ms between glutamate-ergic-mediated neural excitation and GABA-ergic-mediated neural inhibition (see Fig. 12-3a).

The cellular level shows that neural inhibition is dependent on prior neural excitation; there is thus a 'neurophysiological dependence' between glutamate and GABA. In addition there is also a 'biochemical dependence', since the synthesis of GABA depends on glutamate as its direct precursor. How now is such neurophysiological and biochemical dependence between GABA and glutamate manifested on the regional level? The biochemical dependence may be reflected in the positive correlation between GABA and glutamate, as has been reported in Jocham et al. (2012) and Wiebking et al. (2013) (see Chapter 32 for details on the latter).

How about the neurophysiological dependence of neural inhibition on neural excitation? The data show that GABA and glutamate stand in different relation to positive and negative BOLD responses in fMRI. While glutamate seems to increase positive BOLD response, GABA apparently modulates negative BOLD changes (or decreases positive BOLD responses).

Since positive and negative BOLD responses have been associated with neural excitation and inhibition, respectively (see Northoff et al. 2007; Logothetis et al. 2001; Logothetis 2008; Lauritzen et al. 2012; Shmuel et al. 2002, 2006), their differential modulation by glutamate and GABA seems to conform (more or less) to the distinction between neural excitation and inhibition. This is also supported by the findings from Stagg et al. (2011a and b) who, combining MRS and TMS in motor cortex, could directly link glutamate to neural excitation and GABA to neural inhibition (see earlier). Taken together, this suggests that, as on the cellular level, glutamate and

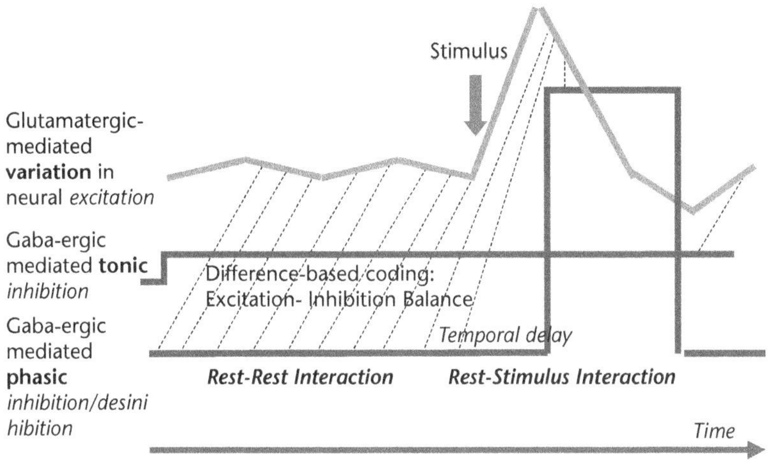

Figure 12-3a GABA, glutamate, and rest–stimulus interaction. The figure illustrates the role of GABA and glutamate in rest–stimulus interaction with regard to the excitation-inhibition balance (*a*) and GABA-ergic-mediated nonlinearity (*b*). (*a*) The figure illustrates the relationship between GABA and glutamate during rest–rest and rest–stimulus interaction. Glutamate mediates fluctuations in the degree of neuronal excitation during both resting-state and stimulus-induced activity (upper line). GABA mediates tonic middle line and phasic lower line above the time axis changes in the degree of neural inhibition during rest–rest and rest–stimulus interaction. Together, GABA and glutamate constitute what is called the excitation-inhibition balance, which is indicated by the thin black dotted lines and is based on difference-based coding, i.e., the encoding of spatial and temporal differences. If the resting-state activity encounters a stimulus (brown arrow), the excitation-inhibition balance is rebalanced between the early glutamatergic-mediated neural excitation and slightly temporally delayed GABA-ergic-mediated phasic neural inhibition. The net effect of both, the degree of change in the excitation-inhibition balance, accounts for the change in or deviation of the stimulus-induced activity (as indicated by the absence of dotted lines) from the resting-state activity level.

GABA mediate neural excitation and inhibition also on a regional level of neural activity.

How about the temporal delay between glutamate-ergic neural excitation and GABA-ergic neural inhibition on a regional level of neural activity? The study by Jocham et al. (2012) observed differential, opposing effects of the resting state concentrations of glutamate and GABA during early and late stages of the BOLD signals; that is, the stimulus-induced activity.

While this provides some initial support for differential temporal effects of glutamate and GABA, it does not address the question of the temporal delay between neural excitation and inhibition on a regional level of neural activity. For that, one would probably need to undertake EEG/MEG and combine it with MRS (and most likely TMS to measure the degrees of cortical excitability and inhibition), which remains to be reported, though.

These findings suggest, though tentatively, that the differential features of glutamate and GABA on the cellular level are somehow preserved and resurface in a not-yet-fully clear way on the regional level of neural activity.

NEURONAL HYPOTHESIS IIIC: GABA-ERGIC EFFECTS ARE DEPENDENT ON STIMULUS-RELATED GLUTAMATE AND RESTING-STATE ACTIVITY

How can we further characterize the effect of GABA on the regional level of neural activity? Due to the need for prior glutamate-ergic-mediated neural excitation, GABA is not independent from glutamate. Instead, the degree of GABA-ergic-mediated neural inhibition very much depends on the degree of prior stimulus-induced glutamate-ergic-mediated neural excitation.

Such dependence on its excitatory counterpart distinguishes GABA-ergic-mediated neural inhibition from glutamate-ergic-mediated neural excitation, which, as described earlier, remains independent of its inhibitory sibling during stimulus-induced activity. Accordingly, there is unilateral dependence of stimulus-related (phasic) GABA from stimulus-related glutamate, but not of stimulus-related glutamate from stimulus-related (phasic) GABA.

In addition, GABA-ergic mediated (phasic) neural inhibition is also very much dependent on the resting-state activity. This is well reflected on a cellular level in the earlier mentioned dependence of the stimulus-related gamma shift and the degree of subsequent GABA-ergic-mediated neural inhibition on the power and timing of the resting state's ongoing gamma cycles.

The same apparently holds true on the regional level. Otherwise, the degree of stimulus-induced negative BOLD response, as related to neural inhibition, would not be predicted and parametrically modulated by the resting state concentration of GABA (see Northoff et al. 2007; Wiebking et al. 2012; Shmuel et al. 2002, 2006).

Neuronal hypothesis IIID: trait versus state GABA

We also need to distinguish between phasic and tonic neural inhibition. GABA-ergic-mediated inhibitory interneurons may exert a continuous and thus tonic inhibitory impact on other neurons that persists more or less throughout the resting-state activity. Since tonic GABA-ergic-mediated neural inhibition is a more persistent feature, it may be regarded as a trait rather than state feature of the resting-state activity.

As such, tonic GABA-ergic inhibition may strongly impact the possible degree of glutamate-ergic-mediated neural excitation. In addition, tonic GABA-ergic inhibition may also modulate the degree to which the stimuli can modulate the more phasic GABA-ergic-mediated neural inhibition during subsequent stimulus-induced activity.

In contrast to tonic inhibition, phasic inhibition may rather be regarded as a state feature of the resting-state activity that reflects the actual state and level of the resting state at a particular point in time. This is manifested in the spontaneous and dynamic fluctuations of the concentration of GABA in the resting state itself. And it is such GABA-ergic-mediated phasic inhibition that is most likely affected by the stimulus and its glutamate-ergic-mediated neural excitation.

How does that stand in relation to the reported results? Due to the low temporal resolution in MRS for GABA (with acquisition times usually at around 15–20 min), the measured resting state concentration may reflect trait-related GABA in the resting state rather than state-related GABA. Future investigations may therefore tackle the question how the spontaneous resting state fluctuations in GABA concentration affect subsequent stimulus-induced activity, including its degree of neural inhibition.

Neuronal hypothesis IVA: glutamate-ergic-mediated neural excitation and GABA-ergic-mediated neural inhibition are difference-based signals

What do these results on glutamate and GABA imply for the encoding of rest–stimulus interaction into neural activity? As demonstrated earlier, both stimulus-induced glutamate-ergic-mediated neural excitation and GABA-ergic-mediated neural excitation must be considered difference-based rather than stimulus-based signals. Although stimulus-induced glutamate-ergic-mediated neural excitation is not dependent upon the degree of stimulus-induced phasic GABA-ergic-mediated neural inhibition, it remains nevertheless dependent upon the resting-state activity: that is, its level, power, and timing (which also include the tonic GABA-ergic effects).

This means that the stimulus-induced glutamate-ergic-mediated neural excitation does not only and exclusively encode the stimulus itself but rather its spatial and temporal relationship to the resting-state activity and its particular spatiotemporal structure. Stimulus-induced glutamate-ergic-mediated neural excitation is thus a difference- rather than stimulus-based signal. Therefore, what we observe and describe as stimulus-induced glutamate-ergic-mediated neural excitation presupposes the encoding of spatial and temporal differences between stimulus and resting-state activity, that is, difference-based coding.

The same applies for the GABA-ergic-mediated neural inhibition. As described earlier GABA-ergic-mediated neural inhibition is dependent upon both the degree of stimulus-induced glutamate-ergic-mediated neural excitation and the resting-state activity itself. Therefore, GABA-ergic-mediated neural inhibition reflects neither the degree of glutamate-ergic-mediated neural excitation alone nor that of the resting-state activity itself. Instead, GABA-ergic-mediated neural inhibition results from their integration and must therefore be considered a difference- rather than stimulus-based signal.

In sum, both stimulus-induced glutamate-ergic-mediated neural excitation and GABA-ergic-mediated neural inhibition must be characterized as difference- rather than stimulus-based signals. This is possible only by encoding spatial and temporal differences amounting to difference-based coding rather than stimulus-based coding.

Neuronal hypothesis IVb: nonlinear effects during rest–stimulus interaction and GABA

How now does such difference-based coding relate to the "need of the stimulus-induced activity" to sufficiently differ from the resting-state activity in order to bring forth the neuronal, behavioral, and phenomenal peculiarities of the stimulus? In order to properly differentiate the stimulus-induced activity from the resting-state activity, the spatial and temporal differences encoded during rest–stimulus interaction need to be sufficiently large.

Only if the stimulus-induced activity differs sufficiently in neuronal terms from the preceding resting-state activity may the stimulus have a "chance" to exert its own and distinct behavioral (and phenomenal) effects (see also the neuroempirical background at the beginning of this chapter). I now propose that GABA and its mediation of nonlinear effects may play a central role in generating sufficiently large spatial and temporal differences during the encoding of rest–stimulus interaction. This in turn allows us to sufficiently distinguish the resulting stimulus-induced activity from the resting-state activity.

Let us recall nonlinearity as one of the central principles guiding both stimulus–stimulus interaction (Chapter 10) and rest–stimulus interaction (see Chapter 11). The principle of nonlinearity states that stimulus-induced activity cannot be considered the result of mere addition or summation of the stimulus on top of the existing resting-state activity level. Instead, the stimulus interacts with the resting-state activity in such way that the latter changes in an exponential, or nonlinear, rather than parametric, or linear, way. This indicates nonlinear rather than linear interaction between resting-state activity and stimulus.

While there is plenty of empirical evidence for the occurrence of such nonlinearity during rest–stimulus interaction, its exact neurophysiological mechanisms remain unclear. This is the moment where GABA and neural inhibition come into play. Following Buzsaki (2006, 63–65), the introduction of GABA-ergic inhibitory interneurons injects nonlinear effects into an otherwise predominantly linear glutamatergic-mediated excitatory system. How does such injection of non-linearity look like? That shall be discussed in the next section.

Neuronal hypothesis IVc: GABA mediates nonlinearity during rest–stimulus interaction

How does GABA introduce nonlinear effects into rest–stimulus interaction? To answer that question, we need to consider the number of pyramidal cells and interneurons (see also Chapters 2 and 6). As detailed in especially Chapter 2 (and Chapter 6), there is an imbalance between glutamatergic pyramidal cells and GABA-ergic interneurons, with the number of the latter exceeding that of the former.

What does this imbalance between glutamatergic pyramidal cells and GABA-ergic interneurons imply for the excitation-inhibition balance (EIB)? GABA-ergic interneurons require glutamatergic excitation in order to get activated. This is further supported on a regional level by the observation of a correlation between intraregional GABA and glutamate concentrations as measured in MRS (Waddell et al. 2011; Schmaal et al. 2012, Wiebking et al. 2013, Jocham et al. 2012).

Once activated by glutamatergic excitation, the GABA-ergic interneurons, due to their large number, increase their degree of neural inhibition in a disproportionately strong way that far exceeds the initial degree of neural excitation (see Kapfer et al. 2007 for empirical support, who demonstrate that two pyramidal cells in rat somatosensory cortex recruit a tenfold number of inhibitory interneurons and thus increase the level of recurrent inhibition disproportionately when compared to the level of excitation).

The disproportionally string increase in the degree of neural inhibition leads to a major shift in the EIB from neural excitation toward neural inhibition (see also Priebe and Ferster 2008, 492–493; as well as Logothetis et al. 2010 for support for nonlinear increase in neural inhibition in visual cortex). The difference-based value of the EIB consequently changes in a nonlinear way, by means of which the resulting degree of neural activity— stimulus-induced activity—can differ in a nonlinear way from the initial level of the preceding activity, the resting-state activity.

This leads me to the following hypothesis. I hypothesize that the degree of the difference between stimulus-induced and resting-state activity is directly proportional to the degree of GABA-ergic-mediated nonlinearity and its encoding of spatial and temporal differences during rest–stimulus interaction: the higher the degree of GABA-ergic-mediated nonlinearity during rest–stimulus interaction, the larger the encoded spatial and temporal differences, and the larger the difference between stimulus-induced activity and resting-state activity (see Fig. 12-3b).

Accordingly, GABA-ergic-mediated neural inhibition may enlarge the spatial and temporal differences that are encoded during rest–stimulus interaction. This in turn allows the resulting stimulus-induced activity to sufficiently differ from the resting-state activity (that is in its power, timing, and level) and thus to "bring out" the distinct behavioral (and phenomenal) effects of the stimulus. I henceforth suggest the distinction between rest and stimulus to be based on GABA and its modulation of the degree of spatial

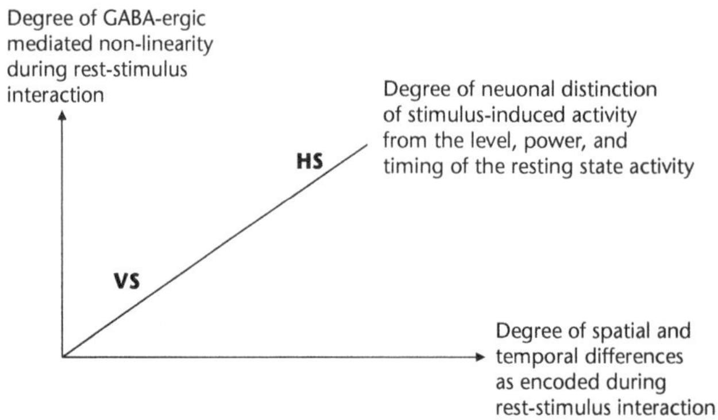

Figure 12.3b **GABA, glutamate, and rest–stimulus interaction. (*b*) The figure illustrates the relationship between the degree of GABA-ergic-mediated nonlinearity (y-axis) and the degree of the encoded spatial and temporal differences during rest–stimulus interaction (x-axis): the higher the degree of GABA-ergic-mediated nonlinearity during rest–stimulus interaction, the larger the encoded spatial and temporal differences during rest–stimulus interaction, and the larger the degree of neuronal distinction between stimulus-induced activity and resting-state activity (its level, timing, and power). Abbreviations: VS = vegetative state, HS = healthy subjects.**

and temporal differences that are encoded into neural activity during rest–stimulus interaction.

NEURONAL HYPOTHESIS IVD: GABA-MEDIATED NONLINEARITY AND CONSCIOUSNESS

What though happens if the degree of GABA-ergic mediated non-linearity is rather low? If the degree of GABA-ergic-mediated nonlinearity during rest–stimulus interaction is rather low, there will at best be linear (i.e., merely additive or summative) but no longer nonlinear differences between stimulus-induced activity and resting-state activity. I consequently suggest that the degree of GABA-ergic-mediated nonlinearity during rest–stimulus interaction is neuronally relevant, in that it determines the degree of stimulus-induced activity and thus its relative difference from the resting-state activity.

In addition to such neuronal relevance, I suggest that GABA-ergic-mediated nonlinearity is also highly relevant for consciousness; that is, phenomenally relevant. In order to associate a phenomenal state, consciousness, with the purely neuronal stimulus-induced activity, the stimulus must interact with the resting-state activity in a nonlinear way to yield sufficiently large differences in stimulus-induced activity when compared to the resting-state activity level.

If, in contrast, there is only linear interaction between stimulus and resting-state activity, the probability that the resulting stimulus-induced activity will be associated with a phenomenal state and thus consciousness is rather low. That may, for instance, be the case in patients with vegetative state, whose loss of consciousness may be related to their loss of GABA-ergic-mediated nonlinearity during rest–stimulus interaction (see Chapters 28 and 29 for details).

Due to their lack of GABA-ergic mediated non-linearity during rest-stimulus interaction, these patients may no longer be able to "bring out" the neuronal, behavioral and phenomenal features associated with the stimulus. This example demonstrates tentative support to the hypothesis that GABA-ergic-mediated nonlinearity during rest–stimulus interaction is not only neuronally but also phenomenally relevant.

NEURONAL HYPOTHESIS VA: GABA MEDIATES SPARSE CODING DURING REST–STIMULUS INTERACTION

Where are we now? I demonstrated various empirical findings that show how the resting state concentrations of GABA and glutamate predict the degree of subsequent intra- or trans-regional stimulus-induced activity. This, as I supposed, is possible only by assuming difference-based coding. Only difference-based coding (as distinct from stimulus-based coding) allows for the encoding of spatial and temporal differences by GABA and glutamate into neural inhibition and excitation whose relative difference constitutes the excitation-inhibition balance.

How can we now further characterize the resulting stimulus-induced activity? We saw in Chapter 2 that GABA-ergic-mediated neural inhibition was closely related to sparse coding on a cellular level of neural activity: the stronger the GABA-ergic-mediated neural inhibition, the higher the degree of temporal and spatial sparsening of the subsequent stimulus-induced activity. After showing that sparse coding also holds on the regional level of neural activity (see Chapter 3), we then demonstrated that the resting state and its spatiotemporal activity pattern can also be characterized by sparse coding and GABA-ergic-mediated neural inhibition (see Chapter 6).

This left open whether GABA-ergic-mediated neural inhibition also drives the temporal and spatial sparsening of neural activity during rest–stimulus interaction and the resulting stimulus-induced activity on a regional level. The earlier suggested difference-based coding of GABA and glutamate during rest–stimulus interaction may consequently entail sparse coding of stimulus-induced activity. Therefore, stimulus-induced activity can be characterized by temporal (lifetime sparseness) and spatial (population sparseness) sparsening, with only a few regions being active in a short time window (see Fig. 12-4a).

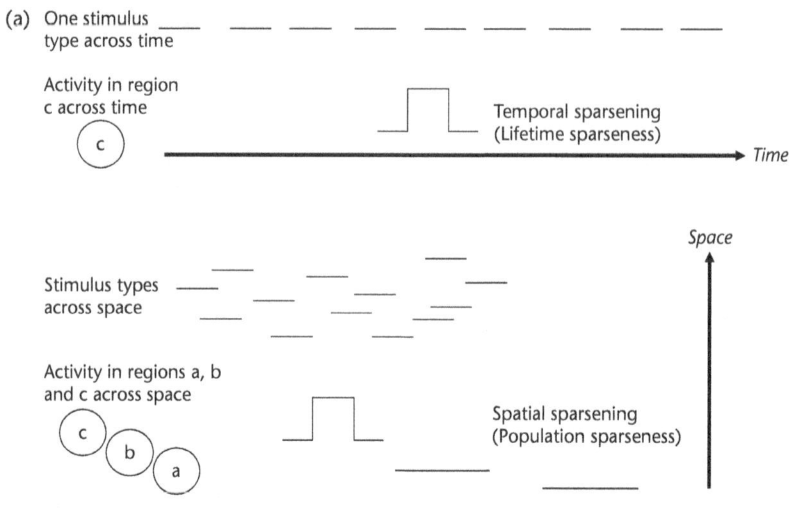

Figure 12-4a **Sparse coding and GABA. The figure illustrates the sparse coding on a regional level (*a*) and how it relates to GABA-ergic-mediated nonlinearity (*b*). (*a*) The figure illustrates how sparse coding operates on the regional level in both temporal (*upper part*) and spatial (*lower part*) regard. If one stimulus occurs several times across time (small horizontal lines), the region c will show activity (bar diagram) at only one discrete point in physical time, thereby integrating the several occurrences of the stimulus across time. Hence, there is what can be described as "temporal sparsening." The same holds for the spatial domain, where different stimulus types occurring at different positions in space (small horizontal lines) do not elicit neural activity in different regions (a, b, c) but only in one of the regions (bar diagram). This amounts to what can be described as "spatial sparsening."**

More specifically, I hypothesize that GABA-ergic-mediated neural inhibition and its nonlinearity are central in the temporal and spatial sparsening of neural activity during rest–stimulus interaction: the higher the degree of GABA-ergic-mediated nonlinearity during rest–stimulus interaction, the higher the degree to which the resulting stimulus-induced activity will be spatially ("population sparseness") and temporally ("lifetime sparseness") sparsened. In short, I propose that GABA-ergic-mediated nonlinearity drives the sparsening of stimulus-induced activity (see Fig. 12-4b).

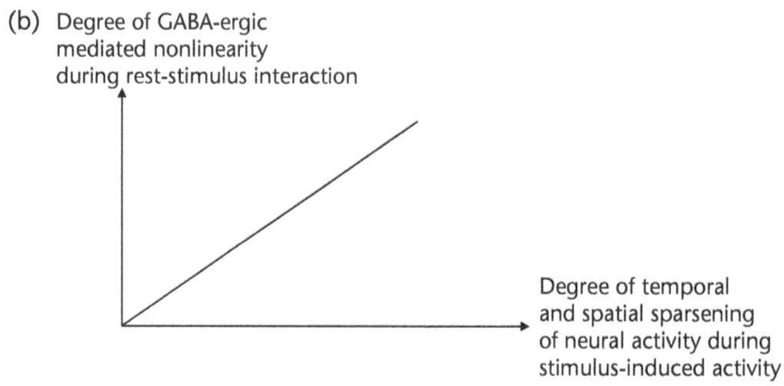

Figure 12-4b **Sparse coding and GABA. (*b*) The figure illustrates the presumed dependence of the degree of temporal and spatial sparsening of stimulus-induced activity (x-axis) on the degree of GABA-ergic-mediated nonlinearity during rest–stimulus interaction (y-axis). The higher the degree of GABA-ergic-mediated nonlinearity during rest–stimulus interaction, the higher the degree of temporal and spatial sparsening in the resulting stimulus-induced activity.**

Neuronal hypothesis Vb: Sparse coding of stimulus-induced activity

If my hypothesis is correct, one would expect that stimulus-induced activity goes along with higher degrees of temporal and spatial sparseness when compared to the resting-state activity. Why is this so? Due to the increased degree of stimulus-induced glutamatergic-mediated neural excitation, the stimulus leads to increased recruitment of GABA-ergic neural inhibition; this in turn increases the likelihood of nonlinearity and consequently the degree of temporal and spatial sparsening in the subsequent stimulus-induced activity.

Is there any empirical support for higher degrees of sparseness during stimulus-induced activity when compared to resting-state activity? Let us recall the investigation by Dan Lloyd (2011) on sparse coding in music, language, and the brain, described in Chapter 6. He applied quantitative measures of sparseness with regard to the number of elements and their combinations actually used.

Thereby, the brain's resting-state activity (with spatiotemporal activity patterns defined at each point in time during scanning/fMRI) showed a degree of sparseness that is comparable to the one in music rather than to the much lower degree of sparseness in language (see Chapter 6 for details). Interestingly, Lloyd included not only resting-state data but also some stimulus-induced data that were acquired during an auditory oddball paradigm in both healthy and schizophrenic subjects.

This showed higher degree of sparseness during stimulus-induced activity when compared to resting-state activity. Lloyd consequently proposes that the stimulus or the task increases the degree of sparse coding in the brain. That is a tentative hypothesis, however, due to the low number of cases included (see also Lee et al. 2011 for further support of increased sparseness during stimulus-induced activity).

What do these findings imply? They provide tentative evidence for the assumption that stimulus-induced activity shows higher degrees of sparseness than resting-state activity. Together with the findings described here, that lends some indirect empirical support to the central role of GABA-ergic-mediated neural inhibition and nonlinearity in increasing the degrees of temporal and spatial sparsening during stimulus-induced activity.

Neuronal hypothesis Vc: Stimulus-induced activity is "hybrid" and difference- and statistically based

Put slightly differently, the encounter with the stimulus provides the brain's resting-state activity with the "opportunity to recruit" higher degrees of GABA-ergic-mediated nonlinearity and to spatially and temporally sparsen its neural activity. Such increased spatial and temporal sparsening is possible only by increased encoding of spatial and temporal differences into neural activity and thus by higher degrees of difference-based coding.

What does such increase in the degree of difference-based coding entail for the different stimuli? The different stimuli—the exteroceptive stimuli from the environment, the interoceptive stimuli from the body, and the neuronal stimuli from the brain itself—have a higher, purely statistically based, chance of getting linked and integrated with each other which makes more likely their encoding in term of spatial and temporal differences. The increase in the encoding of spatial and temporal differences increases, in turn, the degree of temporal and spatial sparsening of the resulting stimulus-induced activity at only a couple of regions at a few points in time. We can thus see a regionally (spatially) and temporally sparse activation pattern which is exactly what we can observe in our results from both EEG and fMRI.

Let us consider the same phenomenon on a slightly more general level. The different stimuli's statistical frequency distributions, their social (exteroceptive stimuli), vegetative (interoceptive stimuli), and neuronal (neuronal stimuli) statistics (see Chapter 8 and 9 for details), are matched and linked and integrated with each other during rest–stimulus interaction when being encoded into neural activity in terms of spatial and temporal differences. The resulting stimulus-induced activity can consequently no longer be said to exclusively originate from either exteroceptive, interoceptive, or neuronal stimuli and thus from either social, vegetative, or neuronal origins. Accordingly, the simulus-induced activity can no longer be associated exclusively with one particular stimulus and its vegetative, social, or neuronal origin.

What does this imply for the characterization of the stimulus-induced activity in positive terms? Instead of being based on the origin of the stimuli; that is, origin- and stimulus-based, the resulting stimulus-induced activity may rather be characterized as statistically and difference-based (see Chapter 25 for extensive discussion of such origin- and stimulus-based coding). The stimulus-induced activity must consequently be regarded rather a statistically and difference-based as well as hybrid where the different stimuli and their respective statistics, social, vegetative, and neuronal, are intrinsically intertwined and indistinguishable.

Accordingly, there is thus no "pure" stimulus-induced activity that reflects one particular stimulus exclusively and by itself. Instead, any stimulus-induced activity must be considered a "hybrid" of neuronal, interoceptive, and exteroceptive stimuli which are always already linked by our brain and its particular encoding strategy.

Neuronal hypothesis VD: Sparse coding and consciousness

Why is the hybrid characterization of stimulus-induced activity as difference- and statistically based so important? First and foremost it is neuronally relevant, since it lets us better understand what stimulus-induced activity is about.

It may explain many findings showing that exteroceptively-related stimulus-induced activity and the associated sensory, motor, or cognitive functions are dependent on both the interoceptive stimuli from the own body, its vegetative state, and the brain's resting-state activity level, its neuronal stimuli (and vice versa) (see Chapter 8). Many of the findings that show context-dependence, as discussed especially in Chapters 8 and 9, may well be explained on a neuronal level by the characterization of stimulus-induced as "hybrid" as well as statistically and difference-based.

Beyond its neuronal relevance, I postulate that the difference- and statistically based as well as hybrid nature of stimulus-induced activity is also behaviorally and especially phenomenally relevant. As will become clear in Volume II, the intrinsic integration and linkage between exteroceptive, interoceptive, and neuronal stimuli and their respective social, vegetative, and neuronal statistics is essential in making possible the association of consciousness and its phenomenal features with the purely neuronal stimulus-induced activity.

What does the relationship between sparse coding and consciousness look like? The better the different stimuli and their respective statistics are linked and integrated and thus encoded into neural activity in terms of spatial and temporal difference, the more hybrid and sparse the resulting purely neuronal stimulus-induced activity, and the higher the likelihood that the latter will be associated with consciousness (see Chapters 28–30). This is well reflected in our subjective experience of consciousness, which can indeed be characterized as a state wherein all three, brain, body, and environment, are integrated in an intrinsic and (more or less) indistinguishable way (see especially Chapter 30) (see Fig. 12-4c).

If, in contrast, the different stimuli are not well integrated and encoded into neural activity in terms of spatial and temporal differences, the resulting stimulus-induced activity will be less hybrid and sparse, which decreases the likelihood of its association with a phenomenal state that is consciousness. This may be the case in vegetative state, where the patients seem to show a less hybrid stimulus-induced activity, which therefore, I would postulate, is no longer associated with the phenomenal features of consciousness (see Chapters 28 and 29).

In that case, brain, body, and environment can no longer be intrinsically linked and integrated; which, I postulate, makes their association with subjective experience and thus consciousness

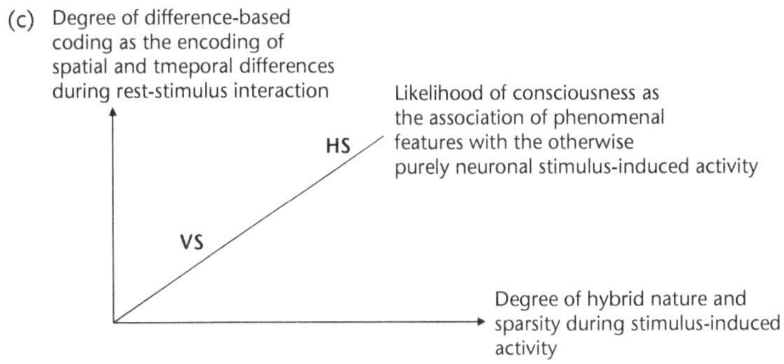

Figure 12-4c Sparse coding and GABA. (*c*) The figure illustrates the presumed dependence of the degree of consciousness on the relationship between the degree of difference-based coding during rest–stimulus interaction (y-axis) and the degree of hybrid nature and sparsity of stimulus-induced activity. The higher the degree of difference-based coding during rest–stimulus interaction, the higher the degree of hybridity and sparsity of stimulus-induced activity, and the higher the likelihood that a phenomenal state will be associated with the otherwise purely neuronal stimulus-induced activity. Abbreviations: VS = vegetative state, HS = healthy subjects.

impossible (see Chapters 28–32). Consciousness must therefore be characterized as intrinsically relational, relating brain, body, and environment in a yet-unclear though intrinsic way. Why is that so, and how does it work? For the answers to these questions, I ask the reader to turn his consciousness to Volume II.

Open Questions

I claim that GABA-ergic-mediated neural inhibition and nonlinearity are central in mediating the degree of sparse coding on a regional level of neural activity. However, there is currently (to my knowledge) no direct empirical support at this point for linking GABA-ergic-mediated neural inhibition and nonlinearity to the degree of sparse coding during rest–stimulus interaction on a regional level of neural activity. My hypothesis must therefore be regarded as tentative.

While there is much support for the hypothesis on the cellular and population level (see Chapter 2), empirical evidence is lacking almost completely on the regional level. Based on the findings described here and in Part I of this volume, one may suggest that the temporal and spatial sparsening of neural activity may be central in bridging the gap from the cellular over the population to the regional level of neural activity. This, however, is a hypothesis that remains to be explored.

Second, one may raise the question of the behavioral, psychological, and phenomenal effects of sparse coding. I focused here on the neuronal effects of sparse coding during different kinds of neural activity; that is, rest–rest and rest–stimulus interaction. But I neglected to explain how such sparse coding impacts behavioral, psychological, and phenomenal functions. One may, for instance, hypothesize that different degrees of sparse coding may go along with differences in the degree of consciousness, as will be discussed in further detail in Chapters 28 and 29.

I am even inclined to go one step further and argue that sparse coding may be central and thus indispensable for predisposing and making possible the constitution of consciousness. If there were no sparse coding, consciousness would remain impossible. This goes beyond the purely neuronal account of the brain as it was the focus of this Volume. I therefore delegate this and the question of its neural predisposition and correlates to Volume II, which concerns consciousness and also focuses on sparse coding (see Chapters 28 and 29).

EPILOGUE: A QUICK GUIDE TO A FUTURE "THEORY OF BRAIN ACTIVITY"

Unlocking the brain? This is the title of this book. I supposed that the brain's neural code, the way it encodes its neural activity, may unlock the brain. "Unlocking" means that the door opens and reveals something like another room that was not visible before. What does this new room look like, which the concept of difference-based coding as the brain's encoding strategy has opened for us?

I postulate that the "new room" puts the brain in the biological context of the rest of the body and the world. In the same way that each organ of the body, like the heart, kidney, or stomach, can be characterized by specific actions and mechanisms, the brain's encoding strategy may reveal its biological role. That is the focus in this short epilogue, which aims to provide a first tentative and rather sketchy outline of a quick guide to a future "theory of brain activity" (see Introduction for the distinction between "theory of brain activity" and "theory of brain function").

What does the brain do?

This question pertains to the kind of action the brain does. Let us first answer this question for other organs of the body, like the stomach, heart, and kidney. What do they do? The stomach segregates the different chemicals from our food by dissociating and extracting them. The heart pumps blood, while the kidneys filter (and detoxify and clean) the blood. These actions—segregating, dissociating, pumping, and filtering—characterize these organs.

What does the brain do? Which kind of action characterizes the brain? I postulate that the brain's action can be characterized by "spatializing" and "temporalizing." "Spatializing" and "temporalizing" describe that extrinsic stimuli and intrinsic activity changes are put into their respective spatial and temporal context.

In the same way that the blood is pumped by the heart and cleaned by the kidney, the extrinsic stimuli are spatialized and temporalized by the brain that is its neural code and intrinsic activity. Accordingly, the brain is a "spatializing" and "temporalizing" organ in very much the same way as the heart is a pumping organ, the kidney a filtering organ, and the stomach a segregating organ.

What do I mean by the terms "spatial context" and "temporal context"? The concept of the spatial context refers here to the co-occurrence of either the same or other stimuli in other neighboring points in space. By putting the single stimulus into its particular spatial context, the stimulus becomes linked and related to other stimuli across different their discrete points in physical space. Applied to all stimuli, this will yield a spatial matrix, grid, or structure that, as statistically based (see later), operates across and supersedes the distinct discrete points in physical space (see Chapter 4).

How about the "temporal context"? The concept of the temporal context describes the occurrence of either the same or other stimuli across different discrete points in physical time. Putting the single stimulus into its particular temporal context makes it possible for the stimulus to becomes linked and related to other stimuli across their different discrete points in physical time. This will ultimately result in the constitution of a temporal matrix, grid, or structure that, as statistically based (see later), operates across and supersedes the distinct discrete points in physical time (see Chapter 5).

Both spatializing and temporalizing result in the constitution of a virtual statistically-based spatial and temporal matrix. Such spatial and temporal matrices are based on the statistical frequency distribution and thus the statistics of the different stimuli, The resulting spatial and temporal matrices are thus statistically based rather than physically based as related to the physical features of the stimuli.

How can the brain construct such statistically based spatial and temporal matrices? I propose that functional connectivity between different regions and thus spaces of the brain is essential; that is, functional connectivity predisposes, or, more technically put, is a necessary and therefore unavoidable condition for, the possible constitution of such spatial matrix. On the temporal side, I hypothesize the brain's frequency fluctuations to be the predisposing or necessary condition for the possible constitution of its temporal counterpart, the temporal matrix.

Neither spatial nor temporal matrix is segregated and processed differently, however. Instead, they are integrated and intrinsically linked to each other. Frequency fluctuations, for example, are supposed to be dependent upon the functional connectivity and vice versa: the lower the frequency ranges of the neuronal fluctuations, the more spatially distant regions can be functionally connected with each other.

Conversely, functional connectivity between spatially closer regions may go along with higher frequency ranges of the neuronal fluctuations. Accordingly, the brain, and especially its intrinsic activity, construct a unified spatiotemporal matrix rather than parallel and separately operating spatial and temporal structures. One should thus better speak of "spatio-temporalizing" rather than "spatializing" and "temporalizing."

Where does the brain operate?

This is the question for the "location" of the brain's action and operation. Let us first answer this question for other organs of the body, like stomach, heart, and kidney.

Where do they operate? The stomach operates in the gastrointestinal tract, which it is part of. Since it supplies energy, though, it acts within the whole body. The same holds for the heart, which acts beyond its own boundaries across the whole body through its pumping of blood. Finally, the kidney also does not limit its action to its own confines but affects the whole body.

Where does the brain act and operate? First and foremost one would say that it acts in the skull where the brain is physically located. However, like the other organs, its actions are not limited to the boundaries of the skull but reach far beyond. This is, as I will argue, is closely related to its action of "spatiotemporalizing."

How does "spatiotemporalizing" relate to the brain's processing of stimuli from different origins as from environment and body? "Spatiotemporalizing" applies to all stimuli, irrespective of their origin. Stimuli originating from the environment, or exteroceptive; from the body, or interoceptive; and from the brain itself, or neuronal, do all become spatiotemporalized: independent of their different origins, they are all put into their respective spatial and temporal context when they are encoded and processed by the brain.

This means that the spatiotemporal matrix is not restricted to the space and time within the brain itself. Instead, it spans in a statistically based and therefore virtual way across the boundaries between brain, body, and environment and their respectively associated (physically based) spatial and temporal frameworks (see Chapters 4, 5, 8, and 9 in Volume I, as well as especially 20 and 21 in Volume II). In the same way, the actions of heart, stomach, and kidney show effects beyond the respective organ itself, in the whole body, the brain's "spatiotemporalizing" reaches even further beyond the skull and its own body to the environment.

Metaphorically, one may want to compare the statistically based spatiotemporal matrix to a hammock in a forest that hangs between different trees called brain, body, and environment. In the same way that a hammock can be abnormally tilted toward any one of these trees, the spatiotemporal matrix can also be abnormally shifted toward either brain, body, or environment.

For instance, psychiatric disorders like depression and schizophrenia show altered "spatializing" and "temporalizing" by the brain. This leads to an abnormal spatiotemporal matrix with abnormal shifts in the relationship between brain, body, and environment, which are manifested in rather bizarre behavioral and phenomenal abnormalities (see Chapters 17, 22, and 27).

Apart from its psychiatric relevance, we will see that the spatiotemporal matrix also provides the "hammock" for consciousness. Consciousness is about our experience of ourselves, others, and events in the environment. That is possible only when there is some kind of basic or prior linkage with the environment. This is provided by the spatiotemporal matrix that links brain, body, and environment in a statistically based way in the same way a hammock in a forest links different trees. Changes in the hammock go along with shifts in your position. Analogously, changes in the spatiotemporal matrix lead to changes and shifts in your consciousness.

How does the brain operate?

This is the question of what kinds of mechanisms enable the brain to perform the kinds of actions it does. Let us first answer this question for other organs of the body like stomach, heart, and kidney.

How do they operate? The stomach operates on the basis of enzymatic reactions to dissociate, segregate, and extract the different chemicals from our food. The heart relies on the mechanism of muscle contraction to pump blood, while the kidneys use an elaborate filter system to filter the blood. These mechanisms—enzymatic reactions, muscle contraction, and filtering system—characterize these organs since they allow them to do their specific action.

How does the brain operate? Which neuronal mechanisms characterize the brain *as* brain such that it allows the brain to do its specific action, the "spatializing" and "temporalizing"? I propose that the central neuronal mechanism here is the kind of coding strategy the brain applies to encode all extrinsic stimuli and intrinsic activity changes into neural activity.

The brain encodes all extrinsic stimuli and intrinsic activity changes in terms of spatial and temporal differences that span across the stimuli's different single discrete points in physical time and space. Rather than encoding the stimuli themselves as in stimulus-based coding, the brain therefore encodes differences between different stimuli into neural activity. This entails what I describe as difference-based coding (see Chapters 1–6).

The encoding of temporal and spatial differences makes possible the encoding of the stimuli's statistical frequency distribution: their statistics. Difference-based coding can thus be described as a statistically based encoding strategy. As such, it proves central for making possible the construction of the statistically based virtual spatiotemporal matrix between brain, body, and environment. This, in contrast, would be impossible in the case of stimulus-based coding.

What do I mean by the concept of "difference"? The concept of difference describes a purely formal metric or measure that applies to distinct levels, functions, and stimuli processed in the brain (see Introduction and Appendix 3 for a more refined conceptual description of the concepts of "difference" and "code"). Taken in this sense, the concept of "difference" remains independent of any concrete feature, content, or function associated with the stimuli that are to be encoded into neural activity.

Nothing is absolute, though, as we all know only too well. This pertains to difference-based coding, too. The brain and its neural processing seem to be characterized by a fine-tuned and flexible balance between the degrees of difference- and stimulus-based coding, with usually the degree of difference-based coding being much higher than the one of stimulus-based coding. I postulate that the brain's intrinsic activity and more specifically its level of resting state activity provides the threshold for the balance between difference- and stimulus-based coding.

That balance, however, as we will see in Volume II, can change in disorders of consciousness like the vegetative state, where the degree of stimulus-based coding increases at the expense of difference-based coding (see Chapter 29). This, as I postulate, may be related to abnormal changes in the resting state which no longer provides the proper threshold. Difference-based coding and its balance to stimulus-based may thus be not only neuronally relevant but also phenomenally; that is, for consciousness.

How does the brain operate? Based on my assumption of difference-based coding, I postulate that the currency or language of the brain consists of spatiotemporal differences between different stimuli rather than of single stimuli themselves and their discrete point in time and space. The brain's general encoding strategy, difference-based coding, is thus the neuronal mechanism that makes possible the brain's action, its spatializing and temporalizing of both extrinsic stimuli and intrinsic activity changes.

How does that stand in relation to the other organs? The stomach's enzymatic reactions, the heart's muscle contractions, and the kidney's filter system allow for their respective actions, that is, dissociation, pumping, and filtering. Analogously, I postulate that difference-based coding allows the brain to "perform" the action that defines the brain as brain; namely, "spatializing" and "temporalizing."

What predisposes the brain to operate in this way?

This is the question of the predisposition or basis that makes possible the brain's action and operation and thus its general encoding strategy by which it generates its own neural activity.

In the case of the heart, it is its nature as one big muscle and its supply of energy that as make it possible for the heart to contract and consequently to pump blood throughout the whole body. For the stomach, it is the presence of the various enzymes that allow the enzymatic reactions, which in turn make possible the extraction and segregation of the chemicals from our food. Finally, in the case of the kidney, its specific architectural design makes it possible for to filter and ultimately detoxify and clean the blood.

Where is the brain's ability of spatializing and temporalizing stimuli via difference-based coding derived from and what is it based on? I propose that the brain's architectonic and energetic design is a predisposing and thus necessary condition of possible spatializing and temporalizing. The brain's architectonic design consists of its anatomical structure that predisposes a particular encoding strategy; that is, difference-based coding.

Let us describe the brain's anatomical structure in both spatial and temporal terms. The brain's anatomical structure can be characterized by mutual and reciprocal structural connections between almost all regions, with the connections being either direct or indirect. Such a structural connectivity pattern predisposes the constitution of functional connectivity between close and distant regions (see Part III). This, in turn, makes possible the encoding of spatial relationships between the different regions' neural activities with the consequent constitution of a statistically based virtual spatial structure (see Chapter 4).

Temporally, the brain itself (its intrinsic activity) can be characterized by low-frequency fluctuations; these are supposed to be segregated and chopped up into higher frequency fluctuations by stimuli arriving at particular time points (see Chapter 5). As in the spatial domain, this leads a particular temporal organization of the neural activity and its constitution of a statistically based virtual temporal structure. Any stimulus, if "it wants to be processed in the brain," must encounter the brain's intrinsic activity and its spatiotemporal structure. This, as I claim, makes possible by default the aforementioned "spatializing" and "temporalizing" of the stimulus, which is thereby put into the spatial and temporal context of the brain itself and its intrinsic activity that is, its spatiotemporal matrix.

In addition to the brain's architectonic design and its spatial and temporal predispositions, we also need to consider the energetic design of the brain. The maintenance of the brain's resting-state activity and its spatiotemporal structure is energetically highly demanding, which resembles the situation in the heart, whose continuous pumping via muscle contractions also requires high levels of energy. To get a sufficient energy supply from the rest of the body, the brain developed a specific way of extracting energy from the blood, the neurometabolic coupling.

The brain's strategy of neurometabolic coupling is reflected in the glutamate-glutamine cycling and the subsequent utilization of glucose and other metabolic processes for generating its own neural activity. This makes it possible for the brain to extract a high level of energy, which in turn predisposes it to encode its own neural activity in terms of difference-based coding and the consecutive "spatializing" and "temporalizing." The brain must thus be considered a neurometabolic rather than purely neuronal device.

This is relevant not only energetically and neuronally but also phenomenally; that is, for consciousness. We will see in Volume II that disruption of the metabolic-energetic supply of the brain can lead to loss of consciousness, as in the vegetative state (see Chapters 28 and 29).

Where can we find the basis of the brain's action? I postulate that the basis can be found in the brain's architectonic design and its neurometabolic coupling. Both architectonic design and neurometabolic coupling predispose the brain to encode its neural activity in terms of difference-based coding. This in turn makes possible the action of the brain; namely, "spatializing" and "temporalizing." Accordingly, in the same way that the muscle structure of the heart and its energetic supply predispose the heart to contract and pump blood, the brain's architectonic and neurometabolic design predispose the brain to spatialize and temporalize both extrinsic stimuli and intrinsic activity.

What is the purpose of the brain's operation?

What is the purpose of the brain for the organism? This is easy to answer for the other organs of the body, while it remains elusive in the case of the brain. Let's start with the easy part, the other organs. The heart's purpose is to distribute oxygen throughout the whole body and its various organs, since otherwise the latter could not survive. The purpose of the stomach is to digest food by means of which the rest of the body is provided with resources for energy. Finally, the purpose of the kidney is to detoxify (and clean) blood, without which the rest of the body would be intoxicated.

What, however, is the brain and what purpose does it serve? As the philosopher John Searle (1992) noted, we currently lack a theory of brain function, meaning we do not yet know what the purpose of the brain is. I here postulated that the brain itself can be characterized by resting-state activity which shows continuous dynamic changes (see Part II). The brain requires a lot of energy to build and maintain its resting-state activity and to continuously change and adapt its spatiotemporal structure to the respective spatial and temporal contexts; namely, body and environment.

Why, though, does the body invest so much energy, 20 percent of its total energy budget, into the brain and its resting state activity? To address this question, we need to characterize the resting-state activity itself in further detail. As detailed in Part II, the brain's resting state activity constitutes a statistically based, virtual, spatiotemporal structure by means of spatial and temporal neuronal measures like functional connectivity and low frequency fluctuations.

This spatiotemporal structure of the brain's intrinsic activity serves as spatiotemporal matrix to process extrinsic stimuli from outside the brain, interoceptive stimuli from the body, and exteroceptive stimuli from the environment. By aligning the extrinsic intero- and/or exteroceptive stimuli to its own intrinsic spatial and temporal neuronal measures; that is, functional connectivity and low frequency fluctuations, the brain's spatiotemporal structure can extend beyond itself and reach out to body and environment. Accordingly, the brain's spatiotemporal matrix makes it possible to link and relate brain, body, and environment in a statistically based and virtual way (see Chapter 20 for more details on that).

Why is it important for the organism to develop such a statistically based spatiotemporal matrix on the basis of its brain? The importance is further underlined by the fact that the body invests 20 percent of its energy resources into an organ that makes up only 2 percent of the total body weight.

As discussed earlier and in full detail in Chapters 4–6, 8, and 9, the spatiotemporal structure is based on the encoding of the statistical frequency distributions of the different stimuli from body and environment: the stimuli's "vegetative, natural, and social statistics" are encoded in relation to the brain's intrinsic activity and its "neuronal statistics" (see Chapters 8 and 9).

What does such statistically based encoding imply for the organism? The brain encodes the stimuli's natural, vegetative, and social statistics in relation to its own neuronal statistics. This makes it possible for the organism to continuously update and adapt its own state in relation to the continuously changing spatial and temporal contexts in both its own body and its environment.

Why is such updating and adapting important for the organism? Such relating, updating, and adapting is important for the organism to sustain and maintain its homeostasis and ultimately to survive. Accordingly, the purpose of the brain may consist in homeostatic regulation of the organism in relation to the continuous changes in its own body and the respective environment. The heart provides the rest of the body with oxygen, the stomach extracts energy for the body, and the kidney cleans and detoxifies the blood and thus the body. This list can now be complemented. The brain relates, updates, and adapts the body to the environment and its continuously changing circumstances.

WHY DO WE HAVE A BRAIN OPERATING IN THIS WAY?

Taken on a most general level, the brain's purpose is the body's survival. The heart's pumping, the kidney's filtering, and the stomach's dissociating each serve the survival of the organism. Though serving distinct purposes and performing different actions, ultimately each organ serves the survival of the organism.

How does the brain's action serve the survival of the organism? The brain's spatializing and temporalizing and the subsequent construction of a statistically based virtual spatiotemporal structure are essential for the organism. Why? The particular encoding strategy, difference-based coding, allows the brain to relate, update, and adapt the organism to the continuously changing spatial and temporal contexts in body and environment.

Without the heart's pumping, the organism dies of heart failure; without the kidney's filtering, the organism dies of blood poisoning; and without the stomach's dissociation, the organism dies of hunger. The same applies in the case of the brain. Without the brain's spatializing and temporalizing during its encoding of neural activity, the organism dies from lacking a relationship to both its own body and its environment. This is exactly what can be observed in minimally conscious state (MCS), vegetative state (VS), coma, and brain death, which reflect greatly decreased if not absent degrees in the organism's relation to its body and environment (see Chapters 28 and 29).

Why is there a brain? The organism needs to detect those events in its body and environment are relevant for it and distinguish them from the ones that remain irrelevant. Only those that are relevant are worth subsequent updating and adapting. In the same way the heart distributes oxygen by pumping, the kidney detoxifies blood, and the stomach digests and extracts, the brain relates to and adapts/updates the organism about and to its actual environment. Since such encoding and therefore relating and adapting/updating are essential for the organism to survive, the brain may be essential for the organism to navigate in its environment.

How is our ability to navigate in the environment manifested in the functions we associate with the brain? This is the point where one would usually discuss the various sensory, motor, affective, cognitive, and social functions of the brain, as investigated these days in the different branches of neuroscience. One would then extend the here-sketched "theory of brain activity" to a "theory of brain function" (see the Introduction for their distinction).

That, however, is to neglect one even more basic function of the brain, one that is sandwiched right in-between the brain's encoding of neural activity on one hand, and the various contents and their related functions, sensory, motor, affective, cognitive, and social on the other.

What is this more basic function? I argue that this is the phenomenal (taken in both a literal and figurative way) function of the brain; that is, consciousness in the sense of phenomenal consciousness. This however extends the purely neuronal focus in this volume. Therefore I refer the reader to the subsequent Volume II. That, as I claim, will not only unlock the secrets of the brain but also the mystery of consciousness.

APPENDICES

I attach three appendices to the main parts of this book. These appendices are proposed to complement the empirical hypotheses by discussing some theoretical issues.

The first appendix discusses how resting-state activity and stimulus-induced activity are related to each other, whether they are principally different or rather reflect distinct points on a commonly underlying continuum of neuronal activity. As suggested by what I describe as the "continuity hypothesis," I opt for the latter.

The second appendix picks up the issue of localization versus holism of functions and their relationship to the brain. I argue that the introduction of the brain's resting-state activity sheds a new light on this long-discussed issue of localization versus holism by rendering both compatible and complementary rather than being incompatible and contradictory.

Finally, the third appendix discusses some epistemological issues: how we as observers can and cannot investigate the brain. More specifically, the question is raised regarding what the brain itself may allow us as observers of the brain to know in principle about it and how it operates. Even more important, by applying difference-based coding and its own intrinsic activity, the brain may also prevent us as observers from accessing and knowing the brain, as it is by itself independent of our brains, on which our own observation of the brain is based. Our brain and its specific encoding strategy, that is, difference-based coding, and its intrinsic activity may thus pose some basic experimental and epistemological constraints on our investigation and knowledge of the brain.

APPENDIX 1
NEUROEMPIRICAL REMARK: RESTING-STATE ACTIVITY VERSUS STIMULUS-INDUCED ACTIVITY—CONTINUITY HYPOTHESIS

Summary

I discussed the neuronal and biochemical mechanisms underlying the transition from resting-state to stimulus-induced activity in Part IV. This showed that the very same neuronal and biochemical mechanisms operating in the resting state are also at work during the transition from resting-state to stimulus-induced activity; that is, rest–stimulus interaction. This leads me on a theoretical level to describe what I call the "continuity hypothesis." The continuity hypothesis is a hypothesis about the relationship between resting-state and stimulus-induced activity. I postulate neuronal continuity between resting state and stimulus-induced activity, with both being continuous and discontinuous in their neural activities at the same time. The co-occurrence of both neuronal continuum and discontinuum between resting-state and stimulus-induced activity is supposed to be made possible by difference-based coding, which in turn is regarded as essential for enabling and predisposing consciousness. The "continuity hypothesis" bridges the often-presupposed divide between intrinsic and extrinsic characterizations of the brain as put forward in the Introduction: both views are no longer considered opposite and contradictory, but rather, two extremes of an underlying continuum of neural activity amounting to an intrinsic-extrinsic view of the brain.

Key Concepts and Topics Covered

Resting-state activity, stimulus-induced activity, neuronal continuum and discontinuum, difference-based versus stimulus-based coding, degree versus origin, neural predisposition versus neural correlate, consciousness

Neuroempirical Remark IA: Difference-Based Coding as Unifying Code Between Resting State and Stimulus-Induced Activity

The brain is often considered an either purely extrinsic or intrinsic organ (see also Introduction). In the case of an extrinsic characterization, the brain is supposed to be characterized by stimulus-induced activity as it is related exclusively to the stimulus itself. In contrast, an intrinsic view proposes intrinsic activity in the brain, that is, resting-state activity, with its function remaining unclear.

How do intrinsic and extrinsic views of the brain stand in relation to each other? Are they mutually exclusive and thus incompatible? Or, rather, are they compatible and complementary? This is the topic here, and it will be discussed in the framework of what I describe as the "continuity hypothesis." The "continuity" hypothesis implies complementarity and compatibility between resting-state activity and stimulus-induced activity rather than incompatibility and opposition.

Let me now sketch the "continuity hypothesis" in more detail. I argued that stimuli of different origins, intero- and exteroceptive and neural, are encoded into neural activity in the same way; namely, in terms of spatial and temporal differences. This implies that both resting-state activity (see Chapters 4–6) and stimulus-induced activity (see Chapters 10–12) are based on difference-based coding rather than stimulus-based coding.

That also entails that the various interactions between different stimuli, that is, stimulus-stimulus interaction (see Chapter 10); between stimuli and resting state, that is rest–stimulus interaction (see Chapter 11); and the interactions within the resting state itself, that is, rest–rest interaction (see Chapter 4 and 5), were encoded in terms of one and the same code; namely, difference-based coding.

What does this tell us about the role of difference-based coding in the brain? I postulate difference-based coding to be the general coding strategy of the brain's neural activity during its different kinds of interactions: that is, rest–rest, rest–stimulus, stimulus–stimulus, and stimulus–rest. Since all neural activity is supposed to arise from these interactions, difference-based coding must be considered *the* neural code of the brain.

This means that rest–rest, rest–stimulus, stimulus–stimulus, and stimulus–rest interactions are linked and united by one coding strategy—difference-based coding. I thus propose that the application of that code to both resting-state and stimulus-induced activity makes their direct interaction possible.

Neuroempirical remark Ib: "Continuity hypothesis" about the neuronal relationship between resting state and stimulus-induced activity

How can we further specify the relationship between the brain's resting-state activity and its stimulus-induced activity? Due to the fact that resting-state and stimulus-induced activity operate on the basis of one and the same neural code, there must be neuronal continuity between them: that is, between and across rest–rest, rest–stimulus, stimulus–stimulus, and stimulus–rest interaction.

Empirically, such assumption is, for example, supported by the observations showing the resting state's strong low-frequency fluctuations and functional connectivity to be carried forth into stimulus-induced activity via rest–stimulus interaction (see Chapters 4, 5, and 11). Conversely, the data also show that the stimulus-induced activity resurfaces in the neural pattern of the subsequent resting-state activity, which is supported by the data on stimulus–rest interaction (see Chapter 11).

I consequently postulate what I describe as a "continuity hypothesis" between resting-state activity and stimulus-induced activity. The continuity hypothesis describes that neuronal activity is continuously carried back and forth between resting-state and stimulus-induced activity (via rest–stimulus and stimulus–rest interaction), resulting in neuronal continuity between both forms of neural activity.

The "continuity hypothesis" is a purely neuronal hypothesis that pertains to the neuronal features and characterization of resting state and stimulus-induced activity. In contrast to the neuronal states of the brain during resting state and stimulus-induced activity, the "continuity hypothesis" does not make any assumptions about the behavioral, psychological, and phenomenal states that are associated with the resting state and stimulus-induced activity. Hence, the neuronal continuity between resting state and stimulus-induced activity does not imply behavioral, psychological, or even phenomenal continuity.

This, however, does not mean that the continuity hypothesis does not carry important implications for behavioral, psychological, and phenomenal states. We will see in Volume II that the neuronal continuity between resting state and stimulus-induced activity is essential in making possible the association of a phenomenal state—consciousness—with the otherwise purely neuronal resting state or stimulus-induced activity (see especially Chapter 30).

Neuroempirical remark Ic: Neuronal continuity between resting state and stimulus-induced activity

The "continuity hypothesis" must be further specified by two aspects, "neuronal continuum" and "neuronal discontinuum." "Neuronal continuum" describes that neural activity in resting state and stimulus-induced activity show similar features, accounting for a neuronal continuum between them. The concept of "neuronal discontinuum" refers to the differences between resting-state and stimulus-induced activity operating across and thus superseding their underlying neuronal continuum.

How can we now describe both neuronal continuum and neuronal discontinuum in further detail? Let me start with the neuronal continuum. The attentive reader may have noticed that I focused on the same kind of neuronal measures when discussing resting-state activity (Part II) and stimulus-induced activity (Part IV). In both cases, I described spatial and temporal measures of neural activity; more specifically, functional connectivity and low- and high-frequency fluctuations.

Functional connectivity and frequency fluctuations are central in constituting both resting-state and stimulus-induced activity; furthermore, they mediate their direct interaction, that is, rest–stimulus and stimulus–rest, via the principles of spatial and temporal coincidence. As such, functional connectivity and frequency fluctuations signify a neuronal continuum between both forms of neural activity.

However, the neuronal continuum went further. Due to the reliance on the same spatial and temporal measures, that is, frequency fluctuations and functional connectivity, both resting-state and stimulus-induced activity are supposed to be linked by a shared and common spatiotemporal structure (see Chapters 4 and 5). Such a spatiotemporal structure operates across and supersedes the purely biophysical-computational features of the brain's space and time in that it is statistically based rather than being exclusively determined by the biophysical-computational features of the brain's neurons (and regions; see Chapters 1, 2, 6, and 11 for details).

The statistically based spatiotemporal structure of the brain's resting state is carried forth to stimulus-induced activity (via rest–stimulus interaction), which in turn impacts the subsequent resting-state activity (via stimulus–rest interaction; see Chapter 11). Such circular movement between resting-state activity and stimulus-induced activity allows for maintaining (and continuously rejuvenating and updating) the brain's intrinsic spatiotemporal structure. One may consequently characterize the brain's intrinsic spatiotemporal structure as the common final functional pathway of both resting-state and stimulus-induced activity. As such, the spatiotemporal structure can provide a neuronal continuum between the two forms of neural activity (see Fig. A1-1a).

Neuroempirical Remark Id: Neuronal Discontinuity Between Resting State and Stimulus-Induced Activity

So far, I have focused on the similarities and thus the neuronal continuum between resting-state and stimulus-induced activity. This, however, should not incline us to brush over their considerable differences accounting for a neuronal discontinuum between the two forms of neural activity. This neuronal discontinuum shall now be further specified. We recall from Chapter 11 that rest–stimulus (and also stimulus–rest) interactions were characterized by non-linearity; non-linearity describes that the resulting stimulus-induced activity does not result from mere linear addition or superposition of both forms of neural activity. The resulting stimulus-induced activity is consequently different both spatially and temporally from the preceding resting-state activity. Hence, there is a neuronal discontinuum on the neuronal level between both forms of neural activity.

The neuronal discontinuum is also visible in the principle of inverse effectiveness (see chapters 10 and 11). In a nutshell, the principle of inverse effectiveness describes that a lower resting-state activity level may lead to stronger rest–stimulus interaction in the presence of a strong stimulus, compared to higher resting-state activity level in the presence of the same stimulus. While empirical support for this principle is mostly pending, it clearly signifies a neuronal discontinuum. A lower resting-state activity turns into a stronger stimulus-induced activity, thus making the latter more discontinuous from the former. In contrast, there is a lower degree of the neuronal discontinuum when the resting-state activity is higher.

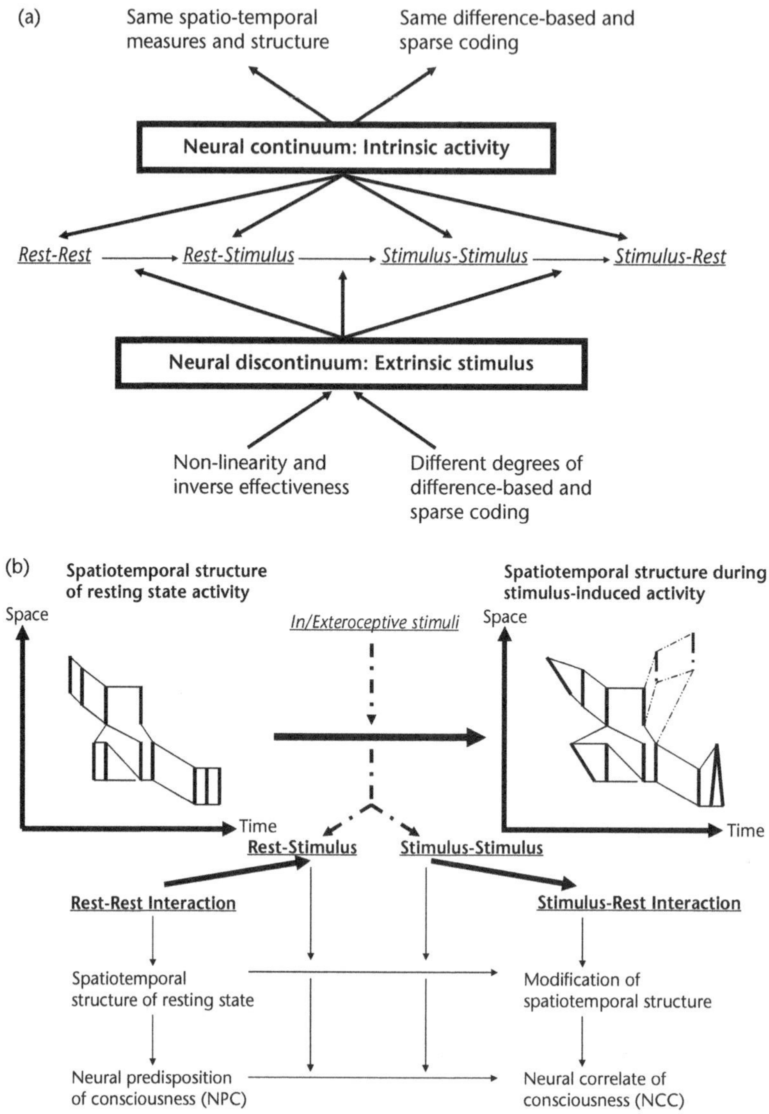

Figure A1-1 **"Continuity hypothesis" between resting state and stimulus-induced activity.**
The figure depicts two central aspects of the continuity hypothesis, the conjunction of both neural continuum and neural discontinuum (a), and the central role of the resting state and its spatiotemporal structure as neural predisposition (b).
(*a*) The figure shows the neural continuum (upper part) and discontinuum (lower part) between resting-state activity and stimulus-induced activity. Both resting-state activity and stimulus-induced activity are based on the same spatiotemporal measures (like functional connectivity and low-frequency fluctuations) and apply the same neural code, difference-based coding and sparse coding (upper part). At the same time, though, there is also neural discontinuum (lower part) between resting-state activity and stimulus-induced activity in that there is non-linearity, inverse effectiveness, and variation in the degrees of difference-based coding and sparse coding.
(*b*) The figure depicts how the stimulus modifies the resting state's spatiotemporal structure, as indicated in the upper part of the figure. However, the degree of modification the stimulus can possibly elicit is predisposed by the resting state itself and its spatiotemporal structure. This means that the resting state provides a neural predisposition, a "spatiotemporal window of opportunity," for the possible degree of subsequent stimulus-induced activity (lower part of the figure).

How can gather further support for the neuronal discontinuum between resting state and stimulus-induced activity? I also demonstrated that the degree of both difference-based coding and sparse coding changes during the encounter with the stimulus. Rest–stimulus interaction may go along with a shift in the balance between difference- and stimulus-based coding toward difference-based coding. There is thus a neuronal discontinuum with regard to the degrees of difference-based coding.

The same holds for the formatting. As tentatively suggested, the degree of sparse coding may increase during stimulus-induced activity when compared to resting-state activity, thereby leading to a neuronal discontinuum on a formatting level (see Chapter 12). Finally, the neuronal discontinuum also extends to the biochemical level, with GABA and glutamate showing different degrees of difference in the excitation-inhibition balance during resting state and stimulus-induced activity (see Chapters 2, 6, and 12).

Neuroempirical remark IIa: continuum of neuronal measures

How are the neuronal continuum and neuronal discontinuum related to each other? I postulate that the neuronal continuum provides the very basis upon which the neuronal discontinuum operates. More specifically, the degrees of the resting state's functional connectivity and high-low frequency fluctuations are varied during subsequent stimulus-induced activity (see Chapter 11).

The same holds for the changes in the degrees of difference-based coding and sparse coding as well as for the degrees of the spatiotemporal structure. As detailed in Chapters 11 and 12, the stimulus may introduce a novel degree of discontinuity into these neuronal measures of the brain's resting-state activity: by varying the resting state's diverse spatial and temporal neuronal measures in their degree, the stimulus introduces a much higher degree of discontinuity compared to the dynamic changes in the resting-state activity itself.

This means that the neuronal discontinuum and thus the neuronal difference between resting-state activity and stimulus-induced activity is a matter of degree. This implies that there is no principal difference between resting-state activity and stimulus-induced activity. Instead of being principally (and qualitatively) different, the stimuli and their associated stimulus-induced activity operate across and supersede resting-state activity and modulate it quantitatively; the stimulus "uses" the resting state's diverse neuronal measures as a starting point to modulate and vary them in their degrees.

Accordingly, the neuronal measures themselves, like functional connectivity and low frequency fluctuations, thus provide the neuronal continuum between resting state and stimulus-induced activity, while their degree signifies neuronal discontinuity. Put differently, stimulus-induced activity can be regarded a discontinuous neuronal extension of the brain's resting-state activity.

This suggests that resting-state and stimulus-induced activity differ only in degree, not in principle. I therefore suggest that the distinction between resting-state and stimulus-induced activity is a matter of degree rather than a matter of principle.

Neuroempirical remark IIb: "matter of degree" versus "matter of principle"

Based on the neuronal continuity, one would suggest that the same kind of neuronal effects that can be observed during stimulus-induced activity should also in principle be possible during resting-state activity; this should be the case in those instances when rest–rest interaction exhibits the same degrees—that is, differences in the diverse measures—that are usually rather associated with rest–stimulus interaction. Let me specify this further in the following.

I demonstrated rest–stimulus interaction during visual or auditory perception to go along with strong activity changes in visual or auditory cortex (see Chapter 11). If the resting state itself, that is, rest–rest interaction, now shows equally strong activity changes in, for instance, auditory cortex, one would expect analogous behavioral and phenomenal states to occur.

This is indeed supported by empirical evidence. For instance, auditory hallucinations in schizophrenia can be characterized by abnormally strong and large rest–rest interaction in auditory cortex, which is then associated with the same phenomenal-perceptual state, the perception of voices, as the same degree of change induced by an external stimulus, a real voice. (see Chapter 22 for details, as well as Northoff and Qin 2011; and Northoff 2011).

Another instance may be dreams. We perceive an external world in our dreams despite the fact that we sleep. And, as in the awake state, we experience emotions and a sense of self. One may consequently propose that the rest–rest interactions in the dreaming state show as strong degrees as the ones during rest–stimulus interaction in the awake state; the rest–rest interaction, then, no longer functions as mere rest–rest interaction but rather as "rest-as-if stimulus interaction" (see Chapter 25 and especially Chapter 26 for details, as well as Northoff 2011). This reaches deeply into the realm of consciousness and is therefore delegated to Volume II (see Part VII in Volume II).

These and various other examples (see Chapters 25 and 26 in Volume II for more details) support my assumption of resting-state and stimulus-induced activity not being principally different. If they were principally different, neither of the behavioral and phenomenal states associated with stimulus-induced activity could possibly be elicited in the resting state itself; that is, during rest–rest interaction. If so, the neuronal difference between resting-state activity and stimulus-induced activity cannot be a principal difference: it is not a "matter of principle" but rather a "matter of degree."

Neuroempirical Remark IIc: "Priority of Degree and Difference" versus "Priority of Origin and Stimulus"

How can we further specify the concept of "matter of degree"? The concept of "matter of degree" describes mere statistical differences, for example, the statistical frequency distribution of neural activity changes across different discrete points in physical time and space. Stronger activity changes are usually associated with rest–stimulus interaction as the interaction between the stimuli's natural statistics and the resting state's neuronal statistics, whereas weaker activity changes occur normally during rest–rest interaction and thus within the resting state's neuronal statistics itself. Accordingly, resting state and stimulus-induced activity are distinguished on the basis of mere statistical differences signifying a "matter of degree" between the resting state's neuronal statistics and the stimuli's natural statistics.

Reliance on mere statistical differences implies that the origin of the stimuli, intero- or exteroceptive or neural, is secondary in determining the associated neuronal, behavioral, and phenomenal states. Any stimulus of whatever origin, whether interoceptive, exteroceptive, or neuronal, can in principle induce and elicit the kind of strong neural activity changes that are usually associated with exteroceptive stimuli. This is so because the resulting neural activity is not primarily based on the origin of the stimulus (see Chapter 12 herein and especially Chapter 25 in Volume II for more details on this point).

Instead, neural activity is based on the degree of the statistically based spatial and temporal differences the stimulus introduces (relative) to the brain's ongoing resting-state activity. If the difference is large, indicating strong rest–stimulus interaction, large neural activity changes will be elicited and accompanied by strong behavioral and phenomenal effects. If, in contrast, the difference is rather small, indicating weak rest–stimulus interaction, the stimulus' effects will be small, too.

Since neural activity is encoded and determined on the basis of statistically based spatial and temporal differences, any stimulus of whatever origin can in principle elicit any kind of stimulus-induced activity, including its associated behavioral and phenomenal (and psychological and mental) effects.

One may consequently speak of "priority of degree" as a "priority of differences" to characterize the relationship between resting-state and stimulus-induced activity. In contrast to the degree of difference, the origin of the stimulus remains secondary: the origin of the stimulus only matters if it leads to statistically based spatial and temporal differences, whereas the origin itself, independent of associated statistical differences, does not matter for determining the degree of neural activity. There is thus no "priority of origin" as a "priority of stimuli" in the brain's resting-state and stimulus-induced activity. There is "priority of difference and degree" rather than "priority of stimulus and origin" in rest–stimulus interaction.

Neuroempirical Remark IId: Resting-State Activity as Neural Predisposition of Stimulus-Induced Activity

I demonstrated that stimulus-induced activity is dependent upon the resting-state activity, as is well reflected in the assumption of a neuronal continuum. However, the neuronal continuum goes hand in hand with a neuronal discontinuum. This means that the resting-state activity is not sufficient but only necessary for stimulus-induced activity.

The resting-state activity is therefore what I describe as the "neural predisposition" for subsequent stimulus-induced activity. Within the present context, the term "neural predisposition" refers to the necessary but not sufficient neuronal conditions of stimulus-induced activity (see Introduction in Volume II for further discussion of the concept of "neural predisposition," as well as Northoff 2013).

As a neural predisposition, the resting-state activity determines the possible and thus available ranges of the degree of subsequent stimulus-induced activity. This was, for instance, indicated in that the resting-state activity sets the ranges for the possible degrees of difference-based coding during subsequent stimulus-induced activity (see Chapter 11). By showing, for instance, strong degrees of functional connectivity in the resting state, the ability of the subsequent stimulus to further increase the degree of functional connectivity is limited, whereas the opposite is the case if the resting state's functional connectivity is rather weak. The resting state thus predisposes the range of possible options that the subsequent stimulus-induced activity can possibly take (see Fig. A1-1b).

Neurometaphorical Excursion Ia: Brain and Supermarket

Let us illustrate the relationship between resting state and stimulus-induced activity by the analogous and metaphorical example of shopping in a supermarket. The supermarket displays various products. What you actually buy depends very much on your own budget and your mood and how that meshes with the products displayed. If you have plenty of money, you may go to the more expensive products. If your mood is gloomy, you may avoid the colorful and shiny products; and so forth. What you actually buy can thus be traced back to what one may want to call "supermarket–customer interaction." Needless to say, that corresponds very well to what I described as rest–stimulus interaction in the brain.

Now, let us assume that the supermarket happens to be in a neighborhood that recently changed considerably, with many rich people moving in. Naturally, these people look for more high-quality high-priced products. The supermarket's previous strategy of offering more low-quality and low-priced products may need to change, considering the neighborhood's influx of rich people. Hence, the supermarket may shift its focus and adapt its products to the new clients by displaying more high-quality and high-priced products. There is thus what can be described as "customer–supermarket interaction." Needless to say, this corresponds well to stimulus–rest interaction in the case of the brain.

Where, though, does the resting state's neural predisposition find its analogue in our example of the supermarket? The supermarket is characterized by certain spatial and temporal features; its building is rather small, and everything is extremely tight. These are the constraints within which the shift in focus, from low-quality to high-quality products, can take place. Beyond that, nothing is possible.

This means that, due to the smallness of its boards, shelves, and display tables in the overall extremely tight space, big high-priced products cannot be displayed, meaning that customers interested in these will not find anything in the supermarket. The supermarket's spatial and temporal structure (its shelves, boards, and tables) thus provides the ground upon which the products can be selected and the customers that can possibly be attracted. In other words, the supermarket's spatial and temporal features provide the predisposition for the range of possible options for subsequent products and customers.

Neurometaphorical excursion Ib: supermarkets and consciousness

Needless to say, the supermarket's spatiotemporal predisposition for certain types of products and customers corresponds to the resting state's spatiotemporal structure, as it predisposes the resting state to process (weaker or stronger) particular stimuli. As the supermarket's spatiotemporal structure allows for certain opportunities and prevents others by means of its spatiotemporal features, so does the brain's resting state and its spatiotemporal structure provide what I described as "spatiotemporal window of opportunity" (see Chapter 11).

The resting state's "spatiotemporal window of opportunity" can thus be characterized as a neural predisposition; that is, a necessary but not sufficient condition, of possible stimulus-induced activity. In addition to its central importance for subsequent stimulus-induced activity, I propose that the resting state's "spatiotemporal window of opportunity" also provides the neural predisposition for the behavioral and phenomenal states associated with the stimulus-induced activity.

More specifically, this means that I consider the resting state and its spatiotemporal structure to be a neural predisposition of possible consciousness (NPC) (which as such must be distinguished from what is currently discussed as neural correlates of consciousness [NCC]). This reaches deeply into the realm of consciousness and will therefore be delegated to Volume II.

How does the brain's predisposition for consciousness relate to our example of the supermarket? This is the point where my analogy finally breaks down, with brain and supermarket parting from each other. In contrast to the brain, supermarkets will never be able to provide a predisposition for consciousness. Accordingly, to put it succinctly, brain is not supermarket and supermarket is not brain. Aren't we lucky that we are owners of a brain that allows us to create supermarkets (on the basis of our consciousness) rather than being owners of a supermarket that (can only) create(s) brains (without consciousness)?

APPENDIX 2 NEUROTHEORETICAL REMARK: LOCALIZATIONISM VERSUS HOLISM

Summary

The assumption of sparse coding holding on the regional level of the brain raises the question of how functions and regions are related to each other. Historically, a one-to-one relationship between function and region has often been assumed, amounting to what is called "localizationism." Alternatively, others have suggested that more than one region or network is recruited during one particular function, and that different functions may recruit the same or at least overlapping regions and network—this has been subsumed under the concept of "holism." I here hypothesize that localizationism and holism are not contradictory but rather complementary. Holism concerns the process level that can be characterized by difference-based coding, while localizationism refers to the outcome or result of the neural processing in terms of differences as described by sparse coding. Since they concern distinct aspects, processes, and the outcome of those processes, holism and localizationism must be regarded as complementary rather than contradictory.

Key Concepts and Topics Covered

Localization, holism, history of neuroscience, overlap of different functions in the same regions/neural networks, sparse coding, difference-based coding, process and outcome, complementarity

Neurohistorical remark Ia: "Localizationism" in past and present neuroscience

One of the main methodological approaches in neuroscience at the beginning of the twentieth century was the investigation of patients with brain lesions. These patients could reveal how their higher-order cognitive functions like consciousness, memory, attention, learning, and so on, were affected by lesions in particular regions.

This was the way that early neurologist Paul Broca found out about a specific region in the brain being in charge of comprehending language—the Broca region. He observed that patients with a lesion in the left lateral prefrontal cortex showed major deficits in uttering words and language, a so-called *aphasia*. From his clinical observations Broca inferred that this region must be in charge of producing words, thus localizing language in the Broca area, as it is called these days.

Observation of patients with lesions and their corresponding mental disturbances has since been a major tool of insight into the function of the brain. From the exact localization of the lesion and the corresponding mental disturbances, one may infer which region in the brain mediates the respectively underlying higher-order cognitive function. Many other higher-order cognitive functions, including consciousness and self, are currently investigated in this way in neurological patients who suffer from specifically localized lesions in the brain (see, for instance, Feinberg

2009; as well as Feinberg and Keenan 2005). This entails what I describe as a "localization-based approach" to the brain.

The concept of the "localization-based approach" can be defined in two ways. First, it implies the neuropsychological assumption that a particular function can be related to the neural activity in a specific brain region, meaning that the former can be localized precisely in the latter. This is a neuronal (or better, neuropsychological) meaning of the concept of "localization-based approach" that pertains to a hypothesis about how the brain's regions are related to psychological functions.

In addition to such neuropsychological meaning, the concept of the "localization-based approach" can also refer to an investigator's particular methodological strategy for approaching the brain. The brain here is approached in terms of regions rather than in terms of, say, processes or codes (see Introduction for such code-based approach to the brain). The methodological approach to the brain in terms of regions is not restricted to the investigation of patients with local brain lesions. It may also extend to the healthy subjects, such as, for instance, those investigated in functional magnetic resonance imaging (fMRI). The use of techniques like fMRI is indeed guided by the search for the localization of particular functions in specific regions of the brain, which it therefore approaches in terms of regions (as distinguished from processes or codes).

Finally, the search for localization of higher-order cognitive functions in patients with brain lesions and functional brain imaging converges with the assumption of modules in cognitive psychology. Cognitive psychology proposed specific functional unities that are in charge of processing and operating such specific cognitive content as attentional content, working memory content, conscious content, self-specific content, and so on. When cognitive psychology entered neuroscience and they were amalgamated into "cognitive neuroscience," the concept of modules was combined with the concept of localization in the brain (see van Eijsden et al. 2009 for a nice description).

What were described as "modules" in cognitive psychology could then be easily transferred to the brain and more specifically to particular brain regions and their connections. Hence, the localization-based view of brain function seems to be intimately coupled with the module-based view of psychological functioning. This resulted in the assumption of the localization of specific cognitive modules in particular regions (or networks of regions) in the brain.

This is still the implicit or explicit presupposition in current neuroscience and especially in cognitive neuroscience (see, for instance, Logothetis 2008), which is often extended to the more recent branches of affective and social neuroscience: "I take the modular organization of many brain systems as a well-established fact, and discuss only how far fMRI can go in revealing the neuronal mechanisms of behavior by mapping different systems modules and their dynamic interrelationships" (Logothetis 2008).

Neurohistorical remark Ib: Holism in past and present neuroscience

However, nothing in the science of the brain goes without the opposite suggestion. A strictly localization-based approach was put into doubt early on by another neurologist, Hughlin Jackson, who suggested a more complex and systematic neural organization with multiple interdependencies between different regions. This paved the way for a more holistic view of brain function, one that relates higher-order cognitive functions to the neural operations in the whole brain and its multiple regions.

Interestingly, Sigmund Freud, the founder of psychoanalysis, who initially was a neuroanatomist, also rejected a localization-based approach to the brain. His reason was that more complex psychological disorders like hysteria or depression could not be confined to alterations in specific brain regions. He instead regarded these disorders as more complex systems disorders where the organization of the "psychic apparatus," as he called it, is abnormal, which is manifested throughout the whole brain and its different regions. One may therefore consider Freud a forerunner of a more holistic view of brain function (see Northoff 2011 and 2012 for details).

Later, neuroscientist Karl Lashley (1943, 1950) observed in his postmortem dissections that the extent of a brain lesion predicts the degree to which higher-order cognitive functions and mental states are disturbed. This let him develop what he called the "Law of Equipotentiality" and the "Law of Mass Action."

Both laws describe the distribution of neural processing across the whole brain during higher-order cognitive functions like consciousness and memory. Different regions were proposed to contribute equally to the generation of complex functions that therefore must be considered the result of "mass action" in the brain. This means that higher-order cognitive functions like memory and consciousness were assumed to result from the neural processing throughout the whole brain, rather than being localized in particular regions or modules within the brain (see also other authors like Koehler and Goldstein as cited in the Introduction).

Analogous observations were made by Russian neuropsychologist A. R. Lurija (1962, 973).

Based on his lesion patients, he suggested that one region in the brain can be involved in various higher-order cognitive functions. Conversely, he postulated that higher-order cognitive functions are mediated not only by one or two regions but by various regions in the brain. Most important, the same higher-order cognitive function may even recruit different regions in different instances, depending on the respective psychological and neuronal contexts. There is thus what Lurija described as "dynamic localization."

This led Lurija to formulate his hypothesis of functional systems as the operating systems of the brain that describe the actual constellation of different regions that mediate a particular function:

> According to this view a function is, in fact, a functional system (...) directed towards the performance of a particular biological task and consisted of a group of interconnected acts that produce the corresponding biological effect. The most significant feature of a functional system is that, as a rule, it is based on a complex dynamic "constellation" of connections, situated at different levels of the nervous system, that in the performance of the adaptive task, may be changed with the task itself may be unchanged. (Lurija 1962)

How about holism in the neuroscience of our days? The earlier-described metabolic approach to the brain by Shulman (van Eijsden et al. 2009) presupposes a more holistic approach to the brain (see Chapter 6). By considering the global metabolic-energetic supply and distribution to the brain as a whole as central for any subsequent neural activity, a holistic, and thus global, component is introduced.

Such a more-holistic view is also promoted in parts of functional brain imaging that focus much more on neural networks spanning across different regions rather than on single regions. This is especially apparent in the functional brain imaging of the resting-state activity (see Chapter 4 for details). However, as we will see further down, even the characterization of the brain by different networks may still presuppose too localizationism.

Finally, the holistic view of the brain also surfaces in the debate about consciousness. As we will see in Volume II, a global workspace of neural activity and information spread is often considered central in constituting consciousness; since such a global workspace allows for global extension and distribution, it implies the involvement of different regions and networks throughout the whole brain (see Introduction and Chapters 18 and 19 in Volume II for details).

Neurohistorical remark Ic: Problems of localizationism in present neuroscience

What is the standing of such a holistic view of brain function these days? The introduction of functional brain imaging has shifted the pendulum back again toward the localization-based view with the assignment of specific regions or networks to particular functions like attention, working memory, and so on (see van Eijsden et al. 2009 for a nice description).

In addition to the various regions and neural networks supposedly serving specific psychological functions, a network particularly involved in mediating resting-state activity, the default-mode network (DMN), has been distinguished in regional and connectional terms. The DMN seems often (though implicitly) to be regarded as the module for the resting state that therefore stands side by side with other networks that function as modules for specific functions such as, for instance, executive functions or salience (see, for instance, Menon 2011).

However, recent imaging studies shed some doubt on the proclaimed localization of specific psychological functions in particular regions or neural networks. The various regions of the DMN, like the anterior and posterior cingulate cortex and the medial prefrontal and parietal cortex, are supposed to serve psychological and mental activity, specifically in the resting state (see especially Chapter 26 for details on that). The same regions are also recruited during a variety of psychological tasks or functions, including contextual association, navigation and spatial processing, episodic memory, decision making, execution errors, self-related processing, mind-reading, emotional processing, and social interaction (see Bar et al. 2007, 2009; Spreng et al. 2009).

This sheds some doubt on the regional or network specificity of the DMN; more specifically, on its specific association with particular psychological functions during either resting-state activity or stimulus-induced activity. Conversely, these observations also argue against region-specific (or network-specific) localization of the various functions themselves, which seem to recruit more or less the same regions and networks.

This situation with the recruitment of the same regions and network by different functions is not peculiar to the DMN. The same pattern can be observed in the case of another neural network that includes the bilateral anterior insula, the dorsal anterior cingulate cortex, and the thalamus as its core regions (these regions are also subsumed under what is described as the "salience network"; see Menon 2011). These regions are active during functions as diverse as interoceptive awareness (Critchley et al. 2004; Wiebking et al. 2010), empathy (Yan et al. 2011), anticipation of emotions (Bermpohl et al. 2006), and aversion (see Hayes and Northoff 2011). The list of regions that are recruited by different functions can easily be extended.

In sum, the observation of the same region and network mediating a variety of different functions sheds some doubt upon the localization-based approach and its attempts to establish a specific one-to-one relationship between regions/networks and functions.

Does this mean that we have to revert to a more holistic view of the brain and its different regions? Based on their data, some neuroscientists—doing either lesion-based studies (Feinberg 2009) or functional imaging using electroencephalography (EEG; John 2006), positron emission tomography (PET; van Eijnsden et al. 2009), or functional magnetic resonance imaging (fMRI; Northoff 2008)—do indeed advocate a more holistic view of brain function. This is further corroborated by neuroanatomy, which considers single regions as hubs or nodes within the neural network of the whole brain rather than as centers or modules by themselves (see Hagmann et al. 2008, Sporns 2011).

Where does this leave us? Do we have to follow the swings between localizationism and holism? My aim in the following discussion is to show how both are very compatible and complementary, rather than being contradictory.

NEUROTHEORETICAL REMARK IA: LOCALIZATION AND SPARSE CODING

While the association of a specific region or network with a specific psychological function must be considered doubtful, the data nevertheless show that only a certain set of regions is recruited during the various tasks or functions. Multiple functions seem to recruit the same set of regions or network entailing a many/multiple-to-one/few relationship between functions and regions. The function–region relationship thus seems to obey the rules of sparseness, with sparse representation of the multiple functions in a few regions/networks of the brain. I consequently hypothesize sparse coding rather than localization to operate and determine the function–region relationship.

The assumption of sparse coding is empirically supported by the data we discussed in

Chapter 3 and especially Chapter 6, which show the spatiotemporal activity pattern during resting-state and stimulus-induced activity to be rather sparse. While these purely neuronal data did not directly address the more neuropsychological relationship between region and function, they nevertheless provide some indirect support for a sparse encoding of functions into the different regions' and networks' neural activities.

More specifically, I propose that what is considered localization of a particular function in a specific region reflects the sparse number of actually activated regions when compared to the total number of regions that could possibly be recruited. The fact that the other regions are not activated does not mean, however, that they do not participate in generating the function in question.

The inactive regions may nevertheless have an important role in that their baseline—that is, resting-state activity—may serve to generate and amplify neural differences (presupposing difference-based coding on a regional level; see Chapter 3). These neural differences may in turn allow the brain to condense and sparsen neural activity in one or a few subsequent regions, yielding those regions that we observe to be activated. Accordingly, sparse coding on a regional level seems to be nicely compatible with the localization of particular functions in specific regions.

How does the assumption of such sparse coding stand in relation to the localization approach? To equate sparse coding with localization is to confuse the underlying processes and their resulting outcomes. The localization-based approach focuses on the outcome while neglecting the process itself; that is, how the apparent localization of a function in a particular region is generated. Instead of considering the process of generating regional localization, the localization-based approach takes the localization of a particular function in a specific region for granted. And it considers the psychological function to be intrinsic or innate to the region itself without further questioning the underlying processes how that function is generated by the region's neural activity.

Such a localization-based approach is, however, to be distinguished from the approach sparse coding takes to the question of localization. Here the focus shifts from the outcome, the observation of a regional localization, to the processes; that is, the rules and principles that generate what we observe as the specific linkage between function and region.

Neurotheoretical remark Ib: Distinction between "activated" and "active" regions

I discussed the processes underlying sparse coding on a regional level of neural activity in detail in Chapter 3. Briefly, I postulated that the activation of a specific region yields from the computing and comparing of neural differences stemming from other regions. These regions, which serve to yield and amplify neural differences, may by themselves either be activated or non-activated. This means that even non-activated or non-recruited regions participate in generating neural differences.

Conceptually, one may therefore want to distinguish between "activated" and "active" regions. "Activated regions" are those regions that show neural activity changes in response to the task we apply. We as observers associate the recruitment of these regions with the function in question and are consequently inclined to localize the latter in the former.

This, however, neglects what I describe as "active regions" that do not show changes in their activity level in response to the task. These regions may nevertheless participate in generating the neural activity changes of the activated regions, more specifically in generating and amplifying neural differences (see what I describe as an "amplification hypothesis" in Chapter 3). They are thus "active" but not "activated." This, however, makes localization of the function in the activated regions impossible, since that would neglect the role of the active regions in generating the neural activity changes in the activated region.

As detailed in Chapter 3, the generation and amplification of neural differences is coupled to the condensation of neural activity (see what I describe as a "condensation hypothesis" in Chapter 3). Rather than each of the original lower order sensory regions' activating a separate higher order cognitive region, the former's neural activity converges in one common region, to which we then attribute localization. This, however, is a false-negative inference that focuses only on the outcome of localization in the higher-order cognitive region, while neglecting its underlying processes in which lower-order sensory regions participate.

More specifically, the outcome of sparse coding does indeed pertain to one particular region, the "activated" region or network as distinguished from all "non-activated" regions/networks. However, the underlying process involves "active" regions/networks (as distinguished from non-active regions/networks) that are essential in yielding and amplifying neural differences.

This means that the function in question cannot be localized exclusively and completely in the "activated" region/network itself. Instead, the function may be associated with both "activated" and "active" regions/networks as distinguished from "non-activated" and "non-active" ones. Accordingly, the regions/networks remaining silent in response to our task, that is, "non-activated," may nevertheless be "active" (rather than "non-active") and may therefore have an important role in processing the function in question (see Fig. A2-1; see also Hayes et al. 2013 for an example of where the density of GABA-A receptors [PET] in ventromedial prefrontal cortex, a non-activated region during an aversive task, modulates the degree of signal changes [fMRI] in an activated region, the sensorimotor cortex; see also Gonzales-Castillo et al.

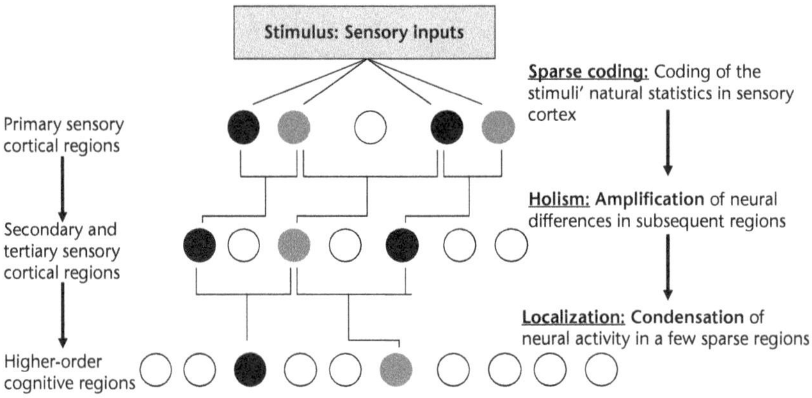

Figure A2-1 Complementarity between holism and localizationism.
***Black*: Activated/recruited regions**
***Gray:* Non-activated but active regions participating in yielding neural differences**
***White:* Non-activated and non-active regions**
The figure depicts the different stages of neural processing. The stimulus is encoded into the sensory cortex's neural activity a sparse way; i.e., as based on its natural statistics as its statistical frequency distribution across different discrete points in time and space. This is possible only if we presuppose difference- rather than stimulus-based coding (upper part). Even if regions are not activated or recruited by themselves, they may still participate in constituting neural differences; they are thus "non-activated" but nevertheless active. The initial neural differences in primary sensory cortex are supposed to be amplified ("amplification hypothesis"; see Chapter 3 in Part I) in subsequent regions, entailing holistic distribution of the initial neural activity changes across different regions of the brain; i.e., holism (middle part). That in turn makes possible the condensation of neural differences ("condensation hypothesis"; see Chapter 3 in Part I) in a few subsequent regions that then do show up as "activated" regions (lower part). These different stages of neural processing across the different regions of the brain are well reflected in changing ratios between "activated" (or recruited) regions, "non-activated" but "active" regions, and "non-activated and non-active" regions.

2012 for the support of active but non-activated regions).

In sum, one may postulate localization of neural activity in specific "activated" regions/networks during particular function. This, as demonstrated, is the outcome of the processes guiding sparse coding on a regional level. However, to infer from such localization (or better, condensation) of neural activity to the localization of the function in question in that particular region/network is to confuse outcome and processes. The function in question must also be associated with regions (and networks) other than the "activated" ones like those that I here described as "active"; that is, actively involved in amplifying neural differences.

Neurotheoretical remark Ic: complementarity between holism and localizationism

We are confronted with two apparently contradicting observations. On one hand, many regions, and ultimately, the whole brain, seem to be implicated in the neural processing of various psychological functions (see earlier). This suggests holism holds true on a psychological level. On the other hand, there is regional sparseness in that different psychological functions seem to recruit similar but at least strongly overlapping regions and networks. This observation, however, contradicts holism and would rather be compatible with localizationism holding true on a neuronal level.

How can we reconcile the contradictory assumptions of localizationism on the neuronal level and holism on the psychological level? The need to reconcile localizationism and holism was already recognized by K. Lashley, as is apparent in the following passage:

> The chief advantage of the strict theories of localization has been their definiteness and comprehensibility. Those of us who have felt the inadequacy of such theories have had to fall back upon expressions like mass action, stress patterns, dynamic effects, melodies of movement, vigilance or nervous energy; all metaphorical and highly unproductive of experimental problems. Yet the facts demand something of this sort. The evidence seems conclusive that in various cortical functions there is every degree of specialization from a limited point-to-point correspondence of cells to a condition of absolute non-specificity. Not only is there diversity in the modes of action of different parts of the cortex but a single area, highly specialized and differentiated for one activity may be wholly undifferentiated for another in which it also participates. We have not a choice between a theory of localization and a theory of decentralization, but must develop a wider view which recognizes the importance and interdependence of both modes of integration. (Lashley 1931, 254)

I hypothesize that we need to set the alternative of localizationism versus holism into the context of sparse coding and difference-based coding in order to reconcile both. There is holism on the process level. As described earlier, even presumably silent, that is, "non-activated" but "active," regions/networks are nevertheless actively participating in generating and amplifying neural differences, thus allowing for difference-based coding. Such difference-based coding is in turn central in condensing and thus sparsening neural activity in a particular region, the "activated" or recruited region, as the manifestation of sparse coding on a regional level.

Many regions, if not (indirectly via the constitution of differences) the whole brain, actively participate in constituting neural differences. One may consequently suggest holism on the level of neuronal processes, whereas the very same neuronal processes, operating throughout different regions, allow and, even stronger, predispose the temporal and spatial sparsening of subsequent neural activity changes in a few highly localized regions as their outcome. The outcome, that is, the changes in the neural activity in a few localized regions, may thus be more localized when compared to the rather holistically operating processes.

What does this entail for the relationship between localizationism and holism? This means that the concepts of localizationism and holism are not opposite and contradictory to each other but rather mutually dependent on each other: As there would be no outcome without a preceding process, localizationism would remain impossible without holism.

Even stronger, the more holistically processes that allow for the amplification of neural differences throughout the whole brain make a more localized outcome, that is, spatial and temporal sparsening of neural activity and the number of "activated" regions, almost necessary. Accordingly, localizationism and holism are bound together as tightly as process and outcome; they remain consequently as inseparable and complementary as yin and yang in the Chinese tradition.

APPENDIX 3 NEUROEPISTEMOLOGICAL REMARK: BRAIN VERSUS OBSERVER

Summary

How are the brain and our observation of it in neuroscientific investigation related to each other? I here distinguish between brain-based and observer-based concepts. "Brain-based concepts" are very much in accordance with the way the brain functions and processes neural activity independently of our observation of it. "Observer-based concepts," in contrast, refer to the dependence of our observations on the observer himself and his particular experimental (and technological and other) requirements. Since in observer-based concepts the observer intrudes into the observations and ultimately into the brain itself, I also speak of "observer-related intrusions." I distinguish between extrinsic and intrinsic observer-related intrusions: extrinsic observer-related intrusions can in principle be avoided and minimized, while intrinsic ones cannot in principle be overcome. Intrinsic observer-related intrusions concern, I claim, intrinsic design features of the brain like its neural code and intrinsic activity that define the brain *qua* brain; since our observation of the brain is necessarily based on both the brain's intrinsic activity and its neural code, we cannot avoid their interfering with and thus confounding and intruding on our observations. Therefore, I conclude that the intrinsic observer-related intrusions pose "neuroexperimental and neuroepistemological constraints" to our possible knowledge of the brain.

Key Concepts and Topics Covered

Brain-based versus observer-based concepts, intrinsic and extrinsic observer-related intrusions, neuroexperimental and neuroepistemological constraints

Neuroepistemological Remark IA: Relationship Between Data/Facts and Concepts

Neuroscience acquires data and ultimately facts to describe the brain (the distinction between data and facts may by itself be worth discussing from a philosophical point of view; see also Northoff 2011). These data and facts are described by concepts that one usually expects to correspond to and thus match the data and facts. In such a case, there is a one-to-one relationship between the data/facts and the contents the concepts describe.

Life is not that easy, though, especially the life of a neuroscientist. Concepts are usually more general and vague than particular data and facts. This means that concepts usually include more than one particular content, thus being more general. That, in turn, makes them more vague and thus less specific when compared to data and facts. The concepts the neuroscientist (and any scientist) uses (or must use) therefore remain unable to completely, 100 percent, match and correspond to the data and facts in a one-to-one way.

Instead, the concepts may also refer to contents other than the ones associated with the particular data and facts in question. This implies a one-to-many relationship where one concept stands for (or "codes") many data/facts. Let us put the relationship between data/facts and concepts in terms of coding, with the former being encoded into the latter. Rather than encoding data and facts in a local (that is one-to-one) (or even sparse in a many-to-one) way, concepts seem to encode data and facts in a rather dense way, with one concept providing the umbrella for different possible data/facts entailing one-to-many relationship. This means that there is almost certainly a certain degree of mismatch between concepts and data/facts, with the former being too unspecific for the single datum/factum.

This all sounds very philosophical, the neuroscientist may want to say. Let the philosophers discuss this, but leave me alone in doing my experiments to generate better data and facts. As I said, life is not that easy. Due to the almost certainly necessary or unavoidable mismatch between concepts and data/facts due to rather dense encoding of the latter by the former, we are prone to confusion.

More specifically, we can never be completely sure (or "know," as the epistemologist may prefer to say) and we thus remain uncertain whether the concept we use to describe our data and facts really matches and corresponds completely and exclusively to the latter. Hence, the possible mismatch between data/facts and concepts goes along with uncertainty in our knowledge about the brain, and therefore is prone to possible confusion.

Neuroepistemological remark Ib: Distinction between brain-based versus observer-based concepts

How can we now describe in more detail and thus alleviate this possible confusion between concepts and data/facts? Concepts are generated by the observer. The very same observer who conducts the experiments also needs to use concepts to describe his data/facts and to formulate his hypothesis. Yielding hypotheses and data/facts is possible only when considering certain requirements that need to be fulfilled within the experimental context.

One such experimental requirement is the careful distinction between different experimental variables that need to be treated in a segregated and independent way. This makes necessary the introduction of concepts describing these segregated and independent variables. The problem starts, however, once the very same concepts that describe the segregated and independent experimental variables are also supposed to describe the brain itself.

More specifically, based on the experimental data/facts, the concepts referring to the respective experimental variables are assumed to describe one to one the processes and mechanisms in the brain itself. Thereby the concept is supposed to match and correspond to the brain's neuronal processes as they are independent of the observer's observation; the concept is thus supposed to refer to the brain as it is by itself.

One such example is the concept of functional connectivity (see later for further examples). It describes an experimental variable, the statistically based correlation between the signal changes in different regions across time amounting to a correlation between two different time series of signals. So far, so good. However, at the same time, the same concept of functional connectivity is also used to describe the neuronal relationship between two (or more) regions' neural activities, thus referring to a purely neuronal feature of the brain independent of our observation.

Does the concept of functional connectivity as an experimental variable match and correspond to the concept as a neuronal feature of the brain itself? As discussed in Chapter 4, we are sure that we can observe statistical correlations between different regions' neural activities and thus functional connectivity in an experimental sense, whereas we are currently unclear about the neuronal features underlying such statistical correlations; i.e., functional connectivity in a neuronal sense.

Let's return to a more general level. One could imagine instances where the concept in an experimental context does not match or correspond to the use of the same concept in the context of the brain's neuronal processes and mechanisms as they are by themselves. In that case, the concept is more related to the observer and her experimental requirements than to the brain itself and its neuronal processes and mechanisms as they are by themselves, independent of our observation. This means the concept is more observer-based than brain-based. I therefore distinguish between what I describe as "observer-based and brain-based concepts" in the following remarks.

The distinction between observer-based and brain-based concepts is not an all-or-nothing distinction but rather a more-or-less distinction. This means a particular concept may be based on both the observer's experimental requirements and the brain's neuronal processes. It may thus be just a matter of degree and balance between the two ingredients, observer and brain, that determines the concept in question. A concept is thus either more or less strongly based on either the observer and her experimental demands, or the brain's neuronal processes.

Accordingly, there is thus a continuum with various shadings and different balances between brain and observer in our concepts is therefore, in the usual case, more or less hybrid. That is to be distinguished from the concepts that reflect the extremes at either end of the continuum between brain and observer that describe purely observer-based and brain-based concepts. Like any scientist, the neuroscientist seeks, of course, concepts where the balance is tilted strongly toward the brain-based end of the continuum and away from the observer-based pole (see Fig. A3-1a).

Neuroepistemological Remark IC: Examples of Observer-Based versus Brain-Based Concepts—GABA and Glutamate

Throughout this volume, we have encountered several examples of suspicious concepts whose balance seemed to be more strongly tilted toward the observer than the brain itself. In the following remarks, I want to briefly mention some of them.

One central issue throughout the whole book was the role of glutamate and GABA in determining the degree of sparse coding (Chapter 2), intrinsic activity (Chapter 6), and rest–stimulus interaction (Chapter 12). Experimentally, we need to segregate glutamate and GABA and correspondingly, neural excitation and inhibition, from each other. For instance, to measure glutamate and neural excitation, we need to experimentally parse both variables from any traces of GABA and neural inhibition. Otherwise, we cannot be sure whether our data really tell us about glutamate and neural excitation themselves. This means ultimately that GABA and glutamate and hence neural inhibition and excitation are treated as segregated and independent experimental variables.

The designation of GABA and glutamate as segregated and independent variables occurs on purely experimental grounds and is therefore strongly observer-based. Based on the data whose acquisition presupposes such experimental segregation and independence, one would suggest GABA and glutamate to also act segregated and independently in the brain itself. One consequently postulates that certain levels of GABA and neural inhibition are necessary for specific kinds of neuronal processes. While these levels may be open to (secondary) modulation by glutamate and neural excitation, they are considered (primarily) as independent and segregated (in a constitutive rather than merely modulatory sense).

What does this assumption imply for our distinction between brain-based and observer-based concepts? This means that now the observer's concepts are transferred to the brain itself. The initially observer-based characterization of GABA and glutamate as independent and segregated experimental variables is now projected onto the brain itself and assumed to describe its neuronal processes. In short, it is no longer treated as observer-based but rather as brain-based.

Does such experimentally based segregation and independence between GABA/neural inhibition and glutamate/neural excitation really

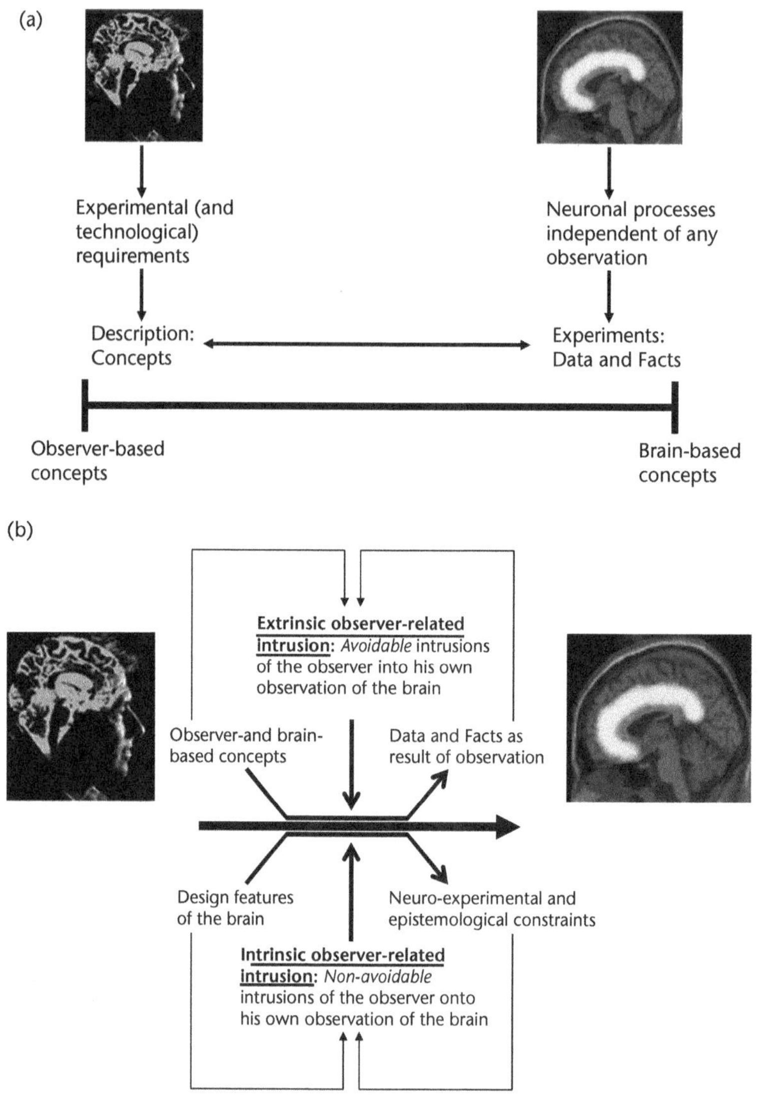

Figure A3-1a and b **Brain, concepts, and observer.**
The figure depicts two key features in the relationship between brain and observer: the continuum between brain-based and observer-based concepts (a), and the distinction between intrinsic and extrinsic observer-related intrusions (b).
(*a*): Observer-based concepts are concepts that describe the brain but rely on us as observers and our abilities to observe the brain. Therefore, we cannot be fully sure whether these concepts are related more to us as observers or to the brain itself, independent of our observation of it. In contrast, "brain-based concepts" are concepts of the brain as it is by itself, independent of our observation of it. This means that our data and facts reflect the brain itself rather than us as observers. I propose a continuum between brain-based and observer-based concepts (lower part), with both being extreme cases in their pure forms on either end of a continuum.
(*b*): Extrinsic observer-related intrusions (upper part) are intrusions of the observer into his/her own observation of the brain's neural activity that can in principle be minimized or even avoided by better experiments, etc. In contrast, intrinsic observer-related intrusions (lower part) are those that cannot in principle be minimized or avoided, because observation is by itself supposed to be possible only on the basis of the brain's intrinsic features, without which observation would remain impossible. Hence, the brain and its intrinsic design features cannot help but intrude in our observation, because otherwise any kind of observation would be impossible.

correspond to the empirical data? I denied that. Instead, I postulated that both GABA and glutamate can be characterized by difference-based coding, with each coding the relative relational difference between the two, rather than their absolute value independent of each other. This was empirically manifested in the excitation-inhibition balance (EIB) that is supposed to provide the measure for the subsequent generation of neural activity.

Such encoding of the difference between GABA and glutamate, rather than encoding both as separate and distinct variables, puts the assumption of (primary and constitutive) segregation and independence between glutamate and GABA in the purely neuronal context (as distinguished from the experimental context) into doubt.

The characterization of GABA and glutamate by (primary and constitutive) segregation and independence may be relevant (and even required) for the observer (and his experimental approach). In contrast, such segregation and independence of GABA and glutamate may as such not apply to the brain as it is by itself, independent of the observer.

This means that such a characterization is more strongly related to the observer and his experimental requirements than to the brain's neuronal processes as they are by themselves independent of the observer's observation. In other words, assuming segregation and independence between GABA and glutamate may turn out to be more observer-based than brain-based.

Neuroepistemological remark ID: Examples of observer-based versus brain-based concepts—stimuli versus differences

Another example is the distinction between different types of stimuli according to their origin in the brain (neuronal stimuli), the body (interoceptive stimuli), or the world (exteroceptive stimuli). Based on these distinct origins, different anatomical structures and pathways have been proposed, as is well reflected in the radial-concentric threefold anatomical organization (see Chapter 1). However, on a functional level, the distinction between the different origins of the stimuli and their respective anatomical structures seems to be blurred. This was, for instance, quite apparent in the observed neural activity, or functional connectivity and low-high frequency fluctuations, and the coding strategy, or difference- rather than stimulus-based coding, that operated across and superseded the underlying anatomical structure and its different stimuli's inputs (see Chapters 4 and 5).

This means, however, that the distinction of stimuli according to their origin, or matter of origin, may be not as relevant for the brain itself and its neuronal processes as it is for us as observers and our experimental requirements. The experimental requirement is not to confuse stimuli of different origins. Otherwise, we cannot say anything about, for instance, exteroceptive stimuli and their underlying neuronal processes and how they are distinguished from the ones related to interoceptive stimuli.

However, as relevant as the distinction of the different stimuli's origins may be for us as observers, it does not seem to be as relevant for the brain itself. The brain seems to be more "interested" in different, more specifically, in different *degrees* of statistically based spatial and temporal differences among different stimuli rather than in the stimuli themselves and their respective origins (see Chapters 2, 6, and 12). Hence, my characterization of the brain's neural activity and its processing by "matter of degrees and differences" rather than as a "matter of its origins and stimuli" (see Appendix 1).

In sum, this means that the characterization of the brain's neural processing by "origin and stimuli" may be more strongly related to the observer himself than the brain itself. In other words, the determination of the brain and its neural activity by the different stimuli and their respective origins—"a matter of origins and stimuli"—may turn out to be observer-based rather than brain-based. This contrast with the characterization of the brain's neural activity as a "matter of degrees and differences" that seems to be tilted more toward the brain-based pole in the continuum between the extremes of purely observer- and brain-based concepts.

Neuroepistemological Remark Ie: Examples of Observer- Versus Brain-Based Concepts—Resting State Versus Stimulus-Induced Activity

Let us provide a final example where brain-based and observer-based concepts may be confused: the distinction between resting-state and stimulus-induced activity. Experimentally, we clearly need to segregate and delineate both, since otherwise we will never be able to know the contributions of the stimulus and those of the brain itself in stimulus-induced activity.

One may therefore postulate segregation between resting-state and stimulus-induced activity. However, as the empirical data suggest (see Chapters 11 and 12), these two cannot principally be distinguished from each other, let alone segregated. Instead of by principal difference and segregation, resting-state activity and stimulus-induced activity can only be distinguished from each other on the basis of degrees. This means, however, that the principal distinction between resting-state and stimulus-induced activity is more strongly based on the observer than on the brain itself. I thus formulated what I describe as the "continuity hypothesis," which includes both neuronal continuum and discontinuum between resting-state and stimulus-induced activity (see Appendix 1).

How can we escape the possible confusion between brain-based and observer-based concepts? To shift concepts away from the observer-based pole toward the brain-based pole, we will need to also shift our perspective. More specifically, we will need to abandon our observer-based perspective and imagine how it is for the brain itself, independent of our observation, to generate the kind of neuronal processes we observe.

We should at least aim to move from the observer's perspective to the ideal (though fictive) case of being able to take the "brain's perspective" (used in a figurative sense, because the brain itself has no "perspective"). Metaphorically, one may therefore say that we need to replace the question of "What it is like for the observer" by the question of "What it is like for the brain."

I have here demonstrated various examples of concepts that seem to be more strongly based on the observer himself and his experimental requirements than on the brain's neuronal processes independent of our observation of them. Thereby, diagnosis of the more strongly observer-based component in these concepts led me to search for other concepts that are presumably more brain-based. This, in turn, was accompanied by a suggestions for future experimental variables and hypotheses in order to test these more brain-based concepts experimentally and lend empirical support to them.

Neuroepistemological Remark IIa: Observer-Related Intrusion

How can we be sure and thus know that the concepts we apply are more brain- than observer-based? The only way for us to know is to develop corresponding hypotheses and conduct the appropriate experiments. If the data are in accordance with the characterization implied by these concepts, the assumption of their being more brain-based than observer-based may be justified. If, in contrast, the data do not support my concepts like difference-based coding, they may turn out to be as observer-based as the ones I replaced.

If the data are in accordance with the concepts, the latter are empirically plausible. They are thus to a higher degree based on the brain than on the observer; while the opposite case of no empirical support suggests that they are more based on the observer than on the brain. Hence, the degree of empirical plausibility—the degree of correspondence or matching of the concept with the empirical data—may be regarded as a measure of the degree to which the concept is brain- or observer-based.

To further test the empirical plausibility and thus the predominantly brain-based nature of our concepts, alternative experimental designs should also be applied using different experimental variables. If they yield the same or analogous results, the likelihood of both data sets being confounded by the experimental requirements of segregation and independence (of experimental variables) is rather low. The data may then provide an excellent basis for being associated with a particular concept that shows a high probability of being brain-based rather than observer-based.

How about the opposite case, with a concept showing low empirical plausibility, which then is more strongly observer-based than brain-based? In that case, the observer and her experimental (and technological and other) requirements seem to intrude too much into the concept and the subsequent experimental design as to yield brain- rather than observer-based concepts. The observer thus intrudes into the brain and imposes herself, thereby manipulating and confounding what she herself can observe from the brain's neuronal processes by her own stance and experimental and technological needs. In short, the observer confounds and intrudes into her own observations, for which reason I speak of "observer-related intrusion."

The concept of "observer-related intrusion" refers to the intrusion or imposition of the observer himself into or onto his own observation of the brain's neuronal processes. Accordingly, observer-related intrusions describe that the observer himself confounds his own observations. Observer-related intrusions do consequently lead to low degrees of empirical plausibility of the respective concepts that are then more observer- than brain-based.

NEUROEPISTEMOLOGICAL REMARK IIB: *EXTRINSIC* OBSERVER-RELATED INTRUSIONS

How can we deal with observer-related intrusions? We can try out alternative concepts and conduct the respective experimental designs. Then we can compare the results from both experimental lines to see how much they accord with the respectively presupposed concept: the experimental line with the higher degree of correspondence between concept and data/facts (empirical plausibility) may then be the line where the concept is less observer- and more brain-based compared to the other line. In other words, we have to try out different alternative concepts and subject them to rigorous experimental testing (see Chapter 3 in Northoff 2011 for a discussion of such methodology, which I describe as "concept-fact iterativity").

This means that we are not completely at the mercy of ourselves and our observer-related intrusions. Instead, we can develop some (methodological) tools to minimize and ultimately avoid them. This means that we can at least minimize the degrees to which an observer intrudes and imposes himself onto his own concepts. In the best case, we can avoid observer-related intrusions altogether—in that case the respective concepts would be strongly brain-based, approaching one extreme of the continuum between brain-based and observer-based concepts.

Since we are in principle able to minimize the degree of observer-related intrusions, I characterize them as *extrinsic*. The concept of "extrinsic observer-related intrusions" means that the observer's intrusion and imposition can in principle be minimized, and ideally, be corrected or even avoided altogether; the intrusion remains therefore extrinsic to both the observation itself and the concepts we use to describe our own observation (see Fig. A3-1b).

NEUROEPISTEMOLOGICAL REMARK IIC: *INTRINSIC* OBSERVER-RELATED INTRUSION

I propose that extrinsic observer-related intrusions can in principle be minimized, and in the best-designed investigations, can be avoided altogether. This is made possible by refining our concepts, as described, and developing better and more precise technological tools for measuring and acquiring data (such as higher-resolution brain scanning). There may be instances, however, where we remain in principle unable to minimize observer-related intrusion. This, to clarify, does not concern the individual observer as distinct from other individual observers; it rather pertains to all possible observers independent of the individual ones.

Let me start with Buzsaki and his emphasis on rhythms and oscillations. He argues in his excellent book *Rhythms of the Brain* (Buzsaki 2006) that rhythms and oscillations are a hallmark feature of the brain. To prove his point of the causal nature of oscillations for certain processes, he would ultimately need to experimentally investigate a brain *without* oscillations and see whether it lacks the kind of effects for which he considers oscillations to be necessary. That remains impossible, however, since we cannot even imagine a brain without oscillations, let alone test it experimentally, as Buzsaki himself remarks (see Buzsaki 2006, 360).

Even pathological cases like schizophrenia, depression, or vegetative states, which may help in overcoming extrinsic observer-related intrusions, do not provide an option in this case. Why is this so? Because even they still show rhythms and oscillations that, despite being distorted, are still present and thus not completely absent as experimentally required. There is thus a principal limit in the possible experimental testing that cannot be overcome and avoided.

How can we describe such a principal limitation in further detail? The limitations consist of the fact that we remain in principle unable to prove whether our concepts, like rhythms and oscillations, are ultimately based on the brain itself and independent of us as observers. Or whether they are more related to us as observers and our ways in which we can (and cannot) observe and experimentally test the brain. We are thus stuck in our own observation, which remains principally unable to tease apart variables that are related to the brain itself from those that are more associated with our observation and its methodological, experimental, and technological demands.

Unlike in the case of extrinsic observer-related intrusion, we here remain principally unable to minimize or even avoid the intrusion by (for instance) the oscillations, without eliminating the observation itself that, as it is brain-based, may require the presence of oscillations (see later). This means that the intrusion is an integral and thus intrinsic feature to the observation, without which the latter would remain impossible. I therefore speak of "intrinsic observer-related intrusion."

NEUROEPISTEMOLOGICAL REMARK IIIA: "INTRINSIC DESIGN FEATURES" OF THE BRAIN

How is it possible that observer-related intrusions are intrinsic rather than extrinsic? This amounts to the question for the different concepts dealt with in intrinsic and extrinsic observer-related intrusions. The concepts of rhythms and oscillations refer to a feature that characterizes the brain's designs and, even more strongly, defines the brain as brain.

Buzsaki for instance cannot even imagine a brain without oscillations, because otherwise he would no longer be talking about a brain (at least not of a human brain), which would be senseless and meaningless. He thus considers rhythms and oscillations to be what I describe as "intrinsic design features" of the brain that define the brain as brain. What are other "intrinsic design features" of the brain besides rhythms and oscillations? Throughout this book, we have already encountered several such "intrinsic design features."

I postulated that difference-based coding, as distinguished from stimulus-based coding, defines the brain's neural code. Since the code very much defines what and how the brain can encode its own activity and stimuli into neural activity, the neural code and thus difference-based coding as suggested here also defines the brain as brain. Since difference-based coding described a coding strategy that results in temporal and spatial sparsening of neural activity, sparse coding must also be regarded as a design feature (see Chapters 1–3). The same holds true for predictive coding, which also seems to be unavoidable once one assumes the presence of difference-based coding (see Chapters 7–9).

Besides the encoding strategy, other, more specific, design features concerned the high- and low-frequency fluctuations of neural activity in both resting-state and stimulus-induced activity, thus mirroring Buzsaki's assumption of rhythms and oscillations. Functional connectivity between different regions during both forms of neural activity was yet another design feature.

Finally, and most important, the brain's intrinsic activity, its resting-state activity, and its consequent constitution of a spatiotemporal structure must also be regarded a design feature of the brain without which the brain would not be a brain (at least not a human brain). Though rather different, all these features share the fact that their absence could not even be imagined without abandoning the ground of the brain. They must therefore be define the brain as (at least a human) brain and are thus what I call the brain's "intrinsic design features."

Neuroepistemological remark IIIb: "Neuroexperimental and neuro-epistemological constraints" in our investigation and knowledge of the brain

We now face a serious problem. The whole book has focused on these "intrinsic design features." And it has aimed to make a case for them, meaning that I proposed them to be more brain-based than other rival concepts that I regarded as more observer-based. To show that these concepts are brain-based, I will need to put them to experimental testing.

That means that I will need to show, not only that the presence of the intrinsic design features induces the kinds of neuronal (see Volume I) and phenomenal (see Volume II) effects I describe, but also that their absence makes the neuronal and phenomenal effects impossible. If I were able to show the latter, I could demonstrate that the brain's "intrinsic design features" are a necessary and henceforth unavoidable condition of the kind of neuronal states we described here in Volume I and also of phenomenal states; that is, of consciousness (see Volume II).

This is the point, however, where the problems start. While I can test the effects of the presence of the brain's "intrinsic design features," the experimental testing of their absence remains in principle impossible.

In the same way Buzsaki cannot even imagine a brain without oscillations, let alone experimentally test its effects, we cannot imagine at all a brain without (for instance) difference-based and sparse coding, a brain without functional connectivity, a brain without intrinsic activity, and a brain without spatiotemporal structure. Why? Because these are design features of the brain that define the brain as (at least human) brain and are therefore intrinsic rather than extrinsic to the brain.

There are principal constraints (and ultimately limits) to how far we can go experimentally. Since these principal constraints (and ultimately limits) can ultimately be traced back to the brain itself and its particular design features, I here speak of "neuroexperimental constraints." The concept of "neuroexperimental constraints" means that we remain principally unable to experimentally manipulate certain neuronal features of the brain like rhythms and oscillations (see later for more examples) without losing the brain as brain.

These neuroexperimental constraints also put some limits on our possible knowledge of the brain; these epistemological constraints— the limits in our possible knowledge of the brain and its empirical function—may therefore be described as "neuroepistemological constraints." The concept of "neuroepistemological constraints" describes principal borders and limits in our possible knowledge of the brain that we cannot pass without losing our own brain as the basis of all our possible knowledge (see later for more detail on the last point, the loss of one's own brain).

Neuroepistemological remark IIIc: "Individual versus general detachment" of our observation from the brain

Let me illustrate this by distinguishing between what I describe as "individual detachment" and "general detachment." "Detachment" means that we as observers are able to distance and thus detach ourselves from the effects of our own brain's operations by means of which the observation of the brain is possible. In other words, the concept of detachment describes the opposite of intrusion; namely, that we are able to pull ourselves, including the effects of our own brain, out of our own observation.

One may now distinguish between two different forms of detachment; namely, "individual detachment" and "general detachment." "Individual detachment" is when we detach ourselves from our own brain and its specific individual level of resting-state activity and its highly specific and individual degree of spatial and temporal differences that are encoded into our brain's stimulus-induced activity.

The detachment here is *individual* because it concerns the level of resting-state activity specific to the particular individual person and the level of the resting-state activity that again is a feature of that individual person. How is such individual detachment possible? This can be done in an *inter*-individual way, with the correction of the individual's observation by another individual with a different level of resting-state activity and different degrees of encoded spatial and temporal differences. Or it can be done in a more *intra*-individual way, by undergoing psychotherapy or real-time fMRI, wherein one receives feedback about one's own neuronal activity level, which then one can modulate by oneself.

Being the positive mirror image of intrusion, such "individual detachment" down-modulates the effects of extrinsic observer-related intrusions, those that can in principle be minimized and avoided. How about intrinsic observer-related intrusion? For that, a different kind of detachment, a more radical one, is needed, which I call "general detachment."

The concept of "general detachment" means that we not only need to detach ourselves from our individual level of resting-state activity, but, more basically, from any kind of resting-state activity itself. One would thus need to achieve a brain without any kind of resting-state activity. Analogously, we would not only need to detach ourselves from the degree of the encoded spatial and temporal differences but, more radically, from the encoding of spatial and temporal differences altogether. One would thus need a brain that applies (for example) 100 percent of stimulus-based coding and zero percent of difference-based coding. Since it applies to the brain in general, I here speak of "general detachment."

Neuroepistemological Remark IIId: Conceptual-Logical and Empirical Implausibility of "General Detachment" of Our Observation from the Brain

Is such a "general detachment" plausible and feasible beyond the merely fictive thought experiment? No: Since both resting-state activity and difference-based coding are supposed to be intrinsic features that define the brain as (at least a human) brain, we would no longer speak of "a brain" in the case of their absence. The case of "general detachment" is thus inconsistent and therefore logically (and conceptually) implausible.

Even worse: Both resting-state activity and difference-based coding may be necessary conditions and thus unavoidable features in making possible observation in general; this means that having a brain without resting-state activity and difference-based coding would make it impossible for the observer to observe anything at all. In other words, "general detachment" implies, not only detachment from one's own brain's resting-state activity and its difference-based coding, but also detachment from observation altogether. Maintaining observation while undergoing "general detachment" remains consequently impossible and therefore logically and empirically implausible.

What does the logical and empirical implausibility of "general detachment" imply for "intrinsic observer-related intrusion"? The impossibility and implausibility of "general detachment" reflects the border that is described by "intrinsic observer-related intrusion"; namely that, by default, we cannot in principle avoid or minimize the possible impact and effects of our brain's resting-state activity and difference-based coding on our observations.

To put it differently, we are caught between Scylla and Charybdis. On one side, we can keep our brain's resting-state activity and its difference-based coding and consequently our ability of observation. This, however, makes it impossible for us as observers to exclude our brain's possible effects on our observation, which makes us prone to intrinsic observer-related intrusion.

Or, on the other side, we can exclude and detach ourselves from both our brain's resting-state activity and its difference-based coding. Since our observation is very much based on our brain's resting-state activity and difference-based coding, however, we are then left without any capacity of observation. This though makes the elimination of the intrinsic observer-related intrusion futile; senseless and meaningless.

We therefore have no choice other than to accept the intrinsic observer-related intrusion as the border of our possible knowledge of the brain—unless we prefer to eliminate our observation altogether, in which case we would no longer be able to observe and thus enjoy the absence of our intrinsic observer-related intrusions.

Neuroepistemological remark IIIe: Probability versus knowledge

How can I prove my hypothesis of difference-based coding and our necessary predisposition to intrinsic observer-related intrusion? General detachment from the brain's resting-state activity and its difference-based coding would ultimately be necessary to experimentally prove or disprove (verify or falsify) my hypothesis of difference-based coding. Due the brain-based nature of observation, which any such experimental demonstration has to rely on, such "general detachment" remains impossible. This, however, as discussed earlier, makes difference-based coding immune to either experimental falsification or verification. All we can say on the basis of our very human brain is that difference-based coding is either more or less likely; thus being a matter of probability.

This is exactly what I have done in this volume. I have provided empirical evidence that makes the assumption of difference-based coding empirically more plausible than the alternative hypothesis of stimulus-based coding. On the basis of that, I hypothesize that difference-based coding has a higher probability of being a brain-based rather than an observer-based concept, compared to stimulus-based coding as the empirical alternative. I thus consider the assumption of difference-based coding an empirically plausible hypothesis whose ultimate proof or falsification remains principally impossible for us, being beyond our brain-based epistemic scope.

More generally, this means that our empirical assumptions about the brain ultimately have to rely on empirical plausibility and probability rather than on knowledge (in a philosophical-epistemological sense). This means that, in the case of the brain, our empirical approach is epistemologically constrained by a border—the border of intrinsic observer-related intrusion, which we remain in principle unable to transgress with our scientific-empirical means and methods. As demonstrated earlier, our brain sets these very epistemological boundaries by itself; this, however, needs to be defined and determined in a more detailed way in future neuroepistemological investigation.

Do we need to be concerned about these principal epistemological borders in our possible knowledge about the brain? No, because empirical plausibility and ultimately statistical probability are all that is needed to gain sufficient empirical-experimental insight into the brain. After all, this is exactly the way the brain itself operates. As demonstrated here, the brain's function itself is ultimately based on empirical plausibility and statistical probability; this is, for instance, well manifested when it encodes the statistical frequency distribution of different stimuli in terms of their spatial and temporal differences into its own neural activity.

Most important, one cannot deny that our brain usually works quite well by encoding the different stimuli's spatial and temporal differences in a statistically based way. And what is seemingly sufficient for the brain should also work well for us in our quest for understanding and knowing the brain and its neural mechanisms and coding strategy. At least in our daily and scientific world that is the natural world we live in, the plausibility and probability of our insights into the brain should be sufficient to survive in our respective environmental contexts. That is, after all, exactly the way brain itself works!

Even if the philosopher still claims there are principal epistemological limits to our possible knowledge of the brain, we may not need to be too concerned about it for our survival. Why? The alleged epistemological limitation can only be revealed by contrasting our natural world of daily life and science with the logical world of the philosopher. But why shall we and our brain "be concerned too much with something," that is like the logical world far beyond the brain's and our own scope, that is, the natural world?

REFERENCES

Albert, N. B., Robertson, E. M., Mehta, P., & Miall, R. C. (2009) Resting state networks and memory consolidation. *Communicative & Integrative Biology*. 2(6), 530–532.

Alcaro, A., Huber, R., & Panksepp, J. (2007), Behavioral functions of the mesolimbic dopaminergic system: an affective neuroethological perspective. *Brain Research Review* 56(2), 283–321. Epub 2007 Aug 21. Review.

Alcaro, A., & Panksepp, J. (2011). The SEEKING mind: Primal neuro-affective substrates for appetitive incentive states and their pathological dynamics in addictions and depression. *Neuroscience & Biobehavioral Reviews*, 35(9), 1805–1820. doi:10.1016/j.neubiorev.2011.03.002

Alcaro, A., Panksepp, J., Witczak, J., Hayes, D. J., & Northoff, G. (2010). Is subcortical-cortical midline activity in depression mediated by glutamate and GABA? A cross-species translational approach. *Neuroscience & Biobehavioral Reviews*, 34(4), 592–605. doi:10.1016/j.neubiorev.2009.11.023

Alink, A., Schwiedrzik, C. M., Kohler, A., Singer, W., & Muckli, L. (2010). Stimulus predictability reduces responses in primary visual cortex. *Journal of Neuroscience*, 30(8), 2960–2966.

Arieli, A., Sterkin, A., Grinvald, A., & Aertsen, A. (1996). Dynamics of ongoing activity: explanation of the large variability in evoked cortical responses. *Science* (New York), 273(5283), 1868–71. Retrieved from http://www.ncbi.nlm.nih.gov/pubmed/8791593.

Arieli, A., Sterkin, A., Grinvald, A., & Aertsen, A. (1996). Dynamics of ongoing activity: Explanation of the large variability in evoked cortical responses. *Science*, 273(5283), 1868–1871.

Assisi, C., Stopfer, M., Laurent, G., & Bazhenov, M. (2007). Adaptive regulation of sparseness by feedforward inhibition. *Nature Neuroscience*, 10(9), 1176–1184. doi:10.1038/nn1947

Augustine, J. R. (1996). Circuitry and functional aspects of the insular lobe in primates including humans. *Brain Research Review* 22(3), 229–244. Review.

Baars, B. J. (2005). Global workspace theory of consciousness: toward a cognitive neuroscience of human experience. *Progress in Brain Research*, 150, 45–53. doi:10.1016/S0079-6123(05)50004-9

Bach, D. R., Weiskopf, N., & Dolan, R. J. (2011). A stable sparse fear memory trace in human amygdala. *Journal of Neuroscience*, 31(25), 1524–11. doi:10.1523/JNEUROSCI.1524-11.2011

Bar, M. (2007). The proactive brain: Using analogies and associations to generate predictions. *Trends in Cognitive Sciences*, 11(9), 280. doi:10.1016/j.tics.2007.08.004

Bar, M. (2009). The proactive brain: Memory for predictions. *Philosophical Transactions of the Royal Society B: Biological Sciences*, 364(1521), 1235–1243. doi:10.1098/rstb.2008.0310

Barlow, H B. (1972). Single units and sensation: a neuron doctrine for perceptual psychology? *Perception*, 1(4), 371–94. Retrieved from http://www.ncbi.nlm.nih.gov/pubmed/4377168.

Barlow, H. (2001). The exploitation of regularities in the environment by the brain. *Behavioral & Brain Sciences*, 24(4), 602–607.

Barlow, Horace B. (2009). Single units and sensation: a neuron doctrine for perceptual psychology? *Perception*, 38(6), 795–8. Retrieved from http://www.ncbi.nlm.nih.gov/pubmed/19806956.

Barry, R. J., Clarke, A. R., Johnstone, S. J., Magee, C. A., & Rushby, J. A. (2007). EEG differences between eyes-closed and eyes-open resting conditions. *Clinical Neurophysiology*, 118(12), 2765–2773. doi:10.1016/j.clinph.2007.07.028

Barry, R. J., Rushby, J. A., Johnstone, S. J., Clarke, A. R., Croft, R. J., & Lawrence, C. A. (2004). Event-related potentials in the auditory oddball as a function of EEG alpha phase at stimulus onset. *Clinical Neurophysiology*, 115(11), 2593–2601. doi:10.1016/j.clinph.2004.06.004

Bechara, A. (2004). The role of emotion in decision-making: Evidence from neurological patients with orbitofrontal damage. *Brain & Cognition*, 55(1), 30–40. doi:10.1016/j.bandc.2003.04.001

Bechara, A., & Naqvi, N. (2004). Listening to your heart: Interoceptive awareness as a gateway to feeling. *Nature Neuroscience*, 7(2), 102–103. doi:10.1038/nn0204-102

Beckmann, C. F., DeLuca, M., Devlin, J. T., & Smith, S. M. (2005). Investigations into resting-state connectivity using independent component analysis. *Philosophical Transactions of the Royal Society B: Biological Sciences*, 360(1457), 1001–1013. doi:10.1098/rstb.2005.1634

Beloozerova, I. N., Sirota, M. G., Swadlow, H. A., Orlovsky, G. N., Popova, L. B., & Deliagina, T. G. (2003). Activity of different classes of neurons of the motor cortex during postural corrections. *Journal of Neuroscience*, 23(21), 7844–53. Retrieved from http://www.ncbi.nlm.nih.gov/pubmed/12944514.

Berkes, P., Orbán, G., Lengyel, M., & Fiser, J. (2011). Spontaneous cortical activity reveals hallmarks of an optimal internal model of the environment. *Science* (New York), 331(6013), 83–7. doi:10.1126/science.1195870

Bermpohl, F., Fregni, F., Boggio, P. S., Thut, G., Northoff, G., Otachi, P. T. M., Rigonatti, S. P., et al. (2006). Effect of low-frequency transcranial magnetic stimulation on an affective go/no-go task in patients with major depression: role of stimulation site and depression severity. *Psychiatry Research*, 141(1), 1–13. doi:10.1016/j.psychres.2005.07.018

Bermpohl, F., Pascual-Leone, A., Amedi, A., Merabet, L. B., Fregni, F., Gaab, N., Alsop, D., et al. (2006a). Attentional modulation of emotional stimulus processing: an fMRI study using emotional expectancy. *Human Brain Mapping*, 27(8), 662–677. doi:10.1002/hbm.20209

Bermpohl, F., Pascual-Leone, A., Amedi, A., Merabet, L. B., Fregni, F., Wrase, J., Schlagenhauf, F., et al. (2008). Novelty seeking modulates medial prefrontal activity during the anticipation of emotional stimuli. *Psychiatry Research*, 164(1), 81–5. doi:10.1016/j.pscychresns.2007.12.019

Bermpohl, F., Walter, M., Sajonz, B., Lücke, C., Hägele, C., Sterzer, P., Adli, M., et al. (2009). Attentional modulation of emotional stimulus processing in patients with major depression—alterations in prefrontal cortical regions. *Neuroscience Letters*, 463(2), 108–13. doi:10.1016/j.neulet.2009.07.061

Berridge, K. C. (2000). Measuring hedonic impact in animals and infants: microstructure of affective taste reactivity patterns. *Neuroscience and Biobehavioral Reviews*, 24(2), 173–198. Review.

Berridge, K. C. (2003). Pleasures of the brain. *Brain and Cognition*,52(1),106–128. Review.

Berridge, K. C. (2004). Motivation concepts in behavioral neuroscience. *Physiology & behavior*81(2), 179–209. Review.

Berridge, K. C. (2007). The debate over dopamine's role in reward: the case for incentive salience. *Psychopharmacology (Berl)*, 191(3), 391–431. Epub 2006 Oct 27. Review.

Berridge, K. C. (2012). From prediction error to incentive salience: mesolimbic computation of reward motivation. *The European Journal of Neuroscience*,35(7), 1124–1143. doi: 10.1111/j.1460-9568.2012.07990.x. Review.

Betzel, R. F., Erickson, M. A., Abell, M., O'Donnell, B. F., Hetrick, W.P., & Sporns, O. (2012). Synchronization dynamics and evidence for a repertoire of network states in resting EEG. *Frontiers in Computational Neuroscience*, 6, 74. doi: 10.3389/fncom.2012.00074. Epub 2012 Sep 28.

Bianciardi, M., van Gelderen, P., Duyn, J. H., Fukunaga, M., & de Zwart, J. A. (2009). Making the most of fMRI at 7 T by suppressing spontaneous signal fluctuations. *NeuroImage*, 44(2), 448–454. doi:10.1016/j.neuroimage.2008.08.037

Biddle, S. (1993). Children, exercise and mental-health. *International Journal of Sport Psychology*, 24(2), 200–216.

Biederlack, J., Castelo-Branco, M., Neuenschwander, S., Wheeler, D. W., Singer, W., & Nikolic, D. (2006). Brightness induction: Rate enhancement and neuronal synchronization as complementary codes. *Neuron*,52(6), 1073–1083. doi:10.1016/j.neuron.2006.11.012 ER

Blakemore, S. J., Wolpert, D. M., & Frith, C. D. (1999a). The cerebellum contributes to somatosensory cortical activity during self-produced tactile stimulation. *Neuroimage*, 10(4), 448–459.

Blakemore, S. J., Wolpert, D. M., & Frith, C. D. (1999b). Central cancellation of self-produced tickle sensation. *Nature Neuroscience*, 1(7), 635–640.

Block, N. (2005). Two neural correlates of consciousness. *Trends in Cognitive Sciences*, 9(2), 46–52. doi:10.1016/j.tics.2004.12.006

Boeker, H., & Northoff, G. (2005). Desymbolisierung in der schweren Depression und das Problem der Hemmung: Ein neuropsychoanalytisches Modell der Störung des emotionalen Selbstbezugs Depressiver. *Psyche2*, 59(9–10), 964–989.

Boeker, H., Budischewski, K., Eppel, A., Hartling, F., Rinnert, J., Schmeling, C., Will, H., et al. (n.d.). Selbstkonzept und Objektbeziehungen bei PatientInnen mit affektiven Störungen: Individuumzentrierte Diagnostik mit der Repertory Grid-Technik. *Psychotherapie, Psychosomatik, Medizinisch Psychologie*, 50, 328–334.

Boeker, Heinz, Kleiser, M., Lehman, D., Jaenke, L., Bogerts, B., & Northoff, G. (n.d.). Executive dysfunction, self, and ego pathology in schizophrenia: an exploratory study of neuropsychology and personality. *Comprehensive Psychiatry*, 47(1), 7–19. doi:10.1016/j.comppsych.2005.04.003

Boeker, Heinz, Northoff, G., Lenz, C., Schmeling, C., Meier, M., & Hell, D. (2000). Untersuchungen des subjektiven Erlebens ehemals katatoner Patienten mittels modifizierter Landfield Kategorien. *Psychiatrische Praxis*, 27(8), 389–396.

Böker, H., & Northoff, G. (2010). Die Entkopplung des Selbst in der Depression: Empirische Befunde und neuropsychodynamische Hypothesen. *Psyche: Zeitschrift für Psychoanalyse und ihre Anwendungen*. Retrieved from https://www.zora.uzh.ch/35772/.

Böker, H., Hell, D., Budischewski, K., Eppel, A., Härtling, F., Rinnert, H., Von Schmeling, F., et al. (2000). Personality and object relations in patients with affective disorders: idiographic research by means of the repertory grid technique. *Journal of Affective Disorders*, 60(1), 53–9. Retrieved from http://www.ncbi.nlm.nih.gov/pubmed/10940448.

Boly, M., Balteau, E., Schnakers, C., Degueldre, C., Moonen, G., Luxen, A., et al. (2007). Baseline brain activity fluctuations predict somatosensory perception in humans. *Proceedings of the National Academy of Sciences USA*, 104(29), 12187–12192. doi:10.1073/pnas.0611404104

Boly, M., Phillips, C., Tshibanda, L., Vanhaudenhuyse, A., Schabus, M., Dang-Vu, T. T., Moonen, G., et al. (2008). Intrinsic brain activity in altered states of consciousness: how conscious is the default mode of brain function? *Annals of the New York Academy of Sciences*, 1129, 119–29. doi:10.1196/annals.1417.015

Bossaerts, P. (2010). Risk and risk prediction error signals in anterior insula. *Brain Structure & Function*, 214(5–6), 645–653. doi:10.1007/s00429-010-0253-1

Brasselet, R., Panzeri, S., Logothetis, N. K., & Kayser, C. (2012). Neurons with stereotyped and rapid responses provide a reference frame for relative temporal coding in primate auditory cortex. *Journal of Neuroscience*, 32(9), 2998–3008. doi:10.1523/JNEUROSCI.5435-11.2012

Brecht, M., Schneider, M., Sakmann, B., & Margrie, T. W. (2004). Whisker movements evoked by stimulation of single pyramidal cells in rat motor cortex. *Nature*, 427(6976), 704–10. doi:10.1038/nature02266

Breiter, H. C., Aharon, I., Kahneman, D., Dale, A., & Shizgal, P. (2001) Functional imaging of neural responses to expectancy and experience of monetary gains and losses. *Neuron*. 2001 May;30(2):619–639.

Brenner, N., Bialek, W., & de Ruyter van Steveninck, R. (2000). Adaptive rescaling maximizes information transmission. *Neuron*, 26(3), 695–702.

Britz, J., Van De Ville, D., & Michel, C. M. (2010). BOLD correlates of EEG topography reveal rapid resting-state network dynamics. *NeuroImage*, 52(4), 1162–70. doi:10.1016/j.neuroimage.2010.02.052

Brown, T. M., & Piggins, H. D. (2007). Electrophysiology of the suprachiasmatic circadian clock. *Progress in Neurobiology*, 82(5), 229–255. doi:10.1016/j.pneurobio.2007.05.002

Broyd, S. J., Demanuele, C., Debener, S., Helps, S. K., James, C. J., & Sonuga-Barke, E. J. S. (2009). Default-mode brain dysfunction in mental disorders: A systematic review. *Neuroscience & Biobehavioral Reviews*, 33(3), 279–296. doi:10.1016/j.neubiorev.2008.09.002 ER

Buckner, R. L., Andrews-Hanna, J. R., & Schacter, D. L. (2008). The brain's default network: anatomy, function, and relevance to disease. *Annals of the New York Academy of Sciences*, 1124, 1–38. doi:10.1196/annals.1440.011

Bullmore, E., & Sporns, O. (2012). The economy of brain network organization. *Nature Reviews Neuroscience*, 13(5). doi:10.1038/nrn3214

Buzsaki, G. (2004). Large-scale recording of neuronal ensembles. *Nature Neuroscience*, 7(5), 446–451. doi:10.1038/nn1233

Buzsáki, G. (2006). *Rhythms of the brain.* Oxford; New York: Oxford University Press. Retrieved from http://www.worldcat.org/title/rhythms-of-the-brain/oclc/63279497&referer=brief_results.

Buzsaki, G. (2007). The structure of consciousness—subjective awareness may depend on neural networks in the brain supporting complex wiring schemes and dynamic patterns of activity. *Nature*, 446(7133), 267–267. doi:10.1038/442267a

Buzsaki, G., & Draguhn, A. (2004). Neuronal oscillations in cortical networks. *Science*, 304(5679), 1926–1929.

Buzsáki, G., Kaila, K., & Raichle, M. (2007). Inhibition and brain work. *Neuron*, 56(5), 771–83. doi:10.1016/j.neuron.2007.11.008

Cabral, J., Hugues, E., Sporns, O., & Deco, G. (2011). Role of local network oscillations in resting-state functional connectivity. *NeuroImage*, 57(1). doi:10.1016/j.neuroimage.2011.04.010

Canolty, R. T., & Knight, R. T. (2010). The functional role of cross-frequency coupling. *Trends in Cognitive Sciences*, 14(11), 506–15. doi:10.1016/j.tics.2010.09.001

Carhart-Harris, R. L., & Friston, K. J. (2010). The default-mode, ego-functions and free-energy: a neurobiological account of Freudian ideas. *Brain*, 133(Pt 4):1265–1283. doi: 10.1093/brain/awq010. Epub 2010 Feb 28. Review.

Chang, C., Metzger, C. D., Glover, G. H., Duyn, J. H., Heinze, H.-J., & Walter, M. (2013). Association between heart rate variability and fluctuations in resting-state functional connectivity. *NeuroImage*, 68, 93–104. doi:10.1016/j.neuroimage.2012.11.038

Cohen, M. R., & Newsome, W. T. (2008). Context-dependent changes in functional circuitry in visual area MT. *Neuron*, 60(1). doi:10.1016/j.neuron.2008.08.007

Coste, C. P., Sadaghiani, S., Friston, K. J., Kleinschmidt, A. (2011). Ongoing brain activity fluctuations directly account for intertrial and indirectly for intersubject variability in Stroop task performance. *Cereb Cortex*, 21(11), 2612–2619. doi: 10.1093/cercor/bhr050. Epub 2011 Apr 6.

Craig, A. D. (2003). Interoception: The sense of the physiological condition of the body. *Current Opinion in Neurobiology*, 13(4), 500–505. doi:10.1016/S0959-4388(03)0090-4

Craig, A. D. (2004). Human feelings: Why are some more aware than others? *Trends in Cognitive Sciences*, 8(6), 239–241.

Craig, A. D. (2005). Forebrain emotional asymmetry: A neuroanatomical basis? *Trends in Cognitive Sciences*, 9(12), 566–571. doi:10.1016/j.tics.2005.10.005

Craig, A. D. (2009a). How do you feel—now? The anterior insula and human awareness. *Nature Reviews. Neuroscience*, 10(1), 59–70. doi: 10.1038/nrn2555

Craig, A. D. (2009b). Emotional moments across time: a possible neural basis for time perception in the anterior insula. *Philosophical Transactions of the Royal Society of London. Series B, Biological Sciences*, 364(1525), 1933–1942. doi: 10.1098/rstb.2009.0008. Review.

Craig, A. D. (2010). The sentient self. *Brain Structure & Function*, 214(5–6), 563–577. doi:10.1007/s00429-010-0248-y

Crick, F. (1995). *The astonishing hypothesis: The scientific search for the soul.* New York: Simon & Schuster.

Crick, F., & Koch, C. (2003). A framework for consciousness. *Nature Neuroscience*, 6(2), 119–26. doi:10.1038/nn0203-119

Critchley, H. D. (2005). Neural mechanisms of autonomic, affective, and cognitive integration. *Journal of Comparative Neurology*, 493(1), 154–166. doi:10.1002/cne.20749

Critchley, H. D., Rotshtein, P., Nagai, Y., O'Doherty, J., Mathias, C. J., & Dolan, R. J. (2005). Activity in the human brain predicting differential heart rate responses to emotional facial expressions. *NeuroImage*, 24(3), 751–762. doi:10.1016/j.neuroimage.2004.10.013

Critchley, H. D., Wiens, S., Rotshtein, P., Ohman, A., & Dolan, R. J. (2004). Neural systems supporting interoceptive awareness. *Nature Neuroscience*, 7(2), 189–195. doi:10.1038/nn1176

Crochet, S., Poulet, J. F. A., Kremer, Y., & Petersen, C. C. H. (2011). Synaptic mechanisms underlying sparse coding of active touch. *Neuron*, 69(1), 1160–1175. doi:10.1016/j.neuron.2011.03.017

Cromwell, H. C. & Panksepp, J. (2011). Rethinking the cognitive revolution from a neural perspective: how overuse/misuse of the term "cognition" and the neglect of affective controls in behavioral neuroscience could be delaying progress in understanding the BrainMind. *Neuroscience & Biobehavioral Reviews*, 35(9), 2026–35.

Damoiseaux, J. S., Rombouts, S. A. R. B., Barkhof, F., Scheltens, P., Stam, C. J., Smith,

S. M., & Beckmann, C. F. (2006). Consistent resting-state networks across healthy subjects. *Proceedings of the National Academy of Sciences USA*, 103(37), 13848–53. doi:10.1073/pnas.0601417103

David, S. V., Vinje, W. E., & Gallant, J. L. (2004). Natural stimulus statistics alter the receptive field structure of V1 neurons. *Journal of Neuroscience*, 24(31), 6991–7006.

Davidson, R. J. (2004). What does the prefrontal cortex "do" in affect: Perspectives on frontal EEG asymmetry research. *Biological Psychology*, 67(1–2), 219–233. doi:10.1016/j.biopsycho.2004.03.008

Davidson, R. J., Jackson, D. C., & Kalin, N. H. (2000). Emotion, plasticity, context, and regulation: Perspectives from affective neuroscience. *Psychological Bulletin*, 126(6), 890–909. doi:10.1037//0033-2909.126.6.890

Davidson, P. R., & Wolpert, D. M. (2005). Widespread access to predictive models in the motor system: a short review. *Journal of Neural Engineering*, 2(3), S313–319. Epub 2005 Aug 31. Review.

De Greck, M., Rotte, M., Paus, R., Moritz, D., Thiemann, R., Proesch, U., Bruer, U., et al. (2008). Is our self based on reward? Self-relatedness recruits neural activity in the reward system. *NeuroImage*, 39(4), 2066–75. doi:10.1016/j.neuroimage.2007.11.006

De Greck, M., Enzi, B., Prösch, U., Gantman, A., Tempelmann, C., & Northoff, G. (2010). Decreased neuronal activity in reward circuitry of pathological gamblers during processing of personal relevant stimuli. *Human Brain Mapping*, 31(11), 1802–12. doi:10.1002/hbm.20981

De Greck, M., Scheidt, L., Bölter, A. F., Frommer, J., Ulrich, C., Stockum, E., Enzi, B., et al. (2011). Multimodal psychodynamic psychotherapy induces normalization of reward related activity in somatoform disorder. *World Journal of Biological Psychiatry*, 12(4), 296–308. doi:10.3109/15622975.2010.539269

De Greck, M., Wang, G., Yang, X., Wang, X., Northoff, G., & Han, S. (2012). Neural substrates underlying intentional empathy. *Social Cognitive & Affective Neuroscience*, 7(2), 135–44. doi:10.1093/scan/nsq093

De Olmos, J. S., & Heimer, L. (1999). The concepts of the ventral striatopallidal system and extended amygdala. *Annals of the New York Academy of Science*, 877, 1–32.

DeCharms, R. C. & Zador, A. (2000). Neural representation and the cortical code. *Annual Review of Neuroscience*, 23, 613–47.

Deco, G., & Corbetta, M. (2011). The dynamical balance of the brain at rest. *Neuroscientist*, 17(1), 107–123. doi:10.1177/1073858409354384

Deco, G., & Jirsa, V. K. (2012). Ongoing cortical activity at rest: Criticality, multistability, and ghost attractors. *Journal of Neuroscience*, 32(10), 3366–3375.

Deco, G., & Romo, R. (2008). The role of fluctuations in perception. *Trends in Neurosciences*, 31(11), 591–598. doi:10.1016/j.tins.2008.08.007

Deco, G., Jirsa, V. K., & McIntosh, A. R. (2011). Emerging concepts for the dynamical organization of resting-state activity in the brain. *Nature Reviews Neuroscience*, 12(1), 43–56. doi:10.1038/nrn2961

Deco, G., Jirsa, V., McIntosh, A. R., Sporns, O., & Koetter, R. (2009). Key role of coupling, delay, and noise in resting brain fluctuations. *Proceedings of the National Academy of Sciences USA*, 106(25), 10302–10307. doi:10.1073/pnas.0901831106

Deco, G., Rolls, E. T., & Romo, R. (2010). Synaptic dynamics and decision making. *Proceedings of the National Academy of Sciences USA*, 107(16), 7545–9. doi:10.1073/pnas.1002333107

Deco, G., Rolls, E., Albantakis, L., & Romo, R. (2013). Brain mechanisms for perceptual and reward-related decision-making.*Progress in Neurobiology*, 103, 194–213. doi: 10.1016/j.pneurobio.2012.01.010. Epub 2012 Feb 2.

Dehaene, S., & Changeux, J.-P. (2005). Ongoing spontaneous activity controls access to consciousness: a neuronal model for inattentional blindness. *PLoS Biology*, 3(5), e141. doi:10.1371/journal.pbio.0030141

Dehaene, S., & Changeux, J.-P. (2011). Experimental and theoretical approaches to conscious processing. *Neuron*, 70(2), 200–27. doi:10.1016/j.neuron.2011.03.018

Dehaene, S., Changeux, J.-P., Naccache, L., Sackur, J., & Sergent, C. (2006). Conscious, preconscious, and subliminal processing: a testable taxonomy. *Trends in Cognitive Sciences*, 10(5), 204–11. doi:10.1016/j.tics.2006.03.007

DeWeese, M. R., Wehr, M., & Zador, A. M. (2003). Binary spiking in auditory cortex. *Journal of Neuroscience*, 23(21), 7940–9.

Diaz-Quesada, M., & Maravall, M. (2008). Intrinsic mechanisms for adaptive gain rescaling in barrel cortex. *Journal of Neuroscience*, 28(3), 696–710. doi:10.1523/JNEUROSCI.4931-07.2008

Duncan, N. W., & Northoff, G. (2013). Overview of potential procedural and participant-related confounds for neuroimaging of the resting state. *Journal of Psychiatry & Neuroscience: JPN*, 38(2), 84–96. doi:10.1503/jpn.120059

Duncan, N. W., Enzi, B., Wiebking, C., & Northoff, G. (2011). Involvement of glutamate in rest-stimulus interaction between perigenual and supragenual anterior cingulate cortex: a combined fMRI-MRS study. *Human Brain Mapping*, 32(12), 2172–82. doi:10.1002/hbm.21179

Duncan, N. W., Wiebking, C., Tiret, B., Marjańska, M., Hayes, D. J., Lyttleton, O., Doyon, J., & Northoff, G. (2013). Glutamate concentration in the medial prefrontal cortex predicts resting-state cortical-subcortical functional connectivity in humans. *PLoS One*, 8(4), e60312. doi: 10.1371/journal.pone.0060312. Epub 2013 Apr 3.

Duncan, N. W., Sherrif, O., Northoff, G. (2013). Resting state and reward - a meta-analysis (in press). *PLoS One*.

Edelman, G. M. (2003). Naturalizing consciousness: a theoretical framework. *Proceedings of the National Academy of Sciences USA*, 100(9), 5520–5524. doi:10.1073/pnas.0931349100

Egner, T., Monti, J. M., & Summerfield, C. (2010). Expectation and surprise determine neural population responses in the ventral visual stream. *Journal of Neuroscience*, 30(49), 16601–16608. doi:10.1523/JNEUROSCI.2770-10.2010

Engel, A. K., & Singer, W. (2001). Temporal binding and the neural correlates of sensory awareness. *Trends in Cognitive Sciences*, 5(1), 16–25.

Engelmann, J. B., & Hein, G. (2013). Contextual and social influences on valuation and choice. *Progress in Brain Research*, 202, 215–237. doi: 10.1016/B978-0-444-62604-2.00013-7

Enzi, B., Duncan, N. W., Kaufmann, J., Tempelmann, C., Wiebking, C., & Northoff, G. (2012). Glutamate modulates resting state activity in the perigenual anterior cingulate cortex—a combined fMRI-MRS study. *Neuroscience*, 227, 102–109. doi:10.1016/j.neuroscience.2012.09.039

Enzi, Bjoern, Doering, S., Faber, C., Hinrichs, J., Bahmer, J., & Northoff, G. (2013). Reduced deactivation in reward circuitry and midline structures during emotion processing in borderline personality disorder. *World Journal of Biological Psychiatry*, 14(1), 45–56. doi:10.3109/15622975.2011.579162

Enzi, Björn, De Greck, M., Prösch, U., Tempelmann, C., & Northoff, G. (2009). Is our self nothing but reward? Neuronal overlap and distinction between reward and personal relevance and its relation to human personality. *PloS One*, 4(12), e8429. doi:10.1371/journal.pone.0008429

Erk, S., Spitzer, M., Wunderlich, A. P., Galley, L., & Walter, H. (2002). Cultural objects modulate reward circuitry. *Neuroreport*, 13(18), 2499–2503. doi:10.1097/01.wnr.0000048542.12213.60

Eryilmaz, H., Van De Ville, D., Schwartz, S., & Vuilleumier, P. (2011). Impact of transient emotions on functional connectivity during subsequent resting state: A wavelet correlation approach. *NeuroImage*, 54(3), 2481–2491. doi:10.1016/j.neuroimage.2010.10.021 ER

Faisal, A. A., Selen, L. P. J., & Wolpert, D. M. (2008). Noise in the nervous system. *Nature Reviews Neuroscience*, 9(4), 292–303. doi:10.1038/nrn2258

Fan, Y., Wonneberger, C., Enzi, B., De Greck, M., Ulrich, C., Tempelmann, C., Bogerts, B., et al. (2011). The narcissistic self and its psychological and neural correlates: an exploratory fMRI study. *Psychological Medicine*, 41(8), 1641–1650. doi:10.1017/S003329171000228X

Farb, N., Segal, Z., & Anderson, A. (2012). Attentional modulation of primary interoceptive and exteroceptive cortices. *Cerebral Cortex*. ePub ahead of print.

Fehr, E., & Camerer, C. F. (2007). Social neuroeconomics: the neural circuitry of social preferences. *Trends in Cognitive Sciences*, 11(10), 419–427. Epub 2007 Oct 2. Review.

Feinberg, I., & Guazzelli, M. (1999). Schizophrenia—a disorder of the corollary discharge systems that integrate the motor systems of thought with the sensory systems of consciousness. *British Journal of Psychiatry*, 174, 196–204.

Feinberg, T. E. (2009). *From axons to identity: Neurological explorations of the nature of the self (Norton Series on Interpersonal Neurobiology)*. New York: W. W. Norton & Company.

Feinberg, T. E. (2011). The nested neural hierarchy and the self. *Consciousness & Cognition*, 20(1), 4–15. doi:10.1016/j.concog.2010.09.016

Feinberg, T. E., Keenan, J. P. (2005) (Eds). *The lost self. Pathologies of Brain and Identity.* Oxford, New York: Oxford University Press.

Feinberg, T. E., Venneri, A., Simone, A. M., Fan, Y., & Northoff, G. (2010). The neuroanatomy of asomatognosia and somatoparaphrenia. *Journal of Neurology, Neurosurgery & Psychiatry*, 81(3), 276–281. doi:10.1136/jnnp.2009.188946

Fell, J., & Axmacher, N. (2011). The role of phase synchronization in memory processes. *Nature Reviews Neuroscience*, 12(2). doi:10.1038/nrn2979

Fiete, I. R., Hahnloser, R. H. R., Fee, M. S., & Seung, H. S. (2004). Temporal sparseness of the premotor drive is important for rapid learning in a neural network model of birdsong. *Journal of Neurophysiology*, 92(4), 2274–82. doi:10.1152/jn.01133.2003

Fingelkurts, A. A., & Fingelkurts, A. A. (2011). Persistent operational synchrony within brain default-mode network and self-processing operations in healthy subjects. *Brain & Cognition*, 75(2). doi:10.1016/j.bandc.2010.11.015

Fingelkurts, A. A., Fingelkurts, A. A., & Kahkonen, S. (2005). Functional connectivity in the brain—is it an elusive concept? *Neuroscience & Biobehavioral Reviews*, 28(8), 827–836. doi:10.1016/j.neubiorev.2004.10.009

Fingelkurts, A. A., Fingelkurts, A. A., & Marchetti, G. (2010a). Brain, mind and language functional architectures. *Open Neuroimaging Journal*, 4, 26–29.

Fingelkurts, A. A., Fingelkurts, A. A., & Neves, C. E. H. (2010b). Natural world physical, brain operational, and mind phenomenal space-time. *Physics of Life Reviews*, 7(2), 195–249. doi:10.1016/j.plrev.2010.04.001

Fingelkurts, A. A., Fingelkurts, A. A., Kivisaari, R., Pekkonen, E., Ilmoniemi, R. J., & Kahkonen, S. (2004a). Enhancement of GABA-related signalling is associated with increase of functional connectivity in human cortex. *Human Brain Mapping*, 22(1), 27–39. doi:10.1002/hbm.20014

Fingelkurts, A. A., Fingelkurts, A. A., Kivisaari, R., Pekkonen, E., Ilmoniemi, R. J., & Kahkonen, S. (2004b). The interplay of lorazepam-induced brain oscillations: Microstructural electromagnetic study. *Clinical Neurophysiology*, 115(3), 674–690. doi:10.1016/j.clinph.2003.10.025

Fingelkurts, A. A., Fingelkurts, A. A., Kivisaari, R., Pekkonen, E., Ilmoniemi, R. J., & Kahkonen, S. (2004c). Local and remote functional connectivity of neocortex under the inhibition influence. *NeuroImage*, 22(3), 1390–1406. doi:10.1016/j.neuroimage.2004.03.013

Fingelkurts, Alexander A, Fingelkurts, A. A., Bagnato, S., Boccagni, C., & Galardi, G. (2011). Life or death: Prognostic value of a resting EEG with regards to survival in patients in vegetative and minimally conscious States. *PloS One*, 6(10), e25967. doi:10.1371/journal.pone.0025967

Fingelkurts, Andrew A, & Fingelkurts, A. A. (2011). Persistent operational synchrony within brain default-mode network and self-processing operations in healthy subjects. *Brain & Cognition*, 75(2), 79–90. doi:10.1016/j.bandc.2010.11.015

Fingelkurts, Andrew A, Fingelkurts, A. A., & Neves, C. F. H. (2010). Natural world physical, brain operational, and mind phenomenal space-time. *Physics of Life Reviews*, 7(2), 195–249. doi:10.1016/j.plrev.2010.04.001

Fingelkurts, Andrew A, Fingelkurts, A. A., Kivisaari, R., Pekkonen, E., Ilmoniemi, R. J., & Kähkönen, S. (2004). Local and remote functional connectivity of neocortex under the inhibition influence. *NeuroImage*, 22(3), 1390–406. doi:10.1016/j.neuroimage.2004.03.013

Fiorillo, C. D., Newsome, W. T., & Schultz, W. (2008). The temporal precision of reward prediction in dopamine neurons. *Nature Neuroscience*, 11(8), 966–973. doi:10.1038/nn.2159

Fiser, J., Chiu, C. Y., & Weliky, M. (2004). Small modulation of ongoing cortical dynamics by sensory input during natural vision. *Nature*, 431(7008), 573–578. doi:10.1038/nature02907

Fliessbach, K., Weber, B., Trautner, P., Dohmen, T., Sunde, U.,... Falk, A. (2007). Social comparison affects reward-related brain activity in the human ventral striatum. *Science*. 318(5854), 1305–1308.

Fox, M. D., & Raichle, M. E. (2007). Spontaneous fluctuations in brain activity observed with functional magnetic resonance imaging. *Nature Reviews Neuroscience*, 8(9), 700–711.

Fox, M. D., Snyder, A. Z., Vincent, J. L., Corbetta, M., Van Essen, D. C., & Raichle, M. E. (2005). The human brain is intrinsically organized into dynamic, anticorrelated functional networks. *Proceedings of the National Academy of Sciences USA*, 102(27), 9673–9678. doi:10.1073/pnas.0504136102

Fox, M. D., Snyder, A. Z., Zacks, J. M., & Raichle, M. E. (2006). Coherent spontaneous activity accounts for trial-to-trial variability in human evoked brain responses. *Nature Neuroscience*, 9(1), 23–25. doi:10.1038/nn1616

Francis, A., Fink, M., Appiani, F., Bertelsen, A., Bolwig, T. G., Bräunig, P., Caroff, S. N., et al.

(2010). Catatonia in *Diagnostic and Statistical Manual of Mental Disorders, Fifth Edition. The Journal of ECT*, 26(4), 246–247. doi:10.1097/YCT.0b013e3181fe28bd

Fransson, P. (2005). Spontaneous low-frequency BOLD signal fluctuations: an fMRI investigation of the resting-state default mode of brain function hypothesis. *Human Brain Mapping*, 26(1), 15–29. doi:10.1002/hbm.20113

Freeman, W. J. (2003). The wave packet: an action potential for the 21st century. *Journal of Integrative Neuroscience*, 2(1), 3–30. Retrieved from http://www.ncbi.nlm.nih.gov/pubmed/15011274.

Freeman, W. J. (2007). Indirect biological measures of consciousness from field studies of brains as dynamical systems. *Neural Networks*, 20(9), 1021–1031. doi:10.1016/j.neunet.2007.09.004

Freeman, W. J. (2011). Understanding perception through neural "codes". *IEEE Transactions on Bio-Medical Engineering*, 58(7), 1884–1890. doi:10.1109/TBME.2010.2095854

Freeman, W. J., Burke, B. C., & Holmes, M. D. (2003). Aperiodic phase re-setting in scalp EEG of beta-gamma oscillations by state transitions at alpha-theta rates. *Human Brain Mapping*, 19(4), 248–272. doi:10.1002/hbm.10120

Freiwald, W. A., Tsao, D. Y., & Livingstone, M. S. (2009). A face feature space in the macaque temporal lobe. *Nature Neuroscience*, 12(9), 1187–96. doi:10.1038/nn.2363

Friedlander, T., & Brenner, N. (2009). Adaptive response by state-dependent inactivation. *Proceedings of the National Academy of Sciences USA*, 106(52). 22558-22563. doi:10.1073/pnas.0902146106

Fries, P., Reynolds, J. H., Rorie, A. E., & Desimone, R. (2001). Modulation of oscillatory neuronal synchronization by selective visual attention. *Science* (New York), 291(5508), 1560–3. doi:10.1126/science.291.5508.1560

Fries, P. (2005). A mechanism for cognitive dynamics: Neuronal communication through neuronal coherence. *Trends in Cognitive Sciences*, 9(10), 474–480. doi:10.1016/j.tics.2005.08.011

Fries, P. (2009). Neuronal gamma-band synchronization as a fundamental process in cortical computation. *Annual Review of Neuroscience*, 32, 209–224. doi:10.1146/annurev.neuro.051508.135603

Fries, P., Nikolic, D., & Singer, W. (2007). The gamma cycle. *Trends in Neurosciences*, 30(7), 309–316. doi:10.1016/j.tins.2007.05.005

Fries, P., Reynolds, J. H., Rorie, A. E., & Desimone, R. (2001). Modulation of oscillatory neuronal synchronization by selective visual attention. *Science*, 291(5508), 1560–1563.

Fries, P. (2005). A mechanism for cognitive dynamics: Neuronal communication through neuronal coherence. *Trends in Cognitive Sciences*, 9(10), 474–480. doi:10.1016/j.tics.2005.08.011

Friston K. J. & Dolan R. J. (2010). Computational and dynamic models in neuroimaging. *NeuroImage*, 52(3), 752–765.

Friston, K. J. (1997). Another neural code? *NeuroImage*, 5(3), 213–220.

Friston, K. J. (2000). The labile brain. I. Neuronal transients and nonlinear coupling. *Philosophical Transactions of the Royal Society of London, Series B: Biological Sciences.*, 355(1394), 215–236.

Friston, K. J. (1995). Neuronal transients. *Proceedings. Biological Sciences/the Royal Society*, 261(1362), 401–405. doi:10.1098/rspb.1995.0166

Friston, K. (2010). The free-energy principle: a unified brain theory? *Nature Reviews. Neuroscience*, 11(2), 127–138. doi: 10.1038/nrn2787. Epub 2010 Jan 13. Review.

Friston, K. J. (2011). Functional and effective connectivity: a review. *Brain and Cognition*, 1(1), 13–36. doi: 10.1089/brain.2011.0008. Review.

Frith, C. D., & Frith, U. (1999). Interacting minds—a biological basis. *Science*, 286(5445), 1692–1695. Review.

Fukushima, M., Saunders, R. C., Leopold, D. A., Mishkin, M., & Averbeck, B. B. (2012). Spontaneous high-gamma band activity reflects functional organization of auditory cortex in the awake macaque. *Neuron*, 74(5), 899–910. doi:10.1016/j.neuron.2012.04.014

Gaetz, W., Edgar, J., Wang, D., & Roberts, T. (2011). Relating MEG measured motor cortical oscillations to resting γ-aminobutyric acid (GABA). concentration. *NeuroImage*, 55(2), 616–621.

Gallese, V., Goldman, A. (1998). Mirror neurons and the simulation theory of mind-reading. *Trends in Cognitive Sciences*, 2(12), 493–501.

Garrett, D. D., Kovacevic, N., McIntosh, A. R., & Grady, C. L. (2010). Blood oxygen level-dependent signal variability is more than just noise. *Journal of Neuroscience*, 30(14), 4914–4921.

Garrett, D. D., Kovacevic, N., McIntosh, A. R., & Grady, C. L. (2011). The importance of being variable. *Journal of Neuroscience*, 31(12), 4496–4503.

Garrido, M. I., Kilner, J. M., Stephan, K. E., & Friston, K. J. (2009). The mismatch negativity: A review of underlying mechanisms. *Clinical Neurophysiology*, 120(3), 453–463. doi:10.1016/j.clinph.2008.11.029

Georgopoulos, A. P., Schwartz, A. B., & Kettner, R. E. (1986). Neuronal population coding of movement direction. *Science*, 233(4771), 1416–1419.

Georgopoulos, A. P., Lurito, J. T., Petrides, M., Schwartz, A. B., & Massey, J. T. (1989). Mental rotation of the neuronal population vector. *Science*, 243(4888), 234–236.

Ghosh, A., Rho, Y., McIntosh, A. R., Kotter, R., & Jirsa, V. K. (2008). Cortical network dynamics with time delays reveals functional connectivity in the resting brain. *Cognitive Neurodynamics*, 2(2), 115–120. doi:10.1007/s11571-008-9044-2 :

Glimcher, P. W. (2011). Understanding dopamine and reinforcement learning: The dopamine reward prediction error hypothesis. *Proceedings of the National Academy of Sciences USA*, 108(42), 17568–17569. doi:10.1073/pnas.1114363108

Goense, J., Merkle, H., & Logothetis, N. K. (2012). High-resolution fMRI reveals laminar differences in neurovascular coupling between positive and negative BOLD responses. *Neuron*, 76(3), 629–639. doi:10.1016/j.neuron.2012.09.019

Goldstein, K. (2000). *The organism. A holistic approach to biology derived from pathological data in men*. New York: Zone Books.

Gonzalez-Castillo, J., Saad, Z. S., Handwerker, D. A., Inati, S. J., Brenowitz, N., & Bandettini, P. A. (2012). Whole-brain, time-locked activation with simple tasks revealed using massive averaging and model-free analysis. *Proceedings of the National Academy of Sciences USA*, 109(14), 5487–92. doi:10.1073/pnas.1121049109

Ghosh, A., Rho, Y., McIntosh, A. R., Kötter, R., & Jirsa, V. K. (2008a). Cortical network dynamics with time delays reveals functional connectivity in the resting brain. *Cognitive Neurodynamics*, 2(2), 115–120. doi: 10.1007/s11571-008-9044-2. Epub 2008 Apr 23.

Ghosh, A., Rho, Y., McIntosh, A. R., Kötter, R., & Jirsa, V. K. (2008b). Noise during rest enables the exploration of the brain's dynamic repertoire. *PLoS Computational Biology*, 4(10), e1000196. doi: 10.1371/journal.pcbi.1000196. Epub 2008 Oct 10.

Grammont, F., & Riehle, A. (2003). Spike synchronization and firing rate in a population of motor cortical neurons in relation to movement direction and reaction time. *Biological Cybernetics*, 88(5), 360–373. doi:10.1007/s00422-002-0385-3

Gray, J. A. (1995). Dopamine release in the nucleus-accumbens—the perspective from aberrations of consciousness in schizophrenia. *Neuropsychologia*, 33(9). doi:10.1016/0028-3932(95)00054-7

Greene, G., Barrett, D. G. T., Sen, K., & Houghton, C. (2009). Sparse coding of birdsong and receptive field structure in songbirds. *Network* (Bristol, England), 20(3), 162–77. doi:10.1080/09548980903108267

Greicius, M. D., & Menon, V. (2004). Default-mode activity during a passive sensory task: Uncoupled from deactivation but impacting activation. *Journal of Cognitive Neuroscience*, 16(9), 1484–1492.

Greicius, M. D., Krasnow, B., Reiss, A. L., & Menon, V. (2003). Functional connectivity in the resting brain: A network analysis of the default mode hypothesis. *Proceedings of the National Academy of Sciences USA*, 100(1), 253–258. doi:10.1073/pnas.0135058100

Greicius, M. D., Srivastava, G., Reiss, A. L., & Menon, V. (2004). Default-mode network activity distinguishes Alzheimer's disease from healthy aging: Evidence from functional MRI. *Proceedings of the National Academy of Sciences USA*, 101(13), 4637–42. doi:10.1073/pnas.0308627101

Greicius, M. D., Supekar, K., Menon, V., & Dougherty, R. F. (2009). Resting-state functional connectivity reflects structural connectivity in the default mode network. *Cerebral Cortex*, 19(1), 72–78. doi:10.1093/cercor/bhn059

Grimm, S., Beck, J., Schuepbach, D., Hell, D., Boesiger, P., Bermpohl, F.,... Northoff, G. (2008). Imbalance between left and right dorsolateral prefrontal cortex in major depression is linked to negative emotional judgment: An fMRI study in severe major depressive disorder. *Biological Psychiatry*, 63(4), 369–376. doi:10.1016/j.biopsych.2007.05.033

Grimm, S., Ernst, J., Boesiger, P., Schuepbach, D., Hell, D., Boeker, H., & Northoff, G. (2009). Increased self-focus in major depressive disorder is related to neural abnormalities in subcortical-cortical midline structures. *Human Brain Mapping*, 30(8), 2617–27. doi:10.1002/hbm.20693

Grimm, S., Schmidt, C. F., Bermpohl, F., Heinzel, A., Dahlem, Y., Wyss, M., Hell, D., et al. (2006). Segregated neural representation of distinct emotion dimensions in the prefrontal cortex-an fMRI study. *NeuroImage*, 30(1), 325–40. doi:10.1016/j.neuroimage.2005.09.006

Guillen, B., Paredes, J. L., & Medina, R. (2011). A sparse based approach for detecting activations in fMRI. *Conf Proc IEEE Eng Med Biol Soc*. 2011, 7816–7819. doi: 10.1109/IEMBS.2011.6091926.

Gusnard, D. A., & Raichle, M. E. (2001). Searching for a baseline: Functional imaging and the resting human brain. *Nature Reviews Neuroscience*, 2(10), 685–694.

Hagmann, P., Cammoun, L., Gigandet, X., Gerhard, S., Grant, P. E., Wedeen, V., . . . Sporns, O. (2010). MR connectomics: Principles and challenges. *Journal of Neuroscience Methods*, 194(1), 34–35. doi:10.1016/j.jneumeth.2010.01.014

Hagmann, P., Cammoun, L., Gigandet, X., Meuli, R., Honey, C. J., Wedeen, V. J., & Sporns, O. (2008). Mapping the structural core of human cerebral cortex. *PloS Biology*, 6(7), 1479–1493. doi:10.1371/journal.pbio.0060159

Haider, B., Krause, M. R., Duque, A., Yu, Y., Touryan, J., . . . McCormick, D. A. (2010). Synaptic and network mechanisms of sparse and reliable visual cortical activity during non-classical receptive field stimulation. *Neuron*, 65(1), 107–121.

Hampton, A. N., Bossaerts, P., & O'Doherty, J. P. (2008). Neural correlates of mentalizing-related computations during strategic interactions in humans. *Proceedings of the National Academy of Sciences of the United States of America*, 105(18), 6741–6746. doi: 10.1073/pnas.0711099105. Epub 2008 Apr 21.

Han, F., Caporale, N., & Dan, Y. (2008). Reverberation of recent visual experience in spontaneous cortical waves. *Neuron*, 60(2), 321–327. doi:10.1016/j.neuron.2008.08.026

Han, S., & Northoff, G. (2008). Culture-sensitive neural substrates of human cognition: A transcultural neuroimaging approach. Nature reviews. *Neuroscience*, 9(8), 646–54. doi:10.1038/nrn2456

Han, S., & Northoff, G. (2009). Understanding the self: A cultural neuroscience approach. *Progress in Brain Research*, 178, 203–12. doi:10.1016/S0079-6123(09)17814-7

Hare, T. A., O'Doherty, J., Camerer, C. F., Schultz, W., & Rangel, A. (2008). Dissociating the role of the orbitofrontal cortex and the striatum in the computation of goal values and prediction errors. *Journal of Neuroscience*, 28(22). doi:10.1523/JNEUROSCI.1309-08.2008

Haynes, J.-D. (2009). Decoding visual consciousness from human brain signals. *Trends in Cognitive Sciences*, 13(5), 194–202. doi:10.1016/j.tics.2009.02.004

Haynes, J. D. (2011). Decoding and predicting intentions. *Annals of the New York Academy of Sciences*, 1224, 9–21. doi: 10.1111/j.1749-6632.2011.05994.x

He, B. J., & Raichle, M. E. (2009). The fMRI signal, slow cortical potential and consciousness. *Trends in Cognitive Sciences*, 13(7), 302–309. doi:10.1016/j.tics.2009.04.004

Heekeren, H. R., Marrett, S., & Ungerleider, L. G. (2008). The neural systems that mediate human perceptual decision making. *Nature Reviews Neuroscience*, 9(6), 467–79. doi:10.1038/nrn2374

Heekeren, H. R., Marrett, S., Bandettini, P. A., & Ungerleider, L. G. (2004). A general mechanism for perceptual decision-making in the human brain. *Nature*, 431(7010), 859–862.

Heimer, L. (2003). A new anatomical framework for neuropsychiatric disorders and drug abuse. *American Journal of Psychiatry*, 160(10), 1726–1739.

Heinzel, A., Schäfer, R., Müller, H.-W., Schieffer, A., Ingenhag, A., Northoff, G., Franz, M., et al. (2010). Differential modulation of valence and arousal in high-alexithymic and low-alexithymic individuals. *Neuroreport*, 21(15), 998–1002. doi:10.1097/WNR.0b013e32833f38e0

Heinzel, A., Steinke, R., Poeppel, T. D., Grosser, O., Bogerts, B., Otto, H., & Northoff, G. (2008). S-ketamine and GABA-A-receptor interaction in humans: an exploratory study with I-123-iomazenil SPECT. *Human Psychopharmacology*, 23(7), 549–54. doi:10.1002/hup.960

Hesselmann, G., Kell, C. A., & Kleinschmidt, A. (2008). Ongoing activity fluctuations in hMT+ bias the perception of coherent visual motion. *Journal of Neuroscience*, 28(53), 14481–5.

Hesselmann, G., Kell, C. A., Eger, E., & Kleinschmidt, A. (2008). Spontaneous local variations in ongoing neural activity bias perceptual decisions. *Proceedings of the National*

Academy of Sciences USA, 105(31), 10984–9. doi:10.1073/pnas.0712043105

Honey, C. J., Sporns, O., Cammoun, L., Gigandet, X., Thiran, J. P., Meuli, R., & Hagmann, P. (2009). Predicting human resting-state functional connectivity from structural connectivity. *Proceedings of the National Academy of Sciences USA*, 106(6), 2035–2040. doi:10.1073/pnas.0811168106

Honey, C. J., Thivierge, J., & Sporns, O. (2010). Can structure predict function in the human brain? *NeuroImage*, 52(3), 766–776. doi:10.1016/j.neuroimage.2010.01.071

Hromádka, T., Deweese, M. R., & Zador, A. M. (2008). Sparse representation of sounds in the unanesthetized auditory cortex. *PLoS Biology*, 6(1), e16. doi:10.1371/journal.pbio.0060016

Hunter, M. D., Eickhoff, S. B., Miller, T. W. R., Farrow, T. F. D., Wilkinson, I. D., & Woodruff, P. W. R. (2006). Neural activity in speech-sensitive auditory cortex during silence. *Proceedings of the National Academy of Sciences USA*, 103(1), 189–94. doi:10.1073/pnas.0506268103

Huth, A. G., Nishimoto, S., Vu, A. T., & Gallant, J. L. (2012). A continuous semantic space describes the representation of thousands of object and action categories across the human brain. *Neuron*, 76(6), 1210–1224. doi:10.1016/j.neuron.2012.10.014

Hyder, F., Patel, A. B., Gjedde, A., Rothman, D. L., Behar, K. L., & Shulman, R. G. (2006). Neuronal-glial glucose oxidation and glutamatergic-GABAergic function. *Journal of Cerebral Blood Flow and Metabolism*, 26(7), 865–877. doi:10.1038/sj.jcbfm.9600263

Jacob, S. N., Vallentin, D., & Nieder, A. (2012). Relating magnitudes: The brain's code for proportions. *Trends in Cognitive Sciences*, 16(3).157–166,doi:10.1016/j.tics.2012.02.002

Jadhav, S. P., Wolfe, J., & Feldman, D. E. (2009). Sparse temporal coding of elementary tactile features during active whisker sensation. *Nature Neuroscience*, 12(6), 792–800. doi:10.1038/nn.2328

Jao, T., Vértes, P. E., Alexander-Bloch, A. F., Tang, I.-N., Yu, Y.-C., Chen, J.-H., & Bullmore, E. T. (2013). Volitional eyes opening perturbs brain dynamics and functional connectivity regardless of light input. *NeuroImage*, 69, 21–34. doi:10.1016/j.neuroimage.2012.12.007

Jaramillo, M., Paavilainen, P., & Naatanen, R. (2000). Mismatch negativity and behavioural discrimination in humans as a function of the magnitude of change in sound duration. *Neuroscience Letters*, 290(2), 101–104.

Jocham, G., Hunt, L. T, Near, J., & Behrens, T. E. (2012). A mechanism for value-guided choice based on the excitation-inhibition balance in prefrontal cortex. *Nature Neuroscience*, 15(7), 960–961. doi: 10.1038/nn.3140.

John, E. R. (2006). The sometimes pernicious role of theory in science. International *Journal of Psychophysiology*, 62(3), 377–383. doi:10.1016/j.ijpsycho.2006.01.007

Jortner, R. A., Farivar, S. S., & Laurent, G. (2007). A simple connectivity scheme for sparse coding in an olfactory system. *Journal of Neuroscience*, 27(7), 1659–1669. doi:10.1523/JNEUROSCI.4171-06.2007

Kant, I. (1998). *Critique of pure reason*. Translated by P.Guyer. Cambridge University Press, Cambridge/UK.

Kapfer, C., Glickfeld, L. L., Atallah, B. V, & Scanziani, M. (2007). Supralinear increase of recurrent inhibition during sparse activity in the somatosensory cortex. *Nature Neuroscience*, 10(6), 743–753. doi:10.1038/nn1909

Kapogiannis, D., Reiter, D. A., Willette, A. A., & Mattson, M. P. (2013). Posteromedial cortex glutamate and GABA predict intrinsic functional connectivity of the default mode network. *NeuroImage*, 64, 112–119. doi:10.1016/j.neuroimage.2012.09.029

Kay, K. N., Naselaris, T., Prenger, R. J., & Gallant, J. L. (2008). Identifying natural images from human brain activity. *Nature*, 452(7185). doi:10.1038/nature06713

Kayser, C. (2009). Phase resetting as a mechanism for supramodal attentional control. *Neuron*, 64(3). doi:10.1016/j.neuron.2009.10.022

Kayser, C. (2010). The multisensory nature of unisensory cortices: A puzzle continued. *Neuron*, 67(2). doi:10.1016/j.neuron.2010.07.012

Kayser, C., & Logothetis, N. K. (2007). Do early sensory cortices integrate cross-modal information? *Brain Structure & Function*, 212(2), 121–132. doi:10.1007/s00429-007-0154-0

Kayser, C., & Remedios, R. (2012). Suppressive competition: how sounds may cheat sight. *Neuron*, 73(4), 627–629. doi:10.1016/j.neuron.2012.02.001

Kayser, C., Petkov, C. I., & Logothetis, N. K. (2008). Visual modulation of neurons in auditory cortex. *Cerebral Cortex*, 18(7). doi:10.1093/cercor/bhm187

Kayser, C., Petkov, C. I., & Logothetis, N. K. (2009). Multisensory interactions in primate auditory cortex: FMRI and electrophysiology. *Hearing Research*, 258(1–2), 80–88. doi:10.1016/j.heares.2009.02.011

Kayser, C., Petkov, C. I., Augath, M., & Logothetis, N. K. (2005). Integration of touch and sound in auditory cortex. *Neuron*, 48(2), 373–384. doi:10.1016/j.neuron.2005.09.018

Kayser, C., Petkov, C., Remedios, R., & Logothetis, N. (2012). Multisensory influences on auditory processing: Perspectives from fMRI and electrophysiology. In M. M. Murray & M. T. Wallace (Eds.), *The neural bases of multisensory processes* (pp. 143–156). Boca Raton, FL: CRC Press.

Kenet, T., Bibitchkov, D., Tsodyks, M., Grinvald, A., & Arieli, A. (2003). Spontaneously emerging cortical representations of visual attributes. *Nature*, 425(6961), 954–956. doi:10.1038/nature02078

Khader, P., Schicke, T., Röder, B., & Rösler, F. (2008). On the relationship between slow cortical potentials and BOLD signal changes in humans. *International Journal of Psychophysiology*, 67(3), 252–261. doi:10.1016/j.ijpsycho.2007.05.018

Kilner, J. M., Friston, K. J., & Frith, C. D. (2007a). Predictive coding: an account of the mirror neuron system. *Cognitive Processing*, 8(3), 159–166. Epub 2007 Apr 12. Review.

Kilner, J. M., Friston, K. J., & Frith, C. D. (2007b). The mirror-neuron system: a Bayesian perspective. *Neuroreport*, 18(6), 619–623. Review.

Kirk, U., Downar, J., & Montague P. R. (2011) Interoception drives increased rational decision-making in meditators playing the ultimatum game. *Frontiers in Neuroendocrinology*, 5:49. doi: 10.3389/fnins.2011.00049.

Kim, D. I., Manoach, D. S., Mathalon, D. H., Turner, J. A., Mannell, M., Brown, G. G., et al. (2009). Dysregulation of working memory and default-mode networks in schizophrenia using independent component analysis, an fBIRN and MCIC study. *Human Brain Mapping*, 30(11), 3795–3811. doi:10.1002/hbm.20807

Kim, J. N., & Shadlen, M. N. (1999). Neural correlates of a decision in the dorsolateral prefrontal cortex of the macaque. *Nature Neuroscience*, 2(2), 176–185. doi:10.1038/5739

Kirk, U., Harvey, A., & Montague, P. R. (2012). Domain expertise insulates against judgment bias by monetary favors through a modulation of ventromedial prefrontal cortex. *Proceedings of the National Academy of Sciences USA*, 108(25), 10332–10336. doi:10.1073/pnas.1205836109

Kleinschmidt, A. (2011). Recovering the contents of consciousness in the noise of neuroimaging. *Medecine Sciences (Paris)*, 27(2), 199–203. doi:10.1051/medsci/2011272199

Kleinschmidt, A., Sterzer, P., & Rees, G. (2012). Variability of perceptual multistability: From brain state to individual trait. *Philosophical Transactions of the Royal Society of London. Series B, Biological Sciences*, 367(1591), 988–1000. doi:10.1098/rstb.2011.0367

Knutson, B., Fong, G. W., Adams, C. M., Varner, J. L., & Hommer, D. (2001). Dissociation of reward anticipation and outcome with event-related fMRI. *Neuroreport*, 12(17), 3683–3687.

Knutson, B., Fong, G. W., Bennett, S. M., Adams, C. M., & Hommer, D. (2003) A region of mesial prefrontal cortex tracks monetarily rewarding outcomes: characterization with rapid event-related fMRI. *Neuroimage*, 18(2), 263–272.

Knutson, B., Taylor, J., Kaufman, M., Peterson, R., & Glover, G. (2005). Distributed neural representation of expected value. *The Journal of Neuroscience*, 25(19), 4806–4812.

Knutson, B., Wimmer, G. E., Rick, S., Hollon, N. G., Prelec, D., & Loewenstein, G. (2008). Neural antecedents of the endowment effect. *Neuron* 58(5), 814–822. doi: 10.1016/j.neuron.2008.05.018

Koch, C. (2004). *The quest or consciousness*. Oxford University Press, Oxford, New York.

Kotz, S. A., & Schwartze, M. (2010). Cortical speech processing unplugged: a timely subcortico-cortical framework. *Trends in Cognitive Sciences*, 14(9), 392–399. doi:10.1016/j.tics.2010.06.005. Epub 2010 Jul 23.

Krebs, J. R., Kacelnik, A., & Taylor,P. (1978). Test of optimal sampling by foraging great tits. *Nature*, 275, 27–31.

Krueger, F., Grafman, J., & McCabe, K. (2008). Neural correlates of economic game playing. *Philosophical Transactions of the Royal Society B: Biological Sciences*, 363(1511). doi:10.1098/rstb.2008.0165

Kruglikov, S. Y., & Schiff, S. J. (2003). Interplay of electroencephalogram phase and auditory-evoked neural activity. *Journal of Neuroscience*, 23(31), 10122–10127.

Langner, R., Kellermann, T., Boers, F., Sturm, W., Willmes, K., & Eickhoff, S. B. (2012) Modality-specific perceptual expectations selectively modulate baseline activity in auditory, somatosensory, and visual cortices. *Cerebral Cortex*, 21(12), 2850–2862. doi: 10.1093/cercor/bhr083. Epub 2011 Apr 28.

Lakatos, P., Chen, C.-M., O'Connell, M. N., Mills, A., & Schroeder, C. E. (2007). Neuronal oscillations and multisensory interaction in primary auditory cortex. *Neuron*, 53(2), 279–292. doi:10.1016/j.neuron.2006.12.011

Lakatos, P., Karmos, G., Mehta, A. D., Ulbert, I., & Schroeder, C. E. (2008). Entrainment of neuronal oscillations as a mechanism of attentional selection. *Science* (New York), 320(5872), 110–113. doi:10.1126/science.1154735

Lakatos, P., O'Connell, M. N., Barczak, A., Mills, A., Javitt, D. C., & Schroeder, C. E. (2009). The leading sense: Supramodal control of neurophysiological context by attention. *Neuron*, 64(3), 419–430. doi:10.1016/j.neuron.2009.10.014 ER

Lakatos, P., Shah, A. S., Knuth, K. H., Ulbert, I., Karmos, G., & Schroeder, C. E. (2005). An oscillatory hierarchy controlling neuronal excitability and stimulus processing in the auditory cortex. *Journal of Neurophysiology*, 94(3), 1904–11. doi:10.1152/jn.00263.2005

Lashley, K. S. (1949). Persistent problems in the evolution of mind. *Quarterly Review of Biology*, 24(1), 28–48.

Laufs, H., Daunizeau, J., Carmichael, D. W., & Kleinschmidt, A. (2008). Recent advances in recording electrophysiological data simultaneously with magnetic resonance imaging. *NeuroImage*, 40(2), 515–528. doi:10.1016/j.neuroimage.2007.11.039

Laurent, G. (2002). Olfactory network dynamics and the coding of multidimensional signals. *Nature Reviews: Neuroscience*, 3(11), 884–895. doi:10.1038/nrn964

Lee, K., Tak, S., & Ye, J. C. (2011). A data-driven sparse GLM for fMRI analysis using sparse dictionary learning with MDL criterion. *IEEE Transactions on Medical Imaging*, 30(5), 1076–1089. doi:10.1109/TMI.2010.2097275

Lehmann, D., Pascual-Marqui, R. D., Strik, W. K., & Koenig, T. (2010). Core networks for visual-concrete and abstract thought content: A brain electric microstate analysis. *NeuroImage*, 49, 1073–1079. doi:10.1016/j.neuroimage.2009.07.054

Lehmann, D., Strik, W. K., Henggeler, B., Koenig, T., & Koukkou, M. (1998). Brain electric microstates and momentary conscious mind states as building blocks of spontaneous thinking: I. Visual imagery and abstract thoughts. *International Journal of Psychophysiology*, 29(1), 1–11. doi:10.1016/S0167-8760(97)00098-6

Lemus, L., Hernandez, A., Luna, R., Zainos, A., & Romo, R. (2010). Do sensory cortices process more than one sensory modality during perceptual judgments? *Neuron*, 67(2). doi:10.1016/j.neuron.2010.06.015

Leopold, D. A., & Maier, A. (2012). Ongoing physiological processes in the cerebral cortex. *NeuroImage*, 62(4), 2190–200. doi:10.1016/j.neuroimage.2011.10.059

Lewicki, M. S. (2002). Efficient coding of natural sounds. *Nature Neuroscience*, 5(4), 356–363. doi:10.1038/nn831

Lewis, C. M., Baldassarre, A., Committeri, G., Romani, G. L., & Corbetta, M. (2009). Learning sculpts the spontaneous activity of the resting human brain. *Proceedings of the National Academy of Sciences USA*, 106(41), 17558–17563. doi:10.1073/pnas.0902455106

Lin, S., Yu, C., & Pai, M. (2006). The occipital white matter lesions in Alzheimer's disease patients with visual hallucinations. *Clinical Imaging*, 30(6), 388–393. doi:10.1016/j.clinimag.2006.09.025

Linkenkaer-Hansen, K., Nikouline, V. V., Palva, J. M., & Ilmoniemi, R. J. (2001). Long-range temporal correlations and scaling behavior in human brain oscillations. *Journal of Neuroscience*, 21(4), 1370–1377.

Liu, X., Zhu, X., & Chen, W. (2011). Baseline BOLD correlation predicts individuals' stimulus-evoked BOLD responses. *NeuroImage*, 54(3), 2278–2286. doi:10.1016/j.neuroimage.2010.10.001

Llinás, R. (2002). *I of the vortex: From neurons to self.* Cambridge, MA: MIT.

Llinas, R. R. (1988). The intrinsic electrophysiological properties of mammalian neurons—insights into central nervous-system function. *Science*, 242(4886), 1654–1664.

Llinas, R., & Ribary, U. (2001). Consciousness and the brain—the thalamocortical dialogue in health and disease. *Annals of the New York Academy of Science*, 929, 166–175.

Llinás, R. R., & Roy, S. (2009). The "prediction imperative" as the basis for self-awareness. *Philosophical Transactions of the Royal Society of London. Series B, Biological Sciences*, 364(1521), 1301–1307. doi: 10.1098/rstb.2008.0309. Review.

Llinás, R., Ribary, U., Contreras, D., & Pedroarena, C. (1998). The neuronal basis for consciousness. *Philosophical Transactions of the Royal Society of London. Series B, Biological Sciences*, 353(1377), 1841–1849. Review.

Lloyd, D. (2011). Mind as music. *Frontiers in Psychology*, 2(63). 2–8, doi:10.3389/fpsyg.2011.00063

Logothetis, N. (2010). Perception and the brain. In: B. M. Glatzeder, V. Goel, & A. Mueller (Eds.), *Towards a theory of thinking* (pp. 161–179). New York: Springer, Heidelberg.

Logothetis, N. K. (2008). What we can do and what we cannot do with fMRI. *Nature*, 453(7197), 869–878.

Logothetis, N. K., Murayama, Y., Augath, M., Steffen, T., Werner, J., & Oeltermann, A. (2009). How not to study spontaneous activity. *NeuroImage*, 45(4), 1080–1089. doi:10.1016/j.neuroimage.2009.01.010

Lörincz, A., Palotai, Z., & Szirtes, G. (2012). Efficient sparse coding in early sensory processing: Lessons from signal recovery. *PloS Computational Biology*, 8(3), e1002372. doi:10.1371/journal.pcbi.1002372

Lörincz, M. L., Geall, F., Bao, Y., Crunelli, V., & Hughes, S. W. (2009). ATP-dependent infra-slow (< 0.1 hz). oscillations in thalamic networks. *PloS One*, 4(2), e4447. doi:10.1371/journal.pone.0004447

Lu, H., Zou, Q., Gu, H., Raichle, M. E., Stein, E. A., & Yang, Y. (2012). Rat brains also have a default mode network. *Proceedings of the National Academy of Sciences USA*, 109(10), 3979–84.. doi:10.1073/pnas.1200506109

Lurija, A. R. (1962). *Higher cortical functions in man*. Moscow University Press.

Lurija, A. R. (1973). *The working brain.,ed.* New York: Basic Books.

Lurilli, G., Ghezzi, D., Olcese, U., Lassi, G., Nazzaro, C., Tonini, R., Tucci, V., Benfenati, F., & Medini, P. (2012). Sound-driven synaptic inhibition in primary visual cortex. *Neuron*, 73(4), 814–828. doi: 10.1016/j.neuron.2011.12.026.

Lutz, A., Lachaux, J. P., Martinerie, J., & Varela, F. J. (2002). Guiding the study of brain dynamics by using first-person data: Synchrony patterns correlate with ongoing conscious states during a simple visual task. *Proceedings of the National Academy of Sciences USA*, 99(3), 1586–1591.

Maandag, N. J., Coman, D., Sanganahalli, B. G., Herman, P., Smith, A. J., Blumenfeld H., et al. (2007). Energetics of neuronal signaling and fMRI activity. *Proceedings of the National Academy of Sciences of the United States of America*, 104(51), 20546–20551. Epub 2007 Dec 13.

Makeig, S., Westerfield, M., Jung, T. P., Enghoff, S., Townsend, J., Courchesne, E., & Sejnowski, T. J. (2002). Dynamic brain sources of visual evoked responses. *Science*, 295(5555), 690–694.

Mannell, M. V., Franco, A. R., Calhoun, V. D., Canive, J. M., Thoma, R. J., & Mayer, A. R. (2010). Resting state and task-induced deactivation: A methodological comparison in patients with schizophrenia and healthy controls. *Human Brain Mapping*, 31(3), 424–437. doi:10.1002/hbm.20876

Mantini, D., Gerits, A., Nelissen, K., Durand, J., Joly, O., Simone, L., et al. (2011). Default mode of brain function in monkeys. *Journal of Neuroscience*, 31(36). doi:10.1523/JNEUROSCI.2318-11.2011

Mantini, D., Perrucci, M. G., Del Gratta, C., Romani, G. L., & Corbetta, M. (2007). Electrophysiological signatures of resting state networks in the human brain. *Proceedings of the National Academy of Sciences USA*, 104(32), 13170–13175. doi:10.1073/pnas.0700668104

Margulies, D. S., Kelly, A. M. C., Uddin, L. Q., Biswal, B. B., Castellanos, F. X., & Milham, M. P. (2007). Mapping the functional connectivity of anterior cingulate cortex. *NeuroImage*, 37(2), 579–88. doi:10.1016/j.neuroimage.2007.05.019

Margulies, D. S., Vincent, J. L., Kelly, C., Lohmann, G., Uddin, L. Q., Biswal, B. B., et al. (2009). Precuneus shares intrinsic functional architecture in humans and monkeys. *Proceedings of the National Academy of Sciences USA*, 106(47), 20069–20074. doi:10.1073/pnas.0905314106

Marx, E., Deutschlander, A., Stephan, T., Dieterich, M., Wiesmann, M., & Brandt, T. (2004). Eyes open and eyes closed as rest conditions: Impact on brain activation patterns. *NeuroImage*, 21(4), 1818–1824. doi:10.1016/j.neuroimage.2003.12.026

Mazzoni, A., Broccard, F. D., Garcia-Perez, E., Bonifazi, P., Ruaro, M. E., & Torre, V. (2007). On the dynamics of the spontaneous activity in neuronal networks. *PloS One*, 2(5), e439. doi:10.1371/journal.pone.0000439

Mazzoni, A., Panzeri, S., Logothetis, N. K., & Brunel, N. (2008). Encoding of naturalistic stimuli by local field potential spectra in networks of excitatory and inhibitory neurons. *PloS Computational Biology*, 4(12), e1000239. doi:10.1371/journal.pcbi.1000239

Mazzoni, A., Whittingstall, K., Brunel, N., Logothetis, N. K., & Panzeri, S. (2010). Understanding the relationships between spike rate and delta/gamma frequency bands of LFPs and EEGs using a local cortical network model. *NeuroImage*, 52(3). doi:10.1016/j.neuroimage.2009.12.040

McAvoy, M., Larson-Prior, L., Nolan, T. S., Vaishnavi, S. N., Raichle, M. E., & d'Avossa, G. (2008). Resting states affect spontaneous BOLD oscillations in sensory and paralimbic cortex. *Journal of Neurophysiology*, 100(2), 922–931. doi:10.1152/jn.90426.2008

McClure, S. M., Li, J., Tomlin, D., Cypert, K. S., Montague, L. M., & Montague, P. R. (2004). Neural correlates of behavioral preference for culturally familiar drinks. *Neuron*, 44(2), 379–387.

McDonnell, M. D., & Ward, L. M. (2011). The benefits of noise in neural systems: Bridging theory and experiment. Nature reviews. *Neuroscience*, 12(7), 415–26. doi:10.1038/nrn3061

McIntosh, A. R., Kovacevic, N., Lippe, S., Garrett, D., Grady, C., & Jirsa, V. (2010). The development of a noisy brain. *Archives italiennes de biologie*, 148(3), 323–37.

Mennes, M., Kelly, C., Zuo, X., Di Martino, A., Biswal, B. B., Castellanos, F. X., & Milham, M. P. (2010). Inter-individual differences in resting-state functional connectivity predict task-induced BOLD activity. *NeuroImage*, 50(4), 1690–1701.

Mennes, M., Zuo, X., Kelly, C., Di Martino, A., Zang, Y., Biswal, B., et al. (2011). Linking inter-individual differences in neural activation and behavior to intrinsic brain dynamics. *NeuroImage*, 54(4). doi:10.1016/j.neuroimage.2010.10.046

Menon, V. (2011). Large-scale brain networks and psychopathology: A unifying triple network model. *Trends in Cognitive Sciences*, 15(10). doi:10.1016/j.tics.2011.08.003

Michel, C. M., & Murray, M. M. (2012). Towards the utilization of EEG as a brain imaging tool. *NeuroImage*, 61(2), 371–85. doi:10.1016/j.neuroimage.2011.12.039

Molotchnikoff, S., & Rouat, J. (2012). Brain at work: Time, sparseness and superposition principles. *Frontiers in Bioscience—Landmark*, 17. doi:10.2741/3946

Montague, P. R., & Berns, G. S. (2002). Neural economics and the biological substrates of valuation. *Neuron*, 36(2), 265–284. Review.

Montague, P. R., King-Casas, B., Cohen, J. D. Imaging valuation models in human choice. *Annual Review of Neuroscience*. 2006;29:417–448.

Montague, D. (2007). Keep your speed down. *Professional Engineering*, 20(12), 17–17.

Montague, G. T. (2007). Temporal oppositions as hermeneutical categories in the epistle to the Hebrews. *Catholic Biblical Quarterly*, 69(3), 588–589.

Montague, M. (2007). Against propositionalism. *Nous*, 41(3), 503–518.

Montague, P. R. (2007a). The first wave. *Trends in Cognitive Sciences*, 11(10), 407–409. doi:10.1016/i.tics.2007.07.005

Montague, P. R. (2007b). Neuroeconomics: A view from neuroscience. *Functional Neurology*, 22(4), 219–234.

Montague, P. R., & King-Casas, B. (2007). Efficient statistics, common currencies and the problem of reward-harvesting. *Trends in Cognitive Sciences*, 11(12), 514–519. doi:10.1016/j.tics.2007.10.002

Morcom, A. M., & Fletcher, P. C. (2007a). Cognitive neuroscience: The case for design rather than default. *NeuroImage*, 37(4), 1097–1099. doi:10.1016/j.neuroimage.2007.07.018

Morcom, A. M., & Fletcher, P. C. (2007b). Does the brain have a baseline? Why we should be resisting a rest. *NeuroImage*, 37(4), 1073–1082. doi:10.1016/j.neuroimage.2006.09.013

Morgane, P. J., & Mokler, D. J. (2006). The limbic brain: Continuing resolution. *Neuroscience & Biobehavioral Reviews*, 30(2), 119–125. doi:10.1016/j.neubiorev.2005.04.020

Morgane, P. J., Galler, J. R., & Mokler, D. J. (2005). A review of systems and networks of the limbic forebrain/limbic midbrain. *Progress in Neurobiology*, 75(2), 143–160. doi:10.1016/j.pneurobio.2005.01.001

Moshe, M. (2009). Research note temporary versus permanent time framing in the Israeli political arena. *Time & Society*, 18(1), 154–171. doi:10.1177/0961463X08099944

Moshe, S. L. (. (2009). Pathophysiology of human absence epilepsy. *Epilepsia*, 50, 4–4.

Murphy, K., Birn, R. M., Handwerker, D. A., Jones, T. B., & Bandettini, P. A. (2009). The impact of global signal regression on resting state correlations: Are anti-correlated networks introduced? *NeuroImage*, 44(3), 893–905. doi:10.1016/j.neuroimage.2008.09.036

Murray, M. M., Molholm, S., Michel, C. M., Heslenfeld, D. J., Ritter, W., Javitt, D. C.,

Schroeder, C. E., & Foxe, J. J. (2005). Grabbing your ear: rapid auditory-somatosensory multisensory interactions in low-level sensory cortices are not constrained by stimulus alignment. *Cerebral Cortex*, 15(7), 963–974. Epub 2004 Nov 10.

Musso, F., Brinkmeyer, J., Mobascher, A., Warbrick, T., & Winterer, G. (2010). Spontaneous brain activity and EEG microstates. A novel EEG/fMRI analysis approach to explore resting-state networks. *NeuroImage*, 52(4).1149–1161, doi:10.1016/j.neuroimage.2010.01.093

Muthukumaraswamy, S. D., & Singh, K. D. (2009). Functional decoupling of BOLD and gamma-band amplitudes in human primary visual cortex. *Human Brain Mapping*, 30(7), 2000–2007. doi:10.1002/hbm.20644

Muthukumaraswamy, S. D., Edden, R. A. E., Jones, D. K., Swettenham, J. B., & Singh, K. D. (2009). Resting GABA concentration predicts peak gamma frequency and fMRI amplitude in response to visual stimulation in humans. *Proceedings of the National Academy of Sciences USA*, 106(20), 8356–8361. doi:10.1073/pnas.0900728106

Muthukumaraswamy, S. D., Evans, C. J., Edden, R. A. E., Wise, R. G., & Singh, K. D. (2012). Individual variability in the shape and amplitude of the BOLD-HRF correlates with endogenous GABAergic inhibition. *Human Brain Mapping*, 33(2). doi:10.1002/hbm.21223

Naatanen, R., Paavilainen, P., Rinne, T., & Alho, K. (2007). The mismatch negativity (MMN) in basic research of central auditory processing: A review. *Clinical Neurophysiology*, 118(12), 2544–2590. doi:10.1016/j.clinph.2007.04.026

Nagai, Y., Critchley, H. D., Featherstone, E., Fenwick, P. B. C., Trimble, M. R., & Dolan, R. J. (2004). Brain activity relating to the contingent negative variation: An fMRI investigation. *NeuroImage*, 21(4), 1232–1241. doi:10.1016/j.neuroimage.2003.10.036

Najib, U., Horvath, J. C., Silvanto, J., & Pascual-Leone, A. (2010). State-dependency effects on TMS: a look at motive phosphene behavior. *Journal of Visualized Experiments*,46. doi:pii: 2273. 10.3791/2273.

Naselaris, T., Prenger, R. J., Kay, K. N., Oliver, M., & Gallant, J. L. (2009). Bayesian reconstruction of natural images from human brain activity. *Neuron*, 63(6), 902–915. doi: 10.1016/j.neuron.2009.09.006.

Naselaris, T., Kay, K. N., Nishimoto, S., & Gallant, J. L. (2011). Encoding and decoding in fMRI. *NeuroImage*, 56(2). doi:10.1016/j.neuroimage.2010.07.073

Naqvi, N. H., & Bechara, A. (2009). The hidden island of addiction: the insula. *Trends in Neurosciences*, 32(1), 56–67. doi: 10.1016/j.tins.2008.09.009. Epub 2008 Nov 3. Review.

Naqvi, N. H., & Bechara, A. (2010). The insula and drug addiction: an interoceptive view of pleasure, urges, and decision-making. *Brain Structure and Function*, 214(5–6), 435–450. doi: 10.1007/s00429-010-0268-7. Epub 2010 May 29.

Naqvi, N. H., Rudrauf, D., Damasio, H., & Bechara, A. (2007). Damage to the insula disrupts addiction to cigarette smoking. *Science*. 315(5811), 531–534.

Neal, A., & Kilner, J. M. (2010). What is simulated in the action observation network when we observe actions? *European Journal of Neuroscience*, 32(10), 1765–1770. doi:10.1111/j.1460-9568.2010.07435.x

Newsome, W. T., Britten, K. H., & Movshon, J. A. (1989). Neuronal correlates of a perceptual decision. *Nature*, 341(6237), 52–4. doi:10.1038/341052a0

Nieuwenhuys, R. (1996). The greater limbic system, the emotional motor system and the brain. *Emotional Motor System*, 107, 551–580.

Nieuwenhuys, R. (1999). The morphological pattern of the vertebrate brain. *European Journal of Morphology*, 37(2–3), 81–4.

Nieuwenhuys, R. (2011). The structural, functional, and molecular organization of the brainstem. *Frontiers in Neuroanatomy*, 5, 5–20. doi:10.3389/fnana.2011.00033

Nieuwenhuys, R. (2012). The insular cortex: A review. *Progress in Brain Research*, 195, 123–163.

Nir, Y., Mukamel, R., Dinstein, I., Fisch, L., Gelbard-Sagiv, H., Arieli, A., et al. (2008a). Inter-hemispheric correlations in spontaneous activity of human sensory cortex during wake and sleep. *Sleep*, 31, 11.

Nir, Y., Mukamel, R., Dinstein, I., Privman, E., Harel, M., Fisch, L., et al. (2008b). Interhemispheric correlations of slow spontaneous neuronal fluctuations revealed in human sensory cortex. *Nature Neuroscience*, 11(9), 1100–1108. doi:10.1038/nn.2177

Nishimoto, S., Vu, A. T., Naselaris, T., Benjamini, Y., Yu, B., & Gallant, J. L. (2011). Reconstructing visual experiences from brain activity evoked by natural movies. *Current*

Biology: CB, 21(19), 1641–1646. doi:10.1016/j.cub.2011.08.031

Noppeney, U. (2008). The neural systems of tool and action semantics: a perspective from functional imaging. *The Journal of Physiology* Paris, 102(1–3), 40–49. doi: 10.1016/j.jphysparis.2008.03.009. Epub 2008 Apr 8. Review.

Northoff, G. (2002a). Neurophysiology, neuropsychiatry and neurophilosophy of catatonia. *Behavioral and Brain Sciences*, 25(5), 592–599.

Northoff, G. (2002b). What catatonia can tell us about "top-down modulation": a neuropsychiatric hypothesis. *Behavioral and Brain Sciences*, 25(5), 555–77; discussion 578-604.

Northoff, G. (2008). What kind of neural coding and self does Hurely's shared circuit model presuppose? *Behavioral and Brain Sciences*, 31(1), 33–43.

Northoff, G. (2010a). Region-based approach versus mechanism-based approach to the brain. *Neuropsychoanalysis*, 12(2), 167–170.

Northoff, G. (2010b). Humans, brains, and their environment: marriage between neuroscience and anthropology? *Neuron*, 65(6), 748–751. doi:10.1016/j.neuron.2010.02.024

Northoff, G. (2011). Self and brain: What is self-related processing? *Trends in Cognitive Sciences*, 15(5), 186–187; author reply 187–188. doi:10.1016/j.tics.2011.03.001

Northoff, G. (2011). *Neuropsychoanalysis in practice. Brain, self, and objects*. New York: Oxford University Press.

Northoff, G., & Bermpohl, F. (2004). Cortical midline structures and the self. *Trends in Cognitive Sciences*, 8(3), 102–7. doi:10.1016/j.tics.2004.01.004

Northoff, G., & Hayes, D. J. (2011). Is our self nothing but reward? *Biol Psychiatry* 69(11), 1019–1025. doi: 10.1016/j.biopsych.2010.12.014. Epub 2011 Jan 31. Review.

Northoff, G., & Panksepp, J. (2008). The trans-species concept of self and the subcortical-cortical midline system. *Trends in Cognitive Sciences*, 12(7), 259–264. doi:10.1016/j.tics.2008.04.007

Northoff, G., Duncan, N. W., & Hayes, D. J. (2010). The brain and its resting state activity—experimental and methodological implications. *Progress in Neurobiology*, 92(4), 593–600. doi:10.1016/j.pneurobio.2010.09.002

Northoff, G., Qin, P., & Feinberg, T. E. (2011). Brain imaging of the self—conceptual, anatomical and methodological issues. *Consciousness & Cognition*, 20(1), 52–63. doi:10.1016/j.concog.2010.09.011

Northoff, G., Qin, P., & Nakao, T. (2010). Rest-stimulus interaction in the brain: A review. *Trends in Neurosciences*, 33(6), 277–84. doi:10.1016/j.tins.2010.02.006

Northoff, G., Heinzel, A., De Greck, M., Bermpohl, F., Dobrowolny, H., & Panksepp, J. (2006). Self-referential processing in our brain—a meta-analysis of imaging studies on the self. *NeuroImage*, 31(1), 440–457. doi:10.1016/j.neuroimage.2005.12.002

Northoff, G., Richter, A., Wahl, C., Grimm, S., Boeker, H., Hell, D., Marquar, V., et al. (2005). NMDA-hypofunction in posterior cingulate as a model for schizophrenia: A ketamine challenge study in fMRI. *Schizophrenia Research* 2(72), 235–248.

Northoff, G., Walter, M., Grimm, S., Boeker, H., Beck, J., Bermpohl, F., & Boesiger, P. (2007). Negative functional MRI response correlates with GABA concentration in human ventromedial prefrontal cortex—A combined fMRI-MRS study. *Nature Neuroscience*, 10(12), 1515–1517.

Northoff, G., Walter, M., Schulte, R. F., Beck, J., Dydak, U., Henning, A., et al. (2007). GABA concentrations in the human anterior cingulate cortex predict negative BOLD responses in fMRI. *Nature Neuroscience*, 10(12), 1515–1517. doi:10.1038/nn2001

Northoff, G., Wiebking, C., Feinberg, T., & Panksepp, J. (2011). The "resting-state hypothesis" of major depressive disorder: A translational subcortical-cortical framework for a system disorder. *Neuroscience & Biobehavioral Reviews*, 35(9), 1929–1945. doi:10.1016/j.neubiorev.2010.12.007

Northoff, G., Witzel, T., Richter, A., Gessner, M., Schlagenhauf, F., Fell, J., Baumgart, F., et al. (2002). GABA-ergic modulation of prefrontal spatio-temporal activation pattern during emotional processing: A combined fMRI/MEG study with placebo and lorazepam. *Journal of Cognitive Neuroscience*, 14(3), 348–370. doi:10.1162/089892902317361895

O'Doherty, J. P. (2004). Reward representations and reward-related learning in the human brain: Insights from neuroimaging. *Current Opinion in Neurobiology*, 14(6), 769–776. doi:10.1016/j.conb.2004.10.016

O'Doherty, J. P. (2011). Contributions of the ventromedial prefrontal cortex to goal-directed action selection. *Annals of the New York Academy of Sciences*, 1239, 118–129. doi: 10.1111/j.1749-6632.2011.06290.x. Review.

Olshausen, B. A., & Field, D. J. (1996). Emergence of simple-cell receptive field properties by learning a sparse code for natural images. *Nature,* 381(6583), 607–609.

Olshausen, B. A., & Field, D. J. (1997). Sparse coding with an overcomplete basis set: a strategy employed by V1? *Vision Research*, 37(23), 3311–3325.

Olshausen, B. A., & Field, D. J. (2004). Sparse coding of sensory inputs. *Current Opinion in Neurobiology*, 14(4), 481–487. doi:10.1016/j.conb.2004.07.007

Olshausen, Bruno A, & O'Connor, K. N. (2002). A new window on sound. *Nature Neuroscience*, 5(4), 292–4. doi:10.1038/nn0402-292

Panksepp, J. (1998). *Affective neuroscience: The foundations of human and animal emotions.* New York: Oxford University Press.

Panksepp, J. (2005). On the embodied neural nature of core emotional affects. *Journal of Consciousness Studies*, 12(8–10), 158–184.

Panksepp, J. (2011a). The basic emotional circuits of mammalian brains: Do animals have affective lives? *Neuroscience & Biobehavioral Reviews*, 35(9), 1791–1804. doi:10.1016/j.neubiorev.2011.08.003

Panksepp, J. (2011b). Cross-species affective neuroscience decoding of the primal affective experiences of humans and related animals. *PloS One*, 6(9), e21236. doi:10.1371/journal.pone.0021236

Panksepp, J., & Northoff, G. (2009). The trans-species core SELF: the emergence of active cultural and neuro-ecological agents through self-related processing within subcortical-cortical midline networks. *Consciousness & Cognition*, 18(1), 193–215. doi:10.1016/j.concog.2008.03.002

Panzeri, S., Brunel, N., Logothetis, N. K., & Kayser, C. (2010). Sensory neural codes using multiplexed temporal scales. *Trends in Neurosciences*, 33(3), 111–120. doi: 10.1016/j.tins.2009.12.001. Epub 2010 Jan 4. Review.

Papadopoulou, M. (2011). Normalization for sparse encoding of odors by a wide-field interneuron. *Science,* 332(6030), 721–725.

Papadopoulou, M., Cassenaer, S., Nowotny, T., & Laurent, G. (2011). Normalization for sparse encoding of odors by a wide-field interneuron. *Science* (New York), 332(6030), 721–5. doi:10.1126/science.1201835

Park, I. H., Kim, J., Chun, J., Jung, Y. C., Seok, J. H., Park, H., & Lee, J. D. (2009). Medial prefrontal default-mode hypoactivity affecting trait physical anhedonia in schizophrenia. *Psychiatry Research—Neuroimaging*, 171(3), 155–165. doi:10.1016/j.pscychresns.2008.03.010

Park, J., Lim, J. H., Choi, H., & Kim, D. (2012a). Predictive coding strategies for developmental neurorobotics. *Frontiers in Psychology*, 3, 134.

Park, S. Q., Kahnt, T., Talmi, D., Rieskamp, J., Dolan, R. J., & Heekeren, H. R. (2012b). Adaptive coding of reward prediction errors is gated by striatal coupling. *Proceedings of the National Academy of Sciences USA*, 109(11), 4285–4289. doi:10.1073/pnas.1119969109

Patel, A. B., de Graaf, R. A., Mason, G. F., Rothman, D. L., Shulman, R. G., & Behar, K. L. (2005). The contribution of GABA to glutamate/glutamine cycling and energy metabolism in the rat cortex in vivo. *Proceedings of the National Academy of Sciences USA*, 102(15), 5588–5893. doi:10.1073/pnas.0501703102

Paulus, M. P. (2007). Decision-making dysfunctions in psychiatry—altered homeostatic processing? *Science*, 318(5850), 602–606. doi:10.1126/science.1142997

Paulus, M. P., & Frank, L. R. (2003). Ventromedial prefrontal cortex activation is critical for preference judgments. *Neuroreport*, 14(10), 1311–1315.

Philiastides, M. G., Auksztulewicz, R., Heekeren, H. R., & Blankenburg, F. (2011). Causal role of dorsolateral prefrontal cortex in human perceptual decision making. *Current Biology*, 21(11). 980–983; doi:10.1016/j.cub.2011.04.034

Philiastides, M. G., Biele, G., & Heekeren, H. R. (2010a). A mechanistic account of value computation in the human brain. *Proceedings of the National Academy of Sciences USA*, 107(20), 9430–9435.

Philiastides, M. G., Biele, G., Vavatzanidis, N., Kazzer, P., & Heekeren, H. R. (2010b). Temporal dynamics of prediction error processing during reward-based decision making. *NeuroImage*, 53(1). doi:10.1016/j.neuroimage.2010.05.052

Poo, C., & Isaacson, J. S. (2009). Odor representations in olfactory cortex: "Sparse" coding, global inhibition, and oscillations. *Neuron,* 62(6), 850–861. doi:10.1016/j.neuron.2009.05.022

Poo, C., & Isaacson, J. S. (2011). Odor representations in olfactory cortex: "sparse" coding, global inhibition, and oscillations. *Neuron*, 62(6), 850–861. doi: 10.1016/j.neuron.2009.05.022

Power, J. D., Fair, D. A., Schlaggar, B. L., & Petersen, S. E. (2010). The development of human functional brain networks. *Neuron,* 67(5), 735–748. doi:10.1016/j.neuron.2010.08.017

Price, J. L. (1999). Prefrontal cortical networks related to visceral function and mood. *Annals of the New York Academy of Science*, 877, 383–396.

Priebe, N. J., & Ferster, D. (2008). Inhibition, spike threshold, and stimulus selectivity in primary visual cortex. *Neuron*, 57(4), 482–497. doi:10.1016/j.neuron.2008.02.005

Pyka, M., Beckmann, C. F., Schoening, S., Hauke, S., Heider, D., Kugel, H., et al. (2009). Impact of working memory load on fMRI resting state pattern in subsequent resting phases. *PloS One*, 4(9), e7198. doi:10.1371/journal.pone.0007198

Qin, P., Grimm, S., Bajbouj, M., Duncan, N. W., & Northoff, G. (in press). Differential rest-stimulus interaction for own and other names. *Frontiers in Neuroscience*, in press.

Qin, P., & Northoff, G. (2011). How is our self related to midline regions and the default-mode network? *NeuroImage*, 57(3), 1221–1233. doi:10.1016/j.neuroimage.2011.05.028

Qin, P., Duncan, N. W., Wiebking, C., Gravel, P., Lyttelton, O., Hayes, D. J., Verhaeghe, J., et al. (2012). GABA(A) receptors in visual and auditory cortex and neural activity changes during basic visual stimulation. *Frontiers in Human Neuroscience*, 6, 337. doi:10.3389/fnhum.2012.00337

Qin, P., Liu, Y., Shi, J., Wang, Y., Duncan, N., Gong, Q., et al. (2013). Dissociation between anterior and posterior cortical regions during self-specificity and familiarity: A combined fMRI-meta-analytic study. *Human Brain Mapping*, 33(1), 154–164. doi:10.1002/hbm.21201

Quiroga, R. Q., Reddy, L., Koch, C., & Fried, I. (2007). Decoding visual inputs from multiple neurons in the human temporal lobe. *Journal of Neurophysiology*, 98(4),. 1997–2007. doi:10.1152/jn.00125.2007

Raichle, M. E. (2009). A brief history of human brain mapping. *Trends in Neurosciences*, 32(2), 118–126. doi:10.1016/j.tins.2008.11.001

Raichle, M. E. (2010). The brain's (dark energy). Scientific American, 302(3), 44–49.

Raichle, M. E., & Gusnard, D. A. (2005). Intrinsic brain activity sets the stage for expression of motivated behavior. *Journal of Comparative Neurology*, 493(1), 167–176. doi:10.1002/cne.20752

Raichle, M. E., & Mintun, M. A. (2006). Brain work and brain imaging. *Annual Review of Neuroscience*, 29, 449–476. doi:10.1146/annurev.neuro.29.051605.112819

Raichle, M. E., MacLeod, A. M., Snyder, A. Z., Powers, W. J., Gusnard, D. A., & Shulman, G. L. (2001). A default mode of brain function. *Proceedings of the National Academy of Sciences USA*, 98(2), 676–82. doi:10.1073/pnas.98.2.676

Rangel, A. (2008). Consciousness meets neuroeconomics: What is the value of stimulus awareness in decision making? *Neuron*, 59(4). doi:10.1016/j.neuron.2008.08.003

Rao, D. G. (2003). A universe of consciousness: How matter becomes imagination. *Journal of the American Psychoanalytic Association*, 51(3), 1030–1034.

Rao, R. P. N. (2010). Decision making under uncertainty: A neural model based on partially observable Markov decision processes. *Frontiers in Computational Neuroscience*, 4, 146. doi:10.3389/fncom.2010.00146

Rao, R. P., Ballard, D. H. (1999). Predictive coding in the visual cortex: a functional interpretation of some extra-classical receptive-field effects. *Nature Neuroscience*, 2(1), 79–87.

Rauss, K., Schwartz, S., & Pourtois, G. (2011). Top-down effects on early visual processing in humans: A predictive coding framework. *Neuroscience & Biobehavioral Reviews*, 35(5), 1237–1253. doi:10.1016/j.neubiorev.2010.12.011

Rieke, F., Bodnar, D. A., & Bialek, W. (1995). Naturalistic stimuli increase the rate and efficiency of information transmission by primary auditory afferents. *Proceedings. Biological Sciences/The Royal Society*, 262(1365), 259–65. doi:10.1098/rspb.1995.0204

Rilling, J. K., Sanfey, A. G., Aronson, J. A., Nystrom, L. E., & Cohen, J. D. (2004). Opposing BOLD responses to reciprocated and unreciprocated altruism in putative reward pathways. *Neuroreport*, 15(16), 2539–2543.

Rilling, J. K., Lacreuse, A., Barks, S. K., Elfenbein, H. A., Pagnoni, G., Votaw, J. R., & Herndon, J. G. (2008). Effect of menstrual cycle on resting brain metabolism in female rhesus monkeys. *Neuroreport*, 19(5), 537–541.

Ringach, D. L. (2003). Neuroscience: states of mind. *Nature*, 425(6961), 912–913.

Rizzolatti, G., & Craighero, L. (2004). The mirror-neuron system. *Annual Review of Neuroscience*, 27, 169–192. Review.

Rodriguez, E., George, N., Lachaux, J. P., Martinerie, J., Renault, B., & Varela, F. J. (1999). Perception's shadow: long-distance synchronization of human brain activity. *Nature*, 397(6718), 430–433.

Rolls, E. T. (2011). Chemosensory learning in the cortex. *Frontiers in Systems Neuroscience*, 5, 78.

Rolls, E. T., & Tovee, M. J. (1995). Sparseness of the neuronal representation of stimuli in the primate temporal visual cortex. *Journal of Neurophysiology*, 73(2), 713–26.

Rolls, E. T., & Treves, A. (2011). The neuronal encoding of information in the brain. *Progress in Neurobiology*, 95(3). doi:10.1016/j.pneurobio.2011.08.002

Rolls, E. T., Tovee, M. J., & Panzeri, S. (1999). The neurophysiology of backward visual masking: Information analysis. *Journal of Cognitive Neuroscience*, 11(3), 300–311.

Romo, R., Hernández, A., Zainos, A., & Salinas, E. (1998). Somatosensory discrimination based on cortical microstimulation. *Nature*, 392(6674), 387–390. doi:10.1038/32891

Romo, R., Hernández, A., Zainos, A., Brody, C. D., & Lemus, L. (2000). Sensing without touching: Psychophysical performance based on cortical microstimulation. *Neuron*, 26(1), 273–8.

Rorie, A. E., Gao, J., McClelland, J. L., & Newsome, W. T. (2010). Integration of sensory and reward information during perceptual decision-making in lateral intraparietal cortex (LIP) of the macaque monkey. *PloS One*, 5(2), e9308. doi:10.1371/journal.pone.0009308

Rothman, D. L., Behar, K. L., Hyder, F., & Shulman, R. G. (2003). In vivo NMR studies of the glutamate neurotransmitter flux and neuroenergetics: implications for brain function. *Annual Review of Physiology*, 65, 401–27. doi:10.1146/annurev.physiol.65.092101.142131

Rozell, C. J., Johnson, D. H., Baraniuk, R. G., & Olshausen, B. A. (2008). Sparse coding via thresholding and local competition in neural circuits. *Neural Computation*, 20(10), 2526–63. doi:10.1162/neco.2008.03-07-486

Rustichini, A. (2009). Neuroeconomics: What have we found, and what should we search for. *Current Opinion in Neurobiology*, 19(6), 672–677..doi:10.1016/j.conb.2009.09.012

Sadaghiani, S., Hesselmann, G., & Kleinschmidt, A. (2009). Distributed and antagonistic contributions of ongoing activity fluctuations to auditory stimulus detection. *Journal of Neuroscience*, 29(42), 13410–13417. doi:10.1523/JNEUROSCI.2592-09.2009

Sadaghiani, S., Scheeringa, R., Lehongre, K., Morillon, B., Giraud, A.-L., & Kleinschmidt, A. (2010). Intrinsic connectivity networks, alpha oscillations, and tonic alertness: a simultaneous electroencephalography/functional magnetic resonance imaging study. *Journal of Neuroscience*, 30(30), 10243–50. doi:10.1523/JNEUROSCI.1004-10.2010

Sapir, A., d'Avossa, G., McAvoy, M., Shulman, G. L., & Corbetta, M. (2005). Brain signals for spatial attention predict performance in a motion discrimination task. *Proceedings of the National Academy of Sciences USA*, 102(49), 17810–17815. doi:10.1073/pnas.0504678102

Sasai, S., Homae, F., Watanabe, H., & Taga, G. (2011). Frequency-specific functional connectivity in the brain during resting state revealed by NIRS. *NeuroImage*, 56(1), 252–257. doi:10.1016/j.neuroimage.2010.12.075

Sauseng, P., & Klimesch, W. (2008). What does phase information of oscillatory brain activity tell us about cognitive processes? *Neuroscience & Biobehavioral Reviews*, 32(5). doi:10.1016/j.neubiorev.2008.03.014

Schaefer M. (2009). Neuroeconomics: in search of the neural representation of brands. *Progress in Brain Research*, 178, 241–252. doi: 10.1016/S0079-6123(09)17817-2.

Schmaal, L., Goudriaan, A. E., van der Meer, J., van den Brink, W., & Veltman, D. J. (2012). The association between cingulate cortex glutamate concentration and delay discounting is mediated by resting state functional connectivity. *Brain Behavior*, 2(5), 553–562. doi: 10.1002/brb3.74. Epub 2012 Jul 16.

Schneider, F., Bermpohl, F., Heinzel, A., Rotte, M., Walter, M., Tempelmann, C., et al. (2008). The resting brain and our self: Self-relatedness modulates resting state neural activity in cortical midline structures. *Neuroscience*, 157(1), 120–131. doi:10.1016/j.neuroscience.2008.08.014

Schoppa, N E. (2009a). Inhibition acts globally to shape olfactory cortical tuning. *Neuron*, 62(6), 750–752. doi:10.1016/j.neuron.2009.06.004

Schoppa, N. E. (2009b). Making scents out of how olfactory neurons are ordered in space. *Nature Neuroscience*, 12(2), 103–104. doi:10.1038/nn0209-103

Schreiner, C. E., & Langner, G. (1997). Laminar fine structure of frequency organization in auditory midbrain. *Nature*, 388(6640), 383–386. doi:10.1038/41106

Schroeder, C. E., & Lakatos, P. (2009a). Low-frequency neuronal oscillations as instruments of sensory selection. *Trends in Neurosciences*, 32(1), 9–18. doi:10.1016/j.tins.2008.09.012

Schroeder, C. E., & Lakatos, P. (2009b). The gamma oscillation: Master or slave? *Brain Topography*, 22(1), 24–26. doi:10.1007/s10548-009-0080-y

Schroeder, C. E., Lakatos, P., Kajikawa, Y., Partan, S., & Puce, A. (2008). Neuronal oscillations and visual amplification of speech. *Trends in Cognitive Sciences*, 12(3), 106–113. doi:10.1016/j.tics.2008.01.002 ER

Schroeder, C. E., Wilson, D. A., Radman, T., Scharfman, H., & Lakatos, P. (2010). Dynamics of active sensing and perceptual selection. *Current Opinion in Neurobiology*, 20(2), 172–176. doi:10.1016/j.conb.2010.02.010

Schütz-Bosbach, S., & Prinz, W. (2007a). Perceptual resonance: action-induced modulation of perception. *Trends in Cognitive Sciences*, 11(8), 349–355. Epub 2007 Jul 12. Review.

Schütz-Bosbach, S., & Prinz, W. (2007b). Prospective coding in event representation. *Cognitive Processing*, 8(2), 93–102. Epub 2007 Apr 4. Review.

Schultz, W. (2006). Behavioral theories and the neurophysiology of reward. *Annual Review of Psychology*, 57, 87–115. doi:10.1146/annurev.psych.56.091103.070229

Schultz, W. (2007a). Behavioral dopamine signals. *Trends in Neurosciences*, 30(5), 203–210. doi:10.1016/j.tins.2007.03.007

Schultz, W. (2007b). Multiple dopamine functions at different time courses. *Annual Review of Neuroscience*, 30, 259–288. doi:10.1146/annurev.neuro.28.061604.135722

Searle, J. R. (1992). *The rediscovery of mind*. Cambridge, MA: MIT Press.

Selezneva, E., Scheich, H., & Brosch, M. (2006). Dual time scales for categorical decision making in auditory cortex. *Current Biology*, 16(24), 2428–2433. doi:10.1016/j.cub.2006.10.027

Seth, A. K., Barrett, A. B., & Barnett, L. (2011). Causal density and integrated information as measures of conscious level. *Philosophical Transactions. Series A, Mathematical, Physical, & Engineering Sciences*, 369(1952), 3748–67. doi:10.1098/rsta.2011.0079

Seth, A. K., Suzuki, K., & Critchley, H. D. (2011). An interoceptive predictive coding model of conscious presence. *Frontiers in Psychology*, 2, 395. doi:10.3389/fpsyg.2011.00395

Seymour, K., Clifford, C. W. G., Logothetis, N. K., & Bartels, A. (2009). The coding of color, motion, and their conjunction in the human visual cortex. *Current Biology*, 19(3), 177–183. doi:10.1016/j.cub.2008.12.050 ER

Seymour, K., Clifford, C. W. G., Logothetis, N. K., & Bartels, A. (2010). Coding and binding of color and form in visual cortex. *Cerebral Cortex*, 20(8), 1946–1954. doi:10.1093/cercor/bhp265 ER

Schaller, B., Mekle, R., Xin, L., Kunz, K., & Gruetter, R. (2013). Net increase of lactate and glutamate concentration in activated human visual cortex detected with magnetic resonance spectroscopy at 7 tesla. *Journal of Neuroscience Research*, in press.

Shadlen, M. N., & Newsome, W. T. (2001). Neural basis of a perceptual decision in the parietal cortex (area LIP) of the rhesus monkey. *Journal of Neurophysiology*, 86(4), 1916–1936.

Sharp, C., Monterosso, J., & Montague, P. R. (2012) Neuroeconomics: a bridge for translational research. *Biological Psychiatry*. 72(2), 87–92. doi: 10.1016/j.biopsych.2012.02.029. Review.

Shmuel, A., & Leopold, D. A. (2008). Neuronal correlates of spontaneous fluctuations in fMRI signals in monkey visual cortex: Implications for functional connectivity at rest. *Human Brain Mapping*, 29(7), 751–761. doi:10.1002/hbm.20580

Shmuel, A., Yacoub, E., Pfeuffer, J., Van de Moortele, P. F., Adriany, G., Hu, X., & Ugurbil, K. (2002). Sustained negative BOLD, blood flow and oxygen consumption response and its coupling to the positive response in the human brain. *Neuron*, 36(6), 1195–1210.

Shmuel, A., Augath, M., Oeltermann, A., & Logothetis, N. K. (2006). Negative functional MRI response correlates with decreases in neuronal activity in monkey visual area V1. *Nature Neuroscience*, 9(4), 569–577. Epub 2006 Mar 19.

Shulman, G. L., Astafiev, S. V., Franke, D., Pope, D. L. W., Snyder, A. Z., McAvoy, M. P., & Corbetta, M. (2009a). Interaction of stimulus-driven reorienting and expectation in ventral and dorsal frontoparietal and basal ganglia-cortical networks. *Journal of Neuroscience*, 29(14), 4392–4407. doi:10.1523/JNEUROSCI.5609-08.2009

Shulman, R. G., Hyder, F., & Rothman, D. L. (2003). Cerebral metabolism and consciousness. *Comptes Rendus Biologies*, 326(3), 253–273.

Shulman, R. G., Hyder, F., & Rothman, D. L. (2009b). Baseline brain energy supports the state of consciousness. *Proceedings of the National Academy of Sciences USA*, 106(27), 11096–11101. doi:10.1073/pnas.0903941106

Shulman, R. G., Rothman, D. L., Behar, K. L., & Hyder, F. (2004). Energetic basis of brain activity: Implications for neuroimaging. *Trends in Neurosciences*, 27(8), 489–495. doi:10.1016/j.tins.2004.06.005

Silvanto J., & Pascual-Leone, A. (2008) State-dependency of transcranial magnetic stimulation. *Brain Topography*, 21(1):1–10. doi: 10.1007/s10548-008-0067-0. Epub 2008 Sep 13. Review.

Silvanto, J., Muggleton, N., & Walsh, V. (2008). State-dependency in brain stimulation studies of perception and cognition. *Trends in Cognitive Sciences*, 12(12), 447–54. doi:10.1016/j.tics.2008.09.004

Simmons, P. J., & Van Steveninck, R. R. de R. (2010). Sparse but specific temporal coding by spikes in an insect sensory-motor ocellar pathway. *Journal of Experimental Biology*, 213(Pt 15), 2629–39. doi:10.1242/jeb.043547

Simoncelli, E. P., & Olshausen, B. A. (2001). Natural image statistics and neural representation. *Annual Review of Neuroscience*, 24, 1193–216. doi:10.1146/annurev.neuro.24.1.1193

Simpson, J. R., Drevets, W. C., Snyder, A. Z., Gusnard, D. A., & Raichle, M. E. (2001). Emotion-induced changes in human medial prefrontal cortex: II. During anticipatory anxiety. *Proceedings of the National Academy of Sciences USA*, 98(2), 688–93. doi:10.1073/pnas.98.2.688

Singer, W. (1999). Neuronal synchrony: A versatile code for the definition of relations? *Neuron*, 24(1), 49–65, 111–25.

Singer, W. (2009). Distributed processing and temporal codes in neuronal networks. *Cognitive Neurodynamics*, 3(3), 189–196. doi:10.1007/s11571-009-9087-z

Smith, S. M., Fox, P. T., Miller, K. L., Glahn, D. C., Fox, P. M., Mackay, C. E.,... Beckmann, C. F. (2009). Correspondence of the brain's functional architecture during activation and rest. *Proceedings of the National Academy of Sciences USA*, 106(31), 13040–13045. doi:10.1073/pnas.0905267106

Sporns, O. (2011). *Networks of the brain*. Cambridge, MA: MIT Press.

Spratling, M. W. (2008). Predictive coding as a model of biased competition in visual attention. *Vision Research*, 48(12), 1391–1408. doi: 10.1016/j.visres.2008.03.009. Epub 2008 Apr 28.

Spratling, M. W. (2010). Predictive coding as a model of response properties in cortical area V1. *Journal of Neurosciences*, 30(9), 3531–3543. doi: 10.1523/JNEUROSCI.4911-09.2010.

Spratling, M. W. (2012a). Predictive coding accounts for V1 response properties recorded using reverse correlation. *Biological Cybernetics*, 106(1), 37–49. doi: 10.1007/s00422-012-0477-7. Epub 2012 Feb 14.

Spratling, M. W. (2012b). Predictive coding as a model of the V1 saliency map hypothesis. *Neural Networks*, 26, 7–28. doi:10.1016/j.neunet.2011.10.002

Spreng, R. N., Mar, R. A., & Kim, A. S. N. (2009). The common neural basis of autobiographical memory, prospection, navigation, theory of mind, and the default mode: A quantitative meta-analysis. *Journal of Cognitive Neuroscience*, 21(3), 489–510.

Sreenivas, S., Boehm, S. G., & Linden, D. E. J. (2012). Emotional faces and the default mode network. *Neuroscience Letters*, 506(2). doi:10.1016/j.neulet.2011.11.012

Stagg, C. J., Bachtiar, V., & Johansen-Berg, H. (2011a). The role of GABA in human motor learning. *Current Biology*, 21(6). doi:10.1016/j.cub.2011.01.069

Stagg, C. J., Bestmann, S., Constantinescu, A. O., Moreno, L. M., Allman, C., Mekle, R., et al. (2011b). Relationship between physiological measures of excitability and levels of glutamate and GABA in the human motor cortex. *Journal of Physiology (London)*, 589(23). doi:10.1113/jphysiol.2011.216978

Stopfer, M. (2007). Olfactory processing: Massive convergence onto sparse codes. *Current Biology: CB*, 17(10), R363–4. doi:10.1016/j.cub.2007.03.019

Strelnikov, K. (2010). Neuroimaging and neuroenergetics: Brain activations as information-driven reorganization of energy flows. *Brain & Cognition*, 72(3), 449–456. doi:10.1016/j.bandc.2009.12.008

Summerfield, C., Egner, T., Greene, M., Koechlin, E., Mangels, J., & Hirsch, J. (2006). Predictive codes for forthcoming perception in the frontal cortex. *Science*, 314(5803). doi:10.1126/science.1132028

Sylvester CM, Shulman GL, Jack AI, Corbetta M. (2007) Asymmetry of anticipatory activity in visual cortex predicts the locus of attention and perception. *Journal of Neurosciences*, 27(52), 14424–14433.

Tamir, D. I., & Mitchell, J. P. (2011). The default network distinguishes construals of proximal versus distal events. *Journal of Cognitive Neuroscience*, 23(10), 2945–55. doi:10.1162/jocn_a_00009

Terashima, H., & Hosoya, H. (2009). Sparse codes of harmonic natural sounds and their modulatory interactions. *Network (Bristol, England)*, 20(4), 253–67. doi:10.3109/0954898090344775l

Theunissen, F. E. (2003). From synchrony to sparseness. *Trends in Neuroscience*, 26(2), 61–64.

Tononi, G. (2004). An information integration theory of consciousness. *BMC Neuroscience*, 5, 42. doi:10.1186/1471-2202-5-42

Tononi, G., & Koch, C. (2008). The neural correlates of consciousness: An update. *Annals of the New York Academy of Sciences*, 1124, 239–61. doi:10.1196/annals.1440.004

Tremblay, S., Beaulé, V., Proulx, S., de Beaumont, L., Marjanska, M., Doyon, J., et al. (2012). Relationship between transcranial magnetic stimulation measures of intracortical inhibition and spectroscopy measures of GABA and glutamate+glutamine. *Journal of Neurophysiology*, 109(5):1343–1349. doi: 10.1152/jn.00704.2012. Epub 2012 Dec 5.

Tricomi, E., Rangel, A., Camerer, C. F., & O'Doherty, J. P. (2010). Neural evidence for inequality-averse social preferences. *Nature*, 463(7284). doi:10.1038/nature08785

Uhlhaas, P. J., Pipa, G., Lima, B., Melloni, L., Neuenschwander, S., Nikolic, D., & Singer, W. (2009). Neural synchrony in cortical networks: History, concept and current status. *Frontiers in Integrative Neuroscience*, 3, 17.

Uhlhaas, P. J., Pipa, G., Neuenschwander, S., Wibral, M., & Singer, W. (2011). A new look at gamma? high- (> 60 hz) gamma-band activity in cortical networks: Function, mechanisms and impairment. *Progress in Biophysics & Molecular Biology*, 105(1–2), 14–28. doi:10.1016/j.pbiomolbio.2010.10.004

Umiltà, M. A., Kohler, E., Gallese, V., Fogassi, L., Fadiga, L., Keysers, C., Rizzolatti, G. (2001). I know what you are doing. a neurophysiological study. *Neuron*, 31(1):155–165.

Van de Ville, D., Britz, J., & Michel, C. M. (2010). EEG microstate sequences in healthy humans at rest reveal scale-free dynamics. *Proceedings of the National Academy of Sciences USA*, 107(42), 18179–18184. doi:10.1073/pnas.1007841107

Van den Heuvel, M. P., Mandl, R. C. W., Kahn, R. S., & Pol, H. E. H. (2009). Functionally linked resting-state networks reflect the underlying structural connectivity architecture of the human brain. *Human Brain Mapping*, 30(10), 3127–3141. doi:10.1002/hbm.20737

Van Duuren, E., Lankelma, J., & Pennartz, C. M. A. (2008). Population coding of reward magnitude in the orbitofrontal cortex of the rat. *Journal of Neuroscience*, 28(34), 8590–8603.

Van Eijsden, P., Hyder, F., Rothman, D. L., & Shulman, R. G. (2009). Neurophysiology of functional imaging. *NeuroImage*, 45(4), 1047–1054. doi:10.1016/j.neuroimage.2008.08.026

Vanhatalo, S., Palva, J. M., Holmes, M. D., Miller, J. W., Voipio, J., & Kaila, K. (2004). Infraslow oscillations modulate excitability and interictal epileptic activity in the human cortex during sleep. *Proceedings of the National Academy of Sciences USA*, 101(14), 5053–5057. doi:10.1073/pnas.0305375101

Vincent, J. L., Patel, G. H., Fox, M. D., Snyder, A. Z., Baker, J. T., Van Essen, D. C., Zempel, J. M., et al. (2007). Intrinsic functional architecture in the anaesthetized monkey brain. *Nature*, 447(7140), 83–86. doi:10.1038/nature05758

Vinck, M., Lima, B., Womelsdorf, T., Oostenveld, R., Singer, W., Neuenschwander, S., & Fries, P. (2010). Gamma-phase shifting in awake monkey visual cortex. *Journal of Neuroscience*, 30(4), 1250–1257. doi:10.1523

Vinje, W. E., & Gallant, J. L. (2000). Sparse coding and decorrelation in primary visual cortex during natural vision. *Science*, 287(5456), 1273–1276.

Vinje, W., & Gallant, J. (2002). Natural stimulation of the nonclassical receptive field increases information transmission efficiency in V1. *Journal of Neuroscience*, 22(7), 2904–15.

Wacongne, C., Labyt, E., van Wassenhove, V., Bekinschtein, T., Naccache, L., & Dehaene, S. (2011). Evidence for a hierarchy of predictions and prediction errors in human cortex. *Proceedings of the National Academy of Sciences USA*, 108(51). doi:10.1073/pnas.1117807108

Waddell, K. W., Zanjanipour, P., Pradhan, S., Xu, L., Welch, E. B., Joers, J. M., et al. (2011). Anterior cingulate and cerebellar GABA and glu correlations measured by H-1 J-difference spectroscopy. *Magnetic Resonance Imaging*, 29(1). 19-24. doi:10.1016/j.mri.2010.07.005

Wang, J., Wang, L., Zang, Y., Yang, H., Tang, H., Gong, Q., Chen, Z., et al. (2009). Parcellation-dependent small-world brain functional networks: A resting-state fMRI study. *Human Brain Mapping*, 30(5), 1511–23. doi:10.1002/hbm.20623

Wang, K., Jiang, T., Yu, C., Li, L. T. J., Liu, Y., Zhou, Y., et al. (2008). Spontaneous activity associated with primary visual cortex: A resting-state fMRI study. *Cerebral Cortex*, 18(3), 697–704. doi:10.1093/cercor/bhm105

Wang, K., Liang, M., Wang, L., Tian, L., Zhang, X., Li, K., & Jiang, T. (2007). Altered functional connectivity in early Alzheimer's disease: A resting-state fMRI study. *Human Brain Mapping*, 28(10), 967–978. doi:10.1002/hbm.20324

Wehr, M., & Zador, A. M. (2003). Balanced inhibition underlies tuning and sharpens spike timing in auditory cortex. *Nature*, 426(6965), 442–446. doi:10.1038/nature02116

Weliky, M., Fiser, J., Hunt, R. H., & Wagner, D. N. (2003). Coding of natural scenes in primary visual cortex. *Neuron*, 37(4), 703–18.

Wicker, B., Ruby, P., Royet, J.-P., & Fonlupt, P. (2003). A relation between rest and the self in the brain? Brain research. *Brain Research Reviews*, 43(2), 224–230.

Wiebking, C., Bauer, A., de Greck, M., Duncan, N. W., Tempelmann, C., & Northoff, G. (2010). Abnormal body perception and neural activity in the insula in depression: An fMRI study of the depressed "material me". *World Journal of Biological Psychiatry*, 11(3), 538–549. doi:10.3109/15622970903563794

Wiebking, C., De Greck, M., Duncan, N. W., Heinzel, A., Tempelmann, C., & Northoff, G. (2011). Are emotions associated with activity during rest or interoception? An exploratory fMRI study in healthy subjects. *Neuroscience Letters*, 491(1), 87–92. doi:10.1016/j.neulet.2011.01.012

Wiebking, C., Duncan, N. W., Qin, P., Hayes, D. J., Lyttelton, O., Gravel, P., Verhaeghe, J., et al. (2012). External awareness and GABA-A multimodal imaging study combining fMRI and [(18) F]flumazenil-PET. *Human Brain Mapping*. doi:10.1002/hbm.22166

Wiebking, C., Duncan, N. W., Tiret, B., Hayes, D. J., Marjańska, M, Doyon, J., et al. (2013), GABA in the insula—a predictor of the neural response to interoceptive awareness. *Neuroimage*. doi:pii: S1053-8119(13)00389-3. 10.1016/j.neuroimage.2013.04.042. [Epub ahead of print]

Willmore, B. D. B., Mazer, J. A., & Gallant, J. L. (2011). Sparse coding in striate and extrastriate visual cortex. *Journal of Neurophysiology*, 105(6). doi:10.1152/jn.00594.2010

Wolfe, J., Houweling, A. R., & Brecht, M. (2010). Sparse and powerful cortical spikes. *Current Opinion in Neurobiology*, 20(3), 306–12. doi:10.1016/j.conb.2010.03.006

Wolpert, D. M., & Miall, R. C. (1996). Forward models for physiological motor control. *Neural Networks*, 9(8), 1265–1279.

Womelsdorf, T., Lima, B., Vinck, M., Oostenveld, R., Singer, W., Neuenschwander, S., & Fries, P. (2012). Orientation selectivity and noise correlation in awake monkey area V1 are modulated by the gamma cycle. *Proceedings of the National Academy of Sciences USA*, 109(11). doi:10.1073/pnas.1114223109

Wunderlich, K., Rangel, A., & O'Doherty, J. P. (2009). Neural computations underlying action-based decision making in the human brain. *Proceedings of the National Academy of Sciences USA*, 106(40). doi:10.1073/pnas.0901077106

Yan, F., Duncan, N. W., De Greck, M., & Northoff, G. (2011). Is there a core neural network in empathy? An fMRI based quantitative meta-analysis. *Neuroscience & Biobehavioral Reviews*, 35(3), 903–11. doi:10.1016/j.neubiorev.2010.10.009

Yan, C., Liu, D., He, Y., Zou, Q., Zhu, C., Zuo, X.,...Zang, Y. (2009). Spontaneous brain activity in the default mode network is sensitive to different resting-state conditions with limited cognitive load. *PloS One*, 4(5), e5743. doi:10.1371/journal.pone.0005743

Young, M. P., & Yamane, S. (1992). Sparse population coding of faces in the inferotemporal cortex. *Science* (New York), 256(5061), 1327–31.

Zentgraf, K., Munzert, J., Bischoff, M., & Newman-Norlund, R. D. (2011). Simulation during observation of human actions—theories, empirical studies, applications. *Vision Research*, 51(8). doi:10.1016/j.visres.2011.01.007

Zhang, X., Guo, L., Li, X., Zhu, D., Li, K., Sun, Z., Jin, C., et al. (2012). Characterization of task-free/task-performance brain states. *Medical Image Computing and Computer-Assisted Intervention: MICCAI...International Conference on Medical Image Computing and Computer-Assisted Intervention*, 15(Pt 2), 237–45.

Zhao, F. Q., Zhao, T. J., Zhou, L., Wu, Q. L., & Hu, X. P. (2008). HOLD study of stimulation-induced neural activity and resting-state connectivity in medetomidine-sedated rat. *NeuroImage*, 39(1), 248–260. doi:10.1016/j.neuroimage.2007.07.063 ER

Zhao, L. (2004). Is sparse and distributed the coding goal of simple cells? *Biological Cybernetics*, 91(6), 408–16. doi:10.1007/s00422-004-0524-0

Zhou, J., Liu, X., Song, W., Yang, Y., Zhao, Z., Ling, F., Hudetz, A. G., et al. (2011). Specific and nonspecific thalamocortical functional connectivity in normal and vegetative states. *Consciousness & Cognition*, 20(2), 257–68. doi:10.1016/j.concog.2010.08.003

Zierhut, K., Bogerts, B., Schott, B., Fenker, D., Walter, M., Albrecht, D., Steiner, J., et al. (2010). The role of hippocampus dysfunction in deficient memory encoding and positive symptoms in schizophrenia. *Psychiatry Research*, 183(3), 187–94. doi:10.1016/j.pscychresns.2010.03.007

Zink, C. F., Pagnoni, G., Martin, M. E., Dhamala, M., Berns, G. S. (2003) Human striatal response to salient nonrewarding stimuli. *Journal of Neurosciences*, 23(22), 8092–8097.

Zink, C. F., Pagnoni, G., Martin-Skurski, M. E., Chappelow, J. C., Berns, G. S. (2004) Human striatal responses to monetary reward depend on saliency. *Neuron,* 42(3):509–517.

Zou, Q., Long, X., Zuo, X., Yan, C., Zhu, C., Yang, Y., et al. (2009). Functional connectivity between the thalamus and visual cortex under eyes closed and eyes open conditions: A resting-state fMRI study. *Human Brain Mapping*, 30(9), 3066–3078. doi:10.1002/hbm.20728

Zuo, X., Di Martino, A., Kelly, C., Shehzad, Z. E., Gee, D. G., Klein, D. F., et al. (2010). The oscillating brain: Complex and reliable. *NeuroImage*, 49(2), 1432–1445. doi:10.1016/j.neuroimage.2009.09.037

Zylberberg, J., Murphy, J. T., & DeWeese, M. R. (2011). A sparse coding model with synaptically local plasticity and spiking neurons can account for the diverse shapes of V1 simple cell receptive fields. *PloS Computational Biology*, 7(10), e1002250. doi:10.1371/journal.pcbi.1002250

INDEX